HOLDEN
763-4111

HANDBOOK OF NEONATOLOGY

Second Edition

Handbook of Neonatology

Second Edition

Rita G. Harper, M.D.
Chief, Division of Perinatal Medicine
North Shore University Hospital
Associate Professor of Pediatrics and Obstetrics and Gynecology
Cornell University Medical College
New York, New York

Jing Ja Yoon, M.D.
Chief, Neonatal Perinatology
Bronx-Lebanon Hospital Center
Associate Professor of Pediatrics
Albert Einstein College of Medicine
New York, New York

YEAR BOOK MEDICAL PUBLISHERS, INC.
Chicago • London

1 2 3 4 5 6 7 8 9 0 CY 91 90 89 88 87

Library of Congress Cataloging-in-Publication Data

Harper, Rita G., 1934–
Handbook of neonatology.

Includes bibliographies and index.
1. Neonatology. I. Yoon, Jing Ja, 1941–
II. Title. [DNLM: 1. Infant, Newborn, Diseases.
WS 420 H295h]
RJ251.H26 1986 618.92′01 85-29520
ISBN 0-8151-4144-0

Sponsoring Editor: Stephany S. Scott
Manager, Copyediting Services: Frances M. Perveiler
Production Project Manager: Max Perez
Proofroom Supervisor: Shirley E. Taylor

To those who devoted their time, talent, and academic careers so that newborns might live.

Preface to the First Edition

In the last 10 years, pediatricians have become increasingly aware that most newborns who die do so within the first 24 hours of life. Thus, the concept of immediate care for the newborn to prevent serious illness has arisen.

Unfortunately, the first physician to see the infant is frequently an intern or resident who is in the training phase of medicine. Emergencies frequently arise when the intern is alone, the hour is late and time is of the essence. Serious clinical changes in the newborn are frequently so minimal and subtle that it is difficult for the intern to determine if and when he has a problem.

This handbook, therefore, was designed to be a functional guide to help the house staff recognize, prevent and treat emerging neonatal problems before the infant becomes seriously ill. It is not a textbook or replacement for a textbook. Although we hope that it will be of value to the general pediatrician, general obstetrician, family physician, nurse midwife, nursery nurse and physician's assistant, it can best be considered as a practical guide for the lonesome intern.

RITA G. HARPER, M.D.
JING JA YOON, M.D.

Preface to the Second Edition

The paper children in the hall,
Pinned against the nursery wall,
Call!   call!   call!
To those still held behind the glass,
The almost-lad and almost-lass
Pass!   pass!   pass!

R.G.H.

In the 13 years that have elapsed since the first edition of this handbook the breadth of perinatal knowledge has become ever more expansive, diagnostic possibilities considerably more complex, and monitoring and therapeutic modalities substantially more sophisticated. The house officer must be able to quickly recognize multiple life-threatening situations, understand a compendium of disease entities, and offer a variety of therapeutic modalities.

To accomplish this Herculean task, the house officer requires a convenient source of information that will rapidly retrieve normal and pathologic data, aid in relating clinical observations to diagnostic possibilities, and suggest current recommendations for supportive or therapeutic modalities. This handbook was developed to be such a guide.

The chapters were purposely designed to be problem-oriented since this is the common method by which the house officer approaches the nursery situation. Chapters are subdivided into general concepts and normal values, common differential diagnoses, disease entities, risk/preventions, clinical/laboratory observations, supportive management, and specific therapy. In some situations, the rapidly changing state of the art only permits controversial therapies to be suggested. We have therefore attempted to provide a knowledge base that will allow the house officer to understand the common problems associated with perinatal illness, support life functions of immediate significance, and handle events until the literature or a senior colleague can be consulted.

This handbook should not be considered a textbook of perinatal medicine. This, like the previous edition, can best be considered a practical guide for the lonesome intern.

Rita G. Harper
Jing Ja Yoon

Acknowledgments

It is with pleasure and gratitude that the authors acknowledge the assistance and support of their many colleagues and associates.

Mervin Silverberg, M.D., Director of the Department of Pediatrics at North Shore University Hospital, and William Caspe, M.D., Chairman of the Department of Pediatrics at Bronx-Lebanon Hospital, were major sources of encouragement throughout the preparation of this manuscript.

We are greatly indebted to our colleagues for their contributions. Concepcion Sia, M.D., assisted in the revision and development of Chapter 5, "Normal Full-term Infants," Mae Hee Kim, M.D., Chapter 14, "Anemia and/or Hemorrhage," Shaista Usmani, M.D., Chapter 15, "Tremors and Convulsions," and Jerrold Schlessel, M.D., Chapter 11, "Respiratory Distress," and Chapter 12, "Cyanosis." Eduvigis Carrera, M.D., Ph.D., reviewed the feeding practices for newborn infants in Chapter 6.

Library research assistants included Bonnie Claire Harper, Andrea Green, Deborah Karp, Roger Villi and Juan Gomez. Their tenacity and capability for finding even obscure references is greatly appreciated.

Our neonatal fellows over several years have been especially helpful. In the past year, the fellows have included Drs. Ronald Saintonge, Ezequiel Cartaya, Shudir Madisetty, Howard Fisher, Pratibha Kabrawala, Ilya Kreynin, Marc de Soler, and Jenny Pan.

Through the many drafts and revisions, our secretarial assistants Florence Harris, Olivia Mosby and Rhoda Seligson have shown unending patience. Without their valuable assistance this book could not have been completed.

Last but not least, we wish to thank our husbands, Richard Harper and Jae Chan Kim, and children, Bonnie Claire, Robin Anne, and Susan Linda Harper, whose love and understanding allowed us to believe that—no matter how many pages—there is an end; there really is an end.

RITA G. HARPER
JING JA YOON

Contents

Chapter 1

Orientation to the Nursery

BEFORE ROTATING THROUGH the nursery, the pediatric house officer should be oriented to the nursery's physical, physiologic, and psychosocial dimensions. The newborn nursery provides care of graded intensity determined by the nature of each newborn's problems. In general, newborns are admitted shortly after birth to the transitional section of the nursery. This area provides intensified surveillance during the first several hours. Normal healthy infants are then placed in the regular nursery where they are observed constantly and have periodic vital signs recorded. Those infants who are considered high risk at birth require specialized monitoring in the immediate postnatal period. The high-risk infant should be seen in the delivery room and followed closely in the neonatal period. Those infants who are potentially infectious should be placed in a specialized area apart from other infants until the presence or absence of infectiousness is determined.

Each infant, whether normal or high risk, should be under continuous medical and nursing surveillance. The pediatric house officer should observe the infant as frequently as necessary. Every infant should receive a physical examination at birth, within 24 hours after birth, and before discharge. A detailed record of the infant's gestation, delivery, and immediate postnatal condition should be made. The results of all examinations should be written on the infant's chart and discussed with the parents.

Many infectious agents are transmitted by the hands of nursery personnel. Therefore, scrupulous attention must be paid to hand washing technique. Pediatric house staff members, students, nursing supervisors, nurses, technicians, and parents must wash their hands to the elbows with an iodoform solution (Betadine) or another cleansing agent before entering the nursery. Proper hand washing before entering the nursery is mandatory, and hands should be considered contaminated unless they are washed just before and just after handling each infant. Wearing a gown is optional and depends upon nursery technique.

All medical instruments should be provided; therefore, no stethoscope, ophthalmoscope, etc., should be brought into the nursery. Instruments should be cleaned with alcohol or Betadine between examinations of infants.

All personnel should realize that if they have even a mild infection, it is important that they do not come in contact with newborns. No staff member should be admitted to the nursery with a respiratory infection, "cold sores," gastroenteritis, or other communicable diseases. It is urged that any person who feels he or she is in the prodromal infectious stage bar himself or herself from admittance. The nurse-in-charge is responsible for ensuring that all nursery personnel, including physicians, follow the policies to protect the newborns from infection.

The neophyte house officer should be acquainted with the physical location of the various areas of the hospital that function in coordination with, or support of, the nursery. The location of the blood gas, microbiologic, and chemistry laboratories; the ante partum and post partum maternal units; and the delivery room and nursery resuscitation areas should all be familiar.

All house officers must be able to recognize a critically ill infant and be able to immediately support the infant's cardiorespiratory status. This requires an understanding of cardiorespiratory physiology, emergency neonatal procedures, and resuscitative drugs. Therefore, before a house officer is left without supervision in the nursery, adequate cardiorespiratory training sessions must be provided.

It is mandatory that the house officer have a basic understanding of the psychosocial aspects of perinatal medicine. The process of mother-infant bonding, the psychosocial aspects of reproduction, the techniques used to cope with an abnormal infant, the stages of grieving, and the concepts of crisis intervention should all be familiar.

For many house officers the neonatal nursery will be exciting and challenging; for some the rapidly changing volume of critically ill infants, the necessity of attending to repetitive detail, and the inability to salvage some infants despite heroic effort will prove frustrating. Orientation should therefore encompass discussion concerning the moral dilemmas inherent in neonatal intensive care.

Chapter 2

The Role of the Pediatrician Before Delivery

THE PEDIATRIC HOUSE officer frequently is on a rotating schedule and knows little about the mother in labor whose infant is soon to come under his or her care. He or she must be acquainted with common obstetric problems and procedures and their effects upon the newborn as well as the common methods of assessing fetal well-being and maturity. The pediatric house officer should contact the obstetric house officer to become aware of potentially sick or high-risk infants before delivery. A pediatric house officer along with a perinatal nurse should attend each high-risk delivery. The obstetric house officer should be able to locate and summon the pediatric house officer at a moment's notice. The following high-risk situations should be discussed with the obstetric house officer before delivery.

COMMON MATERNAL CONDITIONS OR DISEASES DURING PREGNANCY (TABLES 2–1, 8–1)

1. Diabetes mellitus (see chapter 15–XI)
2. History of narcotic addiction (see chapter 15–XIX)
3. Heavy smoking (see chapter 6–III)
4. History of losing a previous infant
5. Hypertensive disease of pregnancy (see chapter 6–III and Table 8–1)
6. Hyperthyroidism (see chapter 15–XVIII)
7. Hypothyroidism (see Table 8–1)
8. Premature rupture of the membranes (see chapter 16)
9. Infection during pregnancy (see chapter 16)
10. Polyhydramnios (see Table 2–1)
11. Oligohydramnios (see Table 2–1)
12. Third trimester bleeding (see chapter 14–VIII and 14–IX)
13. Rh-negative blood type (see chapter 13–VII)
14. Autoimmune thrombocytopenia (see Chapter 14–XIV)

FETAL CONDITIONS (SEE TABLE 2–1)

15. Delivery by cesarean section (see Table 8–1)
16. Delivery by breech presentation (see Table 5–3)
17. Fetal distress or abnormal test result for fetal well-being (see Tables 2–2 and 2–3)
18. Life-threatening congenital malformations (see Chapter 9)
19. Prematurity (see chapter 6–II)
20. Large for gestational age (see chapter 7)
21. Intrauterine growth retardation (see chapter 6–III)
22. Postdate (see chapter 6–III)

TABLE 2–1.—THE ROLE OF THE PEDIATRICIAN FOR MATERNAL AND FETAL HIGH-RISK CONDITIONS BEFORE DELIVERY*

MATERNAL AND FETAL CONDITIONS	FETAL AND NEONATAL RISK	PREPARATIONS BEFORE DELIVERY
Maternal diabetes mellitus (see chapter 15–XI)	Increased perinatal mortality Fetal distress, stillbirth, and perinatal asphyxia Congenital anomalies (hypertrophic cardiomyopathy, transposition of great vessels, ventricular septal defect, sacral agenesis, caudal regression syndrome, hemivertebrae, talipes equinovarus, small left colon syndrome) Macrosomia with or without birth trauma Premature delivery (to prevent stillbirth or due to misjudgment of fetal maturity) Delayed maturation of the lung (respiratory distress syndrome) and possibly other organs Hypoglycemia Hypocalcemia/hypomagnesemia Electrolyte imbalance Polycythemia Hyperbilirubinemia Renal vein thrombosis Meconium plug syndrome Infection Transient tachypnea of the newborn	Discuss with the obstetric house officers the risk of respiratory distress syndrome vs. cesarean section. Ask the obstetric house officer not to give long-acting insulin and by which route last dose of short-acting insulin was given. Obtain obstetric history: Whether maternal diabetes was well controlled with fasting blood glucose <100 mg/dl and 2-hour postprandial value <140 mg/dl and sequential HbA_{1c} 5–10%. Previous fetal or neonatal deaths. The risk of stillbirth increases as pregnancy approaches term (5–10% in the third trimester). Presence of maternal polyhydramnios. Assessment of fetal maturity, fetal size and fetal well-being (see Tables 2–2 and 2–3) Whether steroids were given to accelerate lung maturation Prepare for biochemical and cardiorespiratory monitoring of the infant.
Maternal narcotic addiction (see chapter 15–XIX)	Small-for-date infant Narcotic withdrawal syndrome: CNS irritability Autonomic and GI disturbances Hyperpyrexia and respiratory distress Neonatal infection (e.g., hepatitis, syphilis) Child abuse Exposure to HTLV-III virus	Obtain obstetric history: Type, dose, time, and route of last drug dosage History of hepatitis, syphilis, AIDS, etc. Results of maternal serologic test for syphilis, hepatitis B antigen and antibody, HTLV-III antibody, etc. Apgar score is usually not low. Withdrawal symptoms can occur at birth or anytime during first 2 mo of life. Prepare to observe infant for withdrawal syndrome and treat as necessary.

Maternal smoking	Premature and small-for-date infant Fetal distress Increased perinatal mortality	Obtain obstetric history: Duration and amount of maternal smoking Intrauterine growth pattern Assessment of fetal well-being Prepare for premature or small-for-date infant (see chapter 6)
History of losing a previous infant	Congenital malformations Prematurity Intrauterine growth retardation Maternal diabetes mellitus or hypertension Infection Sudden infant death syndrome (SIDS)	Obtain obstetric history: The cause of previous loss (e.g., congenital malformations, prematurity, intrauterine growth retardation, maternal disease) frequently repeats itself in a subsequent pregnancy.
Maternal hypertensive disease of pregnancy (chronic hypertension, preeclampsia, eclampsia) (see chapter 6–III)	Small-for-date infant with or without hypoglycemia and/or hypocalcemia Fetal distress, perinatal asphyxia, and hypotension Meconium aspiration syndrome Hypermagnesemia secondary to maternal $MgSO_4$ Neutropenia, thrombocytopenia with or without maternal medications Increased perinatal mortality	Obtain obstetric history: Status of maternal hypertension Maternal medication type, dose, time, and route of administration Assessment of fetal well-being Prepare for cardiorespiratory support. Prepare to obtain CBC and glucose, calcium, and magnesium levels of infant and follow closely Prepare to administer 10% calcium gluconate and exchange transfuse infant if depression secondary to $MgSO_4$ occurs.
Maternal hyperthyroidism (see chapter 15–XVIII)	Congenital thyrotoxicosis caused by maternal thyroid stimulating immunoglobulins Congenital goiter caused by maternal ingestion of thyroid inhibitors (e.g., propylthiouracil, methimazole, iodine) Tracheal compression caused by goiter Prematurity Small-for-date infant, often due to propranolol	Obtain obstetric history: Whether mother has associated hypertensive disease of pregnancy Whether maternal hyperthyroidism is well controlled Maternal drug type and dose. When surgery was performed, if done Maternal thyroid stimulating immunoglobulin level (does not always correlate) Be aware of the possibility of congenital hyperthyroidism or hypothyroidism. (see chapters 15–XVIII and 17–XIX) Prepare for tracheostomy and cardiorespiratory support.

(continued).

TABLE 2–1.—*(continued).*

MATERNAL AND FETAL CONDITIONS	FETAL AND NEONATAL RISK	PREPARATIONS BEFORE DELIVERY
Maternal hypothyroidism (see Table 8–1)	Prematurity Occasionally cretinism (?) Outcome of pregnancy is usually good	Obtain obstetric history: Whether maternal hypothyroidism is well controlled Maternal treatment does not affect newborn since thyroid hormone does not cross the placenta. Prepare for respiratory support.
Premature rupture of the membranes (see chapter 16)	Intrauterine pneumonia Omphalitis Septicemia Neonatal meningitis Urinary tract infection	Obtain obstetric history: Whether mother is infected Results of maternal cardiorespiratory rate, temperature, CBC, cervical cultures Whether mother is on treatment Assessment of fetal maturity, e.g., L/S ratio, if fetus is suspected to be premature and fetal well-being (see Tables 2–2 and 2–3) Discuss with the obstetric house officer the risk of respiratory distress syndrome versus the risk of intrauterine infection if fetus is premature. Prepare to get placenta and/or amniotic fluid culture. Prepare for septic infant (cultures, CBC, etc.) Prepare for cardiorespiratory support.
Maternal infection (see chapter 16)	Premature delivery Sepsis Meningitis Pneumonia Urinary tract infection Omphalitis Increased perinatal mortality	Obtain obstetric history: Results of maternal temperature, CBC, and cultures Maternal medication type, dose, time, and route of administration Estimated gestational age of infant Prepare for cardiorespiratory support. Prepare for septic infant (cultures, CBC, etc.) (see chapter 16–III)

Maternal polyhydramnios (>2 L or >2 times normal volume for gestation)	Frequently associated with the following: Tracheoesophageal fistula Intestinal obstruction Anencephaly Exstrophy of the bladder Diaphragmatic hernia Erythroblastosis fetalis Syphilis Twinning Diabetes mellitus (maternal) Hypertensive disease of pregnancy	Obtain obstetric history: Results of maternal pelvic sonogram to determine twinning, hydrops fetalis, or congenital malformations (anencephaly, tracheoesophageal fistula, upper GI obstruction, etc.). Consult surgeon if appropriate. Maternal blood type, Rh, and anti-Rh titer Results of maternal serologic test for syphilis Results of maternal glucose tolerance test or blood pressure to rule out maternal diabetes mellitus or hypertensive disease of pregnancy Results of maternal plasma or amniotic fluid α-fetoprotein Prepare for perinatal asphyxia or congenital malformations. Prepare for immediate exchange transfusion if erythroblastosis fetalis is suspected.
Maternal oligohydramnios (<200 ml or <one-half normal volume for gestation)	Urinary tract anomalies: Potter's syndrome, obstructive uropathy Talipes valgus Fetal death Prolonged rupture of the membranes Postdate Intrauterine growth retardation	Obtain obstetric history: Results of sonogram to evaluate the quantity of amniotic fluid, urinary output, renal or bladder size, or fetal anomalies Signs of fetal death; overlap of skull bones on ultrasonogram or x-ray film and absence of fetal heart tone History of leakage of amniotic fluid Estimation of gestational age Be aware of frequent associations of pulmonary hypoplasia and renal anomalies. Prepare for cardiorespiratory support. Ask the obstetrician to save the placenta to look for amnion nodosum.
Third trimester maternal bleeding (placenta previa, abruptio	Fetal and/or neonatal anemia with or without shock or congestive heart failure Perinatal asphyxia	Obtain obstetric history: Results of assessment of fetal maturity and fetal well-being (see Tables 2–2 and 2–3)

(continued).

TABLE 2–1.—*(continued)*.

MATERNAL AND FETAL CONDITIONS	FETAL AND NEONATAL RISK	PREPARATIONS BEFORE DELIVERY
placenta, or marginal sinus rupture) (see chapter 14–VIII and 14–IX)	Respiratory distress syndrome if infant is premature	Maternal status (blood pressure, acid base balance, or CBC) Whether bleeding is from mother or infant (results of APT test on blood from vagina) Prepare for cardiorespiratory support. Prepare to obtain Hct, blood gas studies, glucose, calcium, blood pressure, central venous pressure, etc. Prepare to transfuse infant immediately with type O Rh-negative blood compatible with maternal serum if necessary.
Rh-negative mothers (see chapter 13–VII)	Anemia, hyperbilirubinemia Hypoalbuminemia Erythroblastosis fetalis Congestive heart failure Generalized edema Kernicterus	Obtain obstetric history: Outcome of previous pregnancies: whether a previous infant developed hyperbilirubinemia, required exchange transfusion, or died because of Rh incompatibility Studies of this pregnancy: maternal anti-Rh titer, optical density of amniotic fluid, sonogram for fetal maturity/condition, amniotic fluid volume or phosphatidylglycerol level, etc. When an infant with erythroblastosis is expected, obtain fetal scalp pH and prepare, before delivery, type O Rh-negative blood compatible with maternal serum for exchange transfusion. Prepare for cardiorespiratory support. Obtain cord Hct, bilirubin, blood group, Rh, and Coombs' test.
Cesarean section (see Table 8–1)	Transient tachypnea of the newborn Problems associated with the indication for the section	Obtain obstetric history: Whether cesarean section is repeat, elective, or emergency section, determine indications for section: cephalopelvic disproportion, breech

		presentation, fetal distress, prior section, maternal active herpes simplex infection, failure to induce labor in the presence of amnionitis, etc. Prepare for cardiorespiratory support.
Breech extraction (see Table 5–3)	Birth trauma: CNS or visceral hemorrhage, spinal cord or peripheral nerve injury, skeletal fractures, soft tissue injury Fetal distress and perinatal asphyxia often associated with cord prolapse Prematurity and congenital malformations	Obtain obstetric history: Results of fetal monitoring or sonogram Whether umbilical cord prolapse was present Whether prematurity or congenital malformations were present Prepare for cardiorespiratory support.
Fetal distress or abnormal test result for fetal well-being (see Tables 2–2 and 2–3)	Perinatal asphyxia and increased perinatal mortality Acidosis Hypothermia Hypoglycemia, hypocalcemia, and hyponatremia Persistant pulmonary hypertension of the newborn CNS edema and hemorrhage Syndrome of inappropriate antidiuretic hormone Acute renal failure Necrotizing enterocolitis Meconium aspiration with or without pulmonary air leak syndrome Congestive heart failure	Obtain obstetric history: Types and results of assessment of fetal well-being and reasons for assessment Scalp pH results Mode of delivery (emergency cesarean section?) Prepare for cardiorespiratory support, asphyxiated infant. (see chapters 3 and 15–IV)
Life-threatening congenital malformations (see chapter 9)	Depends on type of malformations	Obtain obstetric history: Prior history of siblings with congenital malformations or previous abortions Whether mother received genetic counseling if known before delivery
Prematurity (see chapter 6–II)	Fetal distress or perinatal asphyxia Hypoglycemia Hypocalcemia Respiratory distress syndrome: immaturity of lungs Immaturity of other organs (CNS, renal, etc.) Intraventricular hemorrhage Patent ductus arteriosus Infection	Obtain maternal history: Previous preterm delivery Socioeconomic status (low is often associated with prematurity) Cervical incompetence Uterine anomalies Spontaneous rupture of the membrane (ROM) Antepartum hemorrhage Hypertensive disease of pregnancy

(continued).

TABLE 2–1.—*(continued).*

MATERNAL AND FETAL CONDITIONS	FETAL AND NEONATAL RISK	PREPARATIONS BEFORE DELIVERY
Prematurity (see chapter 6–II)–(continued)		Pyelonephritis Peritonitis Pneumonia Obtain fetal history: Growth retardation Malformations of fetus and placenta Hydramnios Estimated fetal weight and gestational age Ultrasonic measurement of crown to rump length before 14 wk gestation Use of tocolytic agents and/or steroids Results of assessment of fetal well-being (see Table 2–2) If born by cesarean section, ask obstetrician the indications for section. Prepare for cardiorespiratory support.
Large for gestational age (see chapter 7)	Birth trauma Hypoglycemia Hypocalcemia Cardiac disease (transposition of great vessels)	Obtain obstetric history: Maternal diabetes and control Large maternal or paternal weight Prior history of macrosomic infant Prepare for cardiorespiratory support. Prepare for infant with cardiac disease (e.g., transposition of great vessels).
Intrauterine growth retardation (small for gestational age) (see chapter 6–III)	Meconium aspiration with or without pulmonary air leak syndrome Fetal and perinatal asphyxia Hypoglycemia Hypocalcemia Thrombocytopenia Hypothermia	Obtain obstetric history: Maternal history of previous infant with low birth weight, congenital anomalies, perinatal death, or spontaneous abortion Maternal history of hypertensive disease of pregnancy, renal disease, infection, diabetes mellitus, cardiopulmonary disease, smoking,

	Polycythemia Hyperbilirubinemia	alcohol consumption, narcotic use, chronic abruptio placentae, etc. Maternal race, stature, address (high altitude), parity, and age Ultrasonic fetal growth pattern or congenital malformations Results of tests for fetal well-being (see Table 2–2), amniocentesis for chromosomal analysis in case of symmetrical growth retardation Color and quantity of amniotic fluid If amniotic fluid is green or yellow, prepare for meconium aspiration syndrome (see Chapter II–XII). Prepare for cardiorespiratory support.
Postdate (>42 wk gestation) (see chapter 6, section on "the small-for-gestational-age infant")	Fetal distress and perinatal asphyxia Meconium aspiration syndrome Oligohydramnios, which may result in difficult delivery, umbilical cord occlusion, thick meconium, etc. Macrosomia, which may result in difficult deliveries, birth trauma, or increased rate of cesarean section Dysmaturity with or without hypoglycemia or hypocalcemia	Obtain obstetric history: Results of tests for fetal well-being (see Table 2–2) If there is a passage of meconium or amniotic fluid is green or yellow, prepare for meconium aspiration, particularly prepare to aspirate meconium from deep pharynx during the process of delivery. Scalp pH results Prepare for cardiorespiratory support.

*L/S ratio, lecithin-sphingomyelin ratio.

REFERENCES

Creasy R.K., Resnik R.: *Maternal-Fetal Medicine.* Philadelphia, W.B. Saunders Co., 1984.

Iffy L., Kaminetzky H.A.: *Principles and Practice of Obstetrics and Perinatology.* New York, John Wiley and Sons, 1981.

TABLE 2–2.—COMMON METHODS USED TO ASSESS FETAL WELL-BEING*

METHOD OR DRUG	COMMENTS
α-Fetoprotein	Fetal malformations are associated with elevated amniotic fluid and maternal blood α-fetoprotein. An elevation of α-fetoprotein at 14–18 wk gestation may indicate multiple gestation, intrauterine growth retardation, intrauterine death, anencephaly, meningomyelocele, meningocele, encephalocele, congenital nephrosis, exstrophy of bladder, exophthalmos, sacrococcygeal teratoma, omphalocele, tracheoesophageal fistula, cirrhosis, maternal causes (toxemia, lupus, liver disease, etc.).
Amniography	Introduction of radiopaque materials into the amniotic fluid by transabdominal amniocentesis can localize the placenta, identify fetal hydrops, and outline GI, GU, CNS, and other physical malformations.
Amnioscopy	A specially designed endoscope permits examination of the amniotic fluid quality (passage of meconium and/or blood) with intact membranes. To perform test, the cervix must be slightly dilated (satisfactory only occasionally in primiparas).
Amniotic fluid	See Tables 2–3 and 2–4.
HbA_{1c} peptide level	Blood HbA_{lc} peptide levels accurately reflect daily net hyperglycemia over a few weeks: perinatal mortality may be reduced if postprandial blood glucose levels are kept below 150 mg/dl, and the range of HbA_{1c} is 5%–10%.
Diagnostic ultrasound (Sonography)	This technique is useful in diagnosing early and abnormal pregnancies, identifying multiple pregnancies, differentiating hydatidiform mole, assessing intrauterine growth rate, and ascertaining fetal gestational age and polyhydramnios or oligohydramnios. Fetal maturity is virtually certain when the biparietal diameter is 9.8 cm (femur length is $>$ 7 cm). Sonography is helpful in in utero diagnosis of anencephaly, ascites, cystic hygroma, diaphragmatic hernia, duodenal atresia, dysplastic kidneys, Ellis-van Creveld syndrome, encephalocele, holoprosencephaly, hydrocephalus, hydronephrosis, hypoplastic right side of heart, ileal volvulus, infantile polycystic kidneys, microcephaly, meningomyelocele, multicystic kidneys, omphalocele, osteogenesis imperfecta, pleural effusion, renal agenesis, Robert's syndrome, sacrococcygeal teratoma, spina bifida, thoracic cysts, tricuspid atresia, ureteral or urethral obstruction, and others.
Fetal blood sampling	Sampling of fetal scalp blood through an endoscope can detect fetal acidosis (which reflects fetal hypoxia). A fall in fetal pH to $<$7.20 is an indicator of fetal compromise and calls for immediate delivery. pH of 7.20–7.25 requires repeat testing in 10–15 min.

Fetal breathing movement (fetal respiration)	Fetal respirations reflect fetal well-being. Fetal breathing movements are episodic, occurring 30 to 70 times/min, 55%–90% of the observation time at term (lower in prematures). Absence of normal fetal breathing movements and the appearance of gasping are associated with subsequent intrapartum fetal distress, fetal demise, and neonatal depression.
Fetal heart rates/ variability	Normal fetal heart rate range: 120–160 beats/min with good baseline fetal heart rate variability. (Changes in the fetal heart rate of 1–8 beats/min with a frequency of 3–10 cycles/min are observed in normal fetuses.) Loss of beat-to-beat variability: Reduced beat-to-beat variability may be due to fetal hypoxia, sedative hypnotics (meperidine, alphaprodine, secobarbital, diazepam, methadone, morphine sulfate), parasympatholytic agents (atropine, scopolamine), general and local anesthetic agents, phenothiazines (Phenergan), magnesium sulfate, fetal sleep, immaturity, hypoxia, fetal tachycardia, and congenital anomalies (anencephaly, microcephaly). A straight line is an extremely ominous sign. Fetal tachycardia: FHR > 160 beats/min Often associated with maternal pyrexia and chorioamnionitis, and reduced fetal beat to beat variability and fetal acidosis. Fetal tachycardia is also associated with fetal movement, maternal anxiety and maternal beta-adrenergic stimulants. Usually there is normal fetal variability and pH. Fetal bradycardia: FHR < 120 beats/min Physiologic (not associated with fetal acidosis): 100–120 beats/min with good variability during the first stage of labor. 85–120 beats/min with good variability during the second stage of labor. < 100 beats/min: Often associated with fetal hypoxia, fetal death (with transmitted maternal signal), fetal myocardial conduction defects (congenital complete heart block) structural heart lesions, fetal CNS anomalies, maternal connective tissue disease (especially SLE present or future in 33%–50%), maternal viral infection, maternal hypothermia and maternal beta adrenergic blocking drug (propranolol).
Fetal heart rate patterns	Early deceleration (Type I dip) A transient decrease in the fetal heart rate in direct response to uterine pressure on the fetal head. This type of pattern is not usually associated with fetal compromise. Variable deceleration Various types of transient fall in fetal heart rate occurring at various times in relation to uterine contractions. Variable deceleration is a common and early sign of acute fetal distress and caused by transient compression of the umbilical cord.

(continued)

TABLE 2–2.—*(continued)*

METHOD OR DRUG	COMMENTS
Fetal heart rate patterns–continued	Late deceleration (type II dip): A transient fall in fetal heart rate occurring after the uterus has begun to relax. This represents an acute reduction in fetal oxygenation and is associated with delivery of asphyxiated and depressed newborns. This pattern is often associated with decreased uterine blood flow from oxytocin, regional anesthesia, maternal hypotension, supine position, or cord prolapse. Other causes include vaginal examination, application of internal fetal scalp electrodes, maternal convulsions, maternal respiratory arrest, and rapid descent of the fetus during expulsion. If late deceleration persists, the fetus should be delivered immediately. Sinusoidal pattern: A sine wave with relatively fixed periodicity of 2–5 cycles/min in 2–10 min. Often associated with fetal anemia and hypoxia. This is an ominous sign and immediate delivery is indicated.
Fetal movements	Each fetus has its own quality and quantity of movement. Decreased or absent fetal movements are associated with intrapartum fetal distress or demise. The presence of normal estrogen values and normal daily fetal movement rate are associated with a good fetal outcome.
Fetoscopy	Fetoscopy for visualization of phenotypic characteristics and blood sampling from placental blood vessels, although quite experimental, hold promise for extending fetal diagnostic testing and surgical procedures.
Human placental lactogen	The level of human placental lactogen is primarily a function of the amount of viable functioning trophoblastic tissue. Low levels may indicate placental insufficiency; high levels may indicate multiple pregnancy, Rh sensitization, and maternal diabetes. Helpful in ruling out sulphatase deficiency, anencephaly, or congenital pituitary or adrenal hypoplasia which all have low E_3.
Maternal serum Estriol (E_3)	Approximately 90% of the E_3 is produced by the fetoplacental unit. A normal E_3 pattern almost always indicates fetal well-being. An abnormal E_3 profile is frequently associated with perinatal morbidity and mortality. Serial determinations are necessary. A low or dropping (>40%) E_3 (unconjugated, total plasma, or 24-hr urinary) suggests intrauterine growth retardation and/or fetal distress (e.g., from maternal diabetes mellitus, preeclampsia, or prolonged gestation). E_3 assays are not of value in Rh isoimmunization, trophoblastic disease, and multiple gestation. Falsely low values are seen in maternal administration of glucocorticosteroids, anencephaly, congenital adrenal hypoplasia, placental sulphatase deficiency, decreased maternal hepatic conjugation, and interruption of maternal enterohepatic circulation (e.g., ampicillin therapy decreases conjugated E_3 only). Impaired maternal renal function increases plasma E_3 levels and decreases urinary E_3 excretion.

Maternal serum Rh antibody titers	Rh antibody titers do not accurately predict the extent of fetal disease in an Rh-sensitized pregnancy. Amniocentesis is required with titers greater than 1:8 (see chapter 13–VII)
NST	Reactive NST: The normal pattern is >2 accelerations of the fetal heart of >15 beats/min above baseline and at least 30-sec duration associated with fetal movement in a 20-min period. Nonreactive NST: Absence of the normal pattern (reactive NST) lasting for 40 min. Seen in fetal sleep, hypoxia, acidosis, fetal anomalies, certain narcotics, and sedatives. With E_3 values, NST helps recognizing false positive oxytocin challenge tests. The NST is particularly useful for patients with contraindications to the OCT (e.g., premature rupture of the membranes, placenta previa, previous classical cesarean section, multiple gestation, and incompetent cervix).
OCT or CST	During spontaneous or oxytocin-induced uterine contractions of at least 3 contractions lasting longer than 40 sec in 10 min, uterine blood flow decreases, which is tolerated in the healthy fetus but not in the compromised fetus. If decelerations are seen (positive test result), they might indicate fetal compromise, which is often seen in maternal diabetes mellitus, hypertension, hyperthyroidism, cyanotic heart disease, hemoglobinopathy, postdate, intrauterine growth retardation, elderly gravida, Rh isoimmunization, etc. Usually evaluations start at 28 wk gestation. The positive OCT is an earlier warning sign of the fetus in jeopardy than the nonreactive NST. False negative results are seen in umbilical cord accidents, abruptio placenta, and sudden maternal metabolic changes (e.g., diabetic ketoacidosis) and false positive results are seen in undiagnosed supine hypotension or excessive uterine activity.
Systolic time intervals	This test is utilized to define gestational age and severity of fetal compromise. The interval between the onset of left ventricular depolarization and the opening of the aortic valve increases with gestational age. The magnitude and duration of the interval is directly related to fetal compromise.

*E_3, estriol; NST, nonstress test; OCT, oxytocin challenge test; CST, contraction stress test.

REFERENCES

Hon E.G.: *An Atlas of Fetal Heart Rate Patterns.* New Haven, Conn., Harty Press, 1968.

Petrie R.H. (ed.): Symposium on fetal monitoring. *Clin. Perinatol.* 9:2, 1982.

TABLE 2–3.—Assessment of Fetal Maturity by Amniotic Fluid Assay*

TEST	RESULT IN NORMAL PREGNANCY	COMMENT
L/S ratio	Sphingomyelin concentration exceeds lecithin until 26th wk. Lecithin concentration exceeds sphingomyelin by 35–36 wk.	L/S ratio >2.0 indicates fetal lung maturity. Falsely high L/S ratio when fluid is contaminated with maternal or fetal blood or vaginal secretions. Respiratory distress syndrome in spite of mature L/S ratio has been seen in diabetic pregnancies or after intrauterine transfusions.
PG	PG detectable beyond 35 wk gestation	Particularly useful in pregnancies complicated by diabetes mellitus. PG can eliminate false maturity by L/S ratio. PG is reliable even when contaminated with blood or vaginal secretions.
Shake test	After 36 wk gestation, complete ring of bubbles present at 1:2 dilution of amniotic fluid in presence of ethanol	A simple, inexpensive, reliable bedside screening test. Contamination with blood or meconium results in a false positive test result.
Foam stability index	At maturity >0.48	Quantitative measure of foam stability of surfactant and ethanol
Lecithin concentration	At maturity lecithin: >3.5 mg/100 ml phosphorus: >0.1 mg/100 ml	Direct measure of primary phospholipid in surfactant
Saturated lecithin	At maturity >500 mg/dl	Measurement after oxidation with osmium tetroxide
Osmolality	Near maternal plasma level (270 mOsm) at <36 wk; value falls as term approaches (250 mOsm).	Value falls as a result of fetal urine contribution; reflects maternal electrolyte level; increases with fetal death.
Creatinine	1.5 mg/100 ml at <36 wk, >2.0 mg/100 ml at 36 wk in 10%, >2.0 mg/100 ml beyond 36 wk.	Values lower in diabetic women. Value depends on renal function of the infant, as well as muscle mass.
Protein	Protein value decreases as gestation progresses.	Value rises with fetal death, anencephaly, and other anomalies.
Bilirubin	13–30 wk gestation, bilirubin remains at highest concentration. Falls to 0 by 36 wk gestation.	Bilirubin in the unconjugated state. Origin a mystery. Elevated in toxemia, hydrops fetalis, GI obstruction, and anencephaly.

*L/S ratio, lecithin-sphingomyelin ratio; PG, phosphatidylglycerol.

REFERENCES

Gabbe S.G.: Recent advances in the assessment of fetal maturity. *J. Reprod. Med.* 23:227, 1979.

Torday J., Carson L., Lawson E.E.: Saturated phosphatidyl choline in amniotic fluid and prediction of respiratory distress syndrome. *N. Engl. J. Med.* 301:1013, 1979.

TABLE 2–4.—CONDITIONS DIAGNOSABLE BY AMNIOCENTESIS

Estimation of gestational age and/or lung maturity (see Table 2–3)	
Estimation of the severity of isoimmune disease (see chapter 13–VII)	
Sex of the fetus and sex-linked recessive disorders	
Chromosomal abnormalities: essentially all significant cytogenetic disorders	
Disorders of amino acid and organic acid metabolism	
Arginase deficiency	Hypervalinemia
Argininosuccinic aciduria	Isovaleric acidemia
Aspartylglycosaminuria	Maple syrup urine disease, severe and intermittent types
Citrullinemia	Methylenetetrahydrolate reductase deficiency
Cystinosis	Methylmalonic acidemia
Cystathioninuria	Ornithine-alpha-keto acid transaminase deficiency
Dihydropteridine reductase deficiency phenylketonuria (PKU) variant	Propionic acidemia (ketotic hyperglycinemia)
Histidinemia	
Homocystinuria (cystathionine synthetase deficiency)	
Mucopolysaccharidoses (types 1–7)	
β-glucuronidase deficiency (VIII)	Morquio's syndrome (IV)
Hunter's syndrome (II A and B)	Sanfilippo's syndrome (III A and B)
Hurler's syndrome (IH)	Scheie's syndrome (IS)
Maroteaux-Lamy syndrome (VI A and B)	
Carbohydrate metabolism disorders	
Fucosidosis	Glycogen storage disease, types II, III, IV, VI, and IX
Galactokinase deficiency	Mannosidosis
Glactosemia	Pyruvate decarboxylase deficiency
Glucose-6-phosphate dehydrogenase deficiency	Sialidosis
Lipid metabolism disorders	
Cholesterol ester storage disease	GM_1 gangliosidosis, types I and II
Fabry's disease	GM_2 gangliosidosis, type I (Tay-Sachs disease)
Familial hypercholesterolemia	GM_2 gangliosidosis, type II (Sandhoff's disease)
Farber's disease	GM_2 gangliosidosis, type III
Gaucher's disease, infantile and adult types	GM_3 gangliosidosis
Krabbe's disease	Refsum's disease
Metachromatic leukodystrophy	Wolman's disease
Niemann-Pick disease, types A, B, and C	
Miscellaneous disorders	
Adenosine deaminase deficiency	Hemophilia
Anencephaly, meningomyelocele, encephalocele	Hemoglobinopathies
Adrenogenital syndrome	Sickle cell anemia
Chédiak-Higashi syndrome	Thalassemia
Chronic granulomatosis disease	Lesch-Nyhan syndrome
Combined immunodeficiency	Lysosomal acid phosphatase deficiency
Congenital erythropoietic porphyria	Lysyl-protocollagen hydroxylase deficiency
Congenital nephrotic syndrome	Marfan's syndrome
Cystic fibrosis	Menkes' syndrome
Erythropoietic porphyria	Xeroderma pigmentosum
Hypophosphatasia	Orotic aciduria
I-cell disease	Porphyria (acute intermittent)

REFERENCES

Golbus M.S., Loughman W.D., Epstein C.J., et al.: Prenatal genetic diagnosis in 3000 amniocentesis. *N. Engl. J. Med.* 300:157, 1979.

Nadler H.L.: Prenatal detection of genetic defects. *Adv. Pediatr.* 22:1, 1976.

TABLE 2–5.—DRUGS GIVEN TO OR TAKEN BY THE MOTHER THAT MAY AFFECT THE FETUS OR NEWBORN*†

DRUG	POSSIBLE EFFECT ON FETUS OR NEWBORN
Accutane	Hydrocephalus, ear, eye, cardiac, skeletal anomalies, cleft palate
Alcohol (ethanol)	Withdrawal syndrome, fetal alcohol syndrome, (retarded growth; craniofacial, limb, and cardiac deformities) (see chapter 15–XX)
Amethopterin (methotrexate), aminopterin	Abortions, congenital defects (see Table 9–4)
Aminophylline	Tachycardia, gagging, vomiting, jitteriness, episthotonos
Ammonium chloride	Acidosis
Amphetamines	Malformations, hepatic calcifications, learning disability, motor incoordination, hypothermia, lethargy
Ampicillin	Decreased maternal urinary and plasma estriol levels
Analgesics	Respiratory depression
Androgens	Masculinization, advanced bone age, cleft lip and palate, congenital heart disease, T-E fistula
Atropine	Intrauterine tachycardia, dilated nonreacting pupils
Barbiturates	Bleeding resulting from deficiency of vitamin-K-dependent factors, withdrawal, cleft lip, cleft palate, congenital heart disease, hernias, chromosome break, large fontanelle, respiratory depression
Betamethasone	Suppressed steroidogenesis in fetal adrenal gland
Bromethol (Avertin)	Intrauterine hypoxia
Caffeine	Increased abortion and prematurity (?)
Carbon monoxide	Stillbirth, fetal brain damage
Cephaloridine	False positive direct Coombs' test result
Chloral hydrate	Intrauterine death with large doses
Chlorambucil	Abortions, congenital defects
Chloramphenicol	Gray baby syndrome, hypoglycemia if used with tolbutamide or phenytoin sodium
Chloroquine phosphate	Deafness, mental retardation, thrombocytopenia, abortion, prematurity, fetal death
Chlorpropamide	Increased fetal mortality, prolonged hypoglycemia
Codeine	Withdrawal syndrome
Cortisone	Congenital malformations (animals only), theoretical adrenal crisis
Curare	Paralysis in utero, position deformities
Coumadin	Nasal bone hypoplasia, long bone epiphyseal stippling
Cyclopropane	Depression
Desmethylimipramine	Breathlessness, cyanosis, tachycardia, tachypnea, irritability, diaphoresis, feeding difficulties
Dexamethasone	Suppressed steroidogenesis in fetal adrenal gland, leukocytosis lasting 1 week
Diazepam	Transient hypotonia, hypothermia, apnea, low Apgar scores, cleft lip and palate, affects beat to beat variability, withdrawal
Diazoxide	Hypertrichosis lanuginosa, alopecia, hyperglycemia

Dicumarol (bishydroxycoumarin)	Bleeding, fetal death, depressed nasal bridge, small nares, upturned nose, flattened midplane facies, stippling of phalanges and vertical column, choanal atresia, optic atrophy, cataracts, macrophthalmia, blindness, mental retardation, cardiac and renal anomalies
Diethylstilbestrol (DES)	Masculinization, vaginal adenocarcinoma
Digitalis	No reported effects
Diphenylhydantoin (Dilantin)	Cleft lip, cleft palate, saddle nose deformity, digital hypoplasia, microcephaly, heart defects, spontaneous abortion
Edrophonium chloride	Transient muscular weakness
Excessive smoking	Low birth weight
Gentamicin sulfate (Garamycin)	Toxic effect on eighth cranial nerve
Halothane	Respiratory depression
Heparin	Apparently safe
Heroin	Withdrawal syndrome, low birth weight, intrauterine death, sudden infant death syndrome
Hexamethonium bromide	Paralytic ileus, perforation, death, platelet dysfunction
Hydralazine	Thrombocytopenia
Indomethacin	Decreased fetal weight, prolonged onset of labor, respiratory distress due to pulmonary hypertension, platelet dysfunction (safe use during pregnancy has not been established)
Iodides	Hypothyroidism, goiter, respiratory distress due to tracheal compression, thrombocytopenia, vascular eruption
Isoniazid	Pyridoxine deficiency with no maternal supplement
IV dextrose and water solution	Hypotonia, lethargy, convulsion caused by hyponatremia
Kanamycin sulfate (Kantrex)	Toxic effect on eighth cranial nerve
Lead, mercury	Abortion, growth retardation, congenital anomalies, cerebral palsy, mental retardation
Lithium carbonate	Respiratory depression, hypotonia, cardiovascular malformations, goiter, neprogenic diabetes insipidus with high maternal levels
LSD	Chromosome breakage in vitro
Magnesium sulfate	CNS depression, respiratory depression, hypotonia by peripheral neuromuscular block, loss of beat-to-beat variability in fetal monitoring
Meperidine hydrochloride	Depression, withdrawal
Mepivacaine hydrochloride	CNS depression, convulsions, bradycardia
Metaproterenol sulfate	Safe use during pregnancy has not been established, possible skeletal abnormalities
Methadone hydrochloride	Withdrawal syndrome, low birth weight, sudden infant death syndrome, thrombocytosis, respiratory alkalosis
Methimazole (Tapazole)	Hypothyroidism
Methonyflurane	Depression
Methotrexate	Abortion, congenital malformation
Morphine (in drug addict)	Withdrawal syndrome, low birth weight, sudden infant death syndrome
Morphine (in labor)	Respiratory depression, bradycardia, death
Naphthalene	Hemolysis in G-6-PD deficients
Nitrofurantoin	Hemolysis in G-6-PD deficients

(continued)

TABLE 2–5.—*(continued)*

DRUG	POSSIBLE EFFECT ON FETUS OR NEWBORN
Nitrous oxide	Depression
Novobiocin	Displacement of bilirubin from albumin binding
Oxytocin	Fetal tachycardia, hyperbilirubinemia, hyponatremia, seizures
Paraldehyde	Apnea, depression
Paramethadione (Paradione)	Fetal death, congenital heart disease, microcephaly, mental retardation
Phencyclidine (PCP)	Lethargy, hypotonia, tremors, poor feeding, triangular facies, spastic quadriparesis
Phenothiazine (chlorpromazine, promethazine)	Hyperbilirubinemia, intrauterine hypoxia, poor temperature regulation, extrapyramidal dysfunction, tremors, increased muscle tone, withdrawal syndrome, CHD
Phenytoin sodium (Dilantin)	see Diphenylhydantoin
Potassium iodide	Goiter, hypothyroidism, hyperthyroidism
Procainamide	Crosses placenta, slow elimination
Propranolol hydrochloride (Inderal)	Fetal growth retardation, prolonged labor, birth asphyxia, respiratory depression, bradycardia, cardiac dysrhythmia for 2 weeks, hypoglycemia, thrombocytopenia
Propylthiouracil	Goiter, hypothyrodism
Progestins	Masculinization, advanced bone age
Quinine	Thrombocytopenic purpura, deafness, CNS anomalies
Radiation	Microcephaly, mental retardation, nondysjunction of chromosomes
Radiopaque media	Elevated protein-bound iodine, depressed ^{131}I uptake, fetal hypothyroidism
Ritodrine	Fetal tachycardia, dysrhythmias, acidosis, irritability, tremors, hyperglycemia or hypoglycemia; hypocalcemia, hypotension, ileus
Reserpine	Nasal congestion, upper respiratory obstruction, respiratory depression, lethargy, hypothermia, bradycardia, abnormal muscle tone
Salicylates (aspirin)	Fetal death, methemoglobinemia, bleeding (prolonged prothrombin time), decreased serum-albumin-binding capacity and platelet adherence
Steroids	Small-for-date infant, immunosuppression, adrenal insufficiency, arrest in replication of DNA, induction of surfactant synthesis
Streptomycin	Deafness resulting from eighth nerve damage
Sulfonamides	Displacement of bilirubin from albumin, hemolysis in G-6-PD deficients, growth retardation, thrombocytopenia
Sulfonylureas	Hypoglycemia, congenital anomalies (?)
Terbutaline sulfate	No apparent adverse effects with regard to fetal growth
Teridax (iophenoxic acid)	Elevated protein-bound iodine and butanol-extractable iodine
Testosterone	Masculinization
Tetracyclines	Staining of teeth, enamel hypoplasia, inhibition of bone growth, congenital cataracts

Thalidomide	Phocomelia, death, hearing loss, heart and GI anomalies
Theophylline	Tachycardia, vomiting, jitteriness
Thiazide diuretics	Thrombocytopenia, bleeding, maternal and fetal acidosis, hyponatremia, hypokalemia, convulsions, hemolysis, respiratory distress
Thiouracil	Goiter, hypothyroidism
Thyroxine	No apparent adverse effects
Tobramycin sulfate (Nebcin)	Toxic effect on eighth cranial nerve
Tolbutamide	Congenital anomalies (?), fetal death, thrombocytopenia
Trichloroethylene	Respiratory depression, caudal regression syndrome (?)
Trimethobenzamide hydrochloride	Extrapyramidal dysfunction
Vaccines	Contraindicated: BCG, measles, mumps, Rubella, small pox and yellow fever, tularemia Only when indicated: Cholera, diphtheria-pertussis-tetanus, polio, rabies, typhoid, influenza, pneumococcal
Vitamin B_6	Withdrawal, convulsions
Vitamin D	Hypercalcemia (?), mental retardation, supravalvular aortic stenosis, elfin facies, lenticular opacities
Vitamin K analogues	Hemolysis, hyperbilirubinemia

*Adapted from McKay R.J., Lucey J.F.: Neonatology. *N. Engl. J. Med.* 270:1231, 1964, and Hill R.M.: *Perinatal Pharmacology.* Evansville, Indiana, Mead Johnson, 1983.

†G-6-PD, glucose-6-phosphate dehydrogenase.

Chapter 3

Delivery Room Resuscitation Procedures

I. PREPARATION

Preparation for resuscitation begins before delivery. Adequately trained personnel and equipment must be available. Every delivery room should be prepared for the worst catastrophe. Sterile equipment should be ready for suction, intermittent positive-pressure breathing (IPPB) by bag and mask, endotracheal intubation, and umbilical vessel catheterization. Prior to arrival in the delivery room, the physician should wash hands and don a sterile gown. The physician responsible for resuscitation should check that all apparatus are available and working. Commonly used drugs should be drawn in syringes ready for immediate use.

A. Personnel

Before delivery, the physician responsible for resuscitation should be trained in resuscitative techniques. Junior house officers should practice resuscitative techniques under senior supervision. A junior house officer should never be allowed to attend a delivery without supervision unless adequately trained by the senior staff. A nurse should be available to help the physician throughout the resuscitative procedure.

B. Equipment

The following equipment should be available at all deliveries:

1. A warmed resuscitation table supplying suction, oxygen, heat, including an overhead radiant heater with servocontrol capability, and procedure light
2. Warmed and humidified oxygen and air
3. Suction apparatus

Bulb syringe, De Lee suction catheter, portable electric suction, and a selection of polyethylene catheters

4. Sterilized straight endotracheal tubes (2.0-, 2.5-, 3.0-, 3.5-, and 4.0-mm internal diameter) or Cole orotracheal tubes (sizes 8, 10, 12, 14 and 16 Fr.) with stylet
5. Oral airways no. 00 and 0
6. Pencil-handled laryngoscope with Miller size 0 and 1 blade
7. Infant stethoscope
8. 250-ml or 500-ml bags, anesthesia bag, and Hope or Cardiff (Penlon) resuscitator bag and masks with connectors
9. Easily seen wall clock with sweep second hand
10. Syringes: 5-ml and 10-ml syringes
11. Umbilical vessel catheterization set
    a. Scissors and iris scissors
    b. Hemostat and needle holder
    c. Cord tie
    d. Forceps: mouse toothed, straight and iris
    e. Several 2 × 2 and 4 × 4 gauzes, 000 and 0000 silk
    f. Fr. 3½, 5, and 8 umbilical vessel catheters
12. Three-way stopcocks
13. Pressure transducers and monitor for vascular pressures
14. Aneroid manometer for observing airway pressure during assisted ventilation
15. Oxygen analyzer
16. Arterial blood gas set (capillary tubes, heparin syringe and butterfly needle)
17. Tape
18. Cardiorespiratory monitor, ECG
19. Tracheostomy set
20. Gloves, sizes 6 to 8½
21. Cord clamp
22. Warm blankets and towels

C. Drugs

1. 4.2% $NaHCO_3$, 0.5 mEq/ml
2. Aqueous epinephrine, 1:10,000 dilution (0.1 mg/ml)
3. Naloxone hydrochloride (Narcan), 0.02 mg/ml
4. Atropine sulfate diluted to 0.1 mg/ml
5. 10% and 5% dextrose in water
6. Blood volume expanders: salt-poor albumin, dextran, Plasmanate (5% plasma protein), normal saline, and/or type O Rh-negative whole blood
7. Calcium gluconate (10% calcium)
8. Heparin sodium, 1000 units/ml
9. Isoproterenol HCl (1:5000), 0.2 mg/ml
10. Dopamine HCl, 40 mg/ml
11. Hydrocortisone, 100 mg/vial

II. GENERAL RESUSCITATIVE MEASURES FOR ALL INFANTS

A. Monitor the Heart

The fetal heart should be monitored constantly to the moment of delivery. A sustained heart rate below 120 or above 160 beats/minute, absence of acceleration, reduced beat to beat variability, the presence of an abnormal fetal heart tracing, a fetal scalp pH less than 7.20, or the presence of meconium-stained amniotic fluid in a vertex presentation are warning signs of fetal distress (see Table 2–2). If these signs develop, the staff should be alerted that an emergency delivery may be indicated.

B. Suction the Nose and Oropharynx

In the vertex presentation after delivery of the head, suction the pharynx and the nose prior to the delivery of the whole body to prevent aspiration. Suction the oropharynx first because nasal suction induces gasping. This is especially important for those infants that have been bathed in meconium.

C. Clamp the Cord

Immediately after delivery, hold the infant head down at the level of the placenta. Clamp the cord and cut within 15 to 20 seconds of birth.

D. Place in Resuscitator

Place the infant at once in 15-degree Trendelenburg's position in a previously warmed resuscitator with an overhead radiant heater. No attempt to remove the clamp and tie the cord should be made at this time. Pat the infant dry to prevent excessive heat loss.

E. Check Heart Rate and Aspirate

An assistant should listen to the heartbeat immediately and indicate the rate by finger movement. The resuscitator aspirates the mouth, pharynx, and nose with a bulb syringe or a suction catheter. This should take less than 15 seconds. Care must be taken not to prolong suctioning, which leads to decreased Pa_{O_2}. To judge the duration of suction time, the physician may hold his or her own breath while suctioning. A suction pressure above 75 cm H_2O should be avoided to prevent bleeding by trauma, if possible. Direct stimulation of the vagal nerve by the catheter tip can cause vasovagal reflex with bradycardia and/or laryngeal spasm with resultant apnea and depression. If this occurs, the more vigorous resuscitation procedures for the moderately or severely depressed infant are required.

For those infants born bathed in meconium, suction the oropharynx with a De

Lee suction catheter while the head is on the perineum. If meconium is present in the oropharynx, visualize and inspect the vocal cords by direct laryngoscopy. If meconium is present at the cords, suction the trachea directly with a De Lee catheter or orotracheal tube. A high suction pressure approximately equal to 75 cm H_2O may be required for thick meconium. Avoid IPPB with bag and mask until visible meconium has been removed from the larynx. If the infant is neurologically depressed and assisted ventilation is required, endotracheal intubation with positive pressure ventilation should be performed.

F. Reinforce Sensory Input

After suctioning, tap the soles of the feet to reinforce sensory input. Avoid traumatic or vigorous physical stimulation.

G. Prevent Undue Exposure

Pat the infant dry to minimize excessive heat loss since chilling predisposes the infant to acidosis, hypoglycemia, and other conditions.

III. CLINICAL CLASSIFICATION AND MANAGEMENT OF THE NEWBORN INFANT BASED ON THE APGAR SCORING SYSTEM

The Apgar score for newborns is a useful aid to evaluate the infant at 1 and 5 minutes after birth. The following five objective signs are evaluated and each given a score of 0, 1, or 2. A score of 10 indicates that the infant is in the best possible condition.

APGAR	SIGN	ACTION TO ASSIGN SCORE	SCORE 0	SCORE 1	SCORE 2
Appearance	Color	Visual assessment	Blue, pale	Body pink, blue extremities	Completely pink
Pulse	Heart rate	Count cord pulse or auscultate heart	Absent	<100/min	>100/min
Grimace	Reflex irritability	Flick sole of foot	No response	Some motion	Cry, sneeze, cough
Activity	Muscle tone	Manipulate extremity	Limp, flaccid	Some flexing of extremities	Well-flexed
Respiration	Respiratory effort	Visual assessment	Absent	Slow, irregular hypoventilation	Good strong cry

Apgar score at 1 minute:
- 7 to 10, normal infants
- 4 to 6, moderately depressed infants
- 0 to 3, severely depressed infants

A. Normal Infants: Apgar Score 7 to 10

Infants are vigorous and cough or cry within seconds of birth. No further procedures are needed after brief suctioning (15 seconds). Elective procedures, for example, tying of the cord or footprinting, should be avoided until after the infant is vigorous and breathing regularly. When the infant's condition is stable, apply one drop of 1% silver nitrate solution in each eye to prevent gonococcal conjunctivitis. Do not rinse silver nitrate solution because rinsing diminishes the effectiveness of the silver nitrate. Erythromycin or tetracycline ophthalmic ointment may be used in place of 1% silver nitrate.

B. Moderately Depressed Newborn Infants: Apgar Score 4 to 6

1. Keep the airway patent by quick and efficient suctioning with negative pressure of 45 to 75 cm H_2O. Administer O_2 IPPB by bag (e.g., Cardiff [Penlon Ltd.] or Hope resuscitator bag) and mask using 30 to 40 cm H_2O pressure at 1.0- to 1.5-second intervals (40 to 60 times/minute) which will stimulate reflex inspiratory effort. Tap soles of feet or rub the skin to stimulate. Keep the infant warm.
2. If spontaneous respirations ensue, no further procedures are necessary.
3. If IPPB by bag and mask does not result in spontaneous respirations by 2 minutes of age, intubate the trachea at once under direct vision and perform the procedure for infants with Apgar scores of 0 to 3.

C. Severely Depressed Newborn Infants: Apgar Score 0 to 3

1. Keep the infant warm. Keep the airway patent by quick and efficient suctioning with negative pressure of 45 to 75 cm H_2O.
2. Institute assisted ventilation immediately. Administer 100% oxygen via an anesthesia or Cardiff (Penlon) bag and mask or an endotracheal tube. While an anesthesia bag can deliver 100% oxygen, it may develop excessive pressure that may result in pulmonary air leaks. Prior practice is necessary. The Hope resuscitator bag, or Cardiff infant inflating bag has a safety pressure valve and does not allow pressure to be greater than 40 cm H_2O. Unfortunately, the Hope resuscitator bag does not allow oxygen concentration to be greater than 40%. Penlon's Cardiff infant inflating bag allows 90% to 100% oxygen and has a safety pressure valve.

   Always intubate the trachea under direct vision. If the intubation procedure lasts longer than 30 seconds because of technical difficulties, ventilate the infant using IPPB by bag and mask until the infant becomes pink. Endotracheal intubation can then be reattempted. IPPB by bag and mask may not improve ventilation in choanal atresia, laryngeal web, tracheoesophageal fistula, diaphragmatic hernia, hypoplastic lungs, pneumothorax, severe pulmonary failure, etc. (see Table 3–1). Monitor the heart rate through the entire procedure. If heart rate is less than 80 beats/minute, initiate closed chest cardiac massage.

a. Technique of endotracheal intubation

1) Select an endotracheal tube. Use a 3.0-mm or larger straight or a Fr. 10 or larger Cole Endotracheal tube because available suction catheters may not fit through smaller bore endotracheal tubes. The only exception applies to the less than 1,000-gm infant where a 2.5-mm straight or Fr. size 8 Cole endotracheal tube is the only size that fits the infant's trachea. Recommended endotracheal tube sizes are 3.0 mm (10 Fr.) for the 1,000 to 1,500-gm infant, 3.5 mm (12 Fr.) for the 1,500- to 2,260-gm infant, and 4.0 mm (14 Fr.) for the 2,260-gm and above infant (see appendix A–6). The tube should not be excessively stiff and should not collapse with negative pressure. If the tube is excessively soft, insert a stylet before intubation. Care should be taken not to extend the stylet beyond the tip of the endotracheal tube. A small amount of air should leak between the endotracheal tube and the vocal cords when IPPB is applied. If the tube fits too tightly without surrounding air leakage, compression of the vocal cords with ensuing destruction, scarring, and stenosis may occur.
2) Place the infant supine with a towel under the neck (Fig 3–1). Do not hyperextend the neck because the trachea can be narrowed.
3) Hold the laryngoscope handle in the left hand above the blade and introduce the blade into the right side of the infant's mouth. Move the laryngoscope blade to the center of the mouth. At this time the laryngoscope blade should be between the base of the tongue and the epiglottis.
4) Tilt the tip of the laryngoscope blade upward to raise the epiglottis anteriorly above the esophagus. To help view the vocal cords, lift the epiglottis with the tip of the straight blade. This exposes the entrance to the trachea (Fig 3–2). The fifth finger of the resuscitator's left hand is used to compress the cricoid cartilage toward the spine, which helps bring the larynx into view.
5) Give quick, brief suction if foreign material such as small blood clots, meconium-stained mucus, or vernix obstructs the larynx.
6) Hold the endotracheal tube in the right hand and pass the tube alongside the laryngoscope blade (not through the groove) under direct vi-

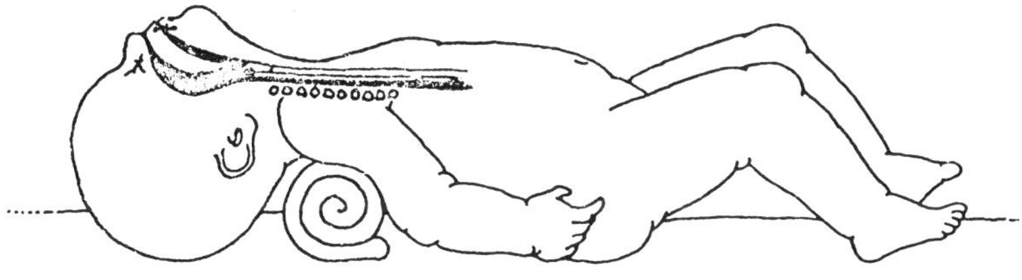

FIG 3–1.
Position of the infant during laryngoscopy. (From Ostheimer G.W.: Newborn resuscitation, in Hersehy S.G. (ed.): *Resuscitation of the Newborn.* ASA Refresher Courses in Anaesthesiology. Vol. 8. Philadelphia, J.B. Lippincott Co., 1980. Used by permission.)

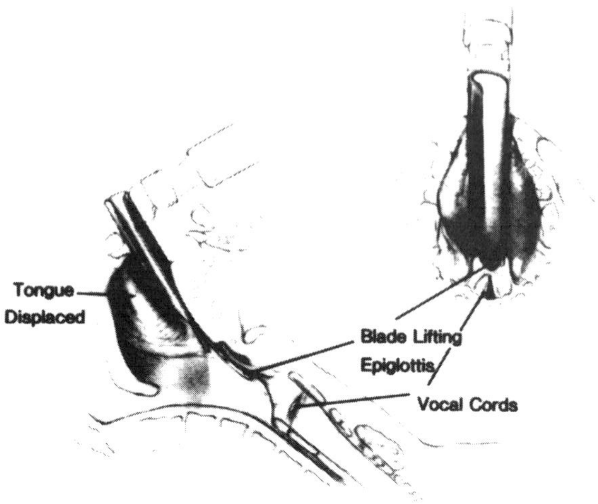

FIG 3–2.
Sagital view *(left)* and laryngoscopist's view *(right)* of upper airway during proper placement of straight laryngoscope blade. (From Natanson C., Shelhamer J.H., Parrillo J.E.: Intubation of the trachea in the critical care setting. *J.A.M.A.* 253: 1160, 1985. Used by permission.)

sion from the right side of the infant's mouth into the tracheal orifice and through the vocal cords to a distance of about 2 cm below the level of the vocal cords and 1 to 2 cm above the carina. The distance to be inserted from the tip of the endotracheal tube to the lip is approximately 7 cm for 1,000-gm, 8 cm for 2,000-gm, and 9 cm for 3,000-gm infants (see appendix A–7).

7) After placing the endotracheal tube, withdraw the laryngoscope carefully while holding the tube with the right hand to avoid displacing the tube. Then remove the stylet and apply short puffs of air fortified with oxygen into the endotracheal tube.
8) Inflate the lungs approximately 40 to 60 times a minute using 30- to 40-cm H_2O pressure. After the lungs have expanded, pressure should be limited to 15 cm H_2O to prevent pneumothorax. Interposing a pressure manometer in the circuit is helpful in assessing the pressure required to inflate the lungs.

   The upper one third of the chest should rise slightly with each inflation. The act of expanding the lungs stimulates respiration (Head's paradox reflex). With the first or second application of positive pressure, some infants make an effort to breathe. The endotracheal tube is removed when the infant is breathing spontaneously and the heart rate is maintained at 120 beats/minute or more.
9) To evaluate the adequacy of ventilation, note the following:
   a) Increased heart rate
   b) Symmetric chest movements of the upper one third of the chest

c) Increased pinkness of the infant's skin
d) Increased muscle tone
e) Presence of breath sounds bilaterally. Listen to the axillary regions as well as the anterior chest. Note that when the esophagus is intubated by mistake in a very small infant, the resuscitator can erroneously think he or she hears breath sounds because the sound of flowing air is well transmitted. If the resuscitator hears breath sounds over the stomach and/or sees stomach distention, the esophagus has been intubated. Remove the tube, ventilate by bag and mask, and reinsert the tube into the trachea.

b. Mouth-to-mouth resuscitation
If the equipment is not available or does not function properly, mouth-to-mouth resuscitation can always be given. Place mouth over the infant's mouth and nose and breathe into the infant's mouth and nose 40 to 60 times/minute. Placing the infant in a semisitting position will facilitate the procedure. Be sure that the airway is patent before beginning mouth-to-mouth resuscitation with air fortified with oxygen.

c. Cardiac massage
In the event of cardiac asystole or severe bradycardia (less than 80 beats/minute), institute cardiac massage. Encircle the infant's thorax with two hands (which increase greater blood pressure) or place two fingers over the heart to the left of the lower sternum. The infant's back should be on a firm surface. Depress the chest wall 1 to 2 cm, 100 to 120 times/minute. Perform ventilation and external cardiac massage in sequence with three to four massages after each insufflation. Recent data indicate that simultaneous ventilation and compression combined with catecholamine administration may increase aortic and carotid as well as cerebral blood flow and improve neurologic outcome. Palpate the infant's pulse to estimate cardiac output.

3. Catheterize the umbilical vessel
When ventilation is established, correct metabolic acidosis and/or shock through the umbilical route. Do not use this route if infant has omphalocele or omphalitis.
   a. Summon an assistant to maintain respirations while the resuscitator catheterizes the umbilical vessel. (One person cannot ventilate the infant and catheterize the umbilical vessel at the same time.)
   b. Sterilely open the umbilical vessel catheterization set.
   c. Don sterile gloves and prepare the umbilicus and the surrounding area with antiseptic solution, e.g., Betadine (The Purdue Frederick Co.), and drape appropriately.
   d. Fill the umbilical catheter with normal saline before inserting the catheter to minimize the possibility of air emboli.
   e. Prepare a 5-ml syringe filled with normal saline or 10% glucose in water solution and connect it to the three-way stopcock. When the catheter is in place, attach the catheter to the stopcock.
   f. Cannulate the umbilical vein or artery. Although arterial blood pressure and

gases can be obtained by arterial catheterization (which also has less complications), do not waste time cannulating the artery. During an emergency, the umbilical vein is much larger and easier to cannulate.

1) Umbilical vein catheterization
   a) Cut the cord with a scalpel to a length of 1.0 cm. Care is required to prevent excessive bleeding.
   b) Apply traction with a mouse-toothed forcep to the umbilical cord stump to facilitate catheter entry. Remove clots with fine iris forcep if present.
   c) Introduce slowly with gentle pressure into the umbilical vein a sterile size 5 or 8 radiopaque polyethylene or Silastic catheter for a length equal to the distance between the umbilical stump and the xyphoid process so that the tip of the catheter lies in the inferior vena cava. (The vein usually appears larger with thinner walls than the artery.) If the catheter cannot advance into the inferior vena cava and some resistance is met, do not force it. Pull the catheter back and readvance. It will frequently enter the inferior vena cava beyond the ductus venosus. A feeding tube may be used as a catheter because it is blunt and nontraumatic.
   d) When blood returns freely through the catheter, it is ready for use.
   e) The umbilical vein is used only for emergencies in the delivery room. Remove when the infant's condition is stabilized.
2) Umbilical artery catheterization
   a) Using a scalpel, cleanly cut through the umbilical cord about 1 cm above the stump.
   b) Overcome the arterial spasm of the selected artery by teasing the artery open with an iris forcep prong. Insert catheter into the dilated artery lumen and remove the forcep prong.
   c) Introduce a size 3½ or 5 Fr. single-end hole saline-filled catheter into and down the lumen of the artery for a length double the distance between the umbilicus and the femoral pulse at the inguinal fold minus 0.5 cm. The catheter end should be at the level of the bifurcation of the aorta (between third and fourth lumbar vertebrae).
   d) Resistance is usually felt at the level of the abdominal wall (where the catheter makes a sharp caudal turn) and at the point where the umbilical artery meets the bladder and turns toward the internal iliac. Resistance can be overcome by rolling the catheter and/or applying gentle pressure for 30 to 45 seconds. *Do not apply strong pressure.*

g. Recheck the catheter length by using normogram for estimation of the proper length when the emergency is over (Fig 3–3).

h. Stabilize the umbilical vessel catheter.
   1) Attach a three-way stopcock to the umbilical vessel catheter so that withdrawal of the blood can be accomplished without opening the system.
   2) If the umbilical vessel catheter is to be left in place, stabilize by placing a suture through the umbilical cord and tying the suture around the

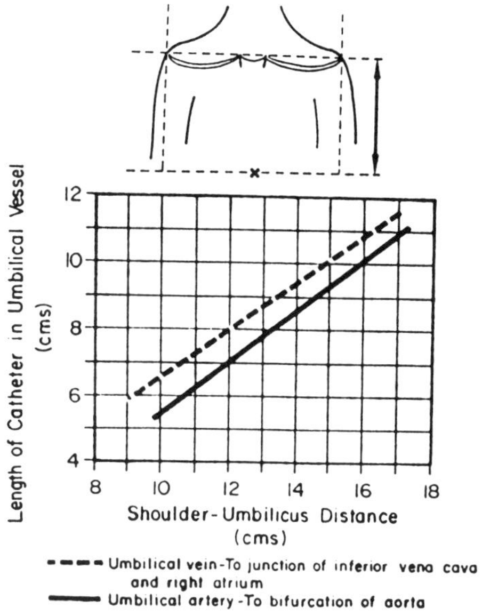

FIG 3–3.
Normogram for estimation of the proper length of umbilical vessel catheter. (Modified from Dunn P.M.: *Arch. Dis. Child.* 41:71, 1966. Used by permission.)

catheter. The catheter can then be taped to the abdomen as in Figure 3–4. Maintain sterility throughout the procedure.

i. When the infant's condition is stabilized, obtain anterior and lateral x-ray films to confirm the catheter's location (Fig 3–5).

j. Complications of umbilical vessel catheterization are the following:

1) Umbilical vein catheterization

Bacteremia, septicemia, venous perforation, thrombosis, bleeding, portal hypertension, necrotizing enterocolitis, omphalitis, bleeding from the umbilical stump, air emboli, cardiac arrhythmias, and others.

2) Umbilical artery catheterization

Arterial spasm (blanching of an extremity, buttock, etc.) or perforation, thrombosis, embolism (e.g., dusky toes) bleeding from the umbilical stump, necrotizing enterocolitis, hypertension with proteinuria or hematuria (possible aortic or renal artery thrombosis), omphalitis, osteomyelitis, gangrene of the buttock, paraplegia, and others.

4. Correct acidosis

If the infant appears severely asphyxiated, attempt to correct acidosis. When the umbilical catheter is filled with blood, attach it to the syringe and give 1 mEq/kg of 4.2% (0.5 mEq/ml) $NaHCO_3$ over the next minute. (Weight may be estimated.) If the heart rate is less than 80 beats/minute, external cardiac massage must be performed during $NaHCO_3$ infusion. Air and clots must not be pushed into the circulation. Correction of acidosis decreases pulmonary vascular resistance, increases cardiac output, and increased Pa_{O_2}. Correction may increase intracerebral blood pressure and osmolarity and may result in intraventricular hemorrhage in premature infants. Do not administer hypertonic

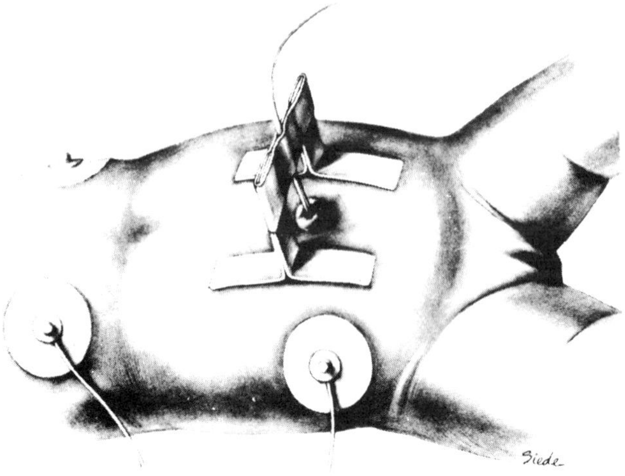

FIG 3–4.
Taping of umbilical vessel catheter. (From Phillips B.L., McQuitty J.: Blood gases: Technical aspects and interpretation, in Goldsmith J.P., Karotkin E.H. (eds.): *Assisted Ventilation of the Neonate.* Philadelphia, W.B. Saunders Co., 1981, p. 223. Used by permission.)

solution rapidly via an umbilical vein catheter to prevent liver damage. *Do not use $NaHCO_3$ unless absolutely necessary.*

5. Expand intravascular volume. Severely asphyxiated infants often (greater than 60%) are volume deficient (hypovolemia and/or shock). When infants have clinical manifestations of hypovolemia (pale, poor perfusion, feeble pulse, poor activity, etc.), administer 10 to 20 ml/kg of fresh 0 negative whole blood, fresh frozen plasma, Plasmanate (or normal saline) or 1 gm/kg of 5% salt-poor albumin or 5% Albumisol.
6. After correction of acidosis and hypovolemia, obtain a blood gas determination. The act of correcting the pH appears to stimulate respiration. Frequently, an infant will make an effort to breathe after $NaHCO_3$ is administered. For those infants who begin to breathe spontaneously, no further procedure in the delivery room is required. The endotracheal tube may be withdrawn when the infant is breathing adequately.
7. Administer other drugs or measures if cardiac output is not restored. If correction of acidosis and hypovolemia and external cardiac massage fail to restore cardiac output, 0.1–0.2 ml/kg of 1:10,000 aqueous epinephrine may be given IV, intratracheal, or intracardiac. Do not use epinephrine to stimulate the heart until the pH has been corrected. Administer 100 to 200 mg/kg of calcium gluconate during cardiac arrest since it increases myocardial contractile force. Atropine may also be used to raise the heart rate (dose, 0.01 to 0.03 mg/kg IV or SQ). If shock persists and endotoxemia is suspected, administer hydro-

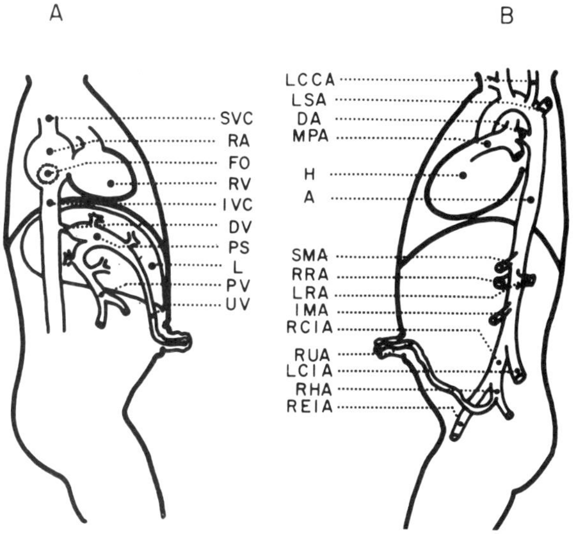

FIG 3–5.
The newborn umbilical venous/arterial systems. **A,** diagram of the newborn umbilical venous system, *SVC,* superior vena cava; *RA,* right atrium; *FO,* foramen ovale; *RV,* right ventricle; *IVC,* inferior vena cava; *DV,* ductus venosus; *PS,* portal sinus; *L,* liver; *PV,* portal vein; *UV,* umbilical vein. **B,** diagram of the newborn arterial system including the umbilical artery. *LCCA,* left common carotid artery; *LSA,* left subclavian artery; *DA,* ductus arteriosus; *MPA,* main pulmonary artery; *H,* heart; *A,* aorta; *SMA,* superior mesenteric artery; *RRA,* right renal artery; *LRA,* left renal artery; *IMA,* inferior mesenteric artery; *RCIA,* right common iliac artery; *RUA,* right umbilical artery; *LCIA,* left common iliac artery; *RHA,* right hypogastric artery; *REIA,* right external iliac artery. (From Kitterman J.A., Phibbs R.H., Tooley W.H.: *Ped. Clin. N. Am.* 17:895, 1970. Used by permission.)

cortisone 35 to 50 mg/kg IV over 10 to 15 minutes, which may be repeated, and naloxone hydrochloride 0.01 mg/kg IV (see chapter 14–IIID7).

Should ventricular fibrillation occur (very rare in newborns), external defibrillation can be achieved with 2 watt-second/kg initially to 3 to 5-watt second/kg subsequently through appropriate paddles.

8. Stabilize the endotracheal tube. The position of the endotracheal tube should be stabilized in the following manner if the infant requires endotracheal intubation and assisted ventilation during transportation to the nursery (Fig 3–6).
   a. Mark the endotracheal tube at the level of the infant's lips to avoid accidental withdrawal or advancement of the tube.
   b. Dry the infant's upper lip and cheeks.
   c. Paint the infant's upper lip, cheeks, and exterior of the tube with tincture of benzoin.
   d. Split a piece of 0.5-inch adhesive tape down the center, almost to the end.

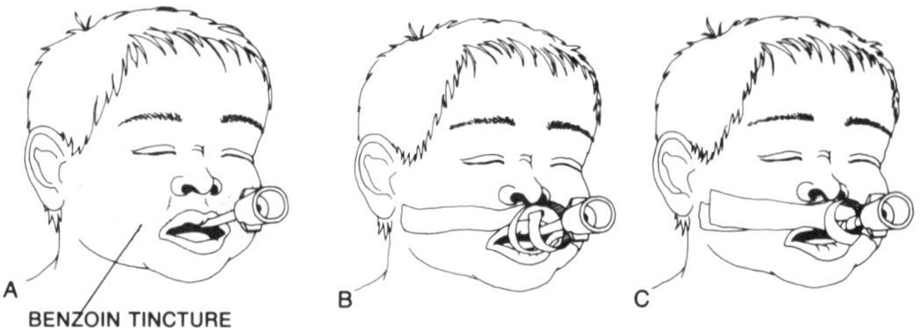

FIG 3–6.
Taping procedure of the endotracheal tube. (From Hughes W.T., Buescher E.S. (eds.): *The Respiratory Tract in Pediatric Procedures.* Philadelphia, W.B. Saunders Co., 1980, p. 221. Used by permission.

e. Place one end of the tape on one cheek; draw it across the upper lip and firmly press it to the skin. Wrap the other end firmly around the tube (2 revolutions) in a counterclockwise direction for the left side and clockwise for the right side and secured to the other cheek.
f. When the endotracheal tube is placed in the middle of the upper lip, cut the tape in the form of an "H" by splitting both ends of the tape leaving the center intact. Place two upper ends across the upper lip, wrap two lower ends around the tube, and secure to cheeks.
g. Change the tube if it is obstructed or extubation occurs.
h. Other causes of respiratory depression are the following:
   1) When depression is secondary to narcotics administered to the mother before delivery (peak fetal narcotic levels occur 1½–2 hours post administration to the mother) or secondary to an excessive quantity of narcotics, give naloxone hydrochloride (Narcan), 0.005 to 0.010 mg/kg, through the umbilical route to reverse the respiratory depressant effect of the narcotics. This drug does not reverse the effect of barbiturates or other sedatives.
   2) When the amniotic fluid is meconium stained (meconium aspiration), the infant's airway should be suctioned and the cords visualized followed by deep pharyngeal suction before positive pressure ventilation is administered.
   3) Other causes of respiratory embarrassment must be rapidly assessed if the infant does not improve or does not have sustained respiration (Table 3–1).

9. Continue postresuscitation care of infants. Resuscitation does *not* end with endotracheal intubation and correction of acidosis and shock in the delivery room; this is only the beginning. Even if the infant no longer needs endotracheal intubation and appears to be in satisfactory condition, the following should be performed on arrival in the nursery:
   a. Completely examine the infant to evaluate any associated congenital malformations, the ventilation status, acid-base balance, and complications of

(continued on page 39)

TABLE 3–1.—RAPID DELIVERY ROOM ASSESSMENT OF THE DISTRESSED NEWBORN TO DETERMINE IMMEDIATE MANAGEMENT*

CLINICAL CONDITION OF THE INFANT AND MATERNAL HISTORY	DIAGNOSIS TO CONSIDER	IMMEDIATE MANAGEMENT
Initial depressed respiratory and motor activity with increasing flaccidity. Color and heart rate improve with positive pressure, but infant fails to breathe spontaneously.	Central nervous system depression	Resuscitate.
Maternal history of recent or excessive narcotics or sedatives	Recent or excessive maternal anesthesia and/or analgesia	If excessive narcotics, treat with Narcan, 0.005–0.010 mg/kg IM or IV stat; repeat as required. Administer cardiorespiratory support.
History of fetal distress, prolonged second stage of labor, difficult delivery with or without abnormal presentation, cord prolapse, etc.	Prolonged perinatal asphyxia	Administer respiratory support. Correct metabolic acidosis. Support cardiac status. Correct shock, if present.
Initial severe suprasternal and/or substernal retractions, flaring alae nasi, and air hunger with progressive respiratory distress and depression; sometimes infant holds head in opisthotonos and keeps mouth open. Normal prenatal history.	Upper airway obstruction	Resuscitate.
Infant continues to deteriorate.	Asphyxia caused by aspiration of clots or meconium, laryngeal web, etc.	Open airway, suction trachea directly. Do not give IPPB by bag and mask until meconium or other material is suctioned from pharynx, larynx, and trachea. Correct metabolic acidosis. Often infants improve with suction. Support cardiac respiratory status.
Infant becomes pink when crying.	Choanal atresia	Open airway with oral airway. If not improved, perform endotracheal intubation. Look for associated malformations.

(continued)

TABLE 3–1.—*(continued)*

CLINICAL CONDITION OF THE INFANT AND MATERNAL HISTORY	DIAGNOSIS TO CONSIDER	IMMEDIATE MANAGEMENT
Progressive cyanosis, respiratory distress, and depression. Decreased unilateral breath sounds. Increased percussion resonance ipsilateral to side of decreased breath sounds. History of aspiration of meconium or blood clots or maternal oligohydramnios.	Pneumothorax	Suction: open airway. Resuscitate as required. Obtain chest AP and lateral film and/or transilluminate the chest. Remove air by needle aspiration and/or placement of chest tube.
No or poor spontaneous respiratory activity, usually pale, occasionally pink, poor perfusion, weak or absent peripheral pulses, increased or decreased heart rate, low central venous pressure and/or blood pressure. Maternal history of bleeding during last trimester.	Anemia with acute hypovolemic shock	Suction: open airway. Resuscitate as required. Obtain central venous and arterial blood pressure; if low, expand intravascular volume. Remember hematocrit can be high even if infant is in shock. In an emergency, blood for transfusion can be obtained from the placenta. Correct metabolic acidosis as required. Monitor central venous pressure, hematocrit, blood gas studies, and temperature. If premature, observe for signs of respiratory distress syndrome.
Tachypneic, pale, hydropic infant. Hepatosplenomegaly and edema. Maternal history of Rh-negative blood type and sensitization.	Erythroblastosis with severe hemolytic anemia.	Suction: open airway; support respiration. Intubate and give IPPB if required. Correct acidosis and/or anemia through umbilical route. Observe heart rate, respiratory rate, and liver for signs of congestive heart failure. If premature, observe for signs of respiratory distress syndrome. Infant may require thoracentesis to remove effusion.
Apnea or tachypnea with retractions and cyanosis. Potter's facies: hypertelorism, epicanthal folds, parrot-beaked nose, large low-set ears. Possible history of oligohydramnios.	Pulmonary hypoplasia, polycystic kidneys, or renal agenesis (Potter's syndrome)	Suction: open airway; resuscitate as required. *Caution:* Give IPPB with the lowest pressure possible and high rate because pneumothorax is common complication of hypoplasia. Resuscitation very difficult because of pulmonary hypoplasia. Palpate kidneys for polycystic masses. Order chest x-ray film, renal sonography. *Remember:* BUN and creatinine are normal at birth in renal agenesis.

At or shortly after birth, cyanosis, severe respiratory distress. Deterioration with IPPB with bag and mask. Diminished breath sounds, frequently on the left and heart sounds heard in the right chest. Scaphoid abdomen. Possible history of polyhydramnios.	Diaphragmatic hernia	Suction: open airway. Intubate: give IPPB via endotracheal tube, but do *not* give IPPB by bag and mask; dilated GI tract will further compress the lung. Support cardiorespiratory status. Decompress GI tract with nasogastric tube. Immediate chest x-ray film to confirm diagnosis. Immediate surgical consult.
Frequently difficult resuscitation. Tachypnea. Excessive secretions from mouth associated with failure to pass nasogastric tube. Possible history of polyhydramnios.	Tracheoesophageal fistula	Suction larynx directly using laryngoscope. Resuscitate as required. Attempt to pass nasogastric tube to test for tracheoesophageal fistula. Leave small catheter in pouch to facilitate drainage. Obtain chest and abdominal x-ray film with nasogastric tube inserted. Consult surgeon immediately. Withhold oral feedings. Look for associated malformations (e.g., VATER syndrome).
Limp, cyanotic infant with ecchymosis and bruising of lower extremities. Nonmolded head. History of difficult breech delivery.	Birth trauma perinatal asphyxia secondary to difficult breech delivery	Suction: open airway. Resuscitate for hypoxic infant as needed. Obtain blood gases. Correct metabolic acidosis. Observe for other signs of CNS damage (convulsions, low Hct, etc.). Obtain head sonography and/or CT scan. Observe for signs of facial nerve palsy, brachial plexus palsy or other types of associated birth injury (see Table 5–3).
Vigorous newborn infant who suddenly stops breathing. Normal maternal history.	Central nervous system bleeding secondary to vascular malformation.	Suction: open airway. Resuscitate as required. Obtain head sonography and/or CT scan as soon as possible.

(continued)

TABLE 3–1.—*(continued)*

CLINICAL CONDITION OF THE INFANT AND MATERNAL HISTORY	DIAGNOSIS TO CONSIDER	IMMEDIATE MANAGEMENT
	Prolonged suction	Stop suctioning; administer IPPB by bag and mask.
	Aspiration of clots, meconium aspiration, etc.	Open airway, suction trachea directly. Do not give IPPB by bag and mask until meconium or other material is suctioned from pharynx, larynx, and trachea. Correct metabolic acidosis. Often infants improve with suction. Support cardiac respiratory status.
Apnea, pale, poor perfusion, flaccid. Infant has putrid smell. History of maternal infection, prolonged rupture of membranes or fetal distress.	Neonatal sepsis	Suction: open airway. Resuscitate as required. Correct metabolic acidosis and shock as required. Start antibiotics after obtaining cultures of blood, CSF, etc. (see chapter 16–III).

*IPPB, intermittent positive-pressure breathing.

REFERENCES

Apgar V.: A proposal for a new method of evaluation of the newborn infant. *Anesth. Analg.* 32:260, 1952.

Brann A.W., Cefalo R.C.: Care of the newborn in the delivery room. *Pediatrics* 64:970, 1979.

Gregory G.A.: Resuscitation of the newborn. *Anesthesiology* 43:225, 1975.

James L.S.: Onset of breathing and resuscitation. *Pediatr. Clin. N. Am.* 13:621, 1966.

Standards of cardiopulmonary resuscitation and emergency cardiac care. *J.A.M.A.* 227(suppl):837, 1974.

Rogers M.C.: New developments in cardiopulmonary resuscitation. *Pediatrics* 71:655, 1983.

Natanson C., Shelhamer J.H., Parrillo J.E.: Intubation of the trachea in the critical care setting. *J.A.M.A.* 253:1160, 1985.

(continued from page 34)

severe asphyxia and resuscitation (especially persistent pulmonary hypertension of the newborn, pneumothorax etc.).

b. Make sure that the airway is patent. Suction as needed.
c. Maintain a rectal temperature at approximately 37.0° C or skin temperature taken on the right upper abdominal quadrant at approximately 36.5° C.
d. Monitor vital signs carefully. Be aware that severe hypoxia can lead to multisystem damage (see Chapter 15–IV).
e. Draw blood for blood gas studies; look for undercorrection and continuing acidosis, overcorrection and continuing acidosis, or overcorrection and alkalosis.
f. Draw blood for hematocrit, calcium, glucose, and electrolyte determinations; remember that excessive $NaHCO_3$ can produce alkalosis, hypocalcemia, hypokalemia, or hypernatremia.
g. Obtain anteroposterior (AP) and lateral chest and abdominal x-ray films to confirm the position of the endotracheal tube (2 cm above the carina) and the tip of the umbilical vessel catheter (artery: vertebrae L-3 to L-4 or T-6 to T-10; vein: intrathoracic portion of the inferior vena cava) if present and to rule out pneumothorax, aspiration pneumonia, or other cardiopulmonary abnormalities.
h. Be sure that the infant has received vitamin K_1, 1.0 mg IM, and one drop of a 1% silver nitrate solution or erythromycin or tetracycline ophthalmic ointment to each eye.
i. Record all details in the infant's chart appropriately.

Chapter 4

Transportation of the Newborn From the Delivery Room

THE NEWBORN SHOULD remain in the delivery room until his or her cardiorespiratory status is stable. Immediate physical examination of the newborn is very important to rule out life-threatening conditions that may require urgent medical or surgical intervention. Care must be taken not to chill the infant by unnecessary procedures such as weighing. Proper identification procedures must be completed before the infant is transferred in a heated incubator to the newborn nursery.

I. TRANSPORTATION REQUIREMENTS

A. Personnel

The person transferring the infant must be prepared to suction the infant, maintain a patent airway, supply oxygen, and support the infant's cardiac status and temperature. Common problems that occur during transportation include apnea, cyanosis, regurgitation, aspiration, and chilling.

B. Equipment

1. Heated transport incubator that allows visibility of the infant
2. Two oxygen tanks (size E) attached to the incubator
3. Small bag (250 or 500 ml) and masks to ventilate the infant artificially by intermittent positive-pressure breathing if the need arises
4. Cardiac monitor with leads to attach to the infant
5. Endotracheal tubes and connectors
6. Laryngoscope
7. Adhesive tape

(continued on page 42)

TABLE 4–1.—PRENATAL AND DELIVERY HISTORY

Obstetrician: Dr. ______
Pediatrician: Dr. ______
Date of Delivery ______ Hour ______ Sex ______ Race ______
Mother's Name ______ Hospital# ______
Date of First Prenatal Visit ______ Number of Visits ______
No Prenatal Care ______

MATERNAL HISTORY

Mother's Age ______ Blood Group & Type ______ Antibody titers ______
Amniocentesis ______
Parity: Full Term ☐ Premature ☐ Abortion ☐ Living ☐
EDC: ______
G.A. by LMP: ______ by Sonogram: ______ by Exam: ______

STS. Pos. ☐ Neg. ☐ If Pos., Treated ☐

PREGNANCY CONDITIONS/DISEASES (Including Drugs)

______

FAMILY HISTORY OF CONGENITAL ANOMALIES OR FAMILIAL DISORDERS

______

PRENATAL TESTS

HbA_{1c} Level ☐ α-FetoProtein ☐ Amniocentesis ☐ Fetal respirations ☐ Fetoscopy ☐
Nonstress Test ☐ Oxytocin Stress Test ☐ Scalp pH ☐ Systolic Time Interval ☐
Sonogram ☐ Fetal Heart Monitor ☐ Biophysical profile ☐
COMMENT: ______

FETAL HEART RATE ABNORMALITIES

Tachycardia ☐ Bradycardia ☐ Loss of Variability ☐
Deceleration: Early ☐ Variable ☐ Late ☐
COMMENT: ______

LABOR HISTORY

1st Stage ______ 2nd Stage ______
Complications of Labor and Delivery ______

Membrane Ruptured: Date ______ Time ______ Spontaneous ☐ Artificial ☐

DELIVERY HISTORY

Position ______
Analgesia ______
Type, time, dose, route
Anesthesia ______
Type, route
Placenta ______
Amniotic Fluid ______

INFANT'S CONDITION AT BIRTH

Apgar Score: 1 min. ______ 5 min. ______

Sign	0	1	2
Heart Rate	Absent	Slow (Below 100)	Over 100
Respiratory Effort	Absent	Slow, Irregular	Good Crying
Muscle Tone	Flaccid	Some Flexion of Extremities	Active Motion
Reflex Irritability	No Response	Cry, weak	Vigorous Cry
Color	Blue, Pale	Body Pink, Ext. Blue	Completely Pink

TYPE DELIVERY

Spontaneous Vertex ☐ Vacuum ☐
Forceps ☐ Low ☐ Mid ☐
Section ☐ Indication ______
Breech ☐ Extraction ☐ Assisted ☐
Pitocin Stimulation ☐

INFANT Vitamin K, Time ______ Not given ☐
Eye care, Time ______ Not given ☐
Passage of urine ☐ Meconium ☐
Resuscitative Measures:
Suction ☐ Oxygen ☐
IPPB ☐ Mask ☐ Intubation ☐
Umbilical Catheterization ☐
Drugs ☐
List: ______
Comment: ______

Signature ______ M.D.

(continued from page 40)

C. Emergency Drugs With Adequate Syringes

1. 4.2% $NaHCO_3$, 0.5 mEq/ml
2. Aqueous epinephrine, 1:10,000
3. Calcium gluconate (10%)

D. Information

A "delivery-room sheet" with the prenatal and delivery histories and the results of brief physical examination should accompany the infant to the newborn nursery (Table 4–1). Table 4–2 explains the reasons for the various items on the delivery-room sheet.

TABLE 4–2.—EXPLANATION OF PRENATAL AND DELIVERY HISTORY*

FACTORS	REASONS
Date and hour of delivery	Medicolegal data. The newborn's physical and chemical status changes rapidly after birth. Some values that are normal at 24 hr of age are totally abnormal at 1 hr of age, e.g., a bilirubin of 5 mg% at 1 hr of age requires an exchange transfusion but is normal at 24 hr of age (see chapter 13–I). Check glucose level (see chapter 15–X), passage of meconium, passage of urine (see appendix A), gas in GI tract (see chapter 17–I), in relation to age in hours.
Sex	Medicolegal data Males have higher incidence of perinatal mortality, respiratory distress syndrome, etc.
Race	Medicolegal data White: e.g., decreased incidence of prematurity (5%) and perinatal mortality. Black: increased incidence of prematurity (8%–15%) and perinatal mortality; increased incidence of G-6-PD deficiency, etc. Oriental: increased incidence of G-6-PD deficiency, cleft palate, etc.
Number of prenatal visits	The number of prenatal visits reflects the maternal degree of interest in the pregnancy as well as the financial and psychosocial ability of the family to afford prenatal care. Those mothers with few or no prenatal visits have a higher perinatal mortality; those with an excessively high number of visits also have a high perinatal mortality.
Maternal age	Best reproductive outcome with maternal ages 20 to 29. Adolescent pregnancy is associated with maternal hypertensive disease of pregnancy, poor nutrition, inadequate perinatal care, child abuse, premature birth, low birth weight, low IQ, etc. Over age 35 associated with higher incidence of perinatal deaths, chromosomal aberrations (e.g., Down's syndrome), congenital malformations, placenta previa, and twinning.
Parity	Number of infants a mother has delivered A previous reproductive problem frequently repeats itself. A woman who has had a stillborn, an infant with congenital malformations, or a premature infant has a high risk of having

TABLE 4–2.—*(continued)*

FACTORS	REASONS
	another infant with the same problem. A history of infertility places the woman at high risk for abortion and perinatal loss.
Gestational age (wk)	Number of weeks after last menstrual period The duration of gestation is directly related to infant's survival: the shorter the gestation the lower the survival rate. Preterm newborns are those with a menstrual age of less than 38 wk; term newborns, 38–42 wk; postterm newborns, > 42 wk.
EDC	Expected date of confinement, i.e., 266 days from the date of conception or 280 days from the date of last menstrual period.
Maternal blood group and type	Medicolegal data The Rh blood group system is of particular importance because of Rh-hemolytic disease (see chapter 13). If fetal Rh-positive cells cross the placenta, the mother produces anti-D Rh antibodies against the fetal red blood cells, the maternal anti-D Rh antibodies cross the placenta, and hemolytic disease ensues. The maternal blood group and antibody titers are recorded so the pediatrician can check if sensitization has occurred. The change in optical density of the amniotic fluid indicates the degree of severity of hemolysis (see chapter 13–VII).
STS	Maternal seriologic test for syphilis As part of maternal prenatal care, syphilis should be ruled out or diagnosed and treated.
Maternal conditions/ complications	Maternal conditions/diseases may affect the fetus and newborn (see chapter 2).
Prenatal tests	Various prenatal tests evaluate fetal growth, development and well-being (see Tables 2–2 and 2–3).
Abnormality of fetal heart rate pattern during labor	See Table 2–2.
Family history of congenital anomalies or familial disorders	A family history of inherited medical illness frequently alerts the physician to the potential for the disease or the effect of the disease in the infant.
Labor history	Duration, 1st stage: from the onset of labor until complete cervical dilation. Primipara, limit of duration: 24.7 hr Multipara, limit of duration: 18.8 hr Duration, 2nd stage: from complete cervical dilation until delivery of the fetus. Primipara, limit of duration: 117 min Multipara, limit of duration: 46 min Values outside the limits of normal indicate abnormal progress and both very short and very long labors result in fetal hypoxia and acidosis.
Complications of labor	Maternal supine position during labor affects aorto-caval compression and decreases uterine perfusion in 28% of laboring women. Amniotomy is associated with an increased risk of prolapsed cord in breech presentation. Prolonged duration of ruptured membranes is associated with neonatal sepsis.

(continued)

TABLE 4–2.—*(continued)*

FACTORS	REASONS
Complications of labor–*(continued)*	Oxytocin infusion can be associated with fetal asphyxia and water intoxication.
Maternal anesthesia and analgesia	All anesthetic agents that depress the CNS of the mother delay the process of labor and also depress the CNS of the infant. Most anesthetics and analgesics given to the mother behaviorally affect the newborn for several days after delivery. Epidural anesthesia: increased incidence of late deceleration, mid forceps delivery, etc. Barbiturates: depressed infant and/or decreased CNS metabolism Spinal anesthesia: associated with a precipitous drop in maternal blood pressure and fetal distress
Vitamin K_1	Newborns have low vitamin K-dependent factors II, VII, IX, X. Vitamin K_1 1.0 mg, prevents hemorrhagic disease of the newborn (see chapter 14–XI).
Amniotic fluid	See Table 2–1 for polyhydramnios and oligohydramnios. Clear: normal. Green: meconium-stained. Consider recent intrauterine anoxia. Yellow: consider intrauterine anoxic episode 1–2 days previously. Clots: consider placental hemorrhage. Green, bile-stained: consider intestinal obstruction (see chapter 17–IV).
Types of delivery	Spontaneous vertex delivery: Associated with best fetal outcome Forceps delivery Outlet forceps: The scalp of the infant is visible at the introitus without separating the labia, the skull has reached the pelvic floor, and the sagittal suture is in the anteroposterior diameter of the pelvis when forceps are applied. Outlet forceps usually do not increase neonatal morbidity. Mid forceps: the head is engaged but indications for outlet forceps have not been met. Any forceps delivery requiring artificial rotation regardless of the status is designated mid forceps and associated with high perinatal mortality and morbidity. High forceps: the application of forceps prior to full engagement of the head is termed high forceps and is never justified. Complications of high forceps include facial bruising, lacerations, cephalohematoma, facial nerve damage, and skull fracture. Vacuum extraction: suction applied to the fetal head to aid delivery. Fetal injuries include a caput, lacerations and/or necrosis of the scalp, cephalohematoma, subgaleal bleeding, retinal hemorrhages, and cerebral damage. Cesarean section: operative delivery. Observe for transient respiratory depression secondary to anesthesia, transient tachypnea of the newborn, etc. Review indications for the section to understand how the infant might be jeopardized. Breech: treacherous method of delivery. Observe infant carefully (see Table 5–3).
Abnormalities of placenta	Large infarcts: associated with fetal growth retardation Placenta previa: associated with premature separation of the placenta and impairment of fetal oxygenation

TABLE 4–2.—*(continued)*

FACTORS	REASONS
	Large placenta: associated with erythroblastosis and maternal diabetes mellitus
	Amnion nodosum: associated with hypoplastic lung and polycystic kidneys, oligohydramnios, etc.
	Small placenta: associated with small-for-gestational age infant
	Calcification of placenta: associated with hypertensive disease of pregnancy, placental insufficiency, etc.
Apgar score	See chapter 3.

*G-6-PD, glucose-6-phosphate dehydrogenase.

REFERENCE

Prichard J.A., McDonald P.C., Gant N.F. (eds.): *William's Obstetrics,* ed. 17. New York, Appleton-Century Crofts, 1985.

II. CLASSIFICATION OF INFANTS ON ARRIVAL IN THE NURSERY

A practical method of grouping infants based on the degree of care required is to divide infants into the following three groups:

A. Normal Fullterm Infants (see Chapter 5)

Infants weighing more than 2,500 grams, of 38 or more weeks of gestational age, and not specifically mentioned in the high-risk category

B. Low Birth Weight Infants (see Chapter 6)

Infants weighing less than 2,500 grams and/or of less than 38 weeks of gestational age. Low birth weight infants may also be grouped in the high-risk category.

C. High-Risk Infants at Birth (see Chapter 8)

Infants who have a statistically high chance of dying or becoming seriously ill in the newborn period.

This grouping allows the infant to be placed with others who require similar nursing care and medical management.

Chapter 5

Normal Fullterm Infants

I. ADMISSION POLICIES FOR NORMAL FULLTERM INFANTS

All healthy fullterm infants should be admitted to the transition section of the nursery where they can be observed while they recover from the shock of being born. Physical examination should be accomplished within 24 hours after delivery.

A. Histories

The prenatal and delivery histories should be reviewed. It is vital that the house officer understand the meaning of all factors on the prenatal and delivery sheets (see Tables 4–1 and 4–2).

B. Physical Examination

Each infant should receive a physical examination and the results should be recorded (see Table 5–1). Junior house officers should examine newborns under senior supervision until they can easily recognize deviations from normal (see Table 5–2). Abnormalities may present singularly or in clusters as a syndrome. When a congenital malformation is noted, careful examination of the infant for associated anomalies is indicated. If infants are born by difficult delivery, abnormal presentation, or cesarean section, observe for birth injury (see Table 5–3).

C. Gestational Age

The gestational age of each infant should be estimated by the following:

1. Obstetric history. The number of weeks from the first day of the mother's last menstrual period until delivery of the infant is determined. This is the gestational age in weeks.
2. Amniotic fluid assay or sonography (see Table 2–3).

(continued on page 65)

TABLE 5–1.—NEWBORN PHYSICAL EXAMINATIONS

NEWBORN PHYSICAL EXAMINATION	DATE ______ LOCATION ______ DOB ______ SEX ______ M.R. NO. ______ NAME ______

EXAMINATION	NURSERY ADMISSION	DISCHARGE
GENERAL CONDITION (COLOR, TONE, CRY, ACTIVITY, MATURITY, B.P., TEMP.)		
SKIN (RASHES, BIRTH MARK, HEMANGIOMA)		
HEAD, FONTANEL, SUTURES, (INCLUDING CEPHALOHEMATOMA, CAPUT SUCCEDANEUM)		
EYES (CATARACT, DISCHARGES, RED REFLEX, ETC.)		
EARS, NOSE, MOUTH, PALATE		
NECK THORAX (INCLUDING BREAST DEVELOPMENT, RETRACTIONS)		
LUNGS (RESP. RATE, AERATION, ETC.)		
HEART (RATE RHYTHM, MURMURS, ETC.)		
FEMORAL PULSES		
ABDOMEN (LIVER, SPLEEN, KIDNEYS, MASSES, ETC.)		
UMBILICAL CORD, UMBIL. ART. 1 OR 2		
GENITALIA (INCLUDING HERNIA)		
ANUS (PATENCY)		
BACK		
EXTREMITIES (INCLUDING CLAVICLES AND HIP)		
REFLEXES (INCLUDING MORO'S, GRASP, SUCK, ETC.)		

PRENATAL COMPLICATIONS		IMPRESSION	WEIGHT	HEAD CIRC.
			LENGTH	BLOOD GROUP
WEIGHT (gm)	HEAD CIRC. (cm)	PLAN: ☐ ROUTINE CARE ☐ OBSERVATION CARE ☐ INTENSIVE CARE	NEONATAL COMPLICATIONS, DISPOSITION:	
LENGTH (cm)	ESTIMATED GESTATION (wks)	SIGNATURE ______ M.D. DATE ______ TIME______	SIGNATURE ______ M.D. DATE ______ TIME______	

TABLE 5–2.—FACTORS TO CONSIDER CONCERNING THE NEWBORN PHYSICAL EXAMINATION

Commonly observed malformations have been cross-referenced to the malformation complexes and syndromes in which they are usually found (Table 9–4).

PHYSICAL EXAMINATION	NORMAL FULL-TERM INFANTS	COMMONLY OBSERVED ABNORMALITIES/MALFORMATIONS
General Appearance		
Color	Pink, acrocyanosis	Generalized cyanosis, pallor, jaundice, plethora
Position	Flexion of extremities	Flaccidity with extension of extremities
Activity	Spontaneous movement	Decreased or absent spontaneous movement
Cry	Vigorous and sustained after stimulation	Weak, high pitched, hoarseness; H7, aphonia, cat-like: C7, growling: D1
Measurements		
Weight	See gestational age chart (Fig 5–1 and 6–2, C)	Small for gestational age: A5, A8, B4, C7, D1, F3, G2, L9, M5, O4, P5, P6, R7, S2, S3, T5, T6 later growth retardation: L3, P8, Z1 Large for gestational age (Chapter 7) Adipose deficiency: L4 Asymmetry: R6 Macrosomia: B2, W2 Obesity: L2, P6 Overgrowth: W2
Length	See normal data (Fig 6–2, C)	Long: Marfan's syndrome Short: A1, A4, B4, C4, D3, E2, F2, H1, L6, M1, M6, M8, N4, O5, P5, P8, R4, R5, R6, S1, S5, T1, T7
Head circumference	See normal data (Fig 6–2, C) Head 1–2 cm greater than chest in full-term infant	Macrocephaly: A4, A7, R4, S4, T1, T2 Microcephaly: A8, B4, C7, D1, F2, F3, R5, S2, S3, T2, T5, T6
Head		
Shape	Molded (secondary to compression in labor) Caput succedaneum	Cephalohematoma Absent calvarium: A10 Acrocephaly: C1 Anencephaly: A10 Asymmetry: K2 Brachycephaly: A5, C1, C4, D1, D5, H1, P1

		Craniosynostosis: A11, C1, C8
		Dolichocephaly: T4
		Encephalocele: A10, M3
		Flat occiput: A11, C1, D5, W2, Z1
		Frontal bossing: B1, C4, C8, G2, T4
		High forehead: A11
		Hydrocephalus: A4, A7, H3, M4, O4, T2
		Large bifrontal diameter: W2
		Narrow bifrontal diameter: P6
		Oxycephaly - see craniosynostosis
		Parietal & occipital bone absence or malformation: A10
		Poorly mineralized cranium: H6, O4
		Prominent occiput wide fontanel: T5
Fontanels	Soft, flat. Open anterior and posterior fontanel	Bulging (caused by increased intracranial pressure) Small: Cranial synostosis or microcephaly Large: H7, O4, P9, T1 Premature closure: A11, C1, C8 Late closure: D5, H6, O4
	Occasionally third fontanel	Third: D5
Face		
Shape	Molded	Asymmetry: facial nerve paralysis, Townes Syndrome (hemifacial microsomia), asymmetric crying facies: A13, facial nuclear agenesis, absent depressor angularioris muscle Broad facies: B1 Coarse facies: G1, G2 Facial telangiectatic erythema: B4 Flat facies: D5, L1, R4, Z1 Hemangioma in a trigeminal facial distribution: S7 Hypoplastic maxilla: A5, C8, F1, F3, R5 Long philtrum—abnormal: F3, W2 Mandible-recessed: H5 Mask-like facies: M7 Micrognathia: A3, A8, D1, H1, H5, M6, M7, P2, P5, T5, T3 Mid-facial hypoplasia: A11, C4

(continued)

TABLE 5–2.—*(continued)*

PHYSICAL EXAMINATION	NORMAL FULL-TERM INFANTS	COMMONLY OBSERVED ABNORMALITIES/MALFORMATIONS
Face—*(continued)*		
		Potter facies: P5
		Prognathism: A11, B1, C8
		Round facies: C7, P6
		Triangular facies: R6
Hair	Silky with visible single strands	Alopecia: P7
		Hirsutism: D1, G2
		Hypotrichosis: H1
		Kinky, twisted and fractured: M5, T4
		Low hairline: C9, N4, S1
		Projection hair onto cheek: T3
Skin		
Color	Pink, acrocyanosis	Generalized cyanosis, mottling, jaundice, petechiae and ecchymosis
Pigmentation	Mongolian spot	Meconium stained
Vernix	Vernix caseosa	Absence of vernix caseosa
Lesions	Milia, erythema toxicum, occasional petechiae	Multiple petechiae
	Telangiectasia	Massive peeling: Postmaturity or congenital ichthyosis
	Mild peeling	Angiomata: K2, T8, X1
		Basal cell nevi: B1
		Café-au-lait (brown pigmentation): B4, F2, M2, N3, R6
		Cutis marmorata: D1, D5, H7, K2
		Dry skin: H7
		Eczema: W3
		Fibrous dysplasia: M2, N3
		Focal dermal hypoplasia: G3
		Hairy multiple nevi: N2
		Hamartomatous skin nodules: T8
		Hemangiomata and telangiectasis: A14, B4, K2, O1, S7, T8, X1
		Hyperhydrosis: R3, R6
		Hyperkeratosis (keratosis): I1, X1
		Hyperpigmentation: F2, X1
		Hypotrichosis: H1

		Insensitivity to pain: R3 Lymphangiomata: K2, T7 Melanomata: N2 Mottled skin (see cutis marmorata) Nevus flammeus: B2 Nevus sebaceous: L7 Partial albinism: C2, W1 Purpura: W3 Skin atrophy: H1 Thick or ichthyotic skin: I1 Thin skin: P7
Eyes		
Shape		Antimongoloid slant: C5, C7, O6, R5, T3 Bushy eyebrows: D1 Epicanthal folds: C7, D5, N4, R5, S3 Hypotelorism: T6 Hypertelorism: A1, A11, C7, C8, D4, F4, L1, L3, L4, O3, W2 Lateral displacement of inner canthi: B3, C1, W1 Long and curved eyelashes: D1, S1 Microphthalmia: H1, R7, T2, T6 Mongoloid slant: D5, L5 Prominent eyes: A8, A11, B2, C8, L4 Shallow orbital ridges: C8 Short palpebral fissure: B3, F3 Synophrys: D1, F3
Eyelids	Lid edema (especially with brow or face presentation)	Edema: congestive heart failure Blepharophimosis: S1 Coloboma: C5, F1, T3, T6 Ectropion: I1 Entropion: Horner's syndrome with or without brachial palsy Ptosis: A1, B3, S3
Conjunctiva	Clear Occasionally subconjunctival hemorrhage	Conjunctivitis: chemical, bacterial or viral
Cornea	Clear	Corneal opacity (cataract): L8, M1, R7, congenital idiopathic hypoparathyroidism

(continued)

TABLE 5–2.—*(continued)*

PHYSICAL EXAMINATION	NORMAL FULL-TERM INFANTS	COMMONLY OBSERVED ABNORMALITIES/MALFORMATIONS
Eyes–*(continued)*		
Ocular		Blue sclera: O4
		Brushfield's spots: D5, Z1
		Cherry-red macular spot: G2
		Glaucoma: R7
		Lack of tearing: R3
		Nystagmus: M1
		Optic atrophy: F4
		Retinal pigmentation/dysplasia: C2, L2, R7
		Strabismus: C7, C8, P6, R5, S3
Ears		
Shape, place, consistency		Crumpled ear: C6
		Deafness: F1, L3, M10, N4, O5, O6, R7, T2, T3, T6, W1
		External ear canal defect: R2
		Large ears: L4, R2, W2
		Low set ears: A8, A11, C7, C8, N4, S1, T5, T6, T7
		Malformed auricles: C9, D3, D4, R2, S2, T3, T6, Z1
		Preauricular tags/pits: F1
		Small ears: D5
Nose		
Patency	Bilateral patency of nares	Choanal atresia (bilateral or unilateral) or "stuffy nose"
Discharge	No discharge	Mucosanguineous discharge of syphilis
Shape		Anteverted nostrils: D1, S3
		Beaked nose: A11, C8, R5, T3
		Broad nasal bridge: A8, B1, G2, W1
		Hypoplasia of nares: C9
		Hypoplastic nasal cartilage: F4
		Low depressed nasal bridge: A3, A4, A5, B3, C4, G2, L1, O4, T1
		Pinched nose: H1
		Prominent nose: R5, S2
		Small or short nose: A1, A5, A11, B4, D1, H1, O4
		Wide nostrils: L4

Mouth		
Lips		Cleft lip: C3 Lower lip pits: P4 Prominent full lips: L4 Hypoplastic philtrum: F3
Palate	Epstein's pearls	Cleft or high-arched palate: A8, A11, C3, N4, O6, P2, P4, S5, T3, T6, T7 High arched palate: C4, D1, H1 Narrow palate: R5, T5 Malar hypoplasia: T3
Tongue	Geographic tongue	Large: B2, H7 Protruding: D5 Glossoptosis with micrognathia: P2
Teeth	None	Ranula, natal teeth: E2 Molar hypoplasia: B4, H1
Mucous membrane	Epithelial pearls (inclusion cysts)	Thrush Epulis
Saliva	Moist mucous membranes	Excessive saliva; esophageal atresia, tracheo-esophageal fistula
Neck		
Shape	Short (head seems to sit on neck)	Web: N4, T7 Excessive tissue back of neck: D5, T7
Masses	No palpable mass	Cystic hygroma, goiter, branchial cysts, hematomas, ectopic thyroid Torticollis
Thorax		
Shape	Symmetric	Asymmetric: pneumothorax, atelectasis, absence of pectoralis, P3 Barrel chest: D2, meconium aspiration pneumonia Broad chest: T7 Pectus excavatum: A1, N4, O6 Pectus carinatum: S1, S5 Short sternum: T5 Small thoracic cage: E2, J1, L9, M6
Clavicles		Hypoplasia: C4, fractures
Breast	> 7 mm palpable breast tissue Engorgement with or without "witches milk"	Mastitis Supernumerary nipples Hyperplasia: L4 Hypoplastic nipple: D1 Nipple absent: P3

(continued)

TABLE 5–2.—*(continued)*

PHYSICAL EXAMINATION	NORMAL FULL-TERM INFANTS	COMMONLY OBSERVED ABNORMALITIES/MALFORMATIONS
Lungs		
Breath Sounds	Presence of breath sound bilaterally	Unilateral absence of breath sounds; pneumothorax or atelectasis Peristaltic sounds: D2
Grunting	Grunting normal during the first hours of life	After first hours of life, grunting abnormal
Rales	Rales normal during the first hours of life	After first hours of life, rales abnormal
Respiratory rate	60/minute for first hours of life, 35–40/minute thereafter	After first hours of life, above 60/minute
Retractions (intercostal, substernal, suprasternal)	Retractions normal during the first hours of life	After the first hour of life, retractions indicate ventilatory insufficiency
Heart		
PMI	Fifth intercostal space on midclavicular line	Shifted to the right, left or displaced downward: dextrocardia, pneumothorax, atelectasis
Rate	After 15 minutes of age, 100–175/minute; can drop to 70/minute during sleep, particularly in prematures	Tachycardia; cardiac, respiratory, metabolic, infectious or hematologic disease, anemia Bradycardia; hypoxia, intracranial disorder, heartblock
Murmurs	Grade I-II/VI systolic murmur in the first 24 hours of life	After 24 hours of life, systolic or diastolic murmurs Aortic arch anomalies: D4 Atrial septal defect: E2, H2, T6 Atrioventricular communis: D5 Coarction of aorta: T7 Conduction defects with arrhythmias: S6 Patent ductus arteriosus: R7, T6, Z1 Pulmonic stenosis: L3, N4, R7 Ventricular septal defect: A13, D5, F3, H2, T5, T6, V1
Abdomen	Flat, not distended	Distended; intestinal obstruction, sepsis, prune-belly syndrome, malrotation, O2 Scaphoid abdomen: D2 Anterior wall defect: E3 Abdominal muscle hypoplasia: A2

Liver	Palpable about 2 cm below the right costal margin	Enlarged: congestive heart failure, sepsis, hepatitis, glycogen-storage disease, G1, K2, R7, Z1 Palpable on the left side in situs inversus
Spleen	Tip palpable in 25% of normal infants	Enlarged: Sepsis, rubella, cytomegalic inclusion disease, etc.
Kidney	Easily palpable bilaterally	Enlarged: Renal vein thrombosis, polycystic kidney, A2, B2, M3, P5, V1
Anus	Patent	Imperforate anus: A13, C5, V1
Inguinal		Hernia: O4, T5
Umbilicus		
Vessels	Two arteries and one vein	Single umbilical artery; gastrointestinal, genitourinary, CNS, cardiovascular system anomalies, T6, V1
Color	Translucent	Green, yellow, meconium-stained resulting from fetal distress Omphalocele: B2, O2
Genitalia		
Male: Testes	Descended into scrotum or palpable in canal. Occasionally undescended testes descend spontaneously later	Testes in abdomen (cryptorchidism): A2, A6, C9, F2, L8, N4, O3, P6, R4, R5, S2, S3, T5, T6
Urethral opening	At center of shaft	Hypospadias: Opening on ventral surface of penis: A6, C9, O3, S3 Micropenis: D5, F2, N4, P6, S3, X2 Enlarged phallus: L4 Hypogonadism: L2, S6, X2 Shawl scrotum: A1
Swelling	Noncommunicating hydrocele	Communicating hydrocele, trauma secondary to breech presentation
Female: vagina		Atresia: C9
Hymen	Hymenal tag	Hydrometrocolpos behind a bulging imperforated hymen
Clitoris	Large clitoris in premature infant	Large clitoris: Adrenogenital syndrome, maternal drug ingestion, hermaphroditism
Discharge	Mucoid vaginal discharge or bleeding caused by maternal hormone withdrawal	
Extremities		
Position and movement	Full range of joint motion Position abnormalities passively corrected are normal	Passive motor limitation Flexion deformities of joints: M6 Hyperflexibility: D5, E1, L8, P8 Joint dislocation: L1

(continued)

TABLE 5–2.—*(continued)*

PHYSICAL EXAMINATION	NORMAL FULL-TERM INFANTS	COMMONLY OBSERVED ABNORMALITIES/MALFORMATIONS
Extremeties–*(continued)*		
		Joint limitation and/or contracture: A12, C6, D3, F3, G1, G2, L5, S1, Z1
		Lower extremities: Talipes or calcaneo equinovarus or valgus: A8, A12, D3, L1, M7
		Flaccidity: spinal cord injury (see Tables 5–3 and 16–4)
		Upper extremities: Brachial plexus injury, clavicular or humerus fracture (see Table 5–3)
Hip	Full abduction of flexed hip	Congenital subluxation or dislocation of hip: Ortolani's sign
Dermatographics		Absence of distal crease on 5th finger: T5
		Low arched dermal ridge: T5
		Simian crease: C7, D5, S2, S3, T6
Hands and Feet		Absence of digit: H5
		Arachnodactyly: C6
		Brachydactyly: A1, C1, D5, L2, M10, R4, R6
		Broad distal phalanx: A11
		Broad thumb and/or toe: L1, L5, P1, R5, W2
		Camptodactyly: T6, W2
		Clenched hand: T5
		Clinodactyly (incurved 5th finger): A1, D5, R6, S2
		Dorsal swelling of hand: N4, T7
		Gap between 1st and 2nd toes: D5, S2
		Hypoplasia of mid phalanx of 5th finger: D5
		Macrodactyly: K2, S4
		Metacarpal hypoplasia: M9
		Nail-hypoplasia or dysplasia: E2, G3, N1, P7, T5, T6
		Narrow hyperconvex: T6, T7
		Short: L1, O6
		Overlapping index finger over 3rd, 4th, 5th finger: T5, T6
		Polydactyly: C1, E2, G4, L2, M3, T6, V1
		Sausage-like fingers: T1
		Short hands and feet: A5, G1
		Spade-like hands: L5

		Syndactyly: A11, C1, G3, P1, P3, S3, V1
		Thumb (hypoplasia to aplasia): F2, H2, V1
		Trident hands: A4
Limbs		Elbow dysplasia: T7
		Multiple fractures: O4
		Patella dysplasia: N1
		Radius hypoplasia to aplasia: A13, F2, H2, R1, V1
		Retarded osseous maturation: R5
		Ring-like constrictions: A9
		Skeletal asymmetry: R6
		Skeletal hypoplasia: P7
		Short distal extremities: E2, G4, L6, R4
		Short femoral neck: A4
		Short limb (amelia, phocomelia): A3, A4, H4, L9, P8, T1
		Small pelvis: T5
Ribs		Bifid: B1
		Flaring of lower rib cage: M8
		Defects: B1, C4, H6, P3, S2, T1, T6
Vertebrae		Caudal narrowing of spine canal: A4, H4
		Defects: A3, A4, A13, S5, T1, V1
		Flattened: O4, O5, P8
		Fused: K1
		Hemivertebrae: F1, K1, R4
		Incomplete ossification of lower spine: A3
		Lordosis: A4
		Scoliosis: B1, D3
		Vertical shortness: S1
Neurological Examinations		
Reflexes	Moro's, sucking, rooting, grasping, walking, pupil, supraciliary tap	Absence of appropriate reflexes Absence of DTR: L8

(continued)

TABLE 5–2.—*(continued)*

PHYSICAL EXAMINATION	NORMAL FULL-TERM INFANTS	COMMONLY OBSERVED ABNORMALITIES/MALFORMATIONS
Neurological Examinations–*(continued)*		
Movement	Spontaneous movement	Ataxia: A14, M1 Cranial nerve compression: A7 Hypertonicity: D1, G2, M4 Hypotonicity: D5, F4, G2, L8, M1, M4, O4, P6, P9, S3, S5, Z1 Incomplete development of forebrain, olfactory, optic nerves: T6 Developmental delay: A5, A11, C1, C7, D1, D5, F1, F4, G2, L2, L7, L8, M1, M7, N4, O6, P6, S2, S3, T5, T6, X2 Seizures: D4, F4, L7, M5, N2, S7, Z1

REFERENCE

Smith D.W.: *Recognizable Patterns of Human Malformations.* Philadelphia, W.B. Saunders Co., 1983.

TABLE 5–3.—COMMON BIRTH INJURIES

PREDISPOSING FACTORS	PROBLEM	CLINICAL MANIFESTATIONS	MANAGEMENT
Breech presentation	CNS hemorrhage (tear of falx cerebri or tentorium, rupture of vein of Galen, subdural or extradural hematoma) (see Chapter 15–VI, VII, VIII.)	Apnea, respiratory depression, lethargy, tremor, convulsion, hypothermia, bradycardia, hypotonia, cyanosis, decreased or absent normal reflexes, quadriplegia or perinatal death	Monitor vital signs, hematocrit, arterial blood gases and ventilatory status. Avoid anoxia or hypoxia. Resuscitate promptly. Support ventilation. Transfuse whole blood as necessary.
	Cervical spine injury (intraspinal hemorrhage, vertebral artery hemorrhage, spinal cord transection)	Flaccid paralysis with loss of sensation below the level of the lesion, priapism, bladder distention caused by neurogenic bladder, bowel incontinence, etc., usually at the level of C6, C7	Immediate neurosurgical consultation for corrective surgical treatment. Administer ventilatory support.
	Peripheral nerve injury		Careful physical examination.
	Bracheal plexus injury Erb's-Duchenne palsy (paralysis of C5-6)	Limp arm held in internal rotation with elbow extended. Asymmetric Moro's reflex. Respiratory distress caused by associated phrenic nerve palsy and diaphragmatic paralysis	Spontaneous recovery is common and the prognosis is better than Klumpke's palsy. Administer gentle full range of joint motion (physical therapy) to prevent contracture after 7–10 days when traumatic neuritis has subsided.
	Klumpke's palsy (paralysis of C8-T1)	Wrist drop. Flaccid paresis of the hand, occasionally associated with Horner's syndrome (ipsilateral miosis, enophthalmos, anhidrosis, etc.)	Keep the wrist in a neutral position with a hand splint and frequent passive range of motion. Prevent contracture.
	Phrenic nerve injury (diaphragmatic palsy acquired eventration) (see Chapter 11–XXVII)	Respiratory distress with paradoxical respiration often associated with brachial plexus injury	Chest x-ray film to see elevated hemidiaphragm. Fluoroscope to confirm the diagnosis with demonstration of paradoxical motion of diaphragm. Complete recovery in 50% in 2–3 mo. and rarely plication may be required after 3 mo.

(continued)

TABLE 5–3.—*(continued)*

PREDISPOSING FACTORS	PROBLEM	CLINICAL MANIFESTATIONS	MANAGEMENT
	Sternocleidomastoid hematoma	Mass over the sternocleidomastoid muscle usually apparent after 1 week of life. Torticollis may develop later as cicatricial contractions occur.	Gentle, passive stretching exercise several times a day as soon as possible. Rule out Sprengel's deformity by x-ray film. Usually completely recovers in 3–6 mo.
	Muscle "crush injury" of lower extremities	Necrosis, ecchymosis, exsanguinating hemorrhage, lower nephron nephrosis Disseminated intravascular coagulopathy, death	Obtain a baseline hematocrit value. Watch for the development of hyperbilirubinemia. Hydrate the infant. Watch for internal hemorrhage, disseminated intravascular coagulation, blood pressure changes.
	Viscera hemorrhage (rupture or subcapsular hematoma)		Monitor vital signs. Obtain sonogram, CT scan.
	Liver or spleen (see chapter 14)	Anemia, shock, abdominal distension	Monitor vitral signs, hematocrit, electrolytes, and urinalysis. Bloody peritoneal tap confirms diagnosis.
	Adrenal (insufficiency)	Shock, anemia, flank mass, death	See Table 17–5 for biomedical data. Correct as required.
	Kidney	Hematuria, flank mass due to enlarged kidney, abdominal distension	Monitor vital signs: hematocrit, electrolytes and urinalysis. Follow renal studies; support blood pressure.
	Fractures		
	Clavicle	Asymmetric Moro's reflex Discontinuity or rarely crepitation of the clavicle found on routine physical examination	If a fracture is suspected, obtain an x-ray film of clavicles. Displaced fractures should be immobilized with a figure-eight bandage to prevent potential bracheal plexus or pleural cavity injury. Usually heals spontaneously with formation of a large callus.

	Humerus (usually middle third)	Asymmetric Moro's reflex Discontinuity or rarely crepitation of the humerus; often associated with clavicular fracture	Obtain an x-ray film and orthopedic consultation. A cast may be necessary.
	Femur	Discontinuity or, rarely, crepitation of the femur	Extension of the leg and flexion of the thigh Maintain position by traction.
Vertex presentation	Caput succedaneum	Edema of the scalp; not limited to any area	Edema disappears spontaneously over several days.
	Cephalohematoma	Swelling caused by subperiosteal hemorrhage and limited to one or both parietal bones. Swelling does not cross the suture line; swelling may not appear at the time of delivery. Rarely, an underlying skull fracture is present.	Swelling disappears gradually over weeks or months. Calcification remains. Observe for hyperbilirubinemia and thrombocytopenia (caused by platelet sequestration), anemia, hypotension (rare). Do not aspirate hemorrhage as aspiration might introduce infection.
	Facial nerve palsy	Paralysis of one side of the face (asymmetry during crying), frequently with inability to close the eye. Differentiate from nontraumatic asymmetry (facial nuclear agenesis, absent depressor anguli oris muscle, etc.).	Spontaneous recovery is the rule. Instill methyl cellulose drops into the affected eye.
	Fracture of the skull	Associated with cephalohematoma and intracranial hemorrhage Scalp discoloration, skull depression	Rarely, surgical open elevation may be necessary if intracranial pressure is increased, bone fragment is within the cerebrum, abnormal neurologic findings or subgaleal CSF is present. Re-evaluate in 2–4 mo. to ascertain growing fracture of the skull associated with leptomeningeal cyst. Hyperventilation, glucocorticoids, fluid restriction, and osmotic diuresis may be used for increased intracranial pressure.

(continued)

TABLE 5–3.—*(continued)*

PREDISPOSING FACTORS	PROBLEM	CLINICAL MANIFESTATIONS	MANAGEMENT
Vacuum extraction, Kielland's forceps, midforcep rotation, prolonged labor	Superficial abrasions or edema on infant's face or scalp	Abrasions, edema Petechiae and/or ecchymosis of the head and neck	Keep abrasions dry and clean. Petechiae and/or ecchymosis clear spontaneously over several days. Observe for signs of hyperbilirubinemia and thrombocytopenia.
	Cephalohematoma	See above.	See above.
	Subgaleal hemorrhage	Hemorrhage between the galea aponeurotica and periosteum from supraorbital ridge to top of ears and nape of neck. Swollen scalp, discoloration, falling hematocrit, pallor, hypotonia	Transfuse whole blood for anemia and shock. Administer fresh frozen plasma and vitamin K for coagulopathy if present.
	CNS hemorrhage	See above and chapter 15–VI, 15–VII, 15–VIII.	See above and chapter 15–VI, 15–VII, 15–VIII.
	Hemorrhage into the eye; conjunctiva or retina	Hemorrhages in the conjunctiva or retina	Hemorrhages clear spontaneously.

Scalp sampling	Broken blade in the scalp		Remove the fragment of blade by probing the wound with a magnet.
	Scalp inflammation or abscess	Inflammation or abscess	Local application of antibiotic ointment after shaving and sterilizing with Betadine. Systemic antibiotic therapy after incision and drainage for abscess.
	Hemorrhage	Bleeding from wound	Apply pressure, a tamponade, or a surgical clip. If there is a family history of coagulation abnormalities, administer appropriate blood component after work-up.
Delivery by cesarean section	Accidental incision of the infant when uterus is incised	Localized, fine incision	Keep the lesion dry and clean. If edges are not approximate, apply suture.

REFERENCE

Faix R.G., Donn S.M.: Immediate management of the traumatized infant. *Clin. Perinatol.* 10:487, 1983.

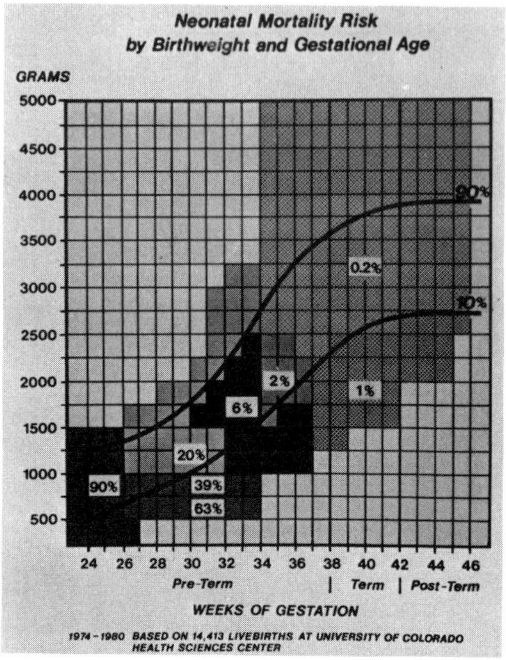

FIG 5–1.
Neonatal mortality risk in relation to birth weight and gestational age. (From Koops B.L., Margon L.J., Battaglia F.C.: *J. Pediatr.* 101:969, 1982. Used by permission.)

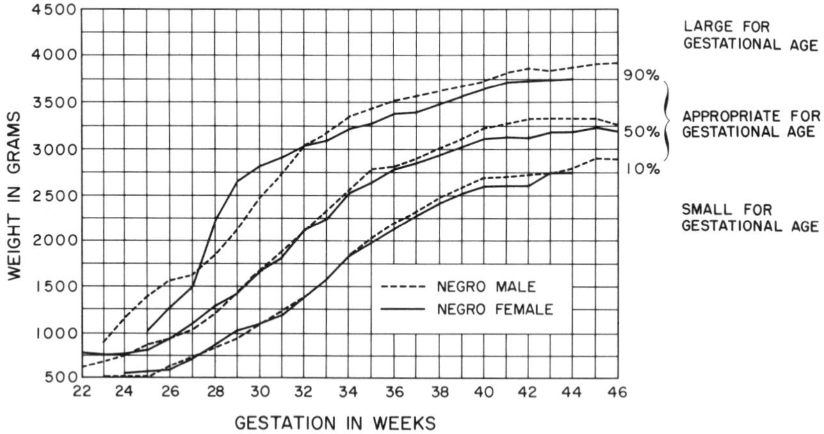

FIG 5–2.
Male and female indigent black weight graphed in percentiles. (From Freeman M.G., Graves W.L., Thompson R.L.: *Pediatrics* 46:9, 1970. Used by permission.)

(continued from page 46)

3. Physical examination of the infant. Various clinical criteria indicate gestational age. (See Figs 6–1 and 6–2 to determine gestational age. Follow the directions on the chart.)

D. Weight

After the gestational age has been estimated, the infant's weight should be plotted against the weeks of gestational age (see Figs 5–1 and 5–2). The infant should then be classified as large for gestational age (>90%), appropriate for gestational age (10%–90%), or small for gestational age (<10%).

E. Suggested Routine Orders for the Normal Full-Term Infant

If the infant has had a normal prenatal history and physical examination and is considered to be appropriate for gestational age, the following care is indicated.

ORDERS	REASONS
1. Maintain a clear airway: suction as required.	Prevent asphyxia and aspiration.
2. Record pulse rate, respiratory rate, blood pressure and temperature on admission to the nursery and every 2 hr until the temperature is stabilized; then record pulse rate, respiratory rate, and temperature every 8 hr.	Changes in vital signs are frequently the first clues to changes in the infant's condition.
3. Bathe the infant on admission to the nursery after the temperature has stabilized. Be sure the infant is not chilled by low environmental temperature.	Minimize skin colonization. Prevent hypothermia and associated hypoglycemia or acidosis.
4. Weigh the infant on admission and daily.	Recognize excessive or inadequate weight gain or loss.
5. Administer vitamin K_1 (AquaMEPHYTON or Konakion), 1.0 mg IM, on admission to the nursery, if the infant did not receive vitamin K_1 in the delivery room.	Prevent hemorrhagic disease of the newborn (see Chapter 14–XI).
6. Make sure the infant has received eye care at birth. If not, 1% $AgNO_3$ or erythromycin or tetracycline ophthalmic ointment may be used.	Prevent gonococcal ophthalmia neonatorum. Erythromycin or tetracycline ophthalmic ointment prevents chlamydial as well as gonococcal ophthalmia.
7. Record time of first passage of urine and stool. Ask the nurse to notify the pediatrician if the infant fails to pass urine or stool by 24 hr of age (see appendix A).	Failure to pass urine or stool is frequently the first sign of urinary tract anomalies or GI obstruction (see appendices A-36, A-37).
8. Ask the nurse to notify the house officer immediately if the mother and/or infant is in the high-risk category (see chapter 8).	Recognize the need for and administer preventive therapy, thus reducing morbidity and mortality.

(continued)

ORDERS	REASONS
9. Observe infants for jaundice, poor feeding, vomiting, diarrhea, dyspnea, tachycardia, tachypnea, grunting, cyanosis, tremors, twitching, convulsion, lethargy, low temperature, pallor, or other problems.	Recognize the need for and administer preventive therapy, thus reducing morbidity and mortality.
10. Maintain the nursery temperature at 25.5° C. Do not place infants in draft, in sunlight, or beside a radiator or air conditioner.	Prevent hypothermia or hyperthermia from convection or radiation.
11. Feeding orders: see Chapter 5–II on feeding the normal fullterm infant.	Prevent overfeeding, underfeeding, or aspiration.
12. Obtain a screening test at the time of discharge for inborn errors of metabolism. (It is best administered after the infant has had 2–3 days of milk feedings.)	Prevent mental retardation resulting from phenylketonuria, branched chain ketonuria, maple syrup urine disease, homocystinuria, histidinemia, galactosemia, adenosine deaminase deficiency, homozygous sickle cell disease, hypothyroidism and other inborn errors of metabolism.
13. Expose the circumcision site (no diapers) for 12 hr if circumcised. Thrombin or an absorbable gauze (Gelfoam or Oxycel) must be available in case the infant bleeds from the circumcision site. If bleeding is excessive, be sure vitamin K_1 has been administered to the infant at birth (see chapter 14–XI). Before circumcising the infant, ask about a family history of bleeding. Obtain coagulation studies as needed. Contraindications for circumcision: a. Hypospadias b. Known bleeding disorders in the family c. Hemorrhagic disease of the newborn d. Infants with thrombocytopenia e. Sick infants	Recognize and treat early. The infant can bleed into a diaper and go into shock before the bleeding is detected.

II. FEEDING OF THE NORMAL FULLTERM INFANT

A. Breast Feeding

Human milk is considered the preferred first food for full term infants because it is known to provide all the required nutrients for infants during the first 4 to 6 months of life.

1. The infant should be fed nothing by mouth for 4 to 6 hours.

2. After 4 to 6 hours, encourage rooming in or bring the infant to the mother for feeding at least every 3 to 4 hours during the day and every 4 hours during the night. The infant may be fed ad libitum.
3. The mother's breasts should be emptied completely, either by the infant's sucking or by a breast pump; regular and complete emptying of the breast is a major stimulus to the secretion of human milk.
4. Wash the nipple with water and dry before and after each nursing. An absorbent pad or a clean cloth may be placed inside the brassiere to absorb milk that leaks.
5. Do not feed supplemental milk to breast-fed infants unless medically indicated; the first 2 weeks of neonatal sucking are crucial for the establishment of an adequate milk supply.
6. Iron, vitamin D, and fluoride should be supplemented by at least 4 months of age because of low transferrin saturation.
7. Note the table of drugs excreted in mother's milk (see Table 5–4). Be careful to determine if the mother is ingesting any of the drugs listed in the table and curtail breast feeding if indicated.
8. Advantages
   a. Convenient and less expensive. Human milk is always at the correct temperature and requires no sterilization.
   b. Fresh and free of contaminative bacteria. Decreased incidence of diarrhea is noted possibly due to antibody (IgA, IgM, IgD and IgE), lactoferrin, more than 20 active enzymes, cells (lymphocytes, macrophages, etc.) and gram-positive intestinal flora passed via milk.
   c. Less incidence of feeding difficulties. High-quality protein, fat, and carbohydrate for easy digestion.
   d. Close mother-to-infant relationship
   e. Protective against the development of allergies.

(continued on page 73)

TABLE 5–4.—DRUGS EXCRETED IN HUMAN MILK*

DRUGS THAT ARE CONTRAINDICATED DURING BREAST FEEDING†‡	
DRUG	REPORTED SIGN OR SYMPTOM IN INFANT OR EFFECT ON LACTATION
Amethopterin†	Possible immune suppression; unknown effect on growth or association with carcinogenesis
Bromocriptine	Suppresses lactation
Cimetidine‡	May suppress gastric acidity in infant, inhibit drug metabolism, and cause CNS stimulation
Clemastine	Drowsiness, irritability, refusal to feed, high-pitched cry, neck stiffness
Cyclophosphamide†	Possible immune suppression; unknown effect on growth or association with carcinogenesis
Ergotamine	Vomiting, diarrhea, convulsions (doses used in migraine medications)
Gold salts	Rash, inflammation of kidney and liver
Methimazole	Potential for interfering with thyroid function
Phenindione	Hemorrhage
Thiouracil	Decreased thyroid function; does not apply to propylthiouracil

(continued)

TABLE 5–4.—*(continued)*

DRUGS THAT REQUIRE TEMPORARY CESSATION OF BREAST FEEDING	
DRUG	RECOMMENDED ALTERATION IN BREAST-FEEDING PATTERN
Metronidazole	Discontinue breast-feeding 12–24 hr to allow excretion of dose
Radiopharmaceuticals	Radioactivity present in milk; consult nuclear medicine physician before performing diagnostic study so that radionuclide that has shortest excretion time in breast milk can be used; prior to study the mother should pump her breast and store enough milk in freezer for feeding the infant; after study the mother should pump her breast to maintain milk production but discard all milk pumped for the required time that radioactivity is present in milk
Gallium 69 (^{69}Ga)	Radioactivity in milk present for 2 wk
Iodine 125 (^{125}I)	Risk of thyroid cancer; radioactivity in milk present for 12 days
Iodine 131 (^{131}I)	Radioactivity in milk present 2–14 days depending on study
Radioactive sodium	Radioactivity in milk present 96 hr
Technetium-99m (^{99m}Tc), ^{99m}Tc macroaggregates, $^{99m}TcO_4$	Radioactivity in milk present 15 hr to 3 days

MATERNAL MEDICATION USUALLY COMPATIBLE WITH BREAST FEEDING‡§	
DRUG	REPORTED SIGN OR SYMPTOM IN INFANT OR EFFECT ON LACTATION
Anesthetics and sedatives	
Alcohol	Drowsiness, diaphoresis, deep sleep, weakness, decrease in linear growth, abnormal weight gain; maternal ingestion of 1 gm/kg daily decreases milk ejection reflex
Barbiturate	None; see antiepileptic drugs
Bromide	Rash, weakness, absence of cry with maternal intake of 5.4 gm/day
Chloral hydrate	Sleepiness
Chloroform	None
Halothane	None
Magnesium sulfate	None
Methyprylon	Drowsiness
Secobarbital	None
Anticoagulants	
Bishydroxycoumarin	None
Warfarin	None
Antiepileptics	
Carbamazepine	None
Ethosuximide	None
Phenobarbital	Methemoglobinemia (1 case); decreased responsiveness, decreased weight gain, excessive sleeping if mother's plasma level ≥30 μg/ml
Phenytoin	Methemoglobinemia (1 case)
Primidone	None
Thiopental	None
Valproic acid	None

TABLE 5–4.—*(continued)*

MATERNAL MEDICATION USUALLY COMPATIBLE WITH BREAST FEEDING‡§	
DRUG	REPORTED SIGN OR SYMPTOM IN INFANT OR EFFECT ON LACTATION
Antihistamines, decongestants, and bronchodilators	
Dexbrompheniramine maleate with *d*-iso-ephedrine	Crying, poor sleeping patterns, irritability
Diphenhydramine	None
Dyphylline‡	None
Iodides	Affects thyroid activity; see miscellaneous, iodine
Theophylline	Irritability
Trimeprazine	None
Tripelennamine	None
Antihypertensive and cardiovascular drugs	
Atenolol	None
Captopril	None
Digoxin	None
Disopyramide	None
Guanethidine	None
Hydralazine	None
Methyldopa	None
Metoprolol‡	None
Nadolol‡	None
Propranolol	None
Quinidine	None
Reserpine	Galactorrhea
Antiinfective drugs (all antibiotics transfer into breast milk in limited amounts)	
Amantadine	Urinary retention, vomiting, skin rash
Cefadroxil	None
Cefazolin	None
Cefotaxime	None
Chloramphenicol	None
Chloroquine	None
Clindamycin	None
Ethambutol	None
Isoniazid	None
Nalidixic acid	Hemolysis in infant with G-6-PD deficiency
Nitrofurantoin	Hemolysis in infant with G-6-PD deficiency
Pyrimethamine	None
Quinine	None
Rifampin	None
Salicylazosulfapyridine (sulfasalazine)	None

TABLE 5–4.—*(continued)*

MATERNAL MEDICATION USUALLY COMPATIBLE WITH BREAST FEEDING‡§	
DRUG	REPORTED SIGN OR SYMPTOM IN INFANT OR EFFECT ON LACTATION
Antiinfective drugs–*(continued)*	
Sulfapyridine	Caution in infant with jaundice or G-6-PD deficiency and ill, stressed, or premature infant
Sulfathiazole	None; nonabsorbable by mother
Sulfisoxazole	Caution in infant with jaundice or G-6-PD deficiency and ill, stressed, or premature infant
Tetracycline	None; negligible absorption by infant
Trimethoprim	None
Antithyroid drugs	
Carbimazole	Goiter
Propylthiouracil	None
Cathartics (drugs that cause abdominal cramping in mother)	Abdominal cramping, colic-like syndrome
Danthron	Increased bowel activity
Diagnostic agents	
Iodine	Goiter; see miscellaneous, iodine
Iopanoic	None
Metrizamide	None
Diuretics	
Bendroflumethiazide	Suppresses lactation, thrombocytopenia (1 case)
Chlorothiazide	May suppress lactation; therefore, avoid prescribing in first month of lactation; this may also apply to other thiazides; questionably dose related
Chlorthalidone	Excreted slowly
Methyclothiazide	None
Spironolactone	None
Hormones	
Chlorotrianisene	None
^{3}H-norethynodrel	None
19-norsteroid	None
Contraceptive pill with estrogen/progesterone	Breast enlargement, dose related; decrease in milk production and protein content
Estradiol	Withdrawal, vaginal bleeding
Muscle relaxants	
Baclofen	None
Carisoprodol	Drowsiness, intestinal upset
Methocarbamol	None
Narcotics, non-narcotic analgesics and antiinflammatory agents	
Acetaminophen	None
Butorphanol	None
Codeine	None
Flufenamic acid	None
Heroin	None
Ibuprofen	None

TABLE 5–4.—*(continued)*

MATERNAL MEDICATION USUALLY COMPATIBLE WITH BREAST FEEDING‡§	
DRUG	REPORTED SIGN OR SYMPTOM IN INFANT OR EFFECT ON LACTATION
Indomethacin	Seizure (1 case)
Mefenamic acid	None
Meperidine	None
Methadone	None if mother receiving $\leq$20 mg/24 hr
Morphine	None
Naproxen	None
Phenylbutazone	None
Prednisolone, prednisone	None
Propoxyphene	None
Salicylates	Metabolic acidosis (dose related); may affect platelet function, rash
Psychotropic agents	
Antianxiety	
Chlordiazepoxide	Conflicting reports of drowsiness
Clorazepate	
Diazepam	
Meprobamate‡	
Oxazepam	
Prazepam‡	
Antidepressants	
Amitriptyline	None
Amoxapine	
Desipramine	
Dothiepin	
Imipramine	
Lithium	
Tranylcypromine	
Antipsychotic	
Chlorpromazine	Galactorrhea in adult; drowsiness and lethargy in infant
Haloperidol	None
Mesoridazine	None
Piperacetazine	
Prochlorperazine	
Thioridazine	
Trifluoperazine	
Other	
Marijuana‡	Unknown, only 1 report literature
Stimulants	
Amphetamine	Irritability, poor sleeping pattern
Caffeine	Irritability, poor sleeping pattern, excreted slowly
Nicotine (excess)	Shock, vomiting, diarrhea, rapid heart rate, restlessness, decreased milk production
Vitamins	
B_1	None
B_{12}	None
D	Increased calcium levels
Folic acid	None
K_1	None

(continued)

TABLE 5–4.—*(continued)*

MATERNAL MEDICATION USUALLY COMPATIBLE WITH BREAST FEEDING‡§	
DRUG	REPORTED SIGN OR SYMPTOM IN INFANT OR EFFECT ON LACTATION
Vitamins–*(continued)*	
Pyridoxine	None
Riboflavin	None
Thiamin	None
Miscellaneous	
Atropine, scopolamine	None
Bethanechol	Abdominal pain, diarrhea
Diphenoxylate with atropine	None
Iodine (povidone-iodine/vaginal douche)	Elevated iodine levels in breast milk, odor of iodine on infant's skin
Tolbutamide	Jaundice

FOOD AND ENVIRONMENTAL AGENTS: EFFECT ON BREAST FEEDING§

AGENT	REPORTED SIGN OR SYMPTOM IN INFANT OR EFFECT ON LACTATION
Aspartame	Caution in patient carrier of phenylketonuria
Bromide (photographic laboratory)	Potential absorption and bromide transfer into milk; see "anesthetics and sedatives"
Chlordane	None reported
Chocolate	Irritability or increased bowel activity if excess amounts (16 oz/day) consumed by mother
Cyclamate	None
DDT, benzenehexachlorides, dieldrin, aldrin, hepatachlorepoxide	None
Fava beans	Hemolysis in patient with G-6-PD deficiency
Fluorides	None
Hexachlorobenzene	Skin rash, diarrhea, vomiting, dark urine, neurotoxicity, death
Hexachlorophene	None; contamination of milk from nipple washing
Lead	Neurotoxicity
Methyl mercury	Affects neurodevelopment
Monosodium glutamate	None
Polychlorinated biphenyls and polybrominated biphenyls	Lack of endurance, hypotonia, sullen expressionless facies
Saccharin	None
Tetrachlorethylene (cleaning fluid)	Obstructive jaundice, dark urine
Vegetarian diet	Signs of B_{12} deficiency

*From Committee on Drugs: The transfer of drugs and other chemicals into human breast milk. *Pediatrics* 72:375, 1983. Used by permission.
†Data not available for other cytotoxic agents.
‡Drug is concentrated in breast milk.
§G-6-PD, glucose-6-phosphate dehydrogenase.

(continued from page 67)

9. Contraindications
   a. Acute illness of the mother: septicemia, nephritis, eclampsia, profuse hemorrhage, active tuberculosis, typhoid fever, or malaria
   b. Chronic illness of the mother: poor nutrition, debility, convulsive disorders, severe neurosis, or psychosis
   c. Illness of the infant
   d. Drug ingestion by the mother (see Table 5–4). Not absolute contraindication; temporary discontinuation should be considered.
10. Late-onset exaggerated unconjugated hyperbilirubinemia may occur at the time when jaundice would normally be abating. Interruption of nursing and substitution of artificial feeding for 2 to 4 days will result in prompt decline of serum bilirubin concentration.

B. Bottle Feeding

1. Withhold oral feeding for 4 to 6 hours.
2. After 4 to 6 hours, give orally 5% dextrose in water, 0.5 to 1.0 oz every 3 to 4 hours for two feedings. (Note: Some neonatologists prefer sterile water in place of 5% dextrose in water to reduce the sequelae from possible aspiration.)
3. If the 5% dextrose in water is tolerated, give a 20-calories/oz formula, 1 to 2 oz every 3 to 4 hours.
4. Bring bottle-fed infants to their mothers at least four times a day for feedings by the mother. If the infant must remain in the nursery, every effort should be made to help the mother hold, feed, and talk to the infant while the infant is in the nursery.
5. Iron-fortified formula for the first year of life is recommended by the American Academy of Pediatrics.

Chapter 6

Low-Birth-Weight Infants

An infant, either premature or fullterm, whose weight is less than 2,500 grams is termed a low-birth-weight (LBW) infant.

I. ADMISSION POLICIES FOR THE LOW-BIRTH-WEIGHT INFANT

All LBW infants should be examined by the pediatric house staff immediately after admission to the nursery regardless of the time, even if they are thought to be in excellent condition. *Remember, LBW infants often become ill shortly after birth and the smaller and more immature they are, the higher the incidence of morbidity.*

A. Responsibilities of the Pediatric House Officer

1. Note whether the infant needs any immediate resuscitative measures, such as suctioning, positioning, or oxygen.
2. Evaluate the infant's prenatal and delivery history (*see* Table 4–1) to determine what factors might be responsible for the infant's low birth weight.
3. Perform an admission physical examination (see Table 5–1) and estimate the infant's gestational age.
   The gestational age of each infant should be estimated by the following:
   a. Obstetric history. The number of weeks from the first day of mother's last menstrual period until delivery of the infant is the gestational age in weeks.
   b. Amniotic fluid assay or serial sonography (see Tables 2–2 and 2–3).
   c. Physical examination of the infant. Various clinical criteria indicate gestational age. (See Figs 6–1 and 6–2 to determine gestational age.)
   The assessment of gestational age by physical criteria can be performed immediately after birth while neurologic evaluation requires the infant to be in a quiet, rested state that may be acquired by the end of first or second day of age. Depressed, asphyxiated, neurologically damaged, or sick in-

fants are difficult to assess because of unpredictable muscle tone. The square window (wrist flexion) is not affected by muscle tone.

4. Classify the infant as a premature infant appropriate for gestational age (AGA), small for gestational age (SGA), or large for gestational age (LGA) or as a fullterm SGA infant (see Figs 5–1 and 5–2). Be aware that SGA infants usually have lost their vernix, have more skin desquamation, more sole creases, and less breast tissue than expected.

II. THE PREMATURE INFANT

The premature infant is an infant born before 38 weeks from the first day of the last menstrual period.

A. Suggested Routine Orders for the Premature Infant

The suggested routine orders listed here are not routine; they are systematized orders designed to recognize and prevent the common preventable complications of the premature infant.

ORDERS	REASONS
1. Maintain a neutral thermal environment (32–34° C, 89.6–93.2° F for newborns) (see Table 6–2).	1. Prevent hypothermia and hyperthermia. Infants kept in a neutral thermal environment have a better chance of survival and grow better.
a. Place all infants weighing under 1,800 gm in an incubator or under a radiant heater. (These units do not work by magic. Check and understand the temperature control mechanisms carefully.) Do not overheat the infant.	a. Hyperthermia may induce tachycardia, tachypnea, irritability, periodic breathing, and apnea. Hypothermia may induce respiratory distress, apnea, acidosis, and/or hypoglycemia.
b. Be careful not to lower the infant's temperature precipitously during procedures, e.g., taking an x-ray film or inserting an IV (this means everybody).	
2. Maintain a clear airway.	2. Prevent asphyxia.
3. Observe the infant continuously for signs of distress. Record the pulse, respiratory rate, and temperature on admission and every hour until the infant's vital signs have stabilized. After stabilization, record pulse, respiratory rate, and temperature at least every 4 hr. Infants requiring intensive care should have hourly vital signs recorded in addition to continuous monitoring. (Note normal data in appendix A.)	3. Changes in the vital signs are frequently the first clue to changes in the infant's condition. Respiratory distress may indicate respiratory distress syndrome, pulmonary edema, patent ductus arteriosus, etc.

(continued)

ORDERS	REASONS
4. Administer vitamin K_1 (AquaMEPHYTON or Konakion), 1.0 mg IM, on admission to the nursery.	4. Prevent hemorrhagic disease of the newborn (See Chapter 14–XI).
5. Weigh the infant on admission to the nursery and daily. Record the infant's weight on the premature growth chart (see Fig 6–3, p. 93). Observe carefully for excessive weight gain or loss. Measure head circumference and plot on head circumference chart (see Figs 6–4 and 6–5).	5. Prevent excessive weight gain or loss. a. Note excessive weight gain: edema, e.g., congestive heart failure, hypoalbuminemia. b. Note excessive weight loss: dehydration, e.g., inadequate fluid intake. c. Note inadequate weight gain, e.g., sepsis, congestive heart failure, renal tubular acidosis, anemia.
6. Wash the infant on admission to the nursery after his or her temperature has stabilized. Many nurseries apply triple dye (Frank W. Kerr Chemical Co.) on the umbilical cord on admission. Bathe the infant daily.	6. Minimize skin and cord colonization.
7. Administer oxygen only when the infant is cyanotic or the PaO_2 is less than 50 mm Hg in room air with or without cyanosis. Measure the ambient oxygen concentration continuously. Note carefully the precautions and contraindications for the use of oxygen for premature infants (see chapter 11–IV).	7. Administer an adequate quantity of oxygen to prevent hypoxia. Avoid oxygen toxicity; retinopathy of prematurity (retrolental fibroplasia), pulmonary hemorrhage, and bronchopulmonary dysplasia. Cyanosis is usually a reliable sign of hypoxia; conversely, hypoxia can be present without cyanosis.
8. Obtain a baseline blood glucose and/or screening test on admission to the nursery and monitor the blood glucose level as needed.	8. Prevent hypoglycemia. Prematures have low carbohydrate stores. Prevent hyperglycemia. Sick prematures, particularly those less than 1,250 gm, may develop hyperglycemia (see chapter 15–X and 15–XII).
9. Obtain a baseline hematocrit value on admission to the nursery, every day until stabilized, and at least once every week.	9. Prevent anemia. Prematures have a higher incidence of maternal history of placenta previa, abruptio placentae, and marginal sinus rupture. They develop hemorrhage (e.g., CNS) more frequently than fullterm infants. Physiologic anemia occurs earlier and more profoundly (see chapter 14–XV).
10. Feeding orders: see chapter 6–II D on feeding "the premature infant."	10. Prevent overfeeding and aspiration, distension, and/or vagal stimulation.
11. Advise the mother and father to see, hold, and talk to the infant as much as possible.	11. Support the family-infant relationship.
12. Notify the social service/psychologist of all premature births. Administer early stimulation for psychosocial development.	12. Psychologically and socially help the infant's family to cope with the crisis of premature birth and preparing for discharge.
13. Administer an IMD (inborn error metabolic disease) screening test at 7	13. Prevent mental retardation caused by IMD as soon as possible.

ORDERS	REASONS
days of age and again at the time of discharge. (The IMD test must be given before the infant receives red blood cell transfusion to detect hemoglobinopathy and after the infant has had 2 to 3 days of milk feedings for the majority of IMD.)	
14. If vitamin intake is inadequate, administer 1 ml of Tri-Vi-Sol (Mead Johnson and Co.) or Vi-Daylin ADC (Ross Laboratories) (Vitamin A, 1,500 IU; D, 400 IU; and C, 35 IU) by mouth daily by the seventh day of life. Vitamin E may be started at birth. Recommended doses and duration of therapy variable: 25 IU/day for 1 week up to 6 weeks has been recommended.	14. Prevent vitamin deficiency.
15. Administer iron supplement. Iron supplement may not be necessary if the infant received multiple transfusions. (See chapter 14, XV.)	15. Build the infant's iron stores. Prevent anemia resulting from low iron.
16. Record head circumference, length, and hematocrit weekly.	16. Ensure adequate growth and hematocrit levels.
17. Discharge orders: see Chapter 10 for discharge policies.	17. Ensure continuous adequate care.

B. Environment for LBW Infants

1. Temperature

   Maintenance of the premature infant's skin temperature at approximately 36.5° C (97.7° F) or the rectal temperature at approximately 37.0° C (98.6° F) is associated with a significant reduction in neonatal mortality. However, normal body temperature does not indicate minimal oxygen consumption since increased metabolic rate may maintain normal body temperature. Minimal metabolism (oxygen consumption that is sufficient to maintain body temperature) is noted in infants nursed in a thermoneutral environment of 32.0° C (89.6° F) operative temperature with 50% relative humidity (ambient water vapor density of 16.9 gm/cu m) and when the gradient between skin and the environmental temperature is less than 1.5° C (2.7° F). Hypothermia is often seen in infants who are LBW, who have intrauterine growth retardation, who have had asphyxia or who have sepsis, intracranial hemorrhage, meningitis, or anomalies. Hyperthermia may be due to an excessive environmental temperature, infection, dehydration, or alterations of central mechanisms of heat control associated with birth trauma or drugs (e.g., withdrawal symptoms).

   a. The effect of acute subthermoneutral (cold) stress

      1) Clinical manifestations: poor feeding; lethargy; "cold to the touch;" cen-

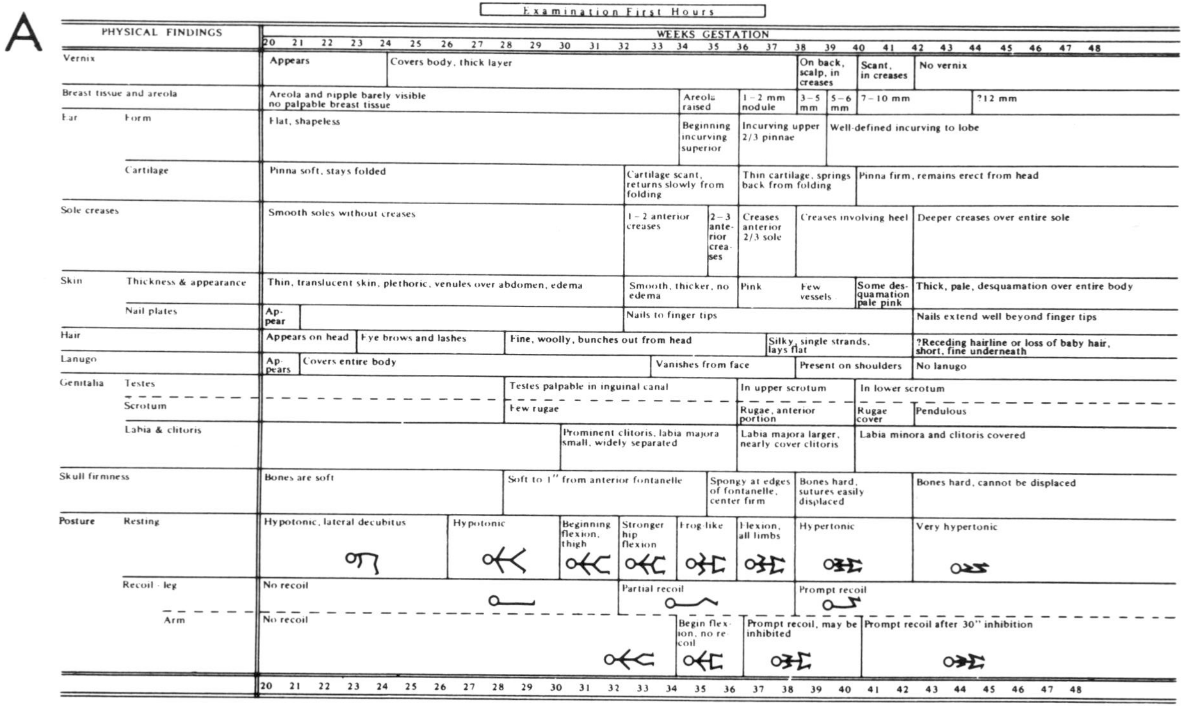

FIG 6–1.

A, clinical estimation of gestational age. (From Kempe C.H., Silver H.K., O'Brien D.: *Current Pediatric Diagnosis and Treatment,* ed. 6. Los Altos, Cal., Lange Medical Publications, 1980. Used by permission.) *(Continued.)*

B

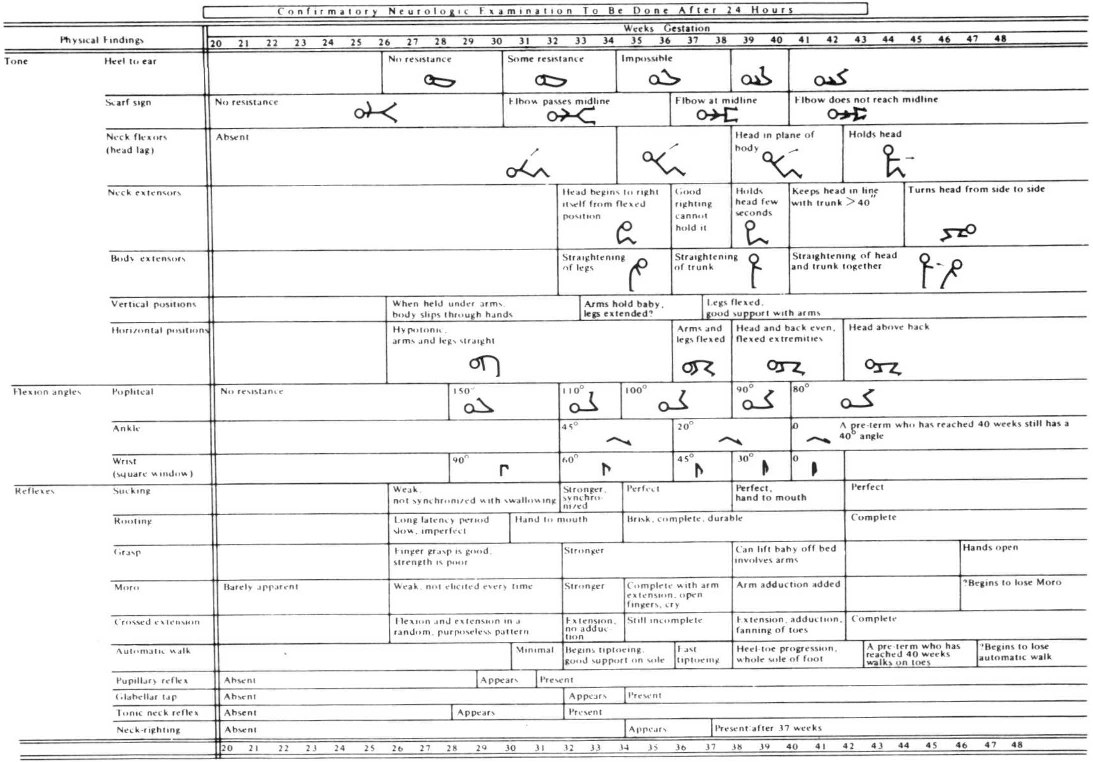

<table>
<tr><th colspan="31">Confirmatory Neurologic Examination To Be Done After 24 Hours</th></tr>
<tr><th colspan="2" rowspan="2">Physical Findings</th><th colspan="29">Weeks Gestation</th></tr>
<tr><th>20</th><th>21</th><th>22</th><th>23</th><th>24</th><th>25</th><th>26</th><th>27</th><th>28</th><th>29</th><th>30</th><th>31</th><th>32</th><th>33</th><th>34</th><th>35</th><th>36</th><th>37</th><th>38</th><th>39</th><th>40</th><th>41</th><th>42</th><th>43</th><th>44</th><th>45</th><th>46</th><th>47</th><th>48</th></tr>
<tr><td rowspan="7">Tone</td><td>Heel to ear</td><td colspan="6"></td><td colspan="5">No resistance</td><td colspan="4">Some resistance</td><td colspan="4">Impossible</td><td colspan="2"></td><td colspan="8"></td></tr>
<tr><td>Scarf sign</td><td colspan="11">No resistance</td><td colspan="6">Elbow passes midline</td><td colspan="4">Elbow at midline</td><td colspan="8">Elbow does not reach midline</td></tr>
<tr><td>Neck flexors (head lag)</td><td colspan="15">Absent</td><td colspan="4"></td><td colspan="4">Head in plane of body</td><td colspan="6">Holds head</td></tr>
<tr><td>Neck extensors</td><td colspan="13"></td><td colspan="4">Head begins to right itself from flexed position</td><td colspan="2">Good righting cannot hold it</td><td colspan="2">Holds head few seconds</td><td colspan="4">Keeps head in line with trunk > 40″</td><td colspan="4">Turns head from side to side</td></tr>
<tr><td>Body extensors</td><td colspan="13"></td><td colspan="4">Straightening of legs</td><td colspan="4">Straightening of trunk</td><td colspan="8">Straightening of head and trunk together</td></tr>
<tr><td>Vertical positions</td><td colspan="6"></td><td colspan="7">When held under arms, body slips through hands</td><td colspan="5">Arms hold baby, legs extended?</td><td colspan="11">Legs flexed, good support with arms</td></tr>
<tr><td>Horizontal positions</td><td colspan="6"></td><td colspan="11">Hypotonic, arms and legs straight</td><td colspan="2">Arms and legs flexed</td><td colspan="4">Head and back even, flexed extremities</td><td colspan="6">Head above back</td></tr>
<tr><td rowspan="3">Flexion angles</td><td>Popliteal</td><td colspan="9">No resistance</td><td colspan="4">150°</td><td colspan="2">110°</td><td colspan="4">100°</td><td colspan="2">90°</td><td colspan="8">80°</td></tr>
<tr><td>Ankle</td><td colspan="13"></td><td colspan="4">45°</td><td colspan="4">20°</td><td colspan="8">0 A pre-term who has reached 40 weeks still has a 40° angle</td></tr>
<tr><td>Wrist (square window)</td><td colspan="9"></td><td colspan="4">90°</td><td colspan="4">60°</td><td colspan="2">45°</td><td colspan="2">30°</td><td colspan="2">0</td><td colspan="6"></td></tr>
<tr><td rowspan="10">Reflexes</td><td>Sucking</td><td colspan="6"></td><td colspan="7">Weak, not synchronized with swallowing</td><td colspan="2">Stronger, synchronized</td><td colspan="4">Perfect</td><td colspan="4">Perfect, hand to mouth</td><td colspan="6">Perfect</td></tr>
<tr><td>Rooting</td><td colspan="6"></td><td colspan="5">Long latency period slow, imperfect</td><td colspan="4">Hand to mouth</td><td colspan="8">Brisk, complete, durable</td><td colspan="6">Complete</td></tr>
<tr><td>Grasp</td><td colspan="6"></td><td colspan="7">Finger grasp is good, strength is poor</td><td colspan="6">Stronger</td><td colspan="4">Can lift baby off bed involves arms</td><td colspan="4"></td><td colspan="2">Hands open</td></tr>
<tr><td>Moro</td><td colspan="6">Barely apparent</td><td colspan="7">Weak, not elicited every time</td><td colspan="2">Stronger</td><td colspan="4">Complete with arm extension, open fingers, cry</td><td colspan="4">Arm adduction added</td><td colspan="4"></td><td colspan="2">?Begins to lose Moro</td></tr>
<tr><td>Crossed extension</td><td colspan="6"></td><td colspan="7">Flexion and extension in a random, purposeless pattern</td><td colspan="2">Extension, no adduction</td><td colspan="4">Still incomplete</td><td colspan="4">Extension, adduction, fanning of toes</td><td colspan="6">Complete</td></tr>
<tr><td>Automatic walk</td><td colspan="11"></td><td colspan="2">Minimal</td><td colspan="4">Begins tiptoeing, good support on sole</td><td colspan="2">Fast tiptoeing</td><td colspan="4">Heel-toe progression, whole sole of foot</td><td colspan="4">A pre-term who has reached 40 weeks walks on toes</td><td colspan="2">?Begins to lose automatic walk</td></tr>
<tr><td>Pupillary reflex</td><td colspan="10">Absent</td><td colspan="2">Appears</td><td colspan="17">Present</td></tr>
<tr><td>Glabellar tap</td><td colspan="13">Absent</td><td colspan="2">Appears</td><td colspan="14">Present</td></tr>
<tr><td>Tonic neck reflex</td><td colspan="9">Absent</td><td colspan="4">Appears</td><td colspan="16">Present</td></tr>
<tr><td>Neck-righting</td><td colspan="15">Absent</td><td colspan="3">Appears</td><td colspan="11">Present after 37 weeks</td></tr>
<tr><td colspan="2"></td><td>20</td><td>21</td><td>22</td><td>23</td><td>24</td><td>25</td><td>26</td><td>27</td><td>28</td><td>29</td><td>30</td><td>31</td><td>32</td><td>33</td><td>34</td><td>35</td><td>36</td><td>37</td><td>38</td><td>39</td><td>40</td><td>41</td><td>42</td><td>43</td><td>44</td><td>45</td><td>46</td><td>47</td><td>48</td></tr>
</table>

FIG 6–1 (cont.).

B, clinical estimation of gestational age. (From Kempe C.H., Silver H.K., O'Brien D.: *Current Pediatric Diagnosis and Treatment,* ed. 6. Los Altos, Cal., Lange Medical Publications, 1980. Used by permission.) *(Continued.)*

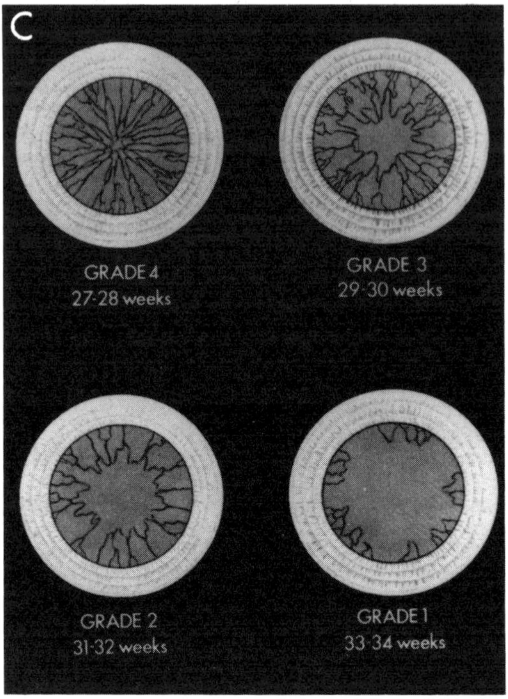

FIG 6–1 (cont.).
C, grading system for assessment of gestational age by examination of the anterior vascular capsule of lens. (From Hittner H.M., Hirsch N.J., Rudolph A.J.: *J. Pediatr.* 91:455, 1977. Used by permission.)

tral cyanosis; pallor; occasionally bright red due to the failure of oxyhemoglobin dissociation at cold temperature; slow, shallow, and irregular respiration; expiratory grunting; occasionally bradycardia; decreased activity; feeble cry; depression; shivering (rarely); abdominal distension; vomiting; edema; and sclerema

2) Metabolic derangements: decreased PaO_2, hypoglycemia, metabolic acidosis, hyperkalemia, elevated blood urea nitrogen (BUN), and oliguria are often associated with acute hypothermia. Hypothermia also increases nonesterified fatty acids that bind with albumin.
3) Decreased pulmonary blood flow and pulmonary hemorrhage are not uncommon.

b. The effect of chronic subthermoneutral (cold) stress
LBW infants exhibit slower weight gain and linear growth.
c. The effect of acute hyperthermia
Hyperthermia induces tachypnea, tachycardia, irritability, periodic breathing, and apnea.

d. Practical considerations concerning the temperature maintenance in the delivery room
   1) Place the infant in a warmed environment, under a radiant heater to minimize heat loss.
   2) Pat the infant dry to prevent heat loss from evaporation.
   3) Remove the infant from the cold environment of the delivery room, which is set for the comfort of the staff, as soon as the infant's cardiovascular status has stabilized.
   4) Support and maintain the infant's temperature by placing the infant in a heated transport incubator during transport to the newborn nursery.
   5) Delay the newborn's initial bath until his or her temperature has stabilized.

e. Practical considerations concerning temperature maintenance in the nursery
   1) Place the infant in a warmed environment and maintain the infant's skin temperature at approximately 36.5° C (97.7° F) and/or rectal temperature at about 37.0° C (98.6° F).
      a) Place the infant in a bassinette if the infant is well and weighs more than 1,800 gm at birth.
      b) Place the infant in an incubator, or under a radiant heater, if the infant is sick or weighs less than 1,800 gm at birth.
      c) Remember that apnea frequently occurs when the infant's temperature rises quickly. The infant should be warmed gradually. Environmental temperature and abdominal skin temperature should not differ greater than 1.5° C (2.7° F) to minimize oxygen consumption.
      d) Inspired oxygen temperature should be set at the same temperature as the incubator. Watch the infant closely during recovery.
   2) The incubator

      The incubator conserves the body temperature by circulating warmed air around the infant. In addition, the incubator permits visualization of the undressed infant and maintenance of the desired gaseous (oxygen) concentration and humidity and helps reduce (through filtration) air pollution and bacterial contamination. To maintain the infant's rectal temperature at 37.0° C (98.6° F) and abdominal skin temperature at 36.5° C (97.7° F), the nurse increases or decreases the temperature of the circulating air (in relation to the infant's temperature). *This requires the constant attention of the nurse.* To maintain the infant's temperature at the desired level on admission to the nursery, set the incubator air temperature at 35 to 36° C (95 to 97° F) for the less than 1,000-gm infant, 34.5 to 35° C (94 to 95° F) for the 1,000- to 1,500-gm infant, and 32° C (89 to 90° F) for the more than 2,500-gm infant (see Table 6–2). The temperature must then be raised or lowered as indicated. In general, the thinner, smaller, and younger the infant, the higher the environment temperature required to achieve the thermoneutral environment. Radiant heat loss may be diminished for the very LBW infant by using a double-walled incubator or a plastic heat shield inside the single-walled

A

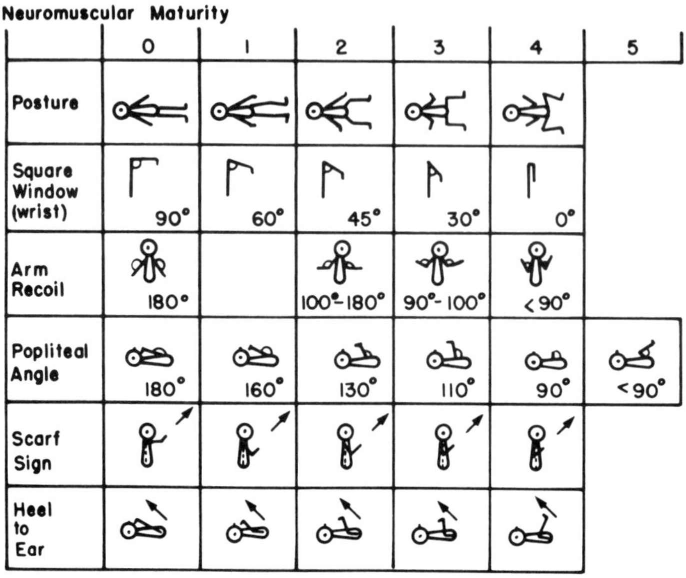

B PHYSICAL MATURITY

Skin	gelatinous red, trans-parent	smooth pink, vis-ible veins	superficial peeling &/or rash few veins	cracking pale area rare veins	parchment deep cracking no vessels	leathery cracked wrinkled
Lanugo	none	abundant	thinning	bald areas	mostly bald	
Plantar Creases	no crease	faint red marks	anterior transverse crease only	creases ant. 2/3	creases cover entire sole	
Breast	barely percept.	flat areola no bud	stippled areola 1–2 mm bud	raised areola 3–4 mm bud	full areola 5–10 mm bud	
Ear	pinna flat, stays folded	sl. curved pinna; soft with slow recoil	well-curv. pinna; soft but ready recoil	formed & firm with instant recoil	thick cartilage ear stiff	
Genitals ♂	scrotum empty no rugae		testes descend-ing, few rugae	testes down good rugae	testes pendulous deep rugae	
Genitals ♀	prominent clitoris & labia minora		majora & minora equally prominent	majora large minora small	clitoris & minora completely covered	

MATURITY RATING

Score	5	10	15	20	25	30	35	40	45	50
Weeks	26	28	30	32	34	36	38	40	42	44

FIG 6–2.
A and **B,** a simplified score for an assessment of fetal maturation of newly born infants. (From Ballard J.L., Novak K.K., Driver M.: *J. Pediatr.* 95:769, 1979. Used by permission.) *(Continued.)*

C

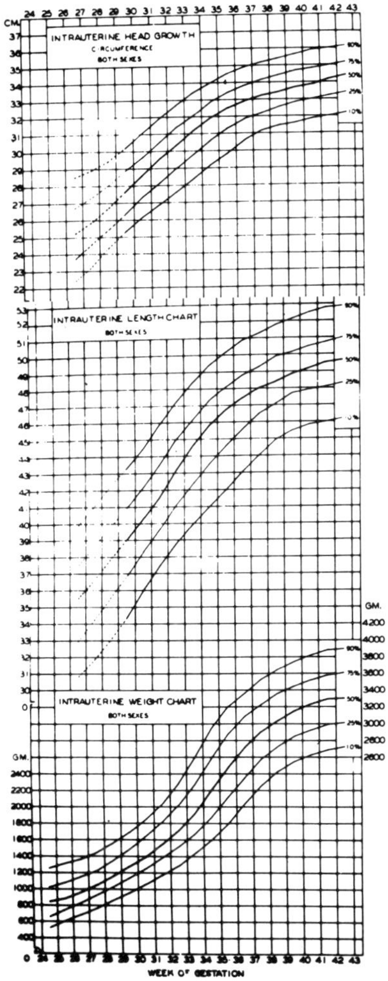

Gest. age by Dates ____________ wks

Gest. age by Exam ____________ wks

B.W. __________ gm. __________ %ile

Length __________ cm. __________ %ile

Head Circum. ________ cm. ______ %ile

Signature ______________________________________ M.D.

FIG 6–2 (cont.).
C, intrauterine head growth, weight, and length chart. (From Lubchenco L.O., Hansman C., Boyd E.: *Pediatrics* 37:403, 1966. Used by permission.)

incubator, but very LBW infants, particularly those less than 750 gm, may still have difficulty maintaining temperature in a double wall incubator.

TABLE 6–1.—SUGGESTED DAILY FLUID REQUIREMENT IN THE NEWBORN PERIOD*

AGE	TERM (ML/KG)	PREMATURE (ML/KG)
Day 1	60–70	60–75
Day 2	75†	80–90
Day 3	80	100–110
Day 4	85†	120–140
Day 5	90	125–150
Week 2, 3, 4	120	150

*From Easter L.B., Halata M.S., Dweck H.S.: Parenteral nutrition in the newborn: A practical guide. *Pediatr. Clin. N. Am.* 29:1171, 1982. Used by permission.

†Interpolated.

TABLE 6–2.—NEUTRAL THERMAL ENVIRONMENTAL TEMPERATURES*

AGE AND WEIGHT	STARTING TEMPERATURE (°C)	RANGE OF TEMPERATURE (°C)
0–6 hr		
Under 1,200 gm	35.0	34.0–35.4
1,200–1,500 gm	34.1	33.9–34.4
1,501–2,500 gm	33.4	32.8–33.8
Over 2,500 gm (and >36 wk)	32.9	32.0–33.8
6–12 hr		
Under 1,200 gm	35.0	34.0–35.4
1,200–1,500 gm	34.0	33.5–34.4
1,501–2,500 gm	33.1	32.2–33.8
Over 2,500 gm (and >36 wk)	32.8	31.4–33.8
12–24 hr		
Under 1,200 gm	34.0	34.0–35.4
1,200–1,500 gm	33.8	33.3–34.3
1,501–2,500 gm	32.8	31.8–33.8
Over 2,500 gm (and >36 wk)	32.4	31.0–33.7
24–36 hr		
Under 1,200 gm	34.0	34.0–35.0
1,200–1,500 gm	33.6	33.1–34.2
1,501–2,500 gm	32.6	31.6–33.6
Over 2,500 gm (and >36 wk)	32.1	30.7–33.5
36–48 hr		
Under 1,200 gm	34.0	34.0–35.0
1,200–1,500 gm	33.5	33.0–34.1
1,501–2,500 gm	32.5	31.4–33.5
Over 2,500 gm (and >36 wk)	31.9	30.5–33.3
48–72 hr		
Under 1,200 gm	34.0	34.0–35.0
1,200–1,500 gm	33.5	33.0–34.0

TABLE 6–2.—*(continued)*

AGE AND WEIGHT	STARTING TEMPERATURE (°C)	RANGE OF TEMPERATURE (°C)
1,501–2,500 gm	32.3	31.2–33.4
Over 2,500 gm (and >36 wk)	31.7	30.1–33.2
72–96 hr		
Under 1,200 gm	34.0	34.0–35.0
1,200–1,500 gm	33.5	33.0–34.0
1,501–2,500 gm	32.2	31.1–33.2
Over 2,500 gm (and >36 wk)	31.3	29.8–32.8
4–12 days		
Under 1,500 gm	33.5	33.0–34.0
1,501–2,500 gm	32.1	31.0–33.2
Over 2,500 gm (and >36 wk)		
4–5 days	31.0	29.5–32.6
5–6 days	30.9	29.4–32.3
6–8 days	30.6	29.0–32.2
8–10 days	30.3	29.0–31.8
10–12 days	30.1	29.0–31.4
12–14 Days		
Under 1,500 gm	33.5	32.6–34.0
1,501–2,500 gm	32.1	31.0–33.2
Over 2,500 gm (and >36 wk)	29.8	29.0–30.8
2–3 wk		
Under 1,500 gm	33.1	32.2–34.0
1,501–2,500 gm	31.7	30.5–33.0
3–4 wk		
Under 1,500 gm	32.6	31.6–33.6
1,501–2,500 gm	31.4	30.0–32.7
4–5 wk		
Under 1,500 gm	32.0	31.2–33.0
1,501–2,500 gm	30.9	29.5–32.2
5–6 wk		
Under 1,500 gm	31.4	30.6–32.3
1,501–2,500 gm	30.4	29.0–31.8

*From *Guidelines for Perinatal Care.* Evanston, Ill., American Academy of Pediatrics, 1983, pp. 228, 229. Reproduced by permission.

3) The Servo-Control

The Servo-Control is a feedback mechanism for automatically regulating the environmental temperature through a thermocouple attached to the infant's abdominal skin (over the liver). When the infant's skin temperature falls, the heating unit adds additional heat; when the infant's skin temperature is at the desired set level, the heating unit automatically shuts off. The infant's abdominal skin temperature is maintained at the Servo-Control point by decreasing or increasing heat output, even if the infant has febrile or hypothermic conditions. The recommended range of the Servo-Control set point is 36.0 to 36.5 C (96.8 to 97.7 F).

4) Common errors occurring with the incubator
   a) The temperature-control mechanism is not regulated by the nurse and the infant's temperature is allowed to fluctuate widely. Maintaining an abdominal skin temperature at 37.2° C (98.9° F) and 35.9° C (96.6° F) increases oxygen consumption by 6% and 10%, respectively.
   b) The infant is placed in the wrong environment. If the incubator temperature drops 2.0° C (3.6° F) or the room temperature falls to 19.0° C (66.2° F), the infant must increase heat production by 35% to prevent a core temperature fall. The infant will lose heat to the cold incubator wall by radiation if the incubator is placed near a cold window or wall or if the nursery is cool (15.6 to 23.8° C; 60 to 75° F). Conversely, the infant will become febrile if the room temperature increases to 31.0° C (87.7° F) or the incubator temperature rises by 2.0° C (3.6° F). The infant will gain heat from the short-wavelength radiant emission if the incubator is placed in the sunlight.
   c) The electric plug is disconnected and no one realizes the infant is chilled.
   d) The temperature-control mechanism is set incorrectly.
   e) The thermocouple wire is pinched by the Isolette window and, therefore, is inaccurate.
   f) The thermocouple falls off the infant and the Isolette overheats.
   g) The thermocouple is placed on the wrong site, e.g., on the foot.
   h) The infant's temperature is maintained at the desired level by the addition of excessive heat or decreasing heat output, but the physician fails to realize that the actual cause of the infant's hypothermia or hyperthermia has not been remedied.
5) The radiant heater

   The radiant heater provides a powerful and direct source of heat (electromagnetic waves transmitting thermal energy directly to the infant's skin) to replace large heat losses. The radiant power density that reaches the exposed skin surface area is regulated automatically by a Servo-Control mechanism. The recommended range for the Servo-Control's set point temperature is 36.0 to 36.5° C (96.8 to 97.7° F). The radiant heater is useful for shortterm use in the delivery room and in the NICU. In addition, since it is usually suspended over an open crib, the radiant heater allows easy accessibility to the infant for the performance of desired procedures, such as umbilical vessel catheterization, exchange transfusion, and others. However, it does not modify the oxygen or humidity level around the infant. An oxygen-enriched environment must be maintained by adding an oxygen hood (see chapter 11–IV). Insensible water loss is increased when infants are under radiant warmers most likely due to low ambient humidity, increased convective air current, and increased evaporative water loss by a direct drying effect. The highest percentage increase in insensible water loss is seen under the Ohio warmer (148%, greater than 1,500 gm), then the KDC warmer (54%, less than 1,500 gm; 43%, 1,000 to 2,000 gm), and least under the IMI warmer (50%, less than 1,500 gm; 82%, greater than 1,500 gm). Insensible water loss is highest under the warmer and phototherapy light combined. Insensible water loss and heat output are increased with decreasing body size because of larger body surface area per kg body weight, larger water composition of body mass, and increased transdermal water loss by a thinner epidermis in more premature and smaller infants. A thin, pliable, clear plastic film blanket significantly reduces insensible water loss, radiant warmer power input demand, and the radiant power density reaching an infant's skin. The infant may be predisposed to handling by persons who have not washed their hands properly as no barrier exists between the newborn and the medical and nursing personnel.

2. Humidity
   If the temperature is controlled properly, the mortality and insensible water loss of premature infants are not affected by the relative humidity, although short periods of increasing ambient water vapor density decrease transepidermal water loss. Super humidification ("rain" in the incubator) is not recommended since no evidence exists that it aids premature infants, but there is evidence that it increases the risk of developing a waterborne infection due to organisms of the *Pseudomonas, Klebsiella, Aerobacter,* and *Proteus* species and others. Extra humidity is of value for those infants who have recently undergone extubation and may have an upper airway obstruction secondary to laryngeal edema.
3. Oxygen therapy (see chapter 11–IV).

REFERENCES

Bruck K.: Temperature regulation in the newborn infant. *Biol. Neonate* 3:65, 1961.

Doyle L.W., Sinclair J.C.: Insensible water loss in newborn infants. *Clin. Perinatol.* 9:453, 1982.

Silverman W.A., Fertig J.W., Berger A.P.: The influence of the thermal environment upon the survival of the newly born premature infants. *Pediatrics* 22:876, 1958.

Sinclair J.C.: Minimizing heat loss from the body after birth. *N. Engl. J. Med.* 284:156, 1971.

C. Nutritional Requirements (see Table 6–4)

1. Calories
   The average enteral caloric intake of 100 to 150 calories/kg/day in a healthy fullterm newborn will result in a weight gain of 20 to 30 gm/day. The average enteral caloric requirement of premature infants is 104 to 129 calories/kg/day; 59 to 84 for the basal metabolic rate, intermittent activity, and cold stress and 45 for specific dynamic action, fecal loss, and allowance for growth (see Table 6–3). Some very LBW infants gain weight of 20 to 30 gm/day with a total parenteral caloric intake of 60 to 90 calories/kg/day. Fullterm infants on breast feeding receive approximately 50% to 55% of total caloric intake as fat, 35% to 40% as carbohydrate, and 5% to 15% as protein.

TABLE 6–3.—Daily Caloric Expenditure and Fluid Loss*

	Caloric Expenditure (Calories/kg/day) 1,000–2,000 gm	3,500 gm		Fluid Loss (ml/kg/day) Premature
Basal metabolic rate			Insensible water loss	17–64
1 day	34	32–37	1,000 gm	64
2–3 days		43	1,001–1,250 gm	56
6 days	42		1,251–1,500 gm	38
2–4 wk	50		1,501–1,750 gm	22
4–6 wk	59		1,750–2,000 gm	17
Intermittent activity	15	15		
Cold stress	10	10		
Specific dynamic action	8	8	Urine (at 300 mOsm/L)	30–72
Fecal loss	12	12	Stool	5–10
Growth allowance	25	25		
Total	104–129	102–113		52–146

*Adapted from Sinclair J.C., Driscoll J.M. Jr., Heird W.C., et al.: Supportive management of the sick neonate: Parenteral calories, water, electrolytes. *Pediatr. Clin. N. Am.* 17:863, 1970, and Rahman N., Boineau F.G., Lewy J.E.: Renal failure in the perinatal period. *Clin. Perinatol.* 8:241, 1981.

2. Fluids

Suggested daily fluid requirement in the newborn period is shown in Table 6–1.

The daily maintenance fluid requirements for the fullterm and LBW infants include the following:

	% of Total Fluid Requirement: Fullterm	LBW
Insensible water loss	20%	32%
Urinary output	50%	56%
Stool losses	10%	6%

Infants require a lower daily fluid intake in the first few postnatal days than later because of lower insensible water loss (lower basal metabolic rates, decreased activity, and normal contraction of extracellular fluid volume). The magnitude of insensible water loss is influenced by the infant's environment, metabolic rate, respiratory rate, gestational maturity, body size, body surface area, and the proportion of body composition composed of water.

a. Conditions requiring greater fluid intake
   1) Very LBW infants less than 30 weeks gestation. Insensible water loss may be increased by as much as 190%, e.g., 1,000-gm infants 3 days of age may require as high as 250 ml/kg/day for insensible water loss.

2) SGA infants in comparison with appropriate for gestational age infants
3) Increased activity (e.g., seizures, respiratory distress, drug withdrawal)
4) Low ambient humidity
5) Cold stress or increased ambient temperature
6) Fever and/or tachypnea
7) Phototherapy
8) Open infant care radiant heater and forced convection
9) Excessive gastrointestinal (GI) losses (fistula, diarrhea, "third space loss" with necrotizing enterocolitis, etc.)
10) Dehydration
11) Hypotension

b. Conditions requiring less fluid intake
   1) Renal failure, congestive heart failure
   2) Increased humidification (intubation, incubator and plastic shield or blanket)
   3) Syndrome of inappropriate antidiuretic hormone: postoperative state, meningitis

Fluids should be administered carefully to the very LBW infant since excessive fluid administration may be associated with the patency of the ductus arteriosus, congestive heart failure, and worsening of bronchopulmonary dysplasia. Each infant must be continuously monitored for hydration status by physical examination of skin turgor, mucous membranes, eyes, and anterior fontanelle, weight, urinary output, and laboratory determinations of hematocrit, plasma sodium, blood urea nitrogen (BUN), plasma osmolality, urine osmolality, and urine specific gravity.

3. Carbohydrate

Human milk and most formulas contain approximately 40% to 50% of total calories as carbohydrates, mainly lactose. Premature infants have relatively low intestinal lactase activity although they can develop well on formulas containing only lactose.

4. Protein

The optimal protein requirement has not been clearly established. The present practice provides protein intake of 2.5 to 4.0 gm/kg/day with protein of 10% to 15% of total caloric intake. LBW infants require cystine, tyrosine, histidine and possibly taurine as essential amino acids. Formula containing protein of 2.25 gm/kg/day with a whey to casein ratio of 60:40 is noted to give the lowest BUN, ammonia, tyrosine, and phenylalanine levels when compared to casein-predominant high-protein (4.5 gm/kg/day) formula. The current recommendation is to use breast milk or whey-predominant protein although breast milk may not contain adequate protein (or calcium and phosphorus) for very LBW premature infants without supplementation. The adequacy of human milk is difficult to assess since the composition varies, the standard for growth is not agreed upon and prospective studies show variable results.

5. Fat

LBW infants have poor fat absorption (malabsorption of as much as 30% of intake), probably due to inadequate pancreatic lipase, immature hepatic synthesis and excretion of bile acids, and insufficient absorptive surface. Human milk and certain mixtures of vegetable fat are better tolerated than butter fat. Medium-chain triglycerides are well tolerated in fullterm infants as well as premature infants.

Fat intake of 2 to 4 gm/kg/day with approximately 40% to 50% of the total calories needs to be provided. Linoleic, linolenic, and arachidonic acids are required since they can not be synthesized although the later two may be synthesized from linoleic acid. Excessive linoleic acid produces excessive peroxidation and increases the vitamin E requirement.

6. Minerals, vitamins, and trace elements

   The daily requirements of minerals, vitamins, and trace elements are shown in Table 6–4.

   a. Sodium

      Premature infants less than 32 weeks' gestation require higher sodium (3 to 4 mEq/kg/day) intake because of relatively high urinary sodium loss, low sodium intake (breast milk or formula), and sodium precipitation in rapidly growing bone. In addition, sodium losses are accentuated in severe respiratory distress syndrome, following diuretic therapy, and in glycosuria.

   b. Vitamin D

      The daily dosage of 400 IU orally or IM corrects increased alkaline phosphatase levels, which may be the earliest signs of rickets.

   c. Vitamin E

      Poly-Vi-Sol, 1.0 ml (5 IU of vitamin E) daily, is recommended to meet the vitamin E requirement in term newborns. Premature infants are born with low serum levels of vitamin E. Vitamin E antioxidant deficiency has been reported to be associated with hemolytic anemia and/or generalized edema at 6 to 10 weeks of age in less than 32-weeks' gestation prematures fed polyunsaturated fat and large amounts of iron (see chapter 14–XV). Recommended doses and duration of therapy are variable: 25 mg/day for 1 week up to 6 weeks has been recommended.

   d. Iron

      Premature infants are born with deficient iron stores because iron is transferred across the placenta in the last trimester. The recommended dose for LBW infants and infants with significant anemia is 2 to 3 mg/kg/day starting at 2 months of age. Iron is not started until the infant is approximately 2 months of age because iron decreases the vitamin E bioavailability and binds with proteins important in bacteriostatic properties; lactoferrin and transferrin. (see chapter 14–XV).

   e. Zinc

      Zinc deficiency is often noted by 5 to 9 weeks of age, particularly in prematures since zinc is transferred across the placenta in the last 10 to 12 weeks of pregnancy. The recommended dosage is 650 mcg/kg/day. Clinical manifestations of zinc deficiency are generalized edema, hypoproteinemia, cutaneous changes, growth failure, and diarrhea. Generalized edema may be noted with feeding of high-solute formulas and in conges-

(continued on page 93)

TABLE 6–4.—Estimated Daily Requirement for Nutrients*

	PREMATURE				FULL-TERM	
	800–1,200 GM		1,200–1,800 GM			
ELEMENTS	DOSE/KG/DAY	DOSE/100 KCAL	DOSE/KG/DAY	DOSE/100 KCAL	DOSE/KG/DAY	DOSE/100 KCAL
Fluid (ml)	65–200	—	65–200	—	65–150	—
Calories (kcal)	114–181	—	114–181	—	90–120	—
Glucose (gm)†	10–20	—	10–20	—	10–20	—
Protein (gm)‡	4.0	3.1	3.5	2–2.5	2.5	1.8
Fat (gm)§	§	§	§	§	2.0	3.3
Na (mEq)	3.5	2.7	3.0	2.3	2–3	—
K (mEq)	2.5	1.9	2.3	1.8	2–3	—
Cl (mEq)	3.1	2.4	2.5	2.0	3–5	—
Ca (mg)	210	160	185	140	20–40	50
PO_4 (mg)	140	108	123	95	20–40	25
Mg (mg)	10.0	7.5	8.5	6.5	5–6	6.0
Iron (mg)	2–3	—	2–3	—	2	0.15
Cu (μg)	117	90	117	90	15–30	60
Zn (μg)	650	500	650	500	350	500
Manganese (μg)	—	5	—	5	—	5
Iodine (μg)	—	5	—	5	—	5

	PREMATURE		FULLTERM	
VITAMINS	DOSE/DAY	DOSE/100 KCAL	DOSE/DAY	DOSE/100 KCAL
A (IU)	1,000	330–660	275–375	250
D (IU)	400	—	400	—
E (IU)	25	2–5	5	3
C (mg)	35	30	35	8
B_6 (mg)	0.25	0.15	0.2	—
B_{12} (μg)	1.0	—	1.0	0.15
Folate (μg)	65	50	30–40	—

(continued)

TABLE 6–4.—*(continued)*

VITAMINS	PREMATURE		FULLTERM	
	DOSE/DAY	DOSE/100 KCAL	DOSE/DAY	DOSE/100 KCAL
Niacin (mg)	6.0	4–6	5–8	—
Riboflavin (mg)	0.5	0.4–0.6	0.4–0.6	—
Thiamine (mg)	0.4	0.3	0.2–0.3	—
K (μg)	4	4	4	4

*Dose/100 kcal is estimated assuming calorie intake of 130 cal/kg/day. Estimated daily requirement/kg is calculated from daily dose/100 kcal assuming body weight of 1,000 gm for the group of infants 800–1,200 gm and assuming body weight of 1,500 gm for the group of infants 1,200–1,800 gm.
†40–50% of total caloric intake as carbohydrate.
‡10–15% of total caloric intake as protein.
§40–50% of total caloric intake as fat.

REFERENCES

American Academy of Pediatrics Committee on Nutrition: Commentary on breast feeding and infant formulas including proposed standards for formulas. *Pediatrics* 57:278, 1976.

American Academy of Pediatrics, Committee on Nutrition: Nutritional needs of LBW infants. *Pediatrics* 75:976, 1985.

Tsang R.: *Vitamin and Mineral Requirements in Preterm Infants.* New York, Marcel Dekker Inc., 1985 tive heart failure, hereditary hypoparathyroidism, and some cases of hypocalcemic tetany as well as in zinc deficiency (see chapter 18–XIII).

f. Calcium and phosphorus

Calcium requirement for premature infants is 185 to 210 mg/kg/day. It is recommended to supplement premature human milk with a formula containing a balanced 2:1 ratio of calcium and phosphorus.

D. Feeding the Premature Infant

The feeding of premature infants requires skillful medical and nursing attention to supply adequate calories and fluids and prevent aspiration. Some neonatologists feel that the aim of feeding should be to keep the infant on the in utero growth curve. Unfortunately, this is extremely difficult to do, and therefore, the aim of feeding is usually to approximate the premature weight curve (see Fig 6–3). The problems associated with enteral feeding of the premature infant include

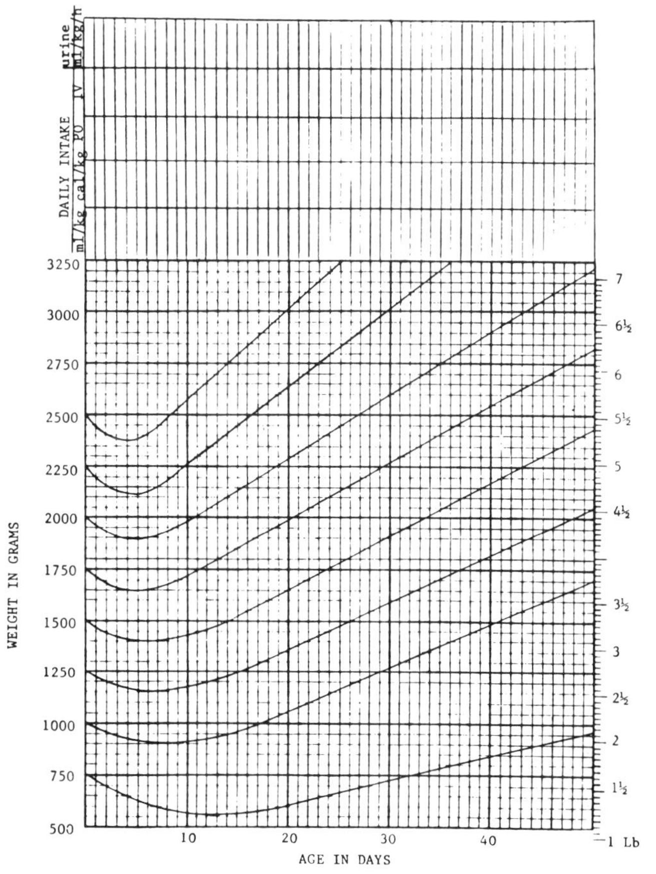

FIG 6–3.
Premature growth chart. (From Dancis J., O'Connell J.R., Holt L.E.: *J. Pediatr.* 33:570, 1948. Used by permission.)

poor suck and swallowing reflexes, relatively high caloric requirement with a small stomach capacity, poor gag reflex leading to aspiration, an incompetent esophageal cardiac sphincter, and decreased absorption of essential nutrients. Prematures digest and absorb dietary carbohydrates and protein well, but fat less efficiently than the older child because of low bile salt synthesis and pool size. Unsaturated fat, in human milk and in commercial formulas, is better absorbed than highly saturated fat. All prematures are given supplemental intravenous feeding until oral intake is adequate.

1. Enteral feedings
   a. Oral feedings
      1) Indications
         a) A premature infant without signs of distress
         b) Infants over 32 to 34 weeks' gestational age and/or 1,500 to 2,000 gm with strong and sustained sucking reflex synchronized with swallowing can be fed by nipple.
         c) Infants less than 32 to 34 weeks' gestational age and/or 1,500 to 2,000 gm can be fed via oro- or nasogastric tube.
      2) Contraindications
         a) Choking, gasping, cyanosis, bradycardia, apnea, or any other type of cardiorespiratory distress
         b) Gastrointestinal obstruction caused by functional disorders (sepsis) or organic diseases (atresia, meconium ileus, etc.)
      3) Oral feeding techniques
         a) A soft premature nipple for bottle feedings
         b) Place the infant at the mother's breast after the infant's weight reaches 1,800 gm for breast feeding.
   b. Tube feedings

      A premature infant who is without distress, less than 34 weeks of gestational age, and/or less than 1,500 gm at birth can have intermittent gavage feeding or continuous nasogastric, nasoduodenal, or nasojejunal tube feedings. The infant should be placed on his or her right side during the feeding if he or she cannot be held, and the infant should be burped with the tube open to the air. When removing the tube, it should be pinched and withdrawn slowly so that milk does not enter the pharynx.
      1) Indwelling tubes are not recommended because they partially obstruct the infant's airway and may induce nasal discharge and infection and hardening of the tube. If, because of bradycardia from vagal response or insufficient nursery personnel, indwelling tubes are used, change the tube frequently.
      2) Complications of nasojejunal or duodenal tube feeding include impaired assimilation of fat, increased bacterial contamination of the jejunum, and duodenal and jejunal perforation.
      3) Give the infant a pacifier during the tube feedings since weight gain is improved with this technique.
   c. Dropper feeding is not recommended; considerable skill is required to avoid aspiration when using this technique.

d. Gastrostomy should not be performed unless indicated (e.g., an infant with a tracheoesophageal fistula).

e. Recommended enteral feeding procedures

1) Withhold oral fluids 4 to 6 hours after birth, then administer sterile water by mouth or by nasogastric tube in the amounts listed in Table 6–5 in relation to the infant's weight and age. The quantity and quality of fluids and calories must be adjusted according to the weight and condition of the infant. Five percent D/W may be used.
2) Advance to a 13-calories/oz formula after the sterile water is tolerated one to two times by the infant. Some neonatologists advance directly to a 20-calories/oz formula.
3) Advance to a 20-calories/oz formula after the 13-calories/oz formula is tolerated three to four times.
4) Advance to a 24 calories/oz formula after the 20-calories/oz formula is tolerated over 5 to 7 days.
   New formulas for prematures and LBW infants from Mead Johnson, Wyeth, and Ross laboratories contain protein with a 60:40 ratio of whey (lactalbumin) to casein, a 2:1 ratio of calcium to phosphorus, better digestability with improved fat, calcium absorption, and a lower osmolality.
5) For prematures, the use of preterm breast milk, which is preferred to mature breast milk and pooled breast milk, may have some benefit, possibly easier digestability, protection from infection and necrotizing enterocolitis.
6) Medium chain triglycerides (MCT) oil may be added to increase caloric intake. Mix thoroughly to prevent sediment and feed carefully to prevent aspiration lipoid pneumonia.

f. Fluid replacement and quantity of enteral feeding

1) In general, premature infants should be started with 65 ml of fluid/kg/day (see Table 6–1). If the infant cannot tolerate all required fluid orally, give the balance of the required fluid IV so that the infant is receiving a total of 65 ml/kg/day (40 calories/kg/day) on the first day of life. Higher or lower quantity may be required.

TABLE 6–5.—SUGGESTED INITIAL QUANTITY OF FLUID TO BE ADMINISTERED BY NIPPLE (N) OR BY NASOGASTRIC (NG) TUBE

BIRTH WEIGHT (GM)	NO. OF ML TO START BY N OR NG	FREQUENCY
<750	0.5–1.0 (NG)	Every 1–2 hr
751–1,000	0.5–1.0 (NG)	Every 1–2 hr
1,001–1,250	2.0 (NG)	Every 2 hr
1,251–1,500	3.0 (NG)	Every 3 hr
1,501–1,750	5.0 (N or NG)	Every 3 hr
1,751–2,000	7.0 (N or NG)	Every 3 hr
>2,001	10.0 (N or NG)	Every 4 hr

2) The quantity of fluid taken orally should be increased daily or every other day in accordance with the infant's ability to tolerate more feeding by mouth. The rest of the fluid requirement should be given IV. Care must be taken to increase the oral intake slowly in very small prematures, particularly with a history of perinatal asphyxia. In a premature infant with a history of perinatal asphyxia, nothing by mouth for 5 to 7 days may be recommended to prevent necrotizing enterocolitis (see chapter 17–XVI).
3) Increase the total quantity of fluid gradually to 120 to 150 ml/kg/day. Daily fluid requirement in the extremely premature infant (less than 1,000 gm of birth weight) may be as much as 200 to 250 ml/kg. Extra fluid of 25 ml/kg/day must be added for radiant heater (warmer) and 25 ml/kg/day for phototherapy. (See Tables 6–1 and 6–3 for daily fluid and caloric requirement.)
4) Watch the infant's weight, physical findings, and urine-specific gravity to determine if the infant requires more or less fluid. Likewise, increase the caloric intake gradually to 100 to 120 calories/kg/day; see the premature weight chart (see Fig 6–3) to keep the infant near the normal weight curve. Obtain daily weight and weekly head circumference and length measurements to evaluate growth (see Figs 6–2,C, 6–3, 6–4, and 6–5). Abdominal skinfold thickness or upper arm skinfold thickness may be utilized for evaluation of fat deposition.

g. The process of refeeding the infant after the infant has had nothing by mouth for a significant duration should progress with caution.
1) The refeeding schedule should be the same as the initial feeding schedule.
2) Breast milk or a formula consisting of protein hydrolysate, glucose, and MCT oil such as Pregestimil may be used.
3) The formula should be diluted to 5 to 10 calories/oz. for the first 1 to 2 days.
4) The progression of feeding may be as slow as 1 to 3 weeks with an alternate increase concentration and volume.
5) Drop back on concentration, decrease volume, or stop feeding again for a short period if abdominal distention or diarrhea develop.

h. Gastrin, cholecystokinin-pancreazymin, and thyroid hormones increase motility while secretin, glucagon, adrenal corticoids, catecholamines, and parathormone decrease motility. The newborns, particularly prematures, are more prone to develop abdominal distention and puddling of intestinal contents because of immature intestinal muscular coat.

i. Stomach emptying time is approximately 1 to 2 hours in healthy prematures and the feedings reach the cecum in 3 to 8 hours and begin to be evacuated by 15 hours.

2. Intravenous fluid administration
a. Indications
Inability to tolerate fluid taken orally or administered by a tube, e.g., respiratory distress, cyanosis, congenital heart disease, apnea, abdominal dis-

A

HEAD CIRCUMFERENCES (CM)			
AGE	GESTATION 30–33 WK (HEALTHY)	GESTATION 34–37 WK (HEALTHY)	GESTATION VARIOUS (SICK)
24 hr	27.0 ± 0.7	32.0 ± 0.7	30.9 ± 0.9
1 wk	28.2 ± 0.7	32.7 ± 0.9	31.3 ± 1.0
2 wk	29.5 ± 0.8	33.8 ± 0.8	31.7 ± 0.8
3 wk	30.8 ± 0.8	35.0 ± 0.7	32.0 ± 0.8
4 wk	32.0 ± 0.9	35.8 ± 0.8	32.4 ± 0.7
6 wk	34.4 ± 0.7	37.1 ± 0.8	32.7 ± 0.8
8 wk	35.8 ± 0.8	38.5 ± 1.0	33.3 ± 0.9
12 wk	38.4 ± 1.1	40.3 ± 1.1	34.0 ± 0.9
16 wk	40.2 ± 1.0	41.8 ± 0.9	34.5 ± 0.9

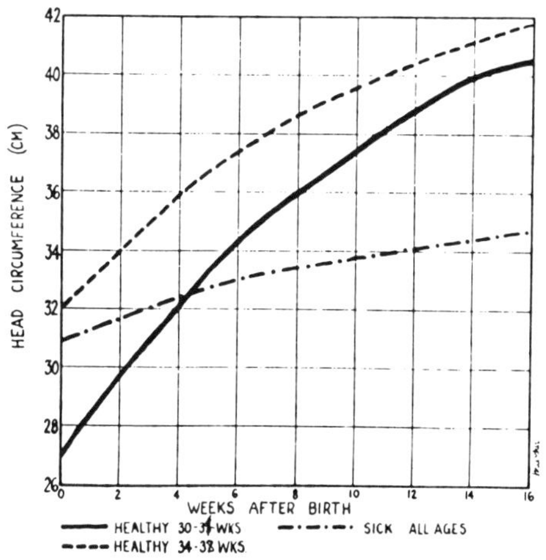

FIG 6–4.
Head circumference in the premature infant from birth to 16 weeks. (From Sher P., Brown S.B.: *Dev. Child. Neurol.* 17:705, 1975. Used by permission.)

tention, hypoglycemia, severe tremors, GI obstruction, and convulsions

b. Contraindications
   A well, premature infant able to tolerate fluid by mouth. Fluids given IV are not without hazard. IV fluids should not be administered if oral fluid intake is adequate.
c. Quantity of fluids given IV
   65 ml/kg/24 hours for the first day of life, then gradually increase fluid quantity to 150 to 200 ml/kg/24 hours in one week
d. Quality of fluids given intravenously
   The quality depends on the infant's condition.
   1) In general, start with one-fourth isotonic solution composed of one-half $NaHCO_3$ and one-half NaCl in 5% to 10% dextrose in water. Omit sodium if the infant received 24-hour sodium requirement already (e.g., $NaHCO_3$ given to correct metabolic acidosis). Remember hyper-

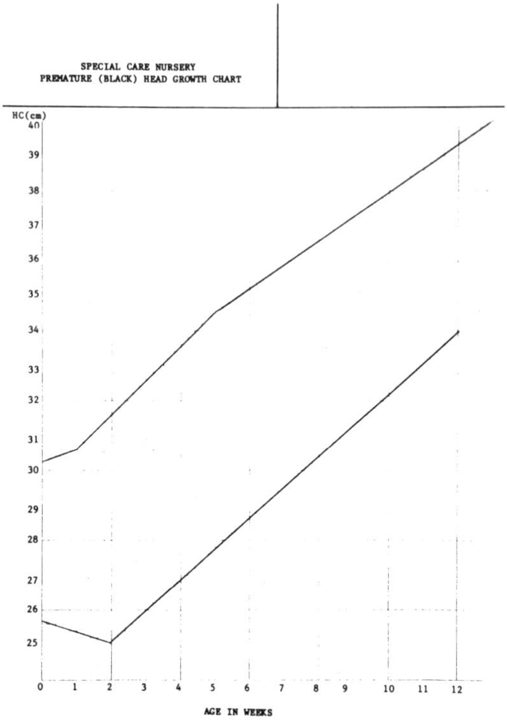

FIG 6–5.
Head growth chart for black premature infants. (From Yoon J.J., Shin K.D., Esquea A.E.: *Ped. Res.* (abstr.) 15:688, 1981. Used by permission.)

glycemia is common in very LBW premature infants (less than 1,250 gm) with glucose infusion greater than 6 to 8 mg/kg/min (0.36 gm/kg/hour).

2) Add maintenance KCl, 2 to 3 mEq/kg/24 hours, by the second or third day of life if the infant is voiding adequately.
3) Add vitamins to the fluids given IV by the first week of life if the infant is not taking formula with a vitamin supplement orally.
4) Administer vitamin K_1, 1 mg once a week, and/or fresh frozen plasma, 10 to 20 ml/kg once a week, if the infant is maintained solely by IV feeding. Some neonatologists would add protein to the IV fluid by the end of the first week of life and fat by the second week of life if the respiratory status permits fat. (See "total or partial parenteral nutrition in the newborn" in this section.)
5) If the fluids given IV are to be used as a vehicle for the administration of drugs, make sure the drugs are compatible, e.g., penicillin and epinephrine, gentamicin and carbenicillin, and heparin and hydrocortisone are incompatible. The combination of chloramphenicol and ampicillin is contraindicated for group B streptococcal meningitis because of antagonism. Ampicillin inactivates rapidly in dextrose. Methicillin is

stable for only 6 hours. Calcium gluconate should not be administered in a $NaHCO_3$ solution. Check with the pharmacist if uncertain.

e. Route
   1) Peripheral veins
      Care must be taken so that the fluid given IV does not infiltrate causing sloughing, ulcers, and infection.
   2) Umbilical vessels
      For instructions on how to place umbilical artery and venous catheter, see Chapter 3–IIIC3.

3. Supplements: see Chapter 6–IIC6
4. Nutritional monitoring
   Feeding the premature by any method is not without hazards.
   a. Evaluation of feeding tolerance
      1) Stool for reducing substance, blood (guaiac test or hematest), and consistency
      2) Abdominal distension
      3) Gastric residual
      4) Vomiting
   b. Evaluation of growth
      1) Daily weight and weekly measurement of length and head circumference (see Figs A–9, 6–3, 6–4 and 6–5)
      2) Daily evaluation of fluid and caloric intake
      3) Weekly measurement of BUN, albumin, calcium, phosphorus, alkaline phosphatase, and zinc if available
5. Total or partial parenteral nutrition (TPN or PPN) in the newborn
   a. Indications
      Infants who are unable to feed enterally or to tolerate enteral feedings for an extended period of time.
      1) Infants with congenital GI anomalies or who had GI surgery, omphalocele, gastroschisis, complicated anastomosis, short gut, and others
      2) Infants unable to be fed orally for prolonged period of time (e.g., intractable diarrhea, necrotizing enterocolitis)
      3) Premature infants beyond 3 to 5 days of age with insufficient caloric intake
   b. Contraindications
      1) Direct hyperbilirubinemia
   c. Procedures
      1) Either peripheral or central lines can be used for parenteral alimentation.
      2) When the central line is necessary:
         a) Obtain written permission for a central venous cutdown or percutaneous central venous catheterization from the mother.
         b) Consult the pediatric surgeon.
         c) Use a Silastic radiopaque catheter or a silicon rubber catheter for a central line.

d) The use of the jugular vein has less complications than the femoral or umbilical veins. The percutaneous central venous line has the least complications.
e) Maintain strict aseptic technique during insertion and maintenance of the catheter.
f) Confirm the catheter tip location by x-ray film. The preferred place is in the superior or inferior vena cava.
g) Sterile dressing on the superficial wound should be changed every 2 to 3 days.
h) The central catheter can remain in place as long as 4 to 6 weeks if there is no sign of infection or phlebitis.

3) Regardless of central or peripheral route, a 0.22 micro-Millipore filter placed in the intravenous line will help prevent infection.
4) The line should be used for only parenteral nutrition, not for any other purpose such as infusion of plasma, blood, medications, or aspiration of blood samples.
5) Lipid should be infused only through a "Y" connector and fluid should not be "piggy-backed."
6) The decision for changing the solution, including volume and constitutions of the solution, should be made by only one "physician in charge" for parenteral nutrition.
7) The solution should be prepared by specially trained personnel, e.g., pharmacist applying aseptic technique in a laminar flow hood according to the physician's prescription (see Table 6–6).
8) Nothing should be added into the infusate bottle on the ward.
9) The bottle, the entire external tubing, and the filter should be changed daily.
10) Only a volumetric continuous infusion pump should be used.

d. Daily requirement and practical method to order total or partial parenteral nutrition for low-birth-weight infants. Requirement for term infants are listed in Table 6–4.

1) Daily calories and fluids (see Table 6–1 and 6–4)
Calculate the 24-hour fluid requirement (65 to 200 ml/kg/day) to be provided by total parenteral nutrition solution. (Remember to subtract fluids administered as the vehicle for drugs or by other routes from the total requirement.)
2) Carbohydrate (see Table 6–4)
Infuse glucose 10 to 20 gm/kg/day as a 5% to 20% solution of glucose to prevent hypoglycemia and hyperglycemia. Blood glucose must be monitored by glucose screening and urine test for glucose particularly when the infant receives IV lipid emulsions since hyperglycemia often develops from altered glucose homeostasis.
Glucose provides approximately 4 calories/gm.
3) Protein (see Tables 6–4 and 6–7)
Calculate starting dose of amino acid solution 0.5 gm/kg/day and increase by 0.5 gm/kg/day to a maximum of 2.0 to 2.5 gm/kg/day over

5 to 10 days. Protein provides approximately 4 calories/gm. Keep 1 gm protein/6 gm dextrose ratio.

Either of two types of amino acid solutions is used.

a) A mixture of pure crystalline amino acids (TrophAmine, Freamine III, Aminosyn, or Travasol)
b) Hydrolysates of fibrin or casein, which has higher preformed ammonia load and the greater ability to vary the composition of the solution (rarely used at this time)

In addition to the eight amino acids essential to the older infants, histidine, cystine, tyrosine, and taurine are essential for newborns. Aminosyn contains cysteine, which is converted in vivo to cystine and taurine. TrophAmine contains cysteine, histidine, taurine and tyrosine. Crystalline amino acid mixtures contain histidine.

4) Minerals (see Table 6–4)
   a) Calculate sodium at 2 to 4 mEq/kg/day using the chloride or acetate salt. Use acetate primarily in hyperchloremic patients to prevent acidosis.
   b) Calculate potassium at 2 to 3 mEq/kg/day, which may be given as the chloride or phosphate salt. If all sodium is given as sodium chloride, potassium phosphate is the only vehicle for providing phosphorus.
   c) Calculate 3 to 5 mEq/kg/day of chloride. (Newborns receiving crystalline amino acids with electrolytes as chloride are prone to metabolic acidosis. Monitor carefully.)
   d) Calculate 30–40 mg/kg/day of phosphorus. Phosphorus may be provided as potassium or sodium phosphate. Phosphate must be administered with caution to prematures in the first postnatal week of life when abnormalities of calcium and phosphorus are common.
   e) Calculate 30–40 mg/kg/day of elemental calcium and adjust based on serum calcium and phosphorus determinations. Do not add calcium to the total parenteral nutrition solution if precipitation occurs; give calcium separately (1 ml 10% Ca gluconate = 9.3 mg elem Ca).
   f) Calculate 15–25 mg/kg/day of magnesium as the sulfate salt. Follow daily serum levels.
5) Trace elements

   Provide 63 μg/kg/day of copper (omit in infants with obstructive biliary disease).

   Provide 438 μg/kg/day of zinc (omit or reduce if infant has reduced renal function).

   Provide chromium, 0.1 to 0.2 μg/kg/day.

   Provide manganese, 5 μg/kg/day.

   Specific recommendations for intravenous iodine, selenium, vanadium, molybdenum, nickel, tin, silicon, and arsenic have not been determined at this time.

6) Vitamins
Add one third total solution/kg of multivitamin infusion (M.V.I. - Pediatric, Armour Pharmaceutical Co.) to each 24 hours of fluid. (This is a very imprecise formulation.)
7) After determining the quantity of each component of the total parenteral nutrition/kg/day, determine the amount in mEq or gm of the stock solution that contains that quantity. This may be done in the pharmacy.
8) Then determine the amount of the stock solution that has to be added to make a 500-ml solution by using the following formula:

$$\frac{\text{mEq}}{\text{Stock solution (ml)}} = \frac{X}{500 \text{ ml}}$$

9) Fat (see Tables 6–4 and 6–7)
Two types of fat emulsions are available: Intralipid, 10% emulsion of soybean oil stabilized with 1.2% egg phospholipid, and Liposyn, derived from safflower oil.
Both linoleic and linolenic acids, essential fatty acids, are provided in the emulsion, and arachidonic acid is derived from the in vivo conversion of linoleic acid. Each emulsion provides approximately 9 calories/gm (1.1 calories/ml).
   a) Administer a test dose of a fat emulsion (Intralipid 10% or Liposyn 10%), 0.4 to 0.5 gm/kg, over a 3- to 4-hour period. Two hours after completion of the therapy, draw and spin a capillary tube, and if the plasma is clear on inspection, therapy can be started.
   b) Calculate 0.5 gm/kg/day of Intralipid as the initial dose and raise the quantity *slowly* to 4 gm/kg/24 hours.
   c) Extra vitamin E is required during treatment with lipid to cover the high serum lipid increasing lipoprotein carrier of vitamin E.
   d) The "do nots" include the following:
   Do not infuse at greater than 0.25 gm/kg/hour.
   Do not exceed 40% of total caloric intake as lipids.
   Do not mix fat emulsion with other solutions. Fat emulsion however, may be run with the total parenteral nutrition solution provided it is at a "Y" connection in the tubing below the in-line filter and immediately before entry into the patient.
   Do not filter 10% fat emulsion.
   Do not leave 10% fat emulsion at room temperature for long periods of time.
   Do not use the solution if there is a layering-out.
   Do not administer 10% fat emulsion to patients with hyperbilirubinemia.
   Do not administer 10% fat emulsion to premature infants in the first week of life.
10) See Table 6–7 for commercially available solutions for parenteral nutrition.

TABLE 6–6.—TOTAL PARENTERAL NUTRITION ORDER SHEET

Birth Weight ________ gm
Gestational Age at Birth ________
Today's Date ________
Weight Today ________ gm

Birthdate ________

	FULLTERM RECOMMENDED DOSE/KG/DAY	TODAY'S ORDER GM OR mEq/KG/DAY	PHARMACY USE
Fluid (ml)	65–200		
Glucose (gm)	5–20		
Protein (gm) (as TrophAmine Freamine III, Aminosyn, or Travasol)	0.5–2.5		
Sodium (mEq) (as 1.5 NaCl & 1.5 Na acetate)	2–3		
Potassium (mEq) (as 1.5 KCl & 0.5–1.5 K_2PO_4)	2–3		
Calcium (mg) (as Calcium Gluconate)	20–40		
Magnesium (mg) (as $MgSO_4$)	5–6		
Phosphorus (mg)	20–40		
Trace Minerals			
Zinc (μg)	350		
Copper (mcg)	15–30		
Chromium (μg)	0.14–0.20		
Manganese (μg)	5		
M.V.I. pediatrics	appropriate dose/ weight		

Signature ________ M.D.

e. Complications

In general, the metabolic complications and catheter-related complications may be reduced by aseptic technique and close monitoring. Cholestasis and mild hepatocellular damage appear in 2 to 3 weeks of total parenteral nutrition in up to 50% of infants and almost always disappear when total parenteral nutrition is stopped.

1) Catheter-related complications

Infection (local and/or generalized), cardiac arrhythmia, air embolus, thrombosis, perforation and/or infusion leak, infusion obstruction (clot, kinking), pneumothorax, hydrothorax, hemothorax, chylothorax, catheter dislodgement

2) Precipitations

Normal requirements of calcium and phosphates will not precipitate

TABLE 6–7.—Commercially Available Amino Acid and Fat Solutions for Total or Partial Parenteral Nutrition Solution Preparation*

Nutritional Requirement	Available Form/Brand Name	Profile	Calories/gm	Doses (Starting to Maximum)
Carbohydrate	Glucose	Glucose	4	5%–20% (increase by 1.0%–2.5%)
Protein	Crystalline amino acids (TrophAmine Freamine III, Aminosyn, and Travasol)	All have eight EAA. Aminosyn also contains cysteine which is converted in vivo to cystine and taurine TrophAmine also contains cysteine, histidine, taurine and tyrosine	4	0.5–2.5 gm (increase by 0.5 gm)
	Hydrolysates of fibrin or casein	Eight EEAs; four EAAs for newborns not provided	4	0.5–2.5 gm (increase by 0.5 gm)
Fat	Intralipid; emulsion of soybean oil and egg phospholipid	Three EFAs; linoleic and linolenic acids in addition to in vivo conversion of linoleic acid to arachidonic acid	9	0.5–2.0 gm (increase by 0.5 gm)
	Liposyn: safflower oil	3 EFAs	9	0.5–2.0 gm (increase by 0.5 gm)

*EAA, essential amino acid; EFA, essential fatty acid.

TABLE 6–8.—PARTIAL OR TOTAL PARENTERAL NUTRITION SURVEILLANCE SCHEDULE

Examinations	
Weight	Daily
Length	Weekly
Head circumference	Weekly
Urine	
Urine dipstick for protein, glucose, blood, ketones; specific gravity and/or osmolality	Every voided specimen for 1 wk, then twice daily
Volume (strict I&O)	Daily
Blood	
Glucose screening	Every 4 hr until stable, then 1–2/wk
Blood glucose	Daily until stable, then weekly
Blood electrolytes & BUN	Daily first wk, then twice weekly
Serum protein, albumin, Ca, Mg, PO_4, pH, NH_4, liver function test	Weekly and as required
CBC	Weekly and as required
Blood gases	As required
Culture for bacteria and fungus	Weekly
For infants receiving fat emulsion	
Lipimin	Daily
Lipid analysis (serum cholesterol, triglycerides, free fatty acids)	First wk, then once in 2 wk

when combined in solution, but larger amounts may, and thus phosphate must be added separately. Providing calcium and phosphorus in alternating solutions over 12-hour periods will prevent precipitation.

3) Carbohydrate-related complications
Hyperglycemia and glucosuria.
Monitor blood glucose, urine glucose and reduce glucose intake if hyperglycemia greater than 125 mg/dl or glycosuria greater than 2+ is present.
4) Protein-related complications
Azotemia, hyperaminoacidemia, isosmolar coma, cholestatic jaundice, hyperammonemia, hyperchloremic acidosis from older formulas, metabolic alkalosis (new generation from the substitution of acetate for chloride to prevent acidosis due to arginine, histidine, and lysine).
Monitor BUN, pH, serum ammonia, and serum and urine amino acids. Discontinue parenteral protein intake when the infant has liver disease.
5) Fat-related complications
Hyperlipidemia with high infusion rate greater than 0.25 gm/kg/hour, reduced bilirubin binding capacity, impaired oxygenation (from intrapulmonary fat deposition possibly due to impaired fatty acid oxidation from carnitine deficiency), hyperglycemia, thrombocytopenia, leuko-

penia, hepatosplenomegaly, transient elevations of liver enzymes, cholestetic jaundice, and immediate reactions, such as hypercoagulability, dyspnea, cyanosis, vomiting, flushing, fever, sweating, and allergic reaction (have not been reported in infants).
Monitor triglycerides and free fatty acids.
Discontinue fat administration if the infant has liver disease, anemia, coagulopathy, or hyperbilirubinemia.

III. THE SMALL-FOR-GESTATIONAL-AGE INFANT

A. Recognition of the SGA Infant

An infant whose weight is less than the tenth percentile for gestational age is classified as a SGA infant. The SGA infant may be proportionately small without wasting or may be dysmature with wasting and signs of intrauterine growth retardation. The SGA infant should be recognized and differentiated from the AGA infant because their perinatal problems differ. The SGA infant may be immature, premature, mature, or postmature, but, regardless of gestational age, the infant is below the expected weight. About one third of LBW infants are SGA although the incidence of SGA infants varies depending upon population and racial and ethnic differences.

B. Factors to Recognize in the SGA Infant

1. The infant's gestational age as determined by physical examination correlates with the infant's age as determined by history and not weight (see Figs 6–1 and 6–2).
   The infant's weight is disproportionate (too low) for his or her gestational age as determined by history or physical examination.
   a. When the infant's weight is plotted against the weeks of gestation, it falls below the tenth percentile (see Figs 5–1 and 5–2).
   b. The infant's maturity appears too advanced for his or her weight.
2. The infant looks long, thin, wasted, alert, and active; seems hungry; has diminished subcutaneous fat and loose, dry, scaling skin; and appears to have recent weight loss. Meconium staining of nails, umbilical cord, and skin is common. While weight is low, often length and head size may be normal. These infants are called dysmature. The vernix caseosa appears minimal or absent in postmature infants.
3. The proportionately small infant without wasting seems to have had intrauterine growth retardation for a long time and looks old for size. Trisomies, genitourinary and GI tract anomalies, fetal infection, and some inborn errors of metabolism are seen frequently.
4. The SGA infant tends not to lose weight in the first days of life and the dys-

mature infant has normal weight gain while the proportionately SGA infant tends not to catch up. If catch-up does not occur by 3 years of age, the child will most likely remain small.

C. Common Causes of the SGA Infant

1. Maternal causes
   a. Vascular disease of pregnancy
      Eclampsia or preeclampsia, renal or adrenal disease, chronic hypertension, diabetes mellitus (classes D, E, F), collagen vascular diseases
   b. Hypoxia
      High altitude, maternal cardiac disease, severe anemia
   c. Maternal infections that affect the fetus
      Cytomegaloviral infection, toxoplasmosis, rubella, etc.
   d. Reduced maternal blood volume
   e. Miscellaneous
      Smoking, severe maternal malnutrition, maternal narcotic addiction, maternal use of alcohol, hydantoin, prednisone, maternal short stature, young primipara, history of previous LBW infant(s)
2. Utero-placental causes
   a. Bicornuate or septate uterus, uterine myomas
   b. Infarcts of placenta, thrombosis of fetal vessels
   c. Premature partial separation of placenta, or twin-to-twin transfusion
   d. Abnormal cord insertion, or circumvallation
3. Fetal causes
   a. Crowding
      Multiple births
   b. Chromosomal aberrations
      Trisomy 13–15, 18, 21 (20%) XO, deletion syndromes
   c. Other congenital malformations
      Seckel's syndrome, Cornelia de Lange's syndrome, osteogenesis imperfecta, single umbilical artery, gastroschisis, Potter syndrome, Russell-Silver syndrome, etc.
   d. Postmaturity
   e. Loss or decreased size of a body part
      Amelia, phocomelia, anencephaly

D. Common Associated Problems in the SGA Infant

1. Asphyxia
   Fetal distress and perinatal asphyxia occur frequently in SGA infants.
2. Meconium aspiration pneumonia and its associated complications (e.g., pulmonary air leak syndrome)

3. Hypothermia most likely due to decreased fat insulation, decreased store of brown fat and carbohydrates (glycogen), and poor lipid metabolism
4. Hypoglycemia (see chapter 15–X)
5. Hypocalcemia (see chapter 15–IX)
6. Polycythemia (see chapter 12–V)
7. Hyperbilirubinemia (see chapter 13)
8. Congenital malformations (see chapter 9)
   The incidence is 10 to 20 times higher (5% to 10%) in SGA infants.
9. High mortality and morbidity
   At the same birth weight, the AGA premature infant has a higher mortality than the SGA infant. At the same gestational age, the SGA infant has a higher mortality rate than the AGA infant. High mortality is mainly due to asphyxia, malformations, and meconium aspiration pneumonia with its associated complications.
   SGA premature infants are shorter and lighter at 5 years of age than AGA premature infants, mainly related to low socioeconomic status, while the incidence of delayed development by 3 years of age is the same as for AGA premature infants. The nonasphyxiated SGA fullterm infants have normal neurologic cognitive development.

E. Admission Policies for the SGA Infant

1. Review the prenatal history to determine if the mother had heart disease, hypertension, malnutrition, severe diabetes, or a history of infection or if the mother was a heavy smoker, lived at a high altitude, or abused drugs.
   Note if the infant is a twin and over 32 weeks' gestation.
2. Examine the infant carefully.
   a. For signs of cytomegaloviral infection, toxoplasmosis, or rubella, particularly with reduced head size (see chapter 16)
   b. For signs of congenital malformation, e.g., trisomy 13–15, trisomy 18, trisomy 21, Cornelia de Lange's syndrome, osteogenesis imperfecta, Seckel's syndrome, genitourinary or alimentary tract anomalies (see chapter 9)
   c. For signs of postmaturity
   d. For loss or decreased size of a body part
   If any of the aforementioned signs are found, provide the proper management as required.
3. Examine the placenta for signs of abnormalities and send the placenta for pathologic examination.
4. If the mother had hypertensive disease of pregnancy, see Table 2–1.
   If intrauterine infection is suspected, see chapter 16.
   If the mother has class D, E, or F diabetes, see chapter 15–XI.
   If maternal history of narcotic addiction is present, see chapter 15–XIX.
   If congenital malformations are present, see chapter 9 and obtain genetic consultation if necessary.

5. SUGGESTED ROUTINE ORDERS FOR THE SGA INFANT

ORDERS	REASONS
a. If the infant is premature, see section on "suggested routine orders for the premature infant" in this chapter.	
b. Maintain the infant's temperature in neutral thermal environment.	b. Prevent hypothermia; SGA infants frequently have a decreased quantity of subcutaneous fat.
c. Maintain a clear airway; suction as required.	c. SGA infants may develop meconium aspiration in utero secondary to fetal distress.
d. Administer vitamin K_1 (AquaMEPHYTON or Konakion), 1.0 mg, on admission to the nursery.	d. Prevent hemorrhagic disease of the newborn.
e. Weigh the infant on admission to nursery and daily. Record the infant's weight on the growth chart.	e. SGA infants may not lose weight during the first few days of life, may gain faster than expected, or may not gain adequately.
f. Wash the infant on admission to the nursery after the infant's temperature has stabilized. Bathe the infant daily.	f. Decrease skin colonization.
g. Obtain a baseline glucose level on admission to the nursery and follow the screening test or blood-glucose level (by the glucose-oxidase method) at 2, 4, 6, 12, and 18 hours of age. Watch for signs of hypoglycemia (see chapter 15–X).	g. Prevent hypoglycemia; SGA infants have low carbohydrate stores and are especially prone to hypoglycemia. Infants of severe diabetics (class D, E, F) may have severe hypoglycemia.
h. Obtain a baseline hematocrit value on admission to the nursery and follow as needed.	h. SGA infants often have polycythemia (see chaper 12–V). The ratio of fetal to adult hemoglobin is greater in SGA infants than in AGA infants since intrauterine hypoxia and hypoglycemia increase fetal hemoglobin synthesis.
i. Obtain a baseline calcium level on admission to the nursery and follow as needed. Watch for signs of hypocalcemia (see chapter 15–IX).	i. Prevent hypocalcemia. SGA infants have a high incidence of hypocalcemia.
j. Observe the infant carefully for signs of intrauterine infection (see Chapter 16).	j. Cytomegaloviral infection, toxoplasmosis, or rubella may be the cause of SGA.
k. If congenital malformations are present, obtain appropriate diagnostic tests and offer emotional support to the family.	k. Malformations are a shock to any family. All families require help through this difficult period.
l. Begin early oral feeding of the vigorous infant. Support the infant's glucose level by the IV route if he or she is unable to tolerate oral feeding. Follow feeding schedule as per premature infants.	l. Prevent hypoglycemia and provide adequate calories and nutrition.

(continued)

5. SUGGESTED ROUTINE ORDERS FOR THE SGA INFANT

ORDERS	REASONS
m. Obtain an IMD screening test at 7 days of age and again at the time of discharge. The IMD test must be given before the infant receives a red blood cell transfusion to detect hemoglobinopathy and after the infant has had 2 to 3 days of milk feedings for the majority of IMD.	m. Prevent mental retardation caused by IMD as soon as possible.
n. Administer Tri-Vi-Sol or Vi-Daylin (vitamins A, D, and C) by the seventh day of life.	n. Prevent vitamin deficiencies.

Chapter 7

Large-for-Gestational-Age Infants

The infant whose weight is above the 90th percentile is considered large for gestational age (LGA). Constitutionally large infants born to constitutionally large mothers usually do not have special problems. Infants with nonimmune hydrops (see chapter 18–XII) are frequently born to mothers with polyhydramnios (75%) and preeclampsia (30% to 50%). Forty percent to 50% of the nonimmune hydropic infants will have a major congenital anomaly; 75% to 98% will die in the perinatal period (approximately one half are stillborn, and one half die in the first 20 days of life). The LGA infants who are not hydropic (infants of diabetics, postterm infants, infants with Beckwith's syndrome etc.) often have a plethora of problems, including hyperbilirubinemia, hypoglycemia, and asphyxia that require immediate care. All LGA infants are at risk for birth injury.

I. COMMON CAUSES OF THE LARGE-FOR-GESTATIONAL-AGE INFANT

A. Infants of Diabetic Mothers (Classes A,B,C)
B. Constitutionally Large Infants (Infants Born to Large Mothers)
C. Large Postterm Infants
D. Infants With Transposition of Great Vessels
E. Infants With Hydrops Fetalis

1. Severe chronic anemia in utero
   Erythroblastosis fetalis, homozygous α-thalassemia, chronic fetomaternal transfusion, chronic twin-to-twin transfusion, glucose-6-phosphate dehydrogenase deficiency (rare)
2. Cardiac failure
   Severe congenital heart disease (paroxysmal atrial tachycardia), large atrio-

venous malformation (hemangioma, choriohemangioma, sacral teratoma), premature closure of foramen ovale, intrauterine arrhythmias
3. Hypoproteinemia
   Renal disease (congenital nephrosis, renal vein thrombosis)
4. Intrauterine infections: Congenital hepatitis, syphilis, erythroblastosis fetalis, toxoplasmosis, cytomegaloviral infection, etc.
5. Pulmonary disease
   Cystic adenomatoid malformation of the lung, pulmonary lymphangiectasis, cardiopulmonary hypoplasia with bilateral hydrothorax
6. Miscellaneous
   Parabiotic syndrome (multiple pregnancy), sublethal umbilical vein or chorionic vein thrombosis, fetal neuroblastomatosis, Chagas' disease, achondroplasia, Gaucher's disease, choriocarcinoma in situ

F. Beckwith's Syndrome

G. Idiopathic (35% of cases, Western hemisphere)

II. ADMISSION POLICIES FOR THE LARGE-FOR-GESTATIONAL-AGE INFANT

A. Review the Prenatal History.

The prenatal history should be reviewed to determine if the mother is constitutionally large; is a known diabetic or has a family history of diabetes; is Rh-negative or has an increased anti-Rh-antibody titer; or has a history of infection, polyhydramnios, or hypertension during pregnancy, or if the delivery date coincides with the expected date of confinement, or if the infant is a twin.

B. Examine and Observe the Infant Carefully for the Possible Cause and Problems Associated with the LGA Infant.

1. Infant of a diabetic mother (classes A,B,C)
   Plethora, "tomato" facies, hepatosplenomegaly, excessive fat, gestational age disproportionate to the infant's size (see chapter 15–XI).
2. A postterm infant (see Table 8–1)
   Long finger and toe nails, alert facies, peeling skin, etc.
3. Transposition of the great vessels (see Table 11–3)
4. Cystic kidney disease (see chapter 18–IX)
5. Edema and/or congestive heart failure (see chapter 11–XXIX)
6. Signs of congenital malformations, e.g., Beckwith-Wiedemann syndrome (see chapter 9)
7. Signs of intrauterine infection (see chapter 16)
8. Signs of birth trauma (Erb's palsy, Kumpke's paralysis, etc.) (see Table 5–3)
9. Any signs of hypoglycemia (see chapter 15–X)

III. SUGGESTED ROUTINE ORDERS FOR THE LARGE-FOR-GESTATIONAL-AGE INFANT

ORDERS	REASONS
A. Weigh the infant on admission to the nursery and daily.	A. LGA infants weigh more than expected for gestational age.
B. Monitor the infant's vital signs.	B. Tachypnea and/or tachycardia frequently indicate congestive heart failure, hypoglycemia, anemia, polycythemia, or lung pathology.
C. Wash the infant on admission to the nursery when his or her temperature has stabilized. Then bathe the infant daily.	C. Decrease skin colonization.
D. Administer vitamin K_1 1.0 mg IM, if not given previously.	D. Prevent hemorrhagic disease of the newborn.
E. Obtain a baseline hematocrit value on admission to the nursery and follow as needed.	E. LGA infants may have chronic anemia in utero, or polycythemia.
F. Obtain a baseline glucose level on admission to the nursery and follow it every hour until 7 hours of age. Then monitor every 3 to 4 hours until 24 hours of age. If the glucose level is low, do stat blood sugar and start IV for treatment (see chapter 15–X). Observe for signs of hypoglycemia.	F. Infants of diabetic mothers or who are postmature, hydropic, infected, or have congenital malformations are at risk for hypoglycemia.
G. Obtain a chest x-ray film and consider carefully the cardiac size, lung vascularity, and any cystic abnormality in the lung.	G. Infants of diabetic mothers frequently have enlarged hearts, structural heart defects, respiratory distress syndrome (see chapter 15–XI). Postterm infants frequently have meconium aspiration syndrome. LGA infants may have congenital heart disease, hydrops with pulmonary edema.
H. Obtain an ECG/echocardiogram if required.	H. Rule out arrhythmias, paroxysmal atrial tachycardia, congenital heart disease.
I. Obtain baseline levels of electrolytes, blood urea nitrogen (BUN), protein, and calcium and repeat as needed.	I. Infants of diabetic mothers frequently develop hypocalcemia. Any infant with hydrops may have an electrolyte imbalance. Infants with severe renal disease can have normal electrolyte and BUN levels on admission to the nursery as the mother has stabilized the infant's electrolytes and BUN status in utero. Protein may be low in those infants with renal disease or hydrops.
J. Record time and quantity of urine passage. Obtain urine analysis.	J. Failure to pass urine during the first day of life is one of the first signs of urinary tract anomalies.

(continued)

III. SUGGESTED ROUTINE ORDERS FOR THE LARGE-FOR-GESTATIONAL-AGE INFANT

ORDERS	REASONS
K. Obtain blood, urine, cerebrospinal fluid culture and sensitivity. Send cerebrospinal fluid for protein, glucose, red blood cells, white blood cells, and differential cell count.	K. LGA infants with hydrops may have intrauterine infection.
L. Obtain serologic test for syphilis (if not obtained on the mother prior to delivery).	L. Rule out syphilis.
M. Follow feeding orders as per gestational age.	M. See chapters 5–II and 6–IID.

Chapter 8

High-Risk Infants

An infant who has a statistically increased chance of dying or becoming seriously compromised in the newborn period is considered a high-risk infant.

All high-risk infants should be observed and monitored appropriately after birth so that the common complications associated with their high-risk status may be recognized, prevented, or treated before the infant becomes seriously ill (see Table 8–1). It is far wiser (and easier) to prevent complications than to treat them. Prior to delivery, the staff must be aware of factors that place an infant in the high-risk category and the neonatal problems that may ensue from this category (see Chapter 2).

I. COMMON CAUSES OF AN INFANT BEING CONSIDERED HIGH RISK

A. Maternal Conditions or Diseases

1. Diabetes mellitus
2. History of addiction or drug intake that may affect the fetus
3. History of heavy smoking
4. History of losing a previous infant(s)
5. Hypertensive disease of pregnancy
6. Hyperthyroidism
7. Hypothyroidism
8. Infection during pregnancy
9. Premature rupture of the membranes
10. Polyhydramnios
11. Oligohydramnios
12. Rh negative blood type
13. Third trimester bleeding

B. Fetal Conditions

1. Delivery by breech presentation
2. Delivery by emergency cesarean section
3. Small for gestational age
4. Large for gestational age
5. Life-threatening congenital malformations
6. Perinatal asphyxia
   a. Fetal distress or abnormal test result for fetal well-being
   b. low Apgar score
7. Postdate
8. Premature

II. PREPARATION

Preparations for a high-risk infant begin before birth. An area should be set aside to observe these infants while they are recovering from the shock of parturition. Adequately trained personnel must be available and equipment ready.

A. Personnel

At least one pediatric house officer should be assigned exclusively to the high-risk unit. The house officer must receive training in resuscitative techniques (see Chapter 3), assisted ventilation (see chapter 11–VI), fluid and electrolyte balance (see chapter 6–IIC), and the recognition and immediate preventive care of the high-risk infant (see chapters 2 and 3). Senior house officers must train juniors before they assume responsibility for the high-risk unit.

A registered professional nurse with education and experience in the recognition, prevention, and care of high-risk infants should be responsible for the area. Supportive personnel include multiple consultants, social workers, respiratory therapists, physical therapists, psychologists, clerical-administrative staff, and others.

B. Equipment

Equipment must be available at all times. It is not enough, however, for the equipment to be present; the house officer must know how to use it at a moment's notice.

1. The following equipment should be available at all times:
   a) Bassinets, incubators, infant warmers, or other units where infants may be placed while being observed
      Transport incubators

b) Suction apparatus
Bulb syringes, De Lee suction traps, portable electric suction, and sizes Fr. 5, 8, and 10 polyethylene suction catheters
c) Adequately available oxygen with the appropriate supporting equipment: O_2 analyzers, O_2 blenders (high and low flow), O_2 pressure gauges and adapters, O_2 hoods, infant respirators, warmed humidifiers, bags (250 and 500 ml) and masks for intermittent positive-pressure breathing (IPPB)
d) Resuscitative apparatus
Laryngoscopes, laryngoscope bulbs, stylets, small McGill forceps, straight endotracheal tubes (2.5, 3.0, 3.5, and 4.0 mm) or Cole endotracheal tubes (no. 8, 10, 12, 14, and 16), 4-mm endotracheal tube adapters, plastic infant airways, face masks for premature and term infants
e) Cardiac and respiratory monitors
f) Blood pressure apparatus (Arterio Sonde or Dinamap)
g) ECG
h) Transcutaneous PO_2, PCO_2 monitors
i) Ultrasound
j) Flashlights and transillumination lights
k) Ophthalmoscopes
l) Sterile tongue blades
m) Infant stethoscopes
n) Easily seen wall clock with sweep second hand
o) Phototherapy lights with eye masks
p) Refrigerator and freezer
q) Urine bags
r) Blood-study kits
Capillary tubes, lancets, slides, and cover glasses
Bilirubin and blood test tubes
s) Feeding tubes, 3.5, 5, and 8 Fr.
t) IV sets
Syringes (TB, 3, 5, 10, 30, and 50 ml), needles (22, 23, and 25 gauge), scalp needles (21, 23, and 25 gauge), angiocaths (22, 23, and 25 gauge), Kling and 4×4's, 2×2's, tourniquets (rubber bands), alcohol sponges, Betadine, arm boards, safety pins, tincture of benzoine, sterile cotton swabs, adhesive tape (½, 1, and 1½ inch), shave sets
u) Infusion pumps with IV extension tubing, three-way stopcocks
v) Sterile drapes and gloves
w) Sterile cord ties and sutures, 4-0, 3-0 silk
x) Sterile sets
Umbilical vessel catheterization sets with umbilical catheters: arterial catheters (3.5 and 5.0 Fr. Argyle) and venous catheters (5.0 and 8.0 Fr. Argyle), thoracotomy set, pleur-evac, cutdown set, tracheostomy set, etc.

III. ADMISSION POLICIES FOR THE HIGH-RISK INFANT

A. General Policies For All Admissions

1. Attend the delivery of all high-risk infants with an experienced perinatal nurse to resuscitate the infant should the need occur (see chapter 3) and prevent further compromise of the infant.
2. After stabilization of the infant's condition in the delivery room, transfer the infant as soon as possible in a heated incubator under direct supervision to the appropriate nursery.
3. Record the pulse rate, respiratory rate, B.P., and temperature on admission and every hour until the infant's vital signs have stabilized. Record the appropriate readings on a flow sheet.
4. Maintain the infant's temperature in the neutral thermal range (see chapter 6–IIB). Keep the infant's abdominal skin temperature at 36.5° C and the infant's rectal temperature at approximately 37° C. Be careful not to lower the infant's temperature precipitously during procedures such as taking an x-ray film, performing a venipuncture, or placing a catheter.
5. Suction as needed to maintain a clear airway.
6. Perform a physical examination and record the results including estimation of the infant's gestational age on admission to the nursery after stabilization of the infant's vital signs (see Tables 5–1, 5–2, and Figs 5–1, 5–2, 6–1, and 6–2).
7. Note the follow-up care for infants who require resuscitation (see chapter 3–IIIC9).
8. Administer oxygen to premature infants if the infant is cyanotic or if the infant's Pa_{O_2} is less than 50 mm Hg in room air (see chapter 11–IV).

B. Specific Admission Policies for High-Risk Infants

The clinical manifestations, appropriate admission studies, and preventive management should be considered for infants in specific high-risk categories (see Table 8–1).

TABLE 8–1.—HIGH-RISK INFANTS: COMMON COMPLICATIONS, CLINICAL MANIFESTATIONS, ADMISSION STUDIES, AND PREVENTIVE MANAGEMENT*

1. INFANTS BORN TO DIABETIC MOTHERS (SEE CHAPTER 15–XI)

COMMON COMPLICATIONS	CLINICAL MANIFESTATIONS	ADMISSION STUDIES AND PREVENTIVE MANAGEMENT
Fetal distress and perinatal asphyxia (increased rates of stillbirth and neonatal mortality)	Abnormal tracing of fetal heart monitor, low Apgar scores <6 at 1 min, poor perfusion, hypotonia, lethargy, shallow and rapid breathing, apnea, convulsions, etc.	Obtain arterial blood gases and prepare for immediate resuscitation and treatment for asphyxia. See chapter 15–IV and Table 8–1, no. 18.
Congenital anomalies (congenital heart disease, musculoskeletal deformity, hydrocephaly, renal anomalies, small left colon syndrome)	See chapter 15–XI.	Perform a careful physical examination. Management depends upon the type of congenital malformation.
Macrosomia with or without birth trauma	Inappropriate size, uneven Moro's reflex, crepitation over clavicle, limp arm with or without wrist drop, asymmetric respiratory movement, pale, poor perfusion	Obtain glucose screening to monitor for hypoglycemia. Perform a careful physical examination. See Table 5–3 for birth trauma.
Hypoglycemia (especially between 2–6 hr of age)	Tremors, lethargy, apnea, convulsions, respiratory distress, sweating, cyanosis, high-pitched weak cry, poor feeding, hypotonia, hypothermia, etc. *Infants can be asymptomatic with severe hypoglycemia. Follow glucose level carefully.*	Obtain a baseline blood sugar level or Dextrostix on admission to the nursery and every hr until the infant is 7 hr of age, then every 4 hr during the first 24 hr of life. The higher the maternal glucose, the faster the glucose disappearance and the lower the plasma glucose level will be. See chapter 15–X. Institute early oral feedings with formula. If oral feedings are not tolerated, administer IV glucose. Follow glucose and treat hypoglycemia promptly.

(continued)

TABLE 8–1.—(*continued*)

1. INFANTS BORN TO DIABETIC MOTHERS (SEE CHAPTER 15–XI)		
COMMON COMPLICATIONS	CLINICAL MANIFESTATIONS	ADMISSION STUDIES AND PREVENTIVE MANAGEMENT
Hypocalcemia	Irritability, tremors, convulsions, apnea, high-pitched cry, cyanosis, hypotonia, hypertonia, and vomiting	Obtain a blood specimen for calcium. At first sign of tremors, obtain an ECG and monitor the QTc interval. If the QTc is prolonged (>0.425) administer 1–5 ml/kg of 10% calcium gluconate slowly while monitoring the ECG to avoid heart block and then maintain the calcium level by administering calcium gluconate, 100–800 mg/kg/day. See chapter 15–IX.
Polycythemia	Plethora, cyanosis, respiratory distress, irritability, poor feeding	Obtain Hct on admission. When central Hct is beyond 65%, partial exchange may be necessary to prevent complications from polycythemia. See chapter 12–V.
Hyperbilirubinemia	Jaundice	Obtain a blood specimen for baseline Hct and bilirubin measurement and monitor appropriately. Supply adequate fluid intake. See chapter 13.
Renal vein thrombosis	Flank mass caused by enlarged kidney, petechiae, edema	Palpate kidneys carefully and follow size. Examine urine for blood and protein. Follow urinalysis. If mass is palpated, determine electrolytes, BUN, and platelet count. Monitor blood pressure. Treat hypertension if present. Discuss with nephrologist and urologist regarding nephrectomy if necessary, anticoagulant therapy (controversial). See chapter 18–VIII.
Respiratory distress syndrome	Respiratory distress (tachypnea, cyanosis in room air, retractions, apnea, expiratory grunting, etc.) See chapter 11–VIII.	Perform a careful physical examination for gestational age and respiratory distress. Resuscitate infant promptly if necessary. Prevent chilling. Support the infant's pH, oxygen requirement, fluids, temperature, gas exchange, etc. See chapter 11–VIII.
Meconium plug syndrome	Failure to pass meconium by 24 hr of age, abdominal distention; rarely, vomiting may present. Hyperactive bowel sounds. Grayish white plug may pass with rectal examination or enema.	Perform rectal examination (plug may pass). Normal saline or Mucomyst enema after making sure there is no bowel perforation or small left colon syndrome. See chapter 17–V.

Infection	Poor feeding, poor cry, abnormal muscle tone, poor reflexes, temperature instability, abdominal distention, vomiting, etc.	Start antibiotic therapy after obtaining cultures of blood, urine, CSF, cord, etc., and a CBC if signs of infection are present. See chapter 16–XIX and Table 8–1, no. 8.

2. INFANTS BORN TO ADDICTED MOTHERS (SEE CHAPTER 15–XIX)

COMMON COMPLICATIONS	CLINICAL MANIFESTATIONS	ADMISSION STUDIES AND PREVENTIVE MANAGEMENT
Small for gestational age	See chapter 6–III and Table 8–1, no. 15.	See chapter 6–III and Table 8–1, no. 15
Withdrawal	Hyperactivity, tremors, convulsions, severe tachypnea, tachycardia, high-pitched cry, dyspnea, sweating, flushing, sneezing, yawning, diarrhea, abdominal distention, poor feeding, vomiting, fever, poor sleep, skin abrasions, etc.	Monitor temperature, pulse, and respiration. Observe the infant's activity for signs of withdrawal. If signs of withdrawal occur, sedate the infant adequately or utilize narcotic replacement therapy. Record intake and output. Feed carefully, prevent aspiration. Observe for diarrhea. Watch intake and record carefully to prevent overfeeding and/or excessive fluid loss.
Neonatal infection (hepatitis, syphilis, AIDS, etc.)	Asymptomatic or jaundice, hepatosplenomegaly, poor feeding, rashes, etc. See chapter 16–X, 16–XII and 16–XXIII.	Obtain result of maternal STS and treatment for syphilis; obtain cord STS if mother's STS is positive. Treat the infant for syphilis if symptomatic or four times higher STS than mother, etc. See chapter 16–X. Screen for HTLV-III antibody. Administer HBIg if mother is a carrier or has hepatitis B after obtaining HB antigens and antibodies. See chapter 16–XII.

3. INFANTS BORN TO MOTHERS WITH A HISTORY OF HEAVY SMOKING

COMMON COMPLICATIONS	CLINICAL MANIFESTATIONS	ADMISSION STUDIES AND PREVENTIVE MANAGEMENT
Intrauterine growth retardation	Small for gestational age with lack of subcutaneous fat (see chapter 6–III)	Estimate gestational age and plot on the intrauterine growth curve. Obtain baseline Hct, blood glucose, calcium and electrolytes and monitor Dextrostix. Observe for signs of hypocalcemia, hypoglycemia, hypothermia, etc. See chapter 6–III and Table 8–1, no. 15.

(continued)

TABLE 8–1.—(*continued*)

3. INFANTS BORN TO MOTHERS WITH A HISTORY OF HEAVY SMOKING

COMMON COMPLICATIONS	CLINICAL MANIFESTATIONS	ADMISSION STUDIES AND PREVENTIVE MANAGEMENT
Prematurity	See Figs 6–1 and 6–2.	Estimate gestational age. Observe for signs of complications. See chapter 6–II and Table 8–1, no. 20.

4. INFANTS BORN TO MOTHERS WHO HAVE LOST A PREVIOUS INFANT(S)

COMMON COMPLICATIONS	CLINICAL MANIFESTATIONS	ADMISSION STUDIES AND PREVENTIVE MANAGEMENT
Complications depend on cause	Symptomotology depends on cause.	Ascertain the reason for previous neonatal death. Preventive management depends on cause.
Prematurity	See chapter 6–II and Table 8–1, no. 20.	See chapter 6–II and Table 8–1, no. 20.
Congenital malformations	Depends upon types of malformation	Depends upon malformation. See chapter 9.
Intrauterine growth retardation	See chapter 6–III and Table 8–1, no. 15.	See chapter 6–III and Table 8–1, no. 15.
Maternal hypertensive disease of pregnancy	See Table 8–1, no. 5.	See Table 8–1, no. 5.
Maternal diabetes	See chapter 15–XI and Table 8–1, no. 1.	See chapter 15–XI and Table 8–1, no. 1.
Infection	See chapter 16 and Table 8–1, no. 8.	See chapter 16 and Table 8–1, no. 8.

5. INFANTS BORN TO MOTHERS WITH HYPERTENSIVE DISEASE OF PREGNANCY

COMMON COMPLICATIONS	CLINICAL MANIFESTATIONS	ADMISSION STUDIES AND PREVENTIVE MANAGEMENT
Intrauterine growth retardation	Small for gestational age, long, thin infant with lack of subcutaneous fat. See chapter 6–III and Table 8–1, no. 15, for signs of small for gestational age.	Estimate gestational age and plot on the intrauterine growth curve. See chapter 6–III and Table 8–1, no. 15.
Fetal distress and perinatal asphyxia (increased stillbirth rate and neonatal mortality rate)	See chapter 15–IV and Table 8–1, no. 18.	See chapter 15–IV and Table 8–1, no. 18. Observe for signs of depression, hypotonia, etc.

6. INFANTS BORN TO MOTHERS WHO HAVE HYPERTHYROIDISM

COMMON COMPLICATIONS	CLINICAL MANIFESTATIONS	ADMISSIONS STUDIES AND PREVENTIVE MANAGEMENT
Congenital thyrotoxicosis	Tachypnea, tachycardia, weight loss, fever, irritability, tremors, plethora, etc. Clinical signs may not be evident for the first 5–10 days of age. See chapter 15–XVIII.	Obtain maternal history whether or when she received antithyroid medications or surgery. Obtain vital signs, CBC, thyroid function tests (T4, FT4, T3, RT3, TSH etc.) and thyroid-stimulating immunoglobulin level if possible. Observe for signs of thyrotoxicosis and congestive heart failure.
Congenital hypothyroidism	Prolonged jaundice, poor feeding, hypotonia, etc. See chapter 17–XIX.	Treat with T4 if necessary.
Goiter with tracheal compression	Inspiratory stridor, air hunger or asphyxia. Enlarged goiter may be palpable.	Intubate promptly. Perform tracheostomy if endotracheal intubation is not possible.
Prematurity	See chapter 6–II and Table 8–1, no. 20.	See chapter 6–II and Table 8–1, no. 20.
Intrauterine growth retardation	Small for gestational age. See chapter 6–III and Table 8–1, no. 15.	Estimate gestational age and plot on the intrauterine growth curve.

7. INFANTS BORN TO MOTHERS WHO HAVE HAD HYPOTHYROIDISM

COMMON COMPLICATIONS	CLINICAL MANIFESTATIONS	ADMISSION STUDIES AND PREVENTIVE MANAGEMENT
Prematurity	See chapter 6–II and Table 8–1, no. 20.	See chapter 6–11 and Table 8–1, no. 20.

(continued)

TABLE 8–1.—(*continued*)

8. INFANTS BORN TO MOTHERS WITH A HISTORY OF INFECTION AND/OR PROLONGED RUPTURE OF MEMBRANES > 24 HOURS (SEE CHAPTER 16)

COMMON COMPLICATIONS	CLINICAL MANIFESTATIONS	ADMISSION STUDIES AND PREVENTIVE MANAGEMENT
Sepsis, meningitis, urinary tract infection, omphalitis, pneumonia	Poor feeding, lethargy, hypotonia, poor weight gain, hepatosplenomegaly, jaundice, petechiae, ecchymoses, chorioretinitis, low Hct. See chapter 16.	Review perinatal history to determine length of prolonged rupture of membranes, type of maternal infection if known, type of therapy, etc. Obtain cultures of blood, CSF and urine. Obtain IgM and CBC. If mother had viral infection, particularly during the first and second trimester, obtain TORCH studies. Obtain maternal culture results, if available. Observe for shock, anemia, hyperbilirubinemia, and treat accordingly. Record infant's vital signs including temperature every 4 hr. Observe the infant's general and neurologic status carefully. Examine the infant at least twice daily to determine if any of the clinical manifestations of sepsis have occurred. Obtain a spinal tap and cultures prior to institution of antibiotics. Treat promptly once signs of sepsis are present. See chapter 16.
Oligohydramnios tetrad	Pulmonary hypoplasia, positional limb defect and facial compression.	See chapter 11–XX.

9. INFANTS BORN TO MOTHERS WITH HISTORY OF POLYHYDRAMNIOS

COMMON ASSOCIATION	CLINICAL MANIFESTATIONS	ADMISSION STUDIES AND PREVENTIVE MANAGEMENT
Tracheoesophageal fistula	See chapter 11–XVIII.	Do not feed until the GI patency is assured and support cardiorespiratory status as required.
Intestinal obstruction	See chapter 17–IV.	
Anencephaly	See Table 9–4.	
Exstrophy of bladder	See Table 9–4.	
Twinning		
Maternal diabetes and hypertension	Also see clinical manifestations of infants of diabetic and hypertensive mothers (see Table 8–1, no. 1 and 5)	See Table 8–1, no. 1 and no. 5.

10. INFANTS BORN TO MOTHERS WITH HISTORY OF OLIGOHYDRAMNIOS

COMMON ASSOCIATION	CLINICAL MANIFESTATIONS	ADMISSION STUDIES AND PREVENTIVE MANAGEMENT
Renal dysgenesis	Potter's syndrome: no urinary output, position defects, fetal compression, Potter's facies. See Table 9–4.	See Table 9–4 and chapter 18–IX.
Pulmonary hypoplasia	Tachypnea, retraction, cyanosis. Often with Potter's syndrome, diaphragmatic hernia, etc.	See Table 9–4 and chapter 11–XX.
Sepsis secondary to prolonged rupture of the membranes	See Table 8–1, no. 8.	See chapter 16 and Table 8–1, no. 8.
Intrauterine growth retardation	Small for gestational age. See chapter 6–III.	See Table 8–1, no. 15.

11. INFANTS BORN TO RH-NEGATIVE MOTHERS (SEE CHAPTER 13–VII)

COMMON COMPLICATIONS	CLINICAL MANIFESTATIONS	ADMISSION STUDIES AND PREVENTIVE MANAGEMENT
Hyperbilirubinemia, anemia	Pallor, jaundice, tachycardia, hepatosplenomegaly, respiratory distress, irritability. See chapter 13–VII.	Obtain the infant's blood group, Rh factor, and a Coombs' test immediately. Obtain a baseline Hct, smear of the peripheral blood and cord bilirubin level. Type and cross match blood if exchange transfusion seems probable. Follow glucose levels, central venous pressure. Exchange transfuse if necessary. See chapter 13–VI.
Hydrops fetalis	Pallor, edema, respiratory distress, tachycardia and poor feeding. Hepatosplenomegaly, increased heart size, petechiae. See chapter 13–VII.	Prepare for exchange transfusion before delivery if severe hemolysis is suspected. Watch carefully for signs of congestive heart failure. Observe cardiac size by x-ray film if hydrops fetalis is present. Digitalize if necessary. See chapters 11–XXIX, 13–VII, and 18–XII.
Kernicterus	Lethargy, hypotonia, poor feeding, opistotonus, spasticity, seizures, chorioathetoid movements, etc. See chapter 13–IV.	Correct factors associated with kernicterus (acidosis, hypothermia, or hypoglycemia, etc.). Exchange transfuse if necessary. See chapter 13–VI.

(continued)

TABLE 8–1.—*(continued)*

12. INFANTS BORN TO MOTHERS WHO HAVE BLED (SEE CHAPTER 14–VIII AND 14–IX)

COMMON COMPLICATIONS	CLINICAL MANIFESTATIONS	ADMISSION STUDIES AND PREVENTIVE MANAGEMENT
Perinatal asphyxia secondary to maternal hypotension and hypoxia, rarely from fetal placental hemorrhage	Pale, poor perfusion, apnea, lethargy, CNS depression, etc. (see chapter 15–IV and Table 8–1, no. 18)	Support cardiorespiratory status. Obtain CBC; type and crossmatch if central venous pressure is low. Monitor arterial blood gases, calcium and glucose (see chapter 15–III and Table 8–1, no. 18).
Fetal placental bleeding, anemia, shock (see chapter 14–VI, 14–VIII and 14–IX)	Pallor, respiratory distress, low blood pressure, low Hct; even infants who look pink on admission to the nursery may be severely anemic. See Table 14–3 to differentiate acute from chronic hemorrhage.	Monitor heart rate, respiratory rate, blood pressure, and Hct on admission and continue to watch closely. Follow arterial blood gases. See chapter 14–III.
Respiratory distress syndrome if the infant is premature	Respiratory distress, apnea, cyanosis, etc. See chapter 11–VIII.	See chapter 11–VIII and Table 8–1, no. 20.

13. INFANTS DELIVERED BY BREECH PRESENTATION (SEE TABLE 5–3)

COMMON COMPLICATIONS	CLINICAL MANIFESTATIONS	ADMISSION STUDIES AND PREVENTIVE MANAGEMENT
Perinatal asphyxia	See chapter 15–IV and Table 8–1, no. 18.	See Table 8–1, no. 18.
CNS hemorrhage	Apnea, respiratory depression, lethargy, tremors, convulsions, hypothermia, bradycardia, decreased or absent Moro's, suck or cry reflex, sudden change in infant's condition. See chapter 15–VI to 15–VIII.	Monitor vital signs, Hct, arterial blood gases, ventilatory status, general activity, neurologic signs; obtain cranial sonogram or CT scan. Replace blood as required. Avoid hypoxia and resuscitate promptly. Restrict fluid intake. Follow platelet and coagulation studies. Start anticonvulsants if convulsions ensue. See chapter 15–III.

13. INFANTS DELIVERED BY BREECH PRESENTATION (SEE TABLE 5–3)

COMMON COMPLICATIONS	CLINICAL MANIFESTATIONS	ADMISSION STUDIES AND PREVENTIVE MANAGEMENT
Spinal cord injury	Normal above the lesion. Flaccid paralysis and loss of sensation below the lesion; later hypertonic. Priapism in males, bladder distension, bowel incontinence	Examine the infant with caution and handle infant gently to minimize trauma. Observe for hypotonic bladder, bowel movements, respiratory distress, etc.
Peripheral nerve injury	Erb's-Duchenne, Klumpke's, and phrenic nerve palsy. See Table 5–3.	Perform a careful physical examination. Obtain neurology consultation if needed. See Table 5–3.
Visceral hemorrhage (liver, spleen, adrenals, kidneys)	Anemia within the first 24–72 hr of life may appear with sudden shock. Abdominal or flank mass may be present. See Table 5–3.	Monitor vital signs, central venous pressure, Hct, electrolytes, and urinalysis See chapter 14–X and Table 5–3.
Skeletal fractures (clavicle, humerus, etc.)	Flaccid extremities often with swelling and crepitations	Obtain x-rays and orthopedic consultation. See Table 5–3.
Soft tissue injury	Ecchymoses, bruising, petechiae (especially of buttock and genitalia)	Monitor vital signs, blood pressure, Hct, platelets, and bilirubin. See Table 5–3.

14. INFANTS DELIVERED BY ELECTIVE CESAREAN SECTION

COMMON COMPLICATIONS	CLINICAL MANIFESTATIONS	ADMISSION STUDIES AND PREVENTIVE MANAGEMENT
Neonatal depression	Hypotonia, poor or absent cry, depressed breathing	Monitor vital signs, blood pressure, and ventilatory status. Assist ventilation if necessary.
Transient tachypnea of the newborn	Tachypnea, grunting, cyanosis with or without dyspnea. See chapter 11–IX.	Obtain chest x-ray film, CBC, arterial blood gases. Oxygen therapy may be necessary. Assist ventilation (rare).

(continued)

TABLE 8–1.—(*continued*)

15. INFANTS WHO ARE SMALL FOR GESTATIONAL AGE (SEE CHAPTER 6–III)

COMMON COMPLICATIONS	CLINICAL MANIFESTATIONS	ADMISSION STUDIES AND PREVENTIVE MANAGEMENT
Hypoglycemia	Tremors, lethargy, apnea, convulsions, respiratory distress, sweating, cyanosis, high-pitched weak cry, poor feeding, hypotonia, and hypothermia. See chapter 15–X.	Obtain a baseline blood-sugar level on admission to the nursery and every hour until 7 hr of age. Institute early oral feeding with or without IV fluid. Treat hypoglycemia promptly. See chapter 15–X.
Hypocalcemia	Irritability, tremors, convulsions, apnea, high-pitched weak cry, cyanosis, hypotonia, hypertonia, and vomiting. See chapter 15–IX.	Obtain blood for calcium studies. At first sign of tremors, obtain QTc interval. If the QTc is >0.425, administer 1–5 ml/kg of 10% calcium gluconate slowly while monitoring ECG to avoid heart block. Then maintain calcium level by administering calcium gluconate maintenance. See chapter 15–IX.
Hypothermia	Low body temperature (below neutral thermal temperature; 37° C of rectal temperature and 36.5° C of abdominal skin temperature).	Record and monitor the infant's temperature. Correct hypothermia promptly and treat concurrent hypoglycemia or acidosis if present. See chapter 6–IIB.
Meconium aspiration syndrome with or without pulmonary air leak syndrome	Yellow or greenish meconium staining of nails or umbilical cord, respiratory distress, cyanosis, barrel chest. See chapter 11–XII.	Perform deep pharyngeal suction while the infant's head is in the perineum and/or before the first breath. Aspirate meconium via an endotracheal tube if meconium at vocal cord. Then assist ventilation. Monitor vital signs. Observe closely for pneumothorax. Obtain a chest x-ray film. See chapter 11–XII.
Polycythemia	Plethoric, cyanosis, respiratory distress, irritability, poor feeding, jaundice, petechiae	Obtain Hct on admission. When central Hct is $>65\%$ partial exchange transfusion may be necessary to prevent complication from polycythemia. Monitor bilirubin and platelets. See chapter 12–V.
Intrauterine infection	Hyperbilirubinemia, anemia, hepatosplenomegaly, petechiae, lethargy, hypotonia, high-pitched weak cry	Review maternal history of infection and treatment. Examine the infant carefully for signs of intrauterine infection. Obtain blood for IgM, CBC, platelets, liver function test, and TORCH study. Obtain skull and long bone x-rays. See chapter 16–III and Table 8–1, no. 8.

15. INFANTS WHO ARE SMALL FOR GESTATIONAL AGE (SEE CHAPTER 6–III)

COMMON COMPLICATIONS	CLINICAL MANIFESTATIONS	ADMISSION STUDIES AND PREVENTIVE MANAGEMENT
High incidence of congenital malformations especially trisomy 13–15, trisomy 21, Cornelia de Lange's syndrome, Seckel's syndrome, osteogenesis imperfecta, etc.	Varies, depends on types of malformations. See chapter 9.	Perform a careful physical examination. See Table 5–2 and chapter 9.

16. INFANTS WHO ARE LARGE FOR GESTATIONAL AGE (SEE CHAPTER 7)

COMMON COMPLICATIONS	CLINICAL MANIFESTATIONS	ADMISSION STUDIES AND PREVENTIVE MANAGEMENT
Birth injuries	See Table 5–3.	See Table 5–3.
Hypoglycemia	See chapter 15–X and Table 8–1, no. 1.	See chapter 15–X and Table 8–1, no. 1.
Hypocalcemia	See chapter 15–IX and Table 8–1, no. 1.	See chapter 15–IX and Table 8–1, no. 1.
Transposition of great vessels	Cyanosis, tachypnea (see Table 11–3)	Obtain arterial blood gases, chest x-ray film, ECG, echocardiogram, and cardiac consult.

17. INFANTS BORN WITH LIFE-THREATENING CONGENITAL ANOMALIES (SEE CHAPTER 9)

COMMON COMPLICATIONS	CLINICAL MANIFESTATIONS	ADMISSION STUDIES AND PREVENTIVE MANAGEMENT
Depends on type of malformations	Depends on type of malformations. See chapter 9.	Determine type of malformation. See chapter 9.

(continued)

TABLE 8–1.—*(continued)*

18. INFANTS BORN WITH PERINATAL ASPHYXIA (SEE CHAPTER 15–IV)

COMMON COMPLICATIONS	CLINICAL MANIFESTATIONS	ADMISSION STUDIES AND PREVENTIVE MANAGEMENT
Acidosis	Pallor with poor perfusion, apnea, respiratory distress, cyanosis, lethargy, CNS depression. See chapter 15–V.	Monitor ventilatory status, heart rate, respiratory rate, temperature. Obtain blood gas studies. Correct base deficit by slow administration of sodium bicarbonate (see chapter 11–IIIB12). Follow infant's ECG for changes in ST segment. After correction of acidosis, check QTc for hypocalcemia. See chapter 15–V.
Hypoglycemia	Tremors, lethargy, apnea, respiratory distress, convulsions, sweating, cyanosis, high-pitched weak cry, poor feeding, hypotonia, hypothermia. See chapter 15–X.	Obtain a baseline blood-sugar level or screening test on admission to the nursery and every 4 hr until 24 hr of age. Institute IV fluids. Treat hypoglycemia promptly. See chapter 15–X.
Hypocalcemia	Irritability, tremors, convulsions, apnea, high-pitched weak cry, cyanosis, hypotonia, hypertonia, vomiting. See chapter 15–IX.	Obtain blood for calcium studies. At first sign of tremors, obtain the QTc interval. If the QTc is prolonged, administer 1–5 ml/kg of 10% calcium gluconate slowly while monitoring the ECG to avoid heart block. Then, maintain the calcium level by administering calcium gluconate maintenance. See chapter 15–IX.
Hypothermia	Low body temperature (below neutral thermal temperature: 37° C rectal temperature and 36.5° C abdominal skin temperature). See chapter 6–IIB.	Record and monitor the infant's temperature. Correct hypothermia promptly and treat concurrent hypoglycemia or acidosis if present.
Persistent pulmonary hypertension of the newborn (persistent fetal circulation)	Cyanosis with >60% O_2, sudden changes of color, retraction, tachypnea, increased chest anteroposterior diameter. See chapter 11–XIII.	Correct acidosis, hypoglycemia, etc. Obtain arterial blood gases and administer hyperventilation. Tolazoline if PaO_2 is still low. See chapter 11–XIII.
CNS edema or hemorrhage	Respiratory depression, lethargy, hypothermia, bradycardia, tremors, apnea, cyanosis, decreased or absent Moro's, suck or cry reflex. Often sudden changes in infant's condition at 24–72 hr of age. See chapter 15–VI to 15–VIII.	Monitor infant's vital signs, Hct, arterial blood gases, ventilatory status, general activity, neurologic status; obtain sonogram and/or CT scan of head. Replace blood loss as required. Restrict fluids. Start anticonvulsant if convulsions occur. See chapter 15–III.

18. INFANTS BORN WITH PERINATAL ASPHYXIA (SEE CHAPTER 15–IV)

COMMON COMPLICATIONS	CLINICAL MANIFESTATIONS	ADMISSION STUDIES AND PREVENTIVE MANAGEMENT
Syndrome of inappropriate antidiuretic hormone	Decreased urinary output, edema, and/or abrupt weight gain. Hyponatremia, hyposmolality, and increased urine specific gravity (osmolality). See chapter 18–XV.	Monitor strict intake and output, urinalysis with specific gravity or osmolality, serum electrolytes. Restrict fluid intake. See chapter 18–XV.
Acute renal failure	Decreased urinary output. Edema and/or abrupt weight gain, seizures. Hyponatremia, increased urine specific gravity, BUN, and creatinine. See chapter 18–IV.	Monitor strict intake and output. Urinalysis with specific gravity and osmolality, serum electrolytes, BUN, creatinine, and serum osmolality. Monitor infant's weight every 8–12 hr. Restrict fluid intake. Monitor blood pressure. See chapter 18–IV.
Necrotizing enterocolitis	Poor feeding, abdominal distension, vomiting, lethargy, hypotonia, hypothermia, apnea, guaiac positive stool, acidosis, shock, leukopenia or leukocytosis, thrombocytopenia. Typical radiologic findings of abdomen. See chapter 17–XVI.	Obtain a detailed prenatal and perinatal history. Give nothing by mouth for the first 3–7 days, particularly prematures with prenatal or perinatal hypoxia. Start, then, breast feeding unless contraindicated. Obtain an abdominal x-ray film and stool for guaiac test if abdominal distension occurs. See chapter 17–XVI for treatment of necrotizing enterocolitis.
Meconium aspiration pneumonia with or without secondary infection	Respiratory distress, meconium staining of nails, umbilical cord. See chapter 11–XII.	Monitor infant's vital signs. Deep pharyngeal suction while the infant's head is in the perineum and/or before the first breathing. Follow vital signs. Thereafter, suction the larynx and trachea. Chest x-ray film to ascertain diagnosis. Observe for pneumothorax. Ventilate as needed. See chapter 11–XII.
Pulmonary air leak syndrome	Increasing respiratory distress: cyanosis, tachypnea, retractions, grunting, muffled heart sounds, frequently asymptomatic or a sudden onset of rapid deterioration. See chapter 11–XIV.	Monitor ventilatory status as above. Obtain chest transillumination and/or x-ray film. Obtain serial chest x-ray films and blood gas studies. Have thoracotomy set ready and immediate underwater drainage if necessary.
Congestive heart failure	Tachypnea without dyspnea, tachycardia, and poor feeding. Increased heart size, hepatosplenomegaly. See chapter 11–XXIX.	Watch carefully for signs of congestive heart failure. Digitalize if necessary. See chapter 11–XXIX.

(continued)

TABLE 8–1.—(*continued*)

19. INFANTS BORN POSTDATE

COMMON COMPLICATIONS	CLINICAL MANIFESTATIONS	ADMISSION STUDIES AND PREVENTIVE MANAGEMENT
Perinatal asphyxia, meconium aspiration syndrome	See Table 8–1, no. 18. Respiratory distress, cyanosis, Increased anteroposterior diameter of chest. Meconium-stained skin, nails and umbilical cord. See chapter 11–XII.	See Table 8–1, no. 18. Monitor vital signs. Deep pharyngeal suction while the infant's head is in the perineum and/or before the first breath. Thereafter, suction the larynx and trachea. Chest x-ray film to ascertain diagnosis. Observe for pneumothorax. See chapter 11–XII.
Macrosomia (large for gestational age)	See Table 8–1, no. 16.	See Table 8–1, no. 16.
Dysmaturity (small for gestational age)	See Table 8–1, no. 15 and chapter 6–III.	See Table 8–1, no. 15.

20. INFANTS BORN PREMATURELY (SEE CHAPTER 6–II)

COMMON COMPLICATIONS	CLINICAL MANIFESTATIONS	ADMISSION STUDIES AND PREVENTIVE MANAGEMENT
Perinatal asphyxia	See Table 8–1, no. 18.	See Table 8–1, no. 18.
Respiratory distress syndrome, congenital atelectasis, aspiration pneumonia	Respiratory distress, tachypnea, cyanosis, retractions, expiratory grunting, etc. See chapter 11–VIII.	Perform a careful assessment of gestational age (see Figs 6–1 and 6–2). Monitor vital signs. Observe for signs of respiratory distress. Resuscitate promptly. Prevent chilling. Suction adequately. Support and monitor oxygen and ventilatory requirements. Obtain chest x-ray film, blood gases, and electrolyte studies as needed. See chapter 11–VIII.
CNS immaturity	Inability to maintain rectal temperature at 37° C or abdominal skin temperature at 36.5° C. Periodic breathing, apnea, bradycardia. Inability to synchronize sucking with swallowing, etc.	Record and monitor infant's vital signs. Avoid chilling. Maintain neutral thermal environment. Treat concurrent acidosis, hypoglycemia and hypocalcemia. Continuous positive airway pressure or aminophylline may be indicated for apnea. Nothing by mouth or nasogastric tube feeding until more mature (>32 wk).
Renal immaturity	Acid-base imbalance, poor weight gain	Weigh the infant daily. Strict intake and output. Follow pH of blood and urine, urine electrolyte and osmolarity.

TABLE 8–1.—(*continued*)

20. INFANTS BORN PREMATURELY (SEE CHAPTER 6–II)		
COMMON COMPLICATIONS	CLINICAL MANIFESTATIONS	ADMISSION STUDIES AND PREVENTIVE MANAGEMENT
Hypoglycemia	Tremors, lethargy, apnea, convulsions, cyanosis, respiratory distress, sweating, high-pitched cry, poor feeding, hypotonia, hypothermia	Monitor serum glucose (Dextrostix) carefully. Support the infant's glucose level; administer fluids orally or intravenously. Treat hypoglycemia promptly. See chapter 15–X.
Hypocalcemia	Irritability, tremors, convulsions, apnea, cyanosis, hypertonia, vomiting	Obtain a blood specimen for calcium. Start maintenance IV calcium gluconate (300 mg/kg/day) and follow serum calcium and QTc. If low, increase calcium maintenance to maintain serum calcium level within normal range. See chapter 15–IX.
CNS hemorrhage	May be asymptomatic or apnea, respiratory depression, lethargy, tremors, convulsions, hypothermia, bradycardia. Often sudden changes in infant's condition at 24–72 hr of age. See chapter 15–VI to 15–VIII.	Monitor vital signs, hematocrit, arterial blood gases, ventilatory status, general activity, neurologic signs; obtain sonogram or CT scan. Avoid anoxia or hypoxia. Resuscitate promptly. Support ventilation. Replace blood loss as required. Restrict fluid intake. Phenobarbital for prevention (?). Start anticonvulsant for convulsions. See chapter 15–VI to 15–VIII.
Patent ductus arteriosus	May be asymptomatic on admission. Apnea. Failure to improve or deterioration of pulmonary function; requirement of higher oxygen concentration and/or CO_2 retention. Hyperactive precordium. Systolic heart murmur. Full or bounding pulses. Widening of the pulse pressure. See chapter 11–XXX.	Perform careful and repeated physical examinations on admission and thereafter, particularly from a few days of age. If symptomatic, obtain a chest x-ray film and echocardiogram. If diagnosed, diuretics, fluid restriction, positive end expiratory pressure, indomethacin, and surgical correction could be performed in order, until corrected. See chapter 11–XXX.
Infection	Lethargy, poor feeding, hypothermia, poor weight gain, jaundice, abdominal distention, weak cry. See chapter 16.	Wash your hands before and after handling infants. Watch carefully for signs of infection. Treat promptly after obtaining cultures of urine, blood and CSF if signs are present. See chapter 16.

REFERENCES

Harper R. G., Yoon J. J.: *Handbook of Neonatology*, ed. 1. Chicago, Year Book Medical Publishers, Inc., 1974.

TABLE 8–2.—Respiratory Sheet for High-Risk Infants

PATIENT'S NAME: ______________ UNIT NUMBER: ______________

		ASSISTED VENTILATION SETTING						BLOOD GASES					TRANSCUTANEOUS			TEMP.		
DATE	TIME	FiO_2	VENT. RATE	INSP. TIME	FLOW RATE	PIP/ PEEP CPAP	MAP	SITE	pH	pCO_2	pO_2	BE/ HCO_3^-	SITE	$tcpO_2$	$tcpCO_2$	INCUB./ NB	NEBUL/ E-T	VENTILATOR CHANGES AND COMMENTS

TABLE 8–3.—LABORATORY FLOW SHEET FOR HIGH-RISK INFANTS

PATIENT'S NAME: ______________________ UNIT NUMBER: ______________________

		CHEMISTRY										CBC WITH DIFFERENTIAL							
DATE	TIME	NA^+/K^+	CL/CO^2	BUN/ CREAT.	SUGAR/ SCRE.*	CA^+/PO_4^-	BIL. TOTAL/ DIR.	TP/ ALB.	SGOT/ SGPT	ALK PHOS/ LDH	CHOL/ CPK	WBC/ RBC	HBG/ HCT	RETIC/ PLTS	POLYS/ BANDS	LYMPHS/ MONOS	EOS/ BASOS	SMEAR NORM/ ABNORM	MEDICATIONS AND COMMENTS

*SCRE. = glucose screening test.

Chapter 9

Infants With Congenital Malformations

Two percent to 4% of all newborns have serious congenital malformations. Etiologic causes include genetic factors, drugs, environmental teratogens, and infectious organisms. Unfortunately, the cause of approximately 30% of major malformations is unknown.

Congenital malformations may be categorized as aberrations of growth, deficiencies in development, or abnormal development including incomplete, accessory, and functional defects. Serious errors in early morphogenesis are almost always fatal in utero; hence, most defects seen in the newborn nursery usually occurred after 23 days' gestation.

I. GLOSSARY

A. Anomaly

A structural abnormality or malformation

B. Malformation Complex

Multiple structural defects without a known cause (e.g., VATER association)

C. Syndrome

A recognized pattern of malformation with a single specific cause (e.g., Holt-Oram syndrome)

D. Major Congenital Malformations

Malformations that interfere with life-sustaining processes or are cosmetically of such significance that the malformation makes a normal life impossible

E. Minor Congenital Malformations

Unusual morphologic features that are of no serious medical or cosmetic consequence to the patient

F. Autosomal Dominant Inheritance

In this type of inheritance, if the gene is present, the patient will be affected. If one parent has an autosomal dominant disease, the infant will have one-out-of-two chance of inheriting the disease (e.g., achondroplasia).

G. Autosomal Recessive Inheritance

In this type of inheritance, both parents do not have the disease but both parents are carriers (e.g., cystic fibrosis). For the infant to be affected, both parents have to give the gene to the infant (one per four pregnancies).

H. Multifactorial Inheritance

In this type of inheritance, many genes from both parents, as well as environmental influences, are necessary before the infant is affected.

I. X-linked Inheritance

In this type of inherited disease, the abnormal gene is present on one of the mother's X chromosomes (e.g., Duchenne's muscular dystrophy).

II. COMMON "AT-RISK" CATEGORIES ASSOCIATED WITH THE DEVELOPMENT OF CONGENITAL MALFORMATIONS

Infants born to parents with the following conditions are at risk.

1. Any malformation in prospective mother or father, their previous offspring, or a near relative. See Table 9–1 for recurrence risks for common congenital malformations.
2. Advanced maternal age (greater than 35 years). See Table 9–2 for estimated rate of chromosomal abnormalities in relation to maternal age.
3. A maternal history of repetitive abortions.
4. A known chromosomal or other genetic aberration in either parent. See Table

9–4 for cause of frequently observed malformation complexes and syndromes.
5. Exposure to infectious or environmental teratogenic agents. See Table 2–5 for drugs and their effect on the fetus and newborn.

For the relative timing and developmental pathology of certain malformations, see Table 9–3.

III. WHAT THE PHYSICIAN SHOULD DO WHEN CONFRONTED WITH AN INFANT WITH CONGENITAL MALFORMATIONS

A. Diagnostic Workup

1. Obtain a detailed history regarding the family history of congenital malformations, past and present pregnancy (speak to the obstetrician!), maternal drugs and illnesses, consanguinity, exposure to teratogens, quantity of smoking, alcohol, etc.
2. Determine if the antenatal diagnosis of structural malformations was made by sonogram (see Table 2–2) or if the antenatal diagnosis of metabolic diseases was made by amniotic fluid assay (see Table 2–4) or biopsy.
3. Examine the infant thoroughly. Record all details accurately. Measure exact dimensions. Do not estimate. Photograph deviations from normal. After obtaining the infant's height, weight, head circumference, fontanelle, and other pertinent measurements, compare against the normal standards (see Figs 5–1, and 5–2, 6–2 C, 6–4, and 6–5 and appendix Figs A8–A16). Formulate a list of possible diagnoses by noting all the findings that the infant exhibits (see commonly observed physical abnormalities, Table 5–2, and cross reference the infant's findings with the common syndromes, Table 9–4). This will facilitate the diagnosis of common syndromes (clusters of congenital malformations). Remember, 90% of infants with three minor anomalies have a major anomaly.
4. If possible, examine the placenta and send it to the pathologist for further study.
5. Formulate a list of possible diagnoses and obtain the specific biochemical, radiographic, sonographic, chromosomal, or other diagnostic tests to corroborate the diagnosis.

B. General Supportive Management for Infants With Congenital Malformations

1. Follow the admission policies for the normal full-term (*see* chapter 5), low-birth-weight (*see* chapter 6), high-risk (*see* chapter 8), or septic newborn (*see* chapter 16) as is indicated by the infant's size or clinical condition.

TABLE 9–1.—RECURRENCE RISKS FOR COMMON CONGENITAL MALFORMATIONS*

MALFORMATION	PERCENTAGE OF RISK FOR EACH SUBSEQUENT CHILD
Cleft lip with or without cleft palate†	
One affected child	4
Two affected children	9
One affected parent	4
One affected parent and one affected child	17
Cleft palate only	
One affected child	2
Two affected children	10
One affected parent	6
One affected parent and one affected child	15
Neural tube defects (anencephaly, myelomeningocele, encephalocele)	
One affected child	4–5
Two affected children	12–15
Congenital heart disease	
Ventricular septal defect	5
Atrial septal defect	3
Patent ductus arteriosus	4
Pulmonic stenosis	3
Aortic stenosis	2
Tetralogy of Fallot	3
Transposition of great vessels	2
Coarctation of aorta	2
Clubfoot	3
Congenital hip dislocation	4–5
Pyloric stenosis	
One affected child	3
Mother affected	16
Father affected	5

*From Nadler H.D., Burton B.J.: Genetics, in Quilligan E.J., Kretchmer N. (eds.): *Fetal and Maternal Medicine.* New York, John Wiley & Sons, 1980, p. 67. Used by permission.

†All the risk figures are somewhat increased if affected individuals are female or if cleft is severe.

2. Speak to the parents.
   a. Inform the parents of the findings noted in the history and physical examination of the infant.
   b. Inform the parents that you will, at a specific time and place, return to discuss the situation further (as you would with a normal child).
   c. Do not explain the intricate details of a disease entity the first time you see the family as it is impossible for a family to cope with more than the basic fundamentals while they recover from the shock of having an abnormal infant.

TABLE 9–2.—ESTIMATED RATE OF CHROMOSOME ABNORMALITIES PER 1,000 LIVE BIRTHS BY 5-YEAR INTERVAL*

MATERNAL AGE† (YR)	DOWN'S SYNDROME	EDWARDS' SYNDROME (TRISOMY 18)	PATAU'S SYNDROME (TRISOMY 13)	XXY	XYY	TURNER'S SYNDROME GENOTYPE
<15	1.0‡	<0.1‡	<0.1–0.1	0.4	0.5	<0.1
20	0.5–0.7	<0.1–0.1	<0.1–0.1	0.4	0.5	<0.1
25	0.7–0.9	<0.1–0.1	<0.1–0.1	0.4	0.5	<0.1
30	0.9–1.2	0.1–0.2	<0.1–0.2	0.5	0.5	<0.1
35	2.5–3.9	0.3–0.5	0.2–0.3	0.9	0.5	<0.1
40	8.5–13.7	0.9–1.6	0.5–1.1	1.8	0.5	<0.1
45	28.7–52.3	2.9–6.0	1.5–4.1	5.1	0.5	<0.1
49	75.8–152.7	7.6–17.6	3.8–11.8	13.8	0.5	<0.1

*Modified from Hook E.B.: Rates of chromosome abnormalities at different maternal ages. *Obstet. Gynecol.* 58:282, 1981. Used by permission.

†Calculation of the total at each age assumes rate for autosomal aneuploidies is at the midpoints of the ranges given.

‡These age-related risk estimates are for women who have no other risk factor except age. They are derived from multiple regression studies of live births of chromosomally abnormal infants.

   d. Repeat the information several times since people in shock frequently do not hear the speaker.
3. In the event that the infant has a structurally repairable lesion, discuss the situation with the family and institute immediate supportive, restorative, or corrective measures as indicated. Obtain the help of specialists as required.
4. In the event that the infant has a structurally irreparable defect, (e.g., trisomy 18, anencephaly) counsel the parents as to the course of the disease process, the usual survival time, and the option for no medical intervention.
5. *Do not run away.* Offer support and reassurance to the family. Regardless of how minimal the malformation seems, the family has just lost its idealized infant. Allow the family to display its culturally normal method of grieving. Remember, the stages of grieving include disbelief, bargaining, anger, and hostility as well as resolution. It takes time to traverse the paths of grieving and it is normal for parents to be angry during this process.
6. In the event that an infant dies in the newborn period:
   a. Allow the family to hold, touch, or caress the dead infant if they desire.
   b. Try to obtain permission for an autopsy as it is important that as much information be obtained as possible.
   c. *Do not abandon the family.* Plan a session at a later date to discuss the pertinent medical complications and autopsy findings. Allow the parents to vent their hostility and anger and come to a resolution for the future. Invite the parents to return during a future pregnancy (or offer to send all information to another physician) so that the information can be applied for that family in the future.

(continued on page 164)

TABLE 9–3.—Relative Timing and Developmental Pathology of Certain Malformations*

TISSUES	MALFORMATION	DEFECT IN	CAUSE PRIOR TO	COMMENT
Central nervous system	Anencephaly	Closure of anterior neural tube	26 days	Subsequent degeneration of forebrain
	Meningomyelocele	Closure in a portion of the posterior neural tube	28 days	80% lumbosacral
Face	Cleft lip	Closure of lip	36 days	42% associated with cleft palate
	Cleft maxillary palate	Fusion of maxillary palatal shelves	10 wk	
	Branchial sinus and/or cyst	Resolution of branchial cleft	8 wk	Preauricular and along the line anterior to sternocleidomastoid
Gut	Esophageal atresia plus tracheoesophageal fistula	Lateral septation of foregut into trachea and foregut	30 days	
	Rectal atresia with fistula	Lateral septation of cloaca into rectum and urogenital sinus	6 wk	
	Duodenal atresia	Recanalization of duodenum	7–8 wk	
	Malrotation of gut	Rotation of intestinal loop so that cecum lies to right	10 wk	Associated incomplete or aberrant mesenteric attachments
	Omphalocele	Return of midgut from yolk sac to abdomen	10 wk	
	Meckel diverticulum	Obliteration of vitelline duct	10 wk	May contain gastric and/or pancreatic tissue
	Diaphragmatic hernia	Closure of pleuroperitoneal canal	6 wk	

(continued)

TABLE 9–3.—*(continued)*

TISSUES	MALFORMATION	DEFECT IN	CAUSE PRIOR TO	COMMENT
Genitourinary system	Extroversion of bladder	Migration of infraumbilical mesenchyme	30 days	Associated müllerian and wolffian duct defects
	Bicornuate uterus	Fusion of lower portion of müllerian ducts	10 wk	
	Hypospadias	Fusion of urethral folds (labia minora)	12 wk	
	Cryptorchidism	Descent of testicle into scrotum	7–9 mo.	
Heart	Transposition of great vessels	Directional development of bulbus cordis septum	34 days	
	Ventricular septal defect	Closure of ventricular septum	6 wk	
	Patent ductus arteriosus	Closure of ductus arteriosus	9–10 mo.	
Limb	Aplasia of radius	Genesis of radial bone	38 days	Often accompanied by other defects of radial side of distal limb
	Severe syndactyly	Separation of digital rays	6 wk	
Complex	Cyclopia, holoprosencephaly	Prechordal mesoderm development	23 days	Secondary defects of midface and forebrain
	Sirenomelia (sympodia)	Development of posterior axis	23 days	Associated defects of cloacal development

*From Smith D.W.: *Recognizable Patterns in Human Malformations, ed. 3.* Philadelphia, W. B. Saunders Co., 1982., p. 550. Used by permission.

TABLE 9–4.—Frequently Observed Malformation Complexes and Syndromes*

Syndrome or Malformation	Ref.†	Clinical Features	Inheritance/Cause	Immediate Management
Aarskog's syndrome	A1	Hypertelorism, brachydactyly, shawl scrotum, short stature, ptosis of eyelids, small nose, clinodactyly, pectus excavatum	X-linked semi-dominant	Rule out other causes of small for gestational age, failure to thrive
Abdominal muscle deficiency (prune belly syndrome)	A2	Abdominal muscle hypoplasia, urinary tract dysplasia, cryptorchidism, hypoplastic or polycystic kidneys, large distended bladder and ureter	Unknown ? abdominal distention in early gestation	Obtain renal sonogram, intravenous pyelogram, barium enema, GI series, BUN, creatinine, apply abdominal binder to improve gas exchange
Achondrogenesis syndrome	A3	Low nasal bridge, very short limbs, incomplete ossification of lower spine, micrognathia, micromelia, short ribs, small flat acetabulae, relatively large liver	Autosomal recessive	Differentiate from other short limb syndromes via skeletal x-ray films; observe for developmental hydrocephalus and neurologic complications (see Table 11–2)
Achondroplasia syndrome	A4	Short limbs, depressed nasal bridge, caudal narrowing of spinal canal, small stature, megacephaly, hydrocephaly, small cuboid-shaped vertebral bodies, lumbar lordosis, short tubular bones, short trident hand, short femoral neck	Autosomal dominant; 80% of cases new mutations	Differentiate from other short limb syndromes via skeletal x-ray films; observe for developmental hydrocephalus and neurologic complications (see Table 11–2)
Acrodysostosis syndrome	A5	Short hands, peripheral dysostosis, small nose, mental deficiency, small for gestational age, brachycephaly, low nasal bridge, hypoplastic maxilla, short with deformity in distal humerus	Unknown	Ophthalmologic consult; neurologic consult
Adrenal cortical hypoplasia (adrenal insufficiency)	A6	Small phallus, hypospadia and cryptorchidism in male, large clitoris, fused labia and thickening, corrugation and pigmentation of labial skin in female suggesting scrotal epidermis	Inborn defect in biosynthesis of adrenocortico-steroids; autosomal recessive	See Table 17–5, 17–6. Follow sodium and electrolytes, urinary 17-ketosteroid, pregnanetriol; R/O other causes of ambiguous genitalia, chromosomal studies.

(continued)

TABLE 9–4.—(*continued*)

SYNDROME OR MALFORMATION	REF.†	CLINICAL FEATURES	INHERITANCE/CAUSE	IMMEDIATE MANAGEMENT
Albers-Schönberg syndrome (osteopetrosis)	A7	Dense, thick, fragile bone, leukocytosis, pancytopenia, cranial nerve compression, marrow compression, hydrocephalus, low calcium, macrocephaly	Autosomal recessive	Obtain skeletal x-ray films, bone marrow studies, rule out hydrocephalus, follow calcium phosphorus level
Aminopterin syndrome	A8	Small for gestational age, microcephaly, hypoplasia of facial bones, wide fontanelles, broad nasal bridge, prominent eyes, micrognathia, cleft palate, low-set ears, mesomelia, talipes equinovarus	Maternal ingestion of aminopterin	Obtain history of maternal drug ingestion, supportive management
Amniotic band anomalies	A9	Partial to complete ring-like constrictions that may result in anomaly of limbs or other parts of the body	Sporadic, early rupture of amnion with formation of amnion and/or chorion strands	Remove constricting band if present; surgical consult for Z-plasty
Anencephaly/encephalocele anomalies	A10	Vascular tissue replaces brain tissue; frontal, parietal and occipital bone absence or malformation; absent calvarium	Neural tube defect (early)	Anencephaly, supportive management; encephalocele, neurologic consult for possible surgical correction
Apert's syndrome	A11	Irregular craniosynostosis, premature closure of anterior fontanelle, hypertelorism, midfacial hypoplasia, low-set ears, small beaked nose, high arched palate, syndactyly, broad distal phalanx, mental deficiency or normal intelligence, high full forehead, flat occiput, prognathia, short fingers, prominent eyes	Autosomal dominant or sporadic	Skull and skeletal x-ray films, neurologic evaluation, plastic surgery consult regarding hand anomalies and facial structure

Arthrogryposis	A12	Contractures of major joints, talipes equinovarus or calcaneovalgus foot deformity or other limb deformities	Variable	Neurologic, orthopedic evaluation, rule out myopathies, connective tissue disease; obtain chromosomal study
Asymmetric crying facies	A13	Ventricular septal defect, vertebral anomalies, anal atresia, radial hypoplasia, renal defects	Partial agenesis of the depressor anguli oris muscle	Rule out congenital heart disease (ventricular septal defect); R/O VATER association, see Table 9–4, V1.
Ataxia-telangiectasia syndrome	A14	Ataxia, telangiectasia, lymphopenia, growth deficiency variable, deficiency in cellular immunity with hypoplasia of thymic, tonsil, and adenoid lymphoid tissue, often low-to-absent IgA and IgE.	Autosomal recessive	Evaluate immune system, prevent infection, neurologic evaluation, rule out Bloom's and Fanconi's syndrome
Basal cell nevus (carcinoma) syndrome	B1	Basal cell nevi, broad facies, rib anomalies, frontoparietal bossing, broad nasal bridge, mild prognathism, short metacarpals, bifid ribs, scoliosis	Autosomal dominant	Supportive management in newborn nursery
Beckwith-Wiedemann syndrome	B2	Macroglossia, omphalocele, macrosomia, ear creases, prominent eyes, capillary nevus flammeus, prominent occiput, large kidneys, pancreatic hyperplasia, fetal adrenocortical cytomegaly, neonatal polycythemia, hypoglycemia	Unknown; polygenic, autosomal, recessive, and dominant	Rule out hypoglycemia and follow closely; repair omphalocele as indicated; support respiration and feedings; treat polycythemia
Blepharophimosis syndrome	B3	Inverted inner canthal fold, short palpebral fissures, lateral displacement of inner canthi, low nasal bridge, ptosis of eyelids	Autosomal dominant	Ophthalmologic consult
Bloom's syndrome	B4	Short stature, malar hypoplasia, small for gestational age, facial telangiectatic erythema butterfly area, café-au-lait spots, microcephaly, small nose, feeding problems, normal intelligence, malignancy (major cause of death)	Autosomal recessive	Obtain chromosome study; support feedings; rule out other causes of short stature

(continued)

TABLE 9–4.—(*continued*)

SYNDROME OR MALFORMATION		CLINICAL FEATURES	INHERITANCE/CAUSE	IMMEDIATE MANAGEMENT
Carpenter's syndrome	C1	Acrocephaly, polydactyly, syndactyly of feet, lateral displacement of inner canthi, mental deficiency, synostosis of coronal, sagittal, lambdoid sutures, brachycephaly, brachydactyly	Autosomal recessive	Rule out cardiac defect; orthopedic consult
Chédiak-Higashi syndrome	C2	Partial albinism, large granules in leukocytes, neutropenia, retinal pigmentation, hepatosplenomegaly	Autosomal recessive	Ophthalmologic consult; EEG; prevent infection; observe leukocytes for inclusions
Cleft lip and palate anomalies	C3	Cleft palate, cleft lip, repeated otitis media	Variable	Feed carefully; prevent and/or treat otitis media; rule out Pierre-Robin syndrome
Cleidocranial dysostosis syndrome	C4	Defect of clavicles, late ossification of cranial sutures, delayed eruption of teeth, short stature, brachycephaly with frontal bossing, midfacial hypoplasia, low nasal bridge, high-arched palate, partial to complete aplasia of clavicle, rib defects, asymmetric length of fingers	Autosomal dominant	Skull and clavicle x-ray films to establish diagnosis; assess hearing; observe for respiratory distress
Coloboma of iris-anal atresia syndrome (cat-eye syndrome)	C5	Coloboma of iris, down-slanting palpebral fissures, anal atresia	Abnormally small acrocentric extra G chromosome	Confirm with chromosome study; neurologic evaluation; ophthalmologic evaluation; surgical consult regarding anal atresia correction
Contractural arachnodactyly syndrome	C6	Joint contractures, arachnodactyly, "crumpled" ear	Autosomal dominant	Supportive management
Cri du chat syndrome	C7	Small for gestational age, slow growth, cat-like cry, mental deficiency, microcephaly, round face, hypertelorism, epicanthal folds, downward slanting of palpebral fissures, strabismus, simian crease, low-set ears	Partial deletion of the short arm of chromosome 5	Confirm with chromosome study; neurologic consult; hearing consult; rule out congenital heart disease

Crouzon's syndrome	C8	Shallow orbits, premature craniosynostosis, maxillary hypoplasia, occular proptosis, strabismus, hypertelorism, frontal bossing, parrot-beaked nose, short anteroposterior and wide lateral cranium, low-set ears, prognathia	Autosomal dominant	Skull x-ray film; follow for craniosynostosis, compression of optic nerve
Cryptophathalmos syndrome (Fraser's syndrome)	C9	Absence of the palpebral fissure or eyelashes or eyebrows, defect of eye, hair growth on lateral forehead, hypoplastic notched nares, ear anomaly, incomplete genitalia development, hypospadias, cryptorchidism, bicornuate uterus, vaginal atresia	Autosomal recessive	Ophthalmologic consult; hearing consult; rule out other causes of ambiguous genitalia
de Lange's syndrome (Cornelia de Lange)	D1	Small for gestational age, mental retardation, hypertonicity, growling cry, microcephaly, microbrachycephaly, bushy eyebrows and synophrys, long, curly eyelashes, small nose, anteverted nostrils, characteristic lips and mouth, high-arched palate, micrognathia, hirsutism, hypoplastic nipples and umbilicus, cutis marmorata, skeletal anomalies	Sporadic occurrence	Neurologic evaluation; feed carefully; correct hand anomalies as indicated; rule out congenital heart disease; rule out deafness
Diaphragmatic hernia	D2	Severe respiratory distress, cyanosis, scaphoid abdomen, decreased breath sounds (left) but barrel chest, peristaltic sound may be audible	Failure of development of posterolateral portion of diaphragm	Immediate chest x-ray film; correct acidosis; immediate surgical repair; see chapter 11–XIX
Diastrophic dwarfism syndrome	D3	Short tubular bones, joint limitation with club foot, hypertrophic auricular cartilage, short stature, scoliosis	Autosomal recessive	Rule out other causes of short stature; skeletal x-ray films; correct talipes equinovarus

(continued)

TABLE 9–4.—(*continued*)

SYNDROME OR MALFORMATION		CLINICAL FEATURES	INHERITANCE/CAUSE	IMMEDIATE MANAGEMENT
DiGeorge's syndrome	D4	Hypoplasia to aplasia of thymus with defect of cellular immunity, hypoplasia to absence of parathyroids, hypocalcemia, seizures, aortic arch anomalies, hypertelorism, ear anomalies	Unknown	Rule out congenital heart disease; prevent infection; follow calcium level; prevent hypocalcemic seizures
Down's syndrome (trisomy 21 syndrome)	D5	Hypotonia, protruding tongue, flat facies, hyperflexibility of joints, brachydactyly, mental deficiency, brachycephaly, late closure of fontanelles, slanted palpebral fissures, Brushfield's spots, hypoplasia of midphalanx of fifth finger, clinodactyly, distal axial triradius, wide gap between first and second toes, hypoplasia with outward lateral flare of iliac wings and shallow acetabular angles, atrioventricular communis, ventricular septal defect, loose folds in posterior neck, fine, soft, sparse hair, relatively small penis, small ears, cutis marmorata, epicanthal folds, simian crease	Trisomy for all or a large part of chromosome 21, translocation or mosaic	Confirm with chromosome study; rule out congenital heart disease; rule out GI anomaly see Table 9–2 for frequency in various age groups
Ehlers-Danlos syndrome	E1	Hyperextensibility of joints, hyperextensibility of skin, poor wound healing, narrow maxilla, easy bruisability	Autosomal dominant	Prevent bruising, skin trauma; observe for aneurysm
Ellis-van Creveld syndrome	E2	Short distal extremities, polydactyly, nail hypoplasia, small stature, fusion of hamate and capitate, small thorax, hypoplasia of upper	Autosomal recessive	Rule out congenital heart disease; differentiate from other causes of short stature; remove neonatal teeth; neurologic consult

		lateral tibia, neonatal teeth, short upper lip, accessory frenula, atrial septal defect		
Exstrophy of bladder anomalies	E3	Anterior abdominal wall defect, widely separate pubic symphysis, stubby penis	Fetal accident	Surgical consult for postnatal primary closure of bladder
Facioauriculo vertebral anomalies (Goldenhar's syndrome)	F1	Coloboma of upper lid, hypoplasia of malar, maxillary and/or mandibular region, microtia, accessory preauricular tags, variable deafness, tongue anomalies, hemivertebrae, mental deficiency	Unknown	Skeletal/vertebral x-ray films; ophthalmologic consult; hearing consult; neurologic consult
Fanconi's pancytopenia syndrome	F2	Radial hypoplasia, hyperpigmentation, pancytopenia, small stature, small cranium, hypoplasia/aplasia of thumb, splenic hypoplasia, brownish pigmentation (café au lait) of skin, small penis, cryptorchidism	Autosomal recessive	Prevent respiratory infections; obtain bone marrow study; differentiate from other causes of ambiguous genitalia; obtain a chromosomal study, CBC, renal function studies, etc.
Fetal alcohol syndrome (see chapter 15–XX)	F3	Small for gestational age, microcephaly, short palpebral fissures, joint contractures, altered palmar crease patterns, congenital heart disease (ventricular septal defect), upturned nose, hypoplastic maxilla, long philtrum, synophrys	Maternal alcoholism	Obtain maternal alcoholism history; rule out congenital heart disease; observe for joint anomalies; neurologic evaluation (see chapter 15–XX)
Fetal warfarin syndrome	F4	Hypoplastic nasal cartilage, stippled epiphyses, hypertelorism, developmental and mental deficiency, hypotonia, seizures, optic atrophy	Warfarin	Skeletal x-ray films; feed carefully; neurologic evaluation
Geleophysic dwarfism syndrome	G1	Coarse, pleasant facies, short hands and feet, joint contractures, thick, long, upper lip, cardiomegaly, hepatomegaly	Autosomal recessive (?)	Skeletal x-ray films; rule out congenital heart disease; prevent respiratory infection; orthopedic consult as indicated

(continued)

TABLE 9–4.—(*continued*)

SYNDROME OR MALFORMATION		CLINICAL FEATURES	INHERITANCE/CAUSE	IMMEDIATE MANAGEMENT
Gangliosidosis (generalized) syndrome, type 1 (severe infantile type)	G2	Coarse facies, joint limitation, kyphosis, slow growth, small for gestational age, delay in development, hypotonia, spasticity, low nasal bridge, broad nose, flaring alae nasi, frontal bossing, hirsutism, cherry red macular spot, large tongue, hepatomegaly	Autosomal recessive	Differentiate from other causes of small for gestational age; neurologic consult; ophthalmologic consult; smear for foamy histiocytes; supportive management
Goldenhar's syndrome		See F1.		
Goltz's syndrome	G3	Focal dermal hypoplasia, syndactyly, dental anomalies, dystrophic and/or hypoplastic nails, hypoplasia of teeth, eye anomalies	Sporadic occurrence	Surgical consult regarding syndactyly; ophthalmologic consult
Grebe's syndrome	G4	Marked distal limb reduction, polydactyly, normal facies, some stillborn	Autosomal recessive	Differentiate other causes of short stature; rule out congenital heart disease
Hallermann-Streiff syndrome	H1	Microphthalmia, small, pinched nose, hypotrichosis, proportionate small stature, brachycephaly, malar hypoplasia, micrognathia, microstomia, high-arched palate, atrophy of skin	Single mutant gene (dominant) (?)	Ophthalmologic consult; differentiate from Seckel's syndrome; differentiate other causes of short stature; neurologic consult
Holt-Oram syndrome (cardiac-limb syndrome)	H2	Upper limb defect, cardiac anomaly, hypoplasia and proximal placement of the thumb, radial hypoplasia, atrial septal defect, ventricular septal defect	Autosomal dominant	Cardiac consult; orthopedic consult; obtain X-rays, ECG, and echocardiogram
Hypochondroplasia syndrome	H4	Short limbs, caudal narrowing of spine, near-normal craniofacies	Autosomal dominant	Rule out other causes of short stature; obtain x-rays
Hydrocephalus	H3	Enlarged head, associated with meningomyelocele, achondroplasia, hydrocephaly, toxoplasmosis	Multiple	Sonogram and/or CT scan; determine cause; consider shunting; neurosurgery consultation

Hypoglossia-hypodactyly syndrome (Hanhart's syndrome)	H5	Hypoglossia, micrognathia, hypodactyly, recessed mandible, partial to complete absence of the digits or limbs	Unknown	Skeletal x-ray films; feed carefully; obtain orthopedic consult
Hypophosphatasia syndrome	H6	Poorly mineralized cranium, late closure of fontanelles, fragile bones, short ribs, incomplete bone mineralization	Autosomal recessive	Rule out craniosynostosis; rule out other causes of poor bone mineralization; support respiratory status; follow calcium level
Hypothyroidism	H7	Feeding problems, decreased activity, constipation; neonatal jaundice, cold to touch, dry skin, mottling, hoarse cry, umbilical hernia, large tongue	Sporadic occurrence	Confirm diagnosis as soon as possible and treat with thyroid replacement if indicated (see chapter 17)
Ichthyosis Lamellar (nonbullous congenital ichthyosiform erythroderma)	I1	Uniform generalized hyperkeratosis of trunk, limb involvement, flexures affected (dry), palms and soles thickened, may have collodion membrane, ectropion present and progressive	Autosomal recessive	Prevent hyperthermia; avoid dry indoor heat; hydrate with water soluble ointment (Aquaphor)
Jeune's syndrome (asphyxiating thoracic dystrophy) (thoracic-pelvic, phalangeal dystrophy)	J1	Small narrow thoracic cage, generalized chondrodystrophy, diaphragm depression, short ribs, hypoplastic iliac crest, irregular costochondrial joint, vertebrae normal (see Table 11–2)	Autosomal recessive	Immediate respiratory support; prevent aspiration; treat pneumonia promptly; obtain chest and long bone x-rays
Klippel-Feil anomalies	K1	Cervical fused vertebrae, hemivertebrae, short neck	Sporadic occurrence	Vertebral x-ray films; passive physiotherapy to neck
Klippel-Trenaunay-Weber syndrome	K2	Congenital or early childhood hypertrophy of usually one, but occasionally more than one limb, hemangiomas vary greatly, unilateral distribution predominates, arteriovenous fistula, lymphangiomatous anomalies, atrophy, macrodactyly, asymmetric facies, visceromegaly, hemangiomas of the GI tract, cutis marmorata	Unknown	Measure affected extremity; determine degree of vascular involvement by CT scan and/or radioactive study; rule out platelet deficiency

TABLE 9–4.—(*continued*)

SYNDROME OR MALFORMATION		CLINICAL FEATURES	INHERITANCE/CAUSE	IMMEDIATE MANAGEMENT
Larsen's syndrome	L1	Multiple joint dislocation, flat facies, hypertelorism, short fingernails, depressed nasal bridge, broad thumbs, talipses equinovalgus or varus	Unknown	Obtain skeletal x-ray films, supportive management.
Laurence-Moon-Biedl syndrome	L2	Obesity, mental deficiency, polydactyly, retinitis pigmentosa, hypogonadism, brachydactyly	Autosomal recessive	Obtain ophthalmologic consult; hearing consult; neurologic consult; rule out other causes of ambiguous genitalia
LEOPARD syndrome (multiple lentigines syndrome)	L3	Lentigines, ECG abnormalities, hypertelorism, pulmonic stenosis, abnormalities of genitalia, growth retardation, deafness	Autosomal dominant	ECG; ophthalmologic consult; rule out congenital heart disease; rule out genital abnormalities; hearing consult
Leprechaunism syndrome (Donohue's syndrome)	L4	Prenatal adipose deficiency, full lips, enlarged phallus, prominent eyes, wide nostrils, large ears, breast hyperplasia in female, hypertelorism	Autosomal recessive	Prevent infection; follow glucose carefully; prevent hypoglycemia; supportive management
Leri's pleonosteosis syndrome	L5	Broad thumb, joint limitation, upward slant to palpebral fissures (mongoloid slant), great toes, short spade-like hand	Autosomal dominant	Supportive management
Leri-Weill dyschondrosteosis	L6	Small sature, short forearm, bowing of radius, altered osseous alignment, partial dislocation of ulna	Autosomal dominant	Skeletal x-ray films
Linear sebaceous nevus anomalies (nevus sebaceous of Jadassohn)	L7	Midfacial nevus sebaceous, seizures, mental deficiency	Unknown	Obtain EEG, neurologic consult, cranial sonogram
Lowe's syndrome (oculo-cerebro-renal syndrome)	L8	Hypotonia, cataract, renal tubular dysfunction, joint hypermotility, absent deep tendon reflexes, mental deficiency, EEG	X-linked recessive	Rule out other causes of hypotonia; EEG; ophthalmologic consult; rule out renal tubular acidosis; follow electrolyte

		abnormality, limited ammonium production, hyperchloremic acidosis, phosphaturia, generalized aminoaciduria, cryptorchidism		
Lymphopenic agammaglobulinemia-short-limbed dwarfism syndrome	L9	Small for gestational age, short limbs, relatively small thorax, short pelvis, large sacrosciatic notch, lymphopenia and agammaglobulinemia with hypoplastic thymus, redundant skin	Autosomal recessive	Rule out other causes of short stature; prevent infection; obtain bone marrow aspirate; rule out immunologic deficiency
Marinesco-Sjögren's syndrome	M1	Cerebellar ataxia, hypotonia, cataracts, growth deficiency, severe mental deficiency, nystagmus, dysarthria	Autosomal recessive	Neurologic consult; ophthalmologic consult
McCune-Albright syndrome	M2	Multiple areas of fibrous dysplasia, irregular brown (cafe au lait) pigmentation, precocious menarche in female, occasional sexual precocity in male	Unknown	Skeletal x-ray films to rule out fibrous dysplasia; triidothyronine, thyroxine, thyroid-stimulating hormone; follow calcium, glucose
Meckel-Gruber syndrome	M3	Dysencephalia splanchnocystica, encephalocele, polydactyly, polycystic kidneys	Autosomal recessive	Supportive management
Meningomyelocele	M4	Associated with hydrocephalus, hypotonia or hypertonia, renal defects, neurogenic bladder, Arnold-Chiarl malformation	Unknown	Immediate neurologic and neurosurgical consult; rule out renal defect; rule out hydrocephalus; treat skeletal defects; physical therapy as indicated. Consider antibiotic therapy for open lesions
Menkes' syndrome	M5	Progressive cerebral deterioration with seizures, twisted and fractured hair, small at birth, pudgy cheeks, sparse and lightly pigmented hair, wormian bones (hair is normal at birth)	X-linked recessive	Obtain EEG, CAT, ceruloplasmin, and serum copper

(continued)

TABLE 9–4.—(*continued*)

SYNDROME OR MALFORMATION		CLINICAL FEATURES	INHERITANCE/CAUSE	IMMEDIATE MANAGEMENT
Metaphyseal chondrodysplasia (Jansen's syndrome)	M6	Short stature, prominent ears, micrognathia, cyst-like areas of metaphyses, small thoracic cage, flexion deformities of joints, bowed legs	Autosomal dominant	Obtain a calcium level; rule out deafness
Moebius' anomalies	M7	Mask-like facies, sixth and seventh nerve palsy, lateral rectus ocular palsy, micrognathia, talipes equinovarus, mental deficiency	Hypoplasia to agenesis of the respective nerve nuclei	Neurologic and ophthalmologic consult; orthopedic consult as indicated; feed carefully; prevent aspiration, obtain CAT
Morquio's syndrome (mucopolysaccharidosis IV)	M8	Flaring of lower rib cage, prominent sternum, frequent upper respiratory infections including otitis media, herniae, and growth deficiency	Autosomal recessive	Ophthalmologic consult; ENT consult; prevent respiratory infections; skeletal x-ray films; ECG; confirm diagnosis with urinary keratosulfate
Multiple exostosis syndrome	M9	Diaphyseal outgrowths leading to limb deformities, with or without short metacarpals	Autosomal dominant	Multiple x-ray films to establish diagnosis
Multiple synostosis syndrome	M10	Hypoplasia of alae nasi, multiple fusion of midphalangeal joints, elbow, and carpal and tarsal bones, variable brachydactyly, distal bone hypoplasia, aplasia in phalanges, fusion of middle ear ossicles, conduction deafness	Autosomal dominant	Hearing evaluation, ENT consult
Myelomeningocele		See meningomyelocele (M4)		
Nail-patella syndrome	N1	Nail dysplasia, patella hypoplasia, iliac spurs, nail splitting, hypoplastic capitellum, small head of radius, spur in midposterior ilium, "clover-leaf" pigmentation in iris, proteinuria	Autosomal dominant	Rule out scoliosis; renal evaluation; ophthalmologic consult; knee and limb x-rays

Neurocutaneous melanosis anomalad	N2	Melanosis of skin and pia arachnoid, CNS deterioration, hairy multiple nevi ("bathing trunk"), seizures	Unknown	Rule out hydrocephalus; obtain EEG, cranial CAT and cranial sonogram
Neurofibromatosis syndrome (von Recklinghausen's disease)	N3	Multiple neurofibromata, café-au-lait spots with or without bone lesions, dysplastic tumors (infant appears normal in nursery)	Autosomal dominant	Observe neurologic development
Noonan's syndrome (Turner-like syndrome)	N4	Webbing of neck, pectus excavatum, cryptorchidism, pulmonic stenosis, short stature, mental retardation, epicanthal folds, antimongoloid slant to eyes, low-set ears, high-arched palate, low posterior hairline, cubitus valgus, small penis, dorsal swelling of hands, nerve deafness	Unknown	Neurologic evaluation; rule out congenital heart disease; rule out other causes of ambiguous genitalia and short stature; ophthalmologic evaluation
Olser hemorrhagic telangiectasia syndrome	O1	Pinpoint, spider, and/or nodular angiectases on tongue, lips, face, conjunctiva, ears, fingertips, nail beds, nasal mucous membrane, GI tract, bladder, vagina, uterus, lungs, liver and/or brain	Autosomal dominant	Rule out arteriovenous fistula; EEG; CAT; ophthalmologic consult
Omphalocele	O2	Small or large midline protruding mass containing malrotated bowel or liver covered by a thin transparent membrane	Variable	Immediate surgical correction; rule out associated defects, i.e., malrotation of intestine, Meckel's diverticulum, patent vitelline duct, cardiovascular abnormalities (see chapter 17–XXI)
Opitz syndrome	O3	Hypertelorism, hypospadias, widow's peak, cryptorchidism, mental retardation	Autosomal dominant (?)	Rule out cardiac defects; rule out ear anomalies
Osteogenesis imperfecta syndrome, type II	O4	Small for gestational age, poorly mineralized soft calvarium with large fontanelles, blue sclerae, small nose, low nasal bridge, multiple fractures and callus	Autosomal recessive (severe neonatal type)	Handle carefully; differentiate from tarda form of syndrome; CT scan to rule out hydrocephalus; obtain appropriate x-ray films

(continued)

TABLE 9–4.—(*continued*)

SYNDROME OR MALFORMATION		CLINICAL FEATURES	INHERITANCE/CAUSE	IMMEDIATE MANAGEMENT
Osteogenesis imperfecta syndrome, type II–(*continued*)		formation, flattened vertebrae, hypotonia, inguinal hernia, variable hydrocephalus, skeletal deformities		
Osteogenesis imperfecta, type I	O5	Small stature in severe cases, flattening of vertebrae, hyperextensible skin and sclerae tend to be thin and translucent, deafness, fragile bone	Autosomal dominant	Handle carefully; feed carefully; orthopedic consult; hearing evaluation; differentiate from type II
Oto-palato-digital syndrome (Taybi's syndrome)	O6	Deafness, cleft palate, hypertelorism, broad distal digits, short nails, mild mental deficiency, small trunk, pectus excavatum, antimongoloid slanted eyes	X-linked semidominant	Hearing evaluation; neurologic evaluation, orthopedic evaluation
Pfeiffer's syndrome	P1	Brachycephaly, mild syndactyly, broad thumb and toes, resembles Apert's syndrome	Autosomal dominant	Rule out choanal atresia; rule out craniosynostosis
Pierre Robin syndrome (Robin anomalies)	P2	Micrognathia, glossoptosis, cleft palate (soft), mandibular hypoplasia	Unknown	Differentiate from cerebro-costomandibular syndrome; nurse on abdomen to allow tongue to fall forward; suction carefully
Poland anomalies	P3	Unilateral absence of the sternal portion of pectoralis major, syndactyly, absence of nipple and areola, rib defects, hypoplasia of hand and arm on ipsilateral side	Sporadic occurrence	Supportive management
Popliteal web syndrome	P4	Popliteal web, cleft palate, lower lip pits, toenail dysplasia	Autosomal dominant	Surgical consult to repair web/cleft palate
Potter's syndrome (oligohydramnios tetrad)	P5	Low or absent urinary output, growth deficiency, Potter facies (low-set ears, small chin, turned-down nose, crease around inner canthi of eyes, wizened look, etc.),	Multiple	Renal sonogram/scan; rule out hypoplastic lungs, follow intake and output carefully; examine placenta; follow blood gases and electrolytes

		chronic leakage of amniotic fluid, pulmonary hypoplasia, fetal compression, limb positioning defects, dysplastic or polycystic kidney, amnion nodosum		
Prader-Willi syndrome	P6	Severe hypotonia, small hands and feet, small at birth, narrow bifrontal diameter, strabismus, mental deficiency, small penis, cryptorchidism	Unknown	Obtain chromosome study with banding; rule out other causes of hypotonia (see Table 16–4); rule out adrenogenital syndrome (see Table 17–5)
Progeria syndrome (Hutchinson-Gilford syndrome)	P7	Alopecia, atrophy of subcutaneous fat, skeletal hypoplasia and dysplasia, thin skin, hypoplasia of nails, periarticular fibrosis, degeneration, metabolic alterations	Unknown	Supportive management
Pseudoachondroplastic spondyloepiphyseal dysplasia syndrome	P8	Short limbs, growth deficiency by second year, "fragmented" epiphyses, variable degrees of flattening of vertebrae, hypermotility of major joints, normal at birth	Apparently autosomal dominant	Supportive management; obtain skeletal x-rays; rule out other forms of dwarfism
Pseudo-vitamin D deficiency (rickets)	P9	Rickets, hypotonia, hypocalcemia, unresponsiveness to usual dosage of vitamin D, growth deficiency, large fontanelles, elevated serum alkaline phosphatase, mild to moderate hypophosphatemia, hyperaminoaciduria, mild renal tubular acidosis, seizures	Autosomal recessive	Rule out other causes of rickets, hypotonia, growth deficiency; obtain skeletal series; monitor blood gases; urinary amino acids
Radial aplasia-thrombocytopenia syndrome (TAR syndrome)	R1	Thrombocytopenia, absence or hypoplasia of megakaryocytes, "leukemoid granulocytosis," eosinophilia, anemia, absence or hypoplasia of radius, ulnar hypoplasia, defects of hands, legs, and/or feet; thumbs are present	Autosomal recessive	Watch platelet level carefully; consider steroid therapy; rule out congenital heart disease; obtain skeletal series

(continued)

TABLE 9–4.—(*continued*)

SYNDROME OR MALFORMATION		CLINICAL FEATURES	INHERITANCE/CAUSE	IMMEDIATE MANAGEMENT
Renal anomalies	R2	Small, large, or absent auricles, low-set ears, atresia of the external auditory canal	Multiple	Rule out ear malformations; observe fluid and electrolytes carefully
Riley-Day syndrome (familial dysautonomia)	R3	Dysautonomia, poor coordination, lack of tearing, swallowing difficulty in infancy, aspiration, cyclic vomiting, diarrhea, temp., emotional lability, breath holding, hyperhidrosis, insensitivity to pain	Autosomal recessive	Prevent aspiration and pneumonia; feed carefully; support growth
Robinow's syndrome (fetal face syndrome)	R4	Flat facial profile, short forearms, hypoplastic genitalia, mild to moderate short stature, macrocephaly, brachydactyly, hemivertebrae, cryptorchidism	Autosomal dominant	Obtain buccal smear and chromosome study; rule out other causes of ambiguous genitalia; monitor electrolytes
Rubinstein-Taybi syndrome	R5	Broad thumbs and toes, antimongoloid slanted palpebral fissures, hypoplastic maxilla, short stature, retarded osseous maturation, small cranium, narrow palate, beaked nose, epicanthal folds, strabismus, cryptorchidism, respiratory infections, feeding difficulties	Unknown	Feed carefully; prevent respiratory infection; obtain neurologic evaluation, skeletal series
Russell-Silver syndrome	R6	Short stature of prenatal onset, skeletal asymmetry, small incurved fifth finger, small triangular facies, cafe-au-lait spots, excess sweating (hyperhydrosis), brachydactyly	Unknown	Prevent hypoglycemia (older infants); observe growth and development; obtain skeletal series
Rubella syndrome (see chapter 16–IV)	R7	Small for gestational age, deafness, cataract, glaucoma,	Rubella virus	Rule out congenital heart disease; ophthalmologic examination;

		microphthalmia, patent ductus arteriosus, peripheral pulmonic stenosis, retinitis pigmentosa, hepatomegaly, etc.		hearing exam; isolate in nursery; watch platelets; obtain specific IgM level (see chapter 16–IV)
Schwartz's syndrome	S1	Myotonia, blepharophimosis, joint limitations, small stature, vertical shortness of vertebrae, pectus carinatum, long eyelashes, low hairline, low-set ears, fixed facies	Autosomal recessive	Rule out other causes of myotonia; orthopedic consult
Seckel's syndrome	S2	Severe small for gestational age, mental deficiency, microcephaly, hypoplasia with prominent nose, low-set malformed auricle, clinodactyly of fifth finger, simian creases, gap between first and second toes, 11 ribs, cryptorchidism	Probable autosomal recessive	Neurologic consult; rule out other causes of small for gestational age
Smith-Lemli-Opitz syndrome	S3	Anteverted nostrils, ptosis of eyelids, epicanthal folds, syndactyly of second and third toes, hypospadias, micropenis, and cryptorchidism in male, small at birth with subsequent failure to thrive, mental deficiency, microcephaly, auricles slanted or low set, strabismus, simian crease, breech birth, feeding difficulty, hypotonic, defects in brain morphogenesis	Autosomal recessive	Feed carefully; prevent aspiration pneumonia; neurologic evaluation. Many affected infants die within first year of life.
Sotos' syndrome (cerebral gigantism)	S4	Cerebral gigantism, large size, large hands and feet, poor coordination, large span, advanced osseous maturation, macrocephaly	Unknown	Neurologic evaluation; EEG; feed carefully; obtain skeletal series

(continued)

TABLE 9–4.—(*continued*)

SYNDROME OR MALFORMATION		CLINICAL FEATURES	INHERITANCE/CAUSE	IMMEDIATE MANAGEMENT
Spondyloepiphyseal dysplasia (SED)	S5	Short trunk, lag in epiphyseal mineralization, myopia, cleft palate, retinal detachment, short spine, flat vertebrae, barrel chest with pectus carinatum, muscle weakness, easy fatigability	Autosomal dominant	Orthopedic consult; ophthalmologic consult; plastic surgical consult; obtain skeletal series
Steinert's myotonic dystrophy syndrome	S6	Myotonia with muscle atrophy, cataract, hypogonadism, testicular atrophy, premature frontal recession, conduction defects with arrhythmias	Autosomal dominant	ECG; muscle biopsy; barium swallow; neurologic evaluation; ophthalmologic evaluation; rule out other causes of ambiguous genitalia
Sturge-Weber anomalad	S7	Facial port-wine hemangioma involving the trigeminal facial distribution, CNS involvement is variable with seizures and intracerebral calcifications and glaucoma	Unknown	Baseline EEG; watch for seizures; neurologic evaluation; obtain CAT (cranial)
Thanatophoric dwarfism syndrome	T1	Short limbs, flat vertebrae, large cranium, low nasal bridge, severe growth deficiency, large fontanelle, sausage-like fingers, short ribs, squarish pelvis	Unknown	Radiologic evaluation to establish diagnosis; respiratory support as indicated
Toxoplasmosis	T2	Microcephaly, microphthalmia, hydrocephaly, deafness, ocular lesions	Toxoplasmosis	See chapter 16–VI
Treacher Collins syndrome (mandibulofacial dysostosis)	T3	Antimongoloid slanting palpebral fissures, malar hypoplasia, mandibular hypoplasia, lower lid coloboma, partial to total absence of lower eyelashes, malformations of auricles, external ear canal defect, deafness, cleft palate,	Autosomal dominant with varying degree of expressivity	Careful feeding; hearing evaluation; plastic surgery evaluation; ophthalmologic evaluation; rule out congenital heart disease; rule out other osseous malformations

		projection of hair onto cheek, beaked nose, micrognathia, preauricular tags		
Trichodento-osseous (TDO) syndrome	T4	Kinky hair at birth, frontal bossing, dolichocephaly, square jaw, increased bone density in the skull	Autosomal dominant	Rule out other causes of craniosynostosis
Trisomy 18 syndrome	T5	Small for gestational age, mental deficiency, microcephaly, prominent occiput, low-set malformed auricles, small oral opening, narrow palatal arch, micrognathia, clenched hand, tendency for overlapping of index finger over third finger and fifth finger over fourth, absence of distal crease on 5th finger, low arch dermal ridge pattern, hypoplasia of nails, short sternum, inguinal or umbilical hernia, small pelvis, cryptorchidism, ventricular septal defect. Most die in <1 year.	Trisomy for all or a large part of the chromosome 18	Confirm with chromosomal study; rule out congenital heart disease; feed carefully; supportive management
Trisomy 13 syndrome (D_1 trisomy syndrome)	T6	Incomplete development of forebrain and olfactory and optic nerves, apneic spells, severe mental defect, deafness, microcephaly, hypotelorism, microphthalmia, coloboma of iris, retinal dysplasia, cleft palate, abnormal helices, low-set ears, capillary hemangiomas, localized scalp defects, simian crease, flexion of fingers with or without overlapping and camptodactyly, hyperconvex hypoplastic nails, rib anomalies, ventricular septal defect, atrial	Trisomy for all or large parts of D group (chromosome 13)	Confirm with chromosome study; rule out congenital heart disease; feed carefully; ophthalmologic exam; rule out deafness; neurologic consult.

(continued)

TABLE 9–4.—(*continued*)

SYNDROME OR MALFORMATION		CLINICAL FEATURES	INHERITANCE/CAUSE	IMMEDIATE MANAGEMENT
Trisomy 13 syndrome (D_1 trisomy syndrome)–(*continued*)		septal defect, patent ductus arteriosus, cryptorchidism, bicornuate uterus, increased frequency of nuclear projections in neutrophils, single umbilical artery, polydactyly. Early infancy death.		
Turner's Syndrome (XO syndrome)	T7	Short female, broad chest, wide spacing of nipples, congenital lymphadema or its residua, ovarian dysgenesis, low posterior hairline, short neck, webbed posterior neck, high arched palate, cubitus valgus, bone dysplasia, narrow hyperconvex nails, horseshoe kidney, coarction of aorta, perceptive hearing impairment, low-set ears, dorsal swelling of hands and feet	XO	Confirm with chromosomal study; rule out other causes of lymphedema; rule out congenital heart disease; hearing evaluation; endocrine evaluation at later age; plastic surgery evaluation
Tuberous sclerosis syndrome (adenoma sebaceum)	T8	Hamartomatous skin nodules, seizures, phakomas, bone lesions, glioma-angioma lesions in cortex and white matter with seizures, cyst-like areas in phalanges, angiomyolipomas	Autosomal dominant	Rule out other causes of angiomatous lesions; hand and skeletal x-ray films; ophthalmologic exam
VATER association	V1	Vertebral anomalies, cardiac defects (ventricular septal defect) anal atresia, with or without fistula, tracheoesophageal fistula, esophageal atresia, radial dysplasia, thumb or radial hypoplasia, preaxial polydactyly, syndactyly, renal anomaly, single umbilical artery	Sporadic occurrence	Skeletal and chest x-ray films; rule out congenital heart disease; confirm tracheoesophageal fistula (see chapter 11–XVIII); rule out renal anomaly with scan or sonar study

Waardenburg's syndrome (type I)	W1	Lateral displacement of inner canthi, broad and high nasal bridge, medial flares of eyebrows that may meet in midline, partial albinism (white forelock), deafness, bicolor iris (at 3 mo.)	Autosomal dominant	Hearing evaluation
Weaver's syndrome	W2	Macrosomia, accelerated skeletal maturation, camptodactyly, unusual facies, large bifrontal diameter, flat occiput, hypertelorism, large ears, long philtrum, broad thumbs, large at birth, accelerated growth	Unknown	Rule out other causes of hypertonia; assess bone age; follow growth pattern
Wiskott-Aldrich syndrome	W3	Thrombocytopenia, eczema, immunological deficiency, melena, purpura, diminished megakaryocytes and lymphocytes, low gamma M with elevated gamma A, elevated gamma E, low isoagglutinins	X-linked recessive	Hematologic consult; evaluate immunoglobulin status; prevent infection, bleeding; observe malignancies; watch for melena, hematuria
Xeroderma pigmentosa	X1	Skin pigmentation, telangiectases, angiomas, keratoses, excessive sensitivity to light	Autosomal recessive	Protect from ultraviolet light
XXY syndrome (Klinefelter's syndrome)	X2	Hypogenitalism, hypogonadism, long legs, mental retardation, small penis and testes	XXY chromosome	Confirm with chromosome study; rule out other causes of ambiguous genitalia
Zellweger's syndrome (cerebrohepatorenal syndrome)	Z1	Hypotonia, high forehead, flat facies, hepatomegaly, growth deficiency, seizures, minor ear anomaly, Brushfield's spots, patent ductus arteriosus, variable contractures	Autosomal recessive	Rule out causes of failure to thrive; rule out congenital heart disease; ophthalmologic evaluation; hepatic evaluation; and auditory evaluation; follow serum iron

†Ref. for Table 5–2.

REFERENCES

Smith D.W.: *Recognizable Patterns in Human Malformation.* Philadelphia, W.B. Saunders Co., 1982.

(continued from page 140)

In the event that the house officer is transient in the nursery, develop a plan as to with whom and how and when future activities will be accomplished.

d. Offer to have the clergy or the social services representative discuss with the family the religious, financial, and cultural aspects of burial.
e. Remember, no one is prepared to handle this situation and everyone needs help.

IV. SPECIFIC MANAGEMENT FOR INFANTS WITH CONGENITAL MALFORMATIONS

The specific management depends on type of malformation (see Table 9–4, p. 143) and specific disease entity.

Chapter 10

Discharge Policies

Discharge planning begins upon admission by encouraging parents to participate in the daily care of their infant.

I. HEALTHY, NORMAL FULLTERM INFANTS

Upon discharge, be certain of the following:

A. The newborn has successfully made the transition from intrauterine existence.
B. The infant feeds well, maintains temperature, and is considered normal on physical examination (e.g., no signs of infection or anemia).
C. No evidence of hemolytic disease due to blood-group incompatibility is present (see chapter 13–VII to 13–IX).
D. The result of the mother's and/or infant's serologic test for syphilis is negative.
E. An inborn metabolic disease screening test has been performed at 3 to 5 days of life.
F. The mother has learned how to care for her infant (e.g., bathing, temperature taking, formula or breast feeding, etc.).
G. The parents are ready for the new baby (e.g., the home has been prepared and the family is interacting well with the infant: holding, cuddling, fondling, and talking with good eye contact).
H. The parents have been instructed to give vitamins, iron, and other medications if needed and feel competent concerning the infant's medical requirements.
I. The mother has received instructions as to how she can obtain medical, nursing, and social help in regard to the infant's well-being.

II. EARLY NEONATAL DISCHARGE

Early neonatal discharge, i.e., within 24 hours of delivery, may be applied on a selective basis. It is necessary that this option be discussed early in the antepartum period.

A. Adequate parental education as to the possible neonatal complications (jaundice, poor feeding, etc.), home preparation, and follow-up care should be delineated prior to delivery. The mother and infant should be hospitalized for a minimum of 6 hours after delivery.
B. All discharge policies listed for the fullterm infant should be carried out.
C. Make an appointment for an inborn metabolic disease screening test to be obtained at 3 to 5 days of age.

III. PREMATURE AND HIGH-RISK/SICK INFANTS

Before discharge, premature and sick newborns should meet the criteria listed for mature, healthy newborns and should have the following:

A. Established adequate fluid and caloric intake independently.
B. Shown a satisfactory pattern of growth and development.
C. Demonstrated thermal stability.
D. Had blood drawn for inborn metabolic disease screening tests at 7 days of age and before discharge.
E. Been referred to community health agencies such as the visiting nurse association, the public health department, or social service for home teaching and support, if necessary.
F. Been referred to an early stimulation program (infant development program) after a thorough developmental assessment, if necessary.
G. Had a medical follow-up appointment with a pediatrician or well-baby clinic. The appointment should be made before discharge.
H. Been referred to the appropriate subspecialty clinic (e.g., neonatology high-risk follow-up, neurology, cardiology, ophthalmology, ENT, if required.

REFERENCE

Guidelines for Perinatal Care. Evanston, Ill., American Academy of Pediatrics, 1983.

Chapter 11

Respiratory Distress

Newborn infants frequently develop respiratory difficulties as the first signs of illness. Respiratory distress in the newborn is nonspecific; it may be the hallmark of diseases of one or many systems, such as the pulmonary, cardiac, metabolic, hematologic, and/or CNS. Respiratory distress can be defined as either (1) respiratory depression with or without apnea or (2) increased respiratory rate (tachypnea) with or without dyspnea (flaring of the alae nasi, subcostal, intercostal or suprasternal retractions, or grunting).

I. NORMAL DATA

A. Respiratory Rate and Pattern

Clinical evaluation of respiratory distress in the newborn infant requires a knowledge of the normal respiratory rate and pattern in relation to the infant's age.

1. First hours of life
   A normal infant may have tachypnea (60 to 80/minute), retractions, peripheral cyanosis (acrocyanosis), rales, and grunting.
2. After the first hours of life
   The respiratory rate should drop to 40/minute. Retractions, rales, and grunting should subside. Peripheral cyanosis can persist for several hours.

B. Blood Gases

Normal blood gas values change rapidly with the first few hours of life. All data must be considered in relation to the infant's gestational and postnatal age (see appendix A–8, A–9).

C. Chest X-ray Films

Retention of fetal lung fluid is sometimes noted in the first few hours after birth. Though most normal newborns show clear lungs by 5 hours after delivery, interlobar fissures are frequently visible. The anterior costophrenic angle is quite shallow; the apex of each hemidiaphragm is anterior and slightly medial to the midpart of the diaphragm. The trachea is deviated to the right of the midline by the left aortic arch. The thymic size varies but may obliterate the border of the heart. The cardiothoracic ratio is 0.55 the first day of life and slightly smaller in subsequent days. The descending aorta can sometimes be identified. The "ductus bump" can be seen occasionally.

D. Types of Respiratory Distress

1. Apnea
   Cessation of breathing associated with cyanosis and a decrease in heart rate and pH. Apnea usually lasts for more than 20 seconds. After 45 seconds of apnea, there is often hypotonia and unresponsiveness
2. Periodic respiration
   Periods of respiration at a rate of 50 to 60/minute lasting about 10 to 15 seconds alternating with cessation of breathing for 5 to 10 seconds usually associated with a normal heart rate and absence of cyanosis
3. Stridor
   A harsh, high-pitched sound that usually occurs during inspiration and is commonly associated with upper airway obstruction
4. Grunting
   Audible sound during the expiratory phase of respiration caused by the infant performing a Valsalva's maneuver and exhaling against it. This is an attempt to maintain positive end expiratory pressure and prevent alveolar collapse
5. Retractions
   The drawing in of the intercostal, substernal, or suprasternal soft tissue during inspiration
6. Tachypnea
   Increased respiratory rate, over 45/minute after the first hours of life

E. Selected Glossary of Terms

1. Laws/relationships/equations
   a. Ideal gas law
      The behavior of an ideal gas is governed by the interdependent relationship of four thermodynamic variables: mass, pressure, volume, and absolute temperature.

$$PV = nRT$$

where:
P = absolute pressure of dry gas in atmospheres

V = volume in liters (L)
n = moles of gas
R = universal gas constant (0.0821 L · atm/mole ° K)
T = absolute temperature in degrees Kelvin (° K)

b. Laplace's relationship

The pressure difference between the inside and outside of a sphere is dependent upon the surface tension of the air/liquid interface and the radius of the sphere.

$$P = \frac{2T}{R}$$

where:
P = transmural pressure difference (dyne/sq cm)
T = surface tension (dyne/cm)
R = radius of sphere (cm)

c. Air flow resistance (Poiseuille's law)

Poiseuille's equation describes the mechanics of laminar flow through a tube and indicates that the pressure difference is directly proportional to the gas flow rate.

$$V = \frac{P\pi r^4}{8nl}$$

where:
V = flow in cu cm/second
P = difference of pressure across the ends of the tube (dyne/sq cm)
π = 3.1416
r = radius of the tube (cm)
l = length of the tube (cm)
n = viscosity in poise (dyne · sec/sq cm)

2. Lung volumes and capacities (in normal fullterm newborns) (Fig 11–1)
   a. Tidal volume (6–8 ml/kg)
      The volume of air inspired and expired at each spontaneous respiratory cycle
   b. Functional residual capacity (30 ml/kg)
      The volume of gas remaining in the lung at the end of tidal exhalation
   c. Anatomic dead space
      The volume of the non-gas-exchanging conducting airways
   d. Alveolar dead space
      Alveoli that continue to be ventilated though deprived of blood flow
   e. Physiologic dead space (2–2.2 ml/kg)
      The anatomic dead space plus the volume of ventilated lung not receiving pulmonary blood flow and thus not participating in gas exchange
   f. Residual volume (23 ml/kg)
      The volume of gas remaining in the lungs after a maximum expiration
   g. Minute ventilation (200–260 ml/kg/min)
      The volume of air inspired and expired in 1 minute

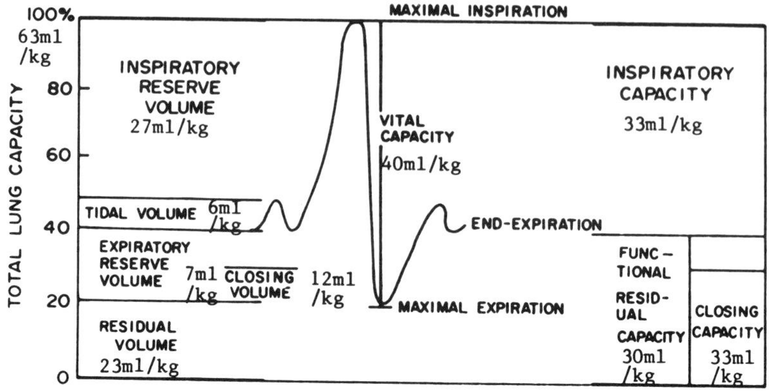

FIG 11–1.
Lung volumes in the infant. (Modified from Smith C.A., Nelson N.M.: *The Physiology of the Newborn Infant,* ed. 4. Springfield, Ill., Charles C Thomas, Publisher, 1976, pp 206 and 207. Used by permission.)

3. Reflexes
   a. Hering-Breuer reflex
      Sustained lung inflation inhibits respiration
   b. Head's paradoxic reflex
      Gasp in response to a rapid lung inflation
4. Other terms
   a. Oxygen saturation (%)
      The amount of oxygen chemically bound to hemoglobin in relation to the maximum amount of oxygen the hemoglobin is capable of carrying
   b. Oxygen tension (mm Hg)
      Partial pressure of oxygen
   c. Oxygen content (volume %)
      The total quantity of oxygen in the blood. This includes the quantity of oxygen dissolved in the plasma plus the quantity of oxygen bound to the hemoglobin.
   d. Oxygen-hemoglobin dissociation curve
      An index of the affinity of hemoglobin for oxygen at various levels of partial pressure of oxygen
   e. Compliance
      A property that describes the elastic behavior of a structure. It quantitates the volume change that results from a change in pressure.
   f. Ventilation-perfusion ratio (Va/Q)
      The relationship between the alveolar ventilation and the perfusion. (The average Va/Q for the lung as a whole is 0.8)
      See index for continuous positive airway pressure (CPAP), positive end expiratory pressure (PEEP), intermittent positive-pressure breathing (IPPB), continuous distending pressure (CDP), inspiratory: expiratory ratio

(I/E ratio), FI_{O_2}, peak inspiratory pressure, intermittent mandatory ventilation, "flip-flop phenomenon," continuous negative pressure (CNP), continuous positive pressure breathing (CPPB), mean airway pressure (MAP)

II. COMMON CAUSES OF RESPIRATORY DISTRESS IN THE NEWBORN INFANT

A. Respiratory

1. Respiratory distress syndrome (RDS)
2. Transient tachypnea of the newborn (TTNB)
3. Apnea
4. Pneumonia
5. Meconium aspiration syndrome (MAS)
6. Persistent pulmonary hypertension of the newborn (persistent fetal circulation (PPHN, PFC)
7. Pulmonary air leak syndrome (ALS)
8. Pulmonary hemorrhage
9. Bronchopulmonary dysplasia (BPD)
10. Wilson-Mikity syndrome
11. Tracheoesophageal fistula (T–E fistula)
12. Diaphragmatic hernia
13. Pulmonary hypoplasia (Potter's syndrome)
14. Atelectasis
15. Upper airway obstruction
    a. Transient mucus plug
    b. Choanal atresia
    c. Pierre Robin syndrome
    d. Subglottic stenosis
    e. Necrotizing tracheobronchitis
    f. Laryngeal web
    g. Laryngotracheomalacia
    h. Extrinsic compression: vascular ring, cystic hygroma, goiter
16. Congenital lobar emphysema (CLE)
17. Lymphangiectasia
18. Cystic adenomatoid malformation of the lung
19. Lung cyst(s)
20. Pleural effusion: chylothorax, hemothorax, pyothorax, etc.
21. Phrenic nerve palsy

B. Cardiovascular

1. Congenital heart disease (CHD) with or without congestive heart failure
2. Congestive heart failure (CHF)
3. Patent ductus arteriosus (PDA)

C. Metabolic

1. Acidosis
2. Hypoglycemia
3. Hyperglycemia
4. Hypocalcemia
5. Hypothermia
6. Hyperthermia
7. Sepsis
8. Hypermagnesemia
9. Congenital hyperthyroidism (neonatal Graves' disease)

D. Hematologic

1. Anemia
2. Hemorrhage
3. Polycythemia

E. Central Nervous System

1. Intracranial hemorrhage:
   a. Periventricular-intraventricular hemorrhage (PVH–IVH)
   b. Subdural hemorrhage (SDH)
   c. Subarachnoid hemorrhage (SAH)
2. Infection
3. Depression caused by drugs (magnesium, analgesics)
4. Narcotics, barbiturate withdrawal
5. Malformation: anencephaly, porencephaly

III. WHAT THE PHYSICIAN SHOULD DO WHEN CONFRONTED WITH AN INFANT WITH RESPIRATORY DISTRESS

A. Diagnostic Workup

1. Suction the infant. Remember, respiratory distress may be secondary to secretions or congenital malformations blocking the upper airway.
2. Take the infant's temperature to ascertain hypothermia or hyperthermia.
3. Review the prenatal and delivery histories for clues to the infant's condition.
4. Examine the infant carefully, considering each of the causes of respiratory distress. Note variations in respiratory rate and rhythm and breath sounds; presence or absence of stridor, apnea, dyspnea, scaphoid abdomen, murmurs, asymmetry of the chest; quantity and quality of retractions; and other physical findings. Obtain vital signs.
5. Obtain arterial blood gases, blood glucose, complete blood count (CBC),

electrolytes, calcium, and blood urea nitrogen (BUN). Obtain magnesium determination if mother received $MgSO_4$. Replace blood drawn for sampling as necessary.

6. Obtain anteroposterior and lateral x-ray films of the chest.
7. If sepsis is suspected, obtain cultures from the blood, cerebrospinal fluid (CSF), and urine. Obtain results of maternal cultures.
8. Obtain ECG and echocardiograph if cardiac abnormalities are suspected.
9. Obtain cranial computerized tomography (CT) scan or sonogram if hemorrhage or anomalies of the central nervous system are suspected.

B. General Supportive Management for the Infant With Respiratory Distress

1. Handle the infant gently (as always).
2. Place the infant in the supine position with a roll under his or her shoulders to extend the neck slightly and open the airway.
3. Suction the infant.
4. Monitor temperature, pulse, respiration, heart rate, blood pressure, and general activity.
5. Maintain the infant's skin temperature at approximately 36.5°C or rectal temperature at approximately 37°C. Work within a warmed environment to avoid precipitous drops in body temperature associated with procedures such as taking an x-ray film or inserting a catheter.
6. Withhold oral feedings to prevent aspiration if the respiratory rate is greater than 60/minute or if apnea or dyspnea is present.
7. Begin an IV infusion of fluids to maintain fluid and electrolyte status and to provide an available IV route in case emergency IV administration of drugs is required (see chapter 6–IID2).
8. Obtain results of arterial blood gas studies.
9. Administer oxygen as required. Judge the infant's oxygen requirements by obtaining serial Pa_{O_2} samples or utilizing transcutaneous P_{O_2}($TcPO_2$.)
10. Correct hypoxia, Pa_{O_2} less than 50 mm Hg, by raising the ambient oxygen concentration gradually.
11. Correct respiratory acidosis, a Pa_{CO_2} greater than 50–60 mm Hg, by assisted ventilation (for each change of Pa_{CO_2} of 10 mm Hg the pH changes approximately 0.1 units). Determine quality and duration of assisted ventilation required by serial blood gas studies and/or $TcPO_2$ and $TcPCO_2$ (see chapter 11–VI). Significant periods of apnea are another indication for assisted ventilation.
12. Correct metabolic acidosis, a pH less than 7.3 and/or a base deficit greater than 6, with sodium bicarbonate. Correct one half of the sodium bicarbonate requirement in 6–12 hours using one of the following formulas:
    a. $NaHCO_3$ = Weight (kg) × Base deficit (mEq)* × 0.3 (one half of the $NaHCO_3$ distribution space)

---

*Base deficit may be calculated from Siggaard-Andersen normogram utilizing pH and P_{CO_2} (see Appendix Fig A–4).

b. $NaHCO_3$ = Weight (kg) × (Desired concentration HCO_3 − Measured concentration HCO_3) × 0.3
c. $NaHCO_3$ = 1 to 2 mEq/kg/0.10 drop in pH below 7.25
   $NaHCO_3$ should be administered slowly as 0.5 mEq (900 mOsm/L/ml/minute.
d. When P_{CO_2} is high, utilize tromethamine in place of bicarbonate. Obtain arterial blood gas 15 to 20 minutes after each correction.
   1) Tromethamine, THAM, 0.3 M solution, 3–5 ml/kg/dose, or
   2) Calculate total requirement to correct base deficit (total dose in ml = weight in kg × base deficit in mEq/L × 1.1)
      Administer ¼ of total dose over 2–5 minutes and give ¾ of total dose according to response.

13. Observe for hypovolemia (shock, pallor) and obtain serial blood pressure readings by using a Doppler flow technique (Arteriosonde), Dynamapp, or a pressure transducer in series or parallel to the umbilical artery catheter. Correct hypovolemia if present. (see chapter 14–IIID).
14. Correct anemia. Infuse whole blood cautiously and slowly (5 to 10 ml/kg over 2 to 4 hours). Maintain the infant's hematocrit at 40% to 45% while on O_2 therapy.
15. After obtaining blood, CSF, and urine cultures, begin antibiotic therapy if the infant is suspected of having sepsis (see chapter 16–III).
16. Begin oral feedings only after the infant's respiratory distress has subsided.

IV. OXYGEN THERAPY

To correct persistently low Pa_{O_2} (less than 50 mm Hg), raise the ambient oxygen concentration. The ambient oxygen concentration is expressed as a percent or fraction of inspired air (F_{IO_2}). The administration of oxygen to premature infants is fraught with danger. While an inadequate quantity of oxygen results in tissue hypoxia, a prolonged high ambient oxygen concentration may lead to bronchopulmonary dysplasia or pulmonary hemorrhage, and an elevated Pa_{O_2} may contribute to the development of retinopathy of prematurity. Unfortunately, the upper limit of safe arterial oxygen tension remains unknown. In addition, the means of attaining, maintaining, and continuously monitoring a reasonable level of tissue oxygenation in the sick, premature, or fullterm infant has not yet been developed to the point of assuring an adequate but nontoxic level of oxygenation without hazard.

A. Recommendations for Administration of Oxygen

1. Do not routinely administer oxygen to well premature or fullterm infants.
2. Administer oxygen to newborn infants when the infant is cyanotic and/or the arterial oxygen tension (Pa_{O_2}) is less than 50 mm Hg in room air with or without cyanosis. Attempt to maintain Pa_{O_2}between 50 and 70 mm Hg.

3. Cyanosis is not the only indication for administering oxygen since hypoxia can be present without cyanosis. The visual perception of "blueness" (cyanosis) may not be observed until the arterial oxygen saturation is 75% to 85%, which represents a Pa_{O_2} level of 33 to 42 mm Hg on the fetal hemoglobin dissociation curve and 42 to 53 mm Hg on the adult hemoglobin dissociation curve (Fig 11–2). Thus, the infant may be significantly hypoxic when cyanosis is first observed. In addition, if the infant is anemic, cyanosis is more difficult to detect since cyanosis only becomes evident when there is 5 gm/dl of deoxygenated hemoglobin.
4. The duration of oxygen administration should be as short as possible consistent with the infant's welfare. Attempt to lower the oxygen concentration as soon as the infant has improved.
5. Do not administer oxygen to premature infants to abolish periodic breathing.
6. One hundred percent oxygen can be used safely for resuscitation; however, an arterial blood gas should be obtained as soon as possible to ascertain the $F_{I_{O_2}}$ required.
7. Warm and humidify the oxygen to 32–37° C and at least 70% saturation with water vapor before administration to prevent heat loss, water loss, excessive oxygen consumption, tracheal mucous membrane irritation, inspissation of secretions, and necrosis of airway mucosa. Commonly used heated humidifiers are Puritan Nebulizer, Puritan-Bennett Co., and Aquapak Nebulizer, Respiratory Care, Inc. In the first, water is added as steam; in the second, water is added as microdroplets.
8. Order oxygen by the percent of oxygen concentration desired and not by flow (L/minute).
9. Standardize the oxygen analyzer against room air (21%) and a known source of oxygen (100% or 40%) every 8 hours. (The nursery personnel should perform this procedure.)

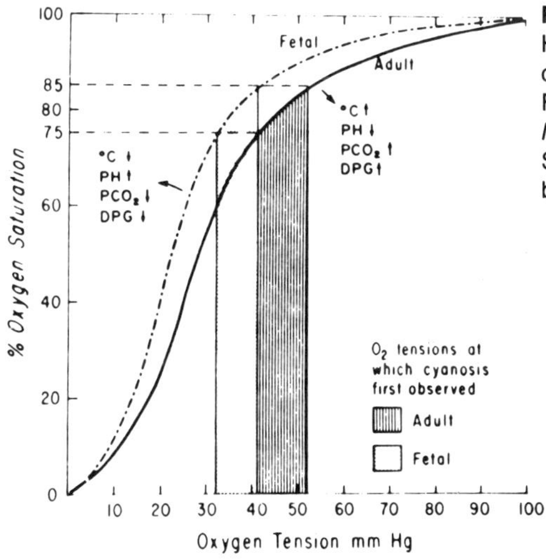

FIG 11–2.
Hemoglobin-oxygen dissociation curves. (Modified from Klaus M., Fanaroff A.: *Care of the High-Risk Neonate,* ed. 3. Philadelphia, W.B. Saunders Co., 1986, p. 173. Used by permission.)

10. Analyze the ambient oxygen concentration at the level of the infant's nose by using the continuous oxygen analyzer and record every hour.
11. Monitor the infant's Pa_{O_2} to keep the Pa_{O_2} level between 50 and 70 mm Hg by adjusting the ambient oxygen concentration.
    a. The ideal Pa_{O_2} sampling sites are the right radial, brachial, or superficial temporal arteries. However, sampling is frequently performed through an indwelling umbilical artery because repeated sampling from peripheral arteries is difficult. The frequency of need for sampling is unknown. In addition, retinal Pa_{O_2} may be higher than the Pa_{O_2} measured in the descending aorta if there is a right-to-left shunt through the patent ductus arteriosus. Arterialized capillary blood is not as reliable for the determination of Pa_{O_2} as arterial blood but may be used when an arterial sample is not available. Sampling may be reduced by $TcPCO_2$ and $TcPCO_2$ monitoring (correlate with Pa_{O_2} and Pa_{CO_2}). There is poor correlation when there is poor perfusion, e.g., acidosis, shock, sepsis, etc.
    b. Utilize the right-left shunt curves as a guide for decreasing or increasing ambient oxygen concentration (Fig 11–3).
        1) Determine the percent of right-left shunt by noting the Pa_{O_2} and FI_{O_2} administered to the infant.
        2) Then assuming the shunt to remain steady, note the FI_{O_2} that can be decreased or increased to obtain the desired Pa_{O_2}.
        3) Remember that the degree of right-to-left shunt varies as the infant's condition changes.

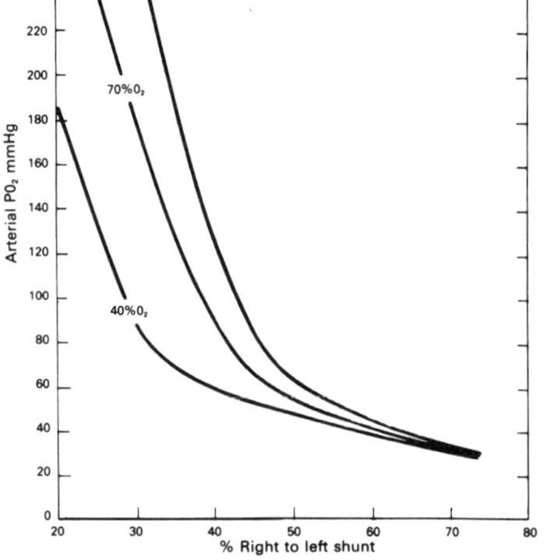

FIG 11–3.
Right-left shunt curves. (From Barnett H. (ed.): *Pediatrics* ed. 15. New York, Appleton-Century-Crofts, 1972. Used by permission.)

B. Methods of Providing an Oxygen-Enriched Environment

1. Hood
   The hood is a plastic container that surrounds the infant's head and maintains the desired atmospheric concentration without impairing the visibility of the infant's face. It is the simplest, most economical, and most effective way to maintain an ambient oxygen concentration. When the hood is opened, the oxygen concentration falls. Care must be taken to supply an adequate flow through the system and not overheat the infant.
2. Incubator
   The ambient oxygen concentration is regulated by the quantity of oxygen inflow into the closed incubator. Routine checking of the ambient oxygen concentration with an oxygen analyzer must be a standard procedure. The oxygen temperature is raised to the proper level as it passes over the heater. Maintaining a stable $F_{I_{O_2}}$ is difficult in the face of the need for frequent nursing care since the closed incubator environment is often entered. The authors do not recommend this mode of oxygen administration.

C. Complications of Oxygen Therapy

1. Pulmonary hemorrhage (see chapter 11–XV)
2. Bronchopulmonary dysplasia (see chapter 11–XVI)
3. Retinopathy of prematurity (see chapter 11–V)

REFERENCE

Klaus M., Meyer B.P.: Oxygen therapy for the newborn. *Pediatr. Clin. Am.* 13:731, 1966.

V. RETINOPATHY OF PREMATURITY (ROP): RETROLENTAL FIBROPLASIA (RLF)

Retinopathy of prematurity (ROP) is an ocular disorder of premature infants resulting in retinal dysfunction. Factors such as the length of exposure of the infant to high Pa_{O_2}, degree of immaturity of the retinal vessels, high Pa_{CO_2}, deficiency of vitamin E, and adult blood transfusion may be important etiologically. The spectrum of retinal dysfunction may range from complete recovery to mild myopia or blindness.

A. Prevention

1. See the section on oxygen therapy. Follow recommendations (see Chapter 11–IV).
2. Administer oxygen to premature infants only when the infant's Pa_{O_2} is less than 50 mm Hg in room air with or without cyanosis. Oxygen tension of arterial blood should be maintained between 50 and 70 mm Hg.

3. Some data suggest that vitamin E, with a serum level of 1.3 to 3.0 mg/dl, is effective in the prevention of ROP (under investigation).
4. Some data suggest that D-penicillamine may reduce the incidence and severity of ROP (under investigation).

B. Who Is at Risk?

1. Premature infants, particularly with birth weights less than 1,500 gm. The incidence of ROP is inversely related to birth weight and gestational age. Active disease was reported to be 38% to 54% in less than 1,000-gm infants and 2% to 15% in 1,000- to 1,500-gm infants. Blindness from ROP is reported to be 5% to 11% in infants less than 1,000 gm and 0.3% to 1.1% in 1,000 to 1,500-gm infants.
2. Premature infants receiving prolonged oxygen therapy. The peak Pa_{O_2} level and duration of O_2 therapy that prevent ROP are not yet established.
3. Premature infants who have never received oxygen therapy may still develop ROP possibly due to an exaggerated response of the immature retinal vessels to the normal Pa_{O_2} rise after birth.
4. Prematures with hypoxia and apnea
5. Premature infants in the following situations are considered at risk, but data is still controversial: Those with high Pa_{CO_2}, those with a patent ductus arteriosus and indomethacin therapy, twins, or those who received exchange transfusion.
6. Fullterm infants with Down's syndrome, anencephaly, other congenital anomalies, or maternal severe anemia are at risk for congenital ROP.
7. Fullterm infants with isolated retinal immaturity
8. Infants born to mothers with complications of pregnancy possibly due to intrauterine hypoxia
9. Premature infants exposed to bright light may be at risk.

C. Clinical Manifestations

The international classification of ROP (1984) allows the examiner to describe the location of the disease in the retina and the extent of the developing vasculature involved. See Figure 11–4 for the examination record.

1. Location of ROP

   Zone I (posterior pole or inner zone) consists of a circle the radius of which extends from the disc to twice the distance from the disc to the center of the macula and subtends an angle of 30 degrees. Zone II extends from the edge of zone I peripherally to a point tangential to the nasal ora serrata and around to an area near the temporal anatomic equator. Zone III is the residual crescent of retina anterior to zone II. This is the zone that is the least vascularized in the premature eye and is the zone, by common agreement of clinicians, most frequently involved with ROP.

BIOGRAPHICAL DATA

Name ______________________ Hospital # __ __ __ __ __ __ __

Birthdate (MM/DD/YY) __ __/__ __/__ __ Sex (M=1, F=2) __

Birthweight (grams) __ __ __ __ Gestational Age (weeks) __ __

Multiple Births (Single=1, Twin=2, Triplet=3) __

EXAMINATION

Date of Exam __ __/__ __/__ __ Examiner's Initials or # __ __ __

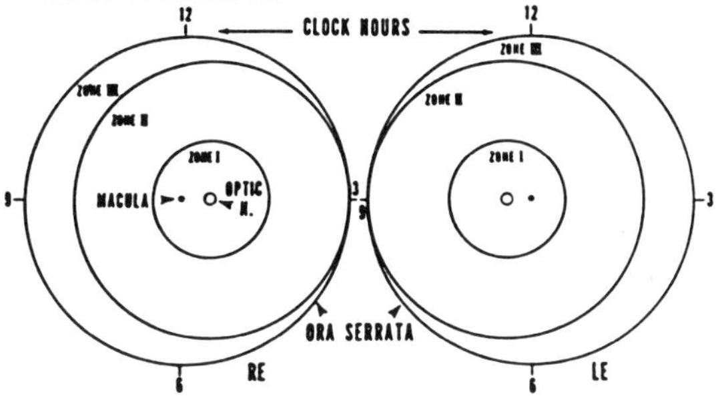

ZONE
Mark with 'X'

RE Z 1	RE Z 2	RE Z 3	LE Z 1	LE Z 2	LE Z 3
☐	☐	☐	☐	☐	☐

STAGE AT CLOCK HOURS

Blank=normal
1=Demarcation line
2=Ridge
3=2+Extraret prolif
4=3+Retinal detach
9=No information

(Grids for each eye, clock hours 12, 11, 10, 9, 8, 7, 6 on left and 12, 1, 2, 3, 4, 5, 6 on right)

Mark highest stage at every clock hour

☐ If Stage 3: 1=mild, 2=moderate, 3=severe ☐

☐ If Stage 4: 1=exudative, 2=tractional, 3= combined ☐

Other Findings
Mark with 'X'

O.D.			O.S.
☐	A	Dilatation/tortuosity posterior vessels	☐
☐	B	Iris vessel dilatation	☐
☐	C	Pupil rigidity	☐
☐	D	Vitreous haze	☐
☐	E	Hemorrhages	☐

Cicatricial RLF (Reese, 1953)
Mark with 'X'

O.D.			O.S.
☐	I.	Small mass opaque tissue in periphery without detachment	☐
☐	II.	Larger mass opaque tissue in periphery with localized detachment	☐
☐	III.	Larger mass in periphery with traction fold to disc	☐
☐	IV.	Retrolental tissue covering part of pupil	☐
☐	V.	Retrolental tissue covering entire pupillary area	☐

COMMENTS:

FIG 11–4.
Retinopathy of prematurity: ophthalmic examination record. (From Garner A.: *Pediatrics* 74:127, 1984. Used by permission of *Pediatrics.*)

2. Extent of the disease
   This is specified as hours of the clock.
3. Staging the disease (Fig 11–5)
   The level of abnormal vasculature response is divided into four stages. Each stage is defined as follows, and the extent of each stage by clock hours and location as listed here is recorded.
   a. Stage 1
      There is a demarcation line that is white, thin, and relatively flat and lies within the plane of the retina and separates the avascular anterior from the vascularized posterior retina. There are recognizable abnormal branching or arcading vessels leading up to the demarcation line.
   b. Stage 2
      The line of stage 1 has grown, has height and width, and occupies volume that extends up out of the retinal plane. Vessels may leave the plane of the retina to enter the demarcation line. Small isolater tufts of new vessels on the surface of retina may be seen posterior to the demarcation line.
   c. Stage 3
      The thicker and wider demarcation line now has extraretinal fibrovascular proliferative tissue. The characteristic locations are the following:
      1) Continuous with the posterior aspect of the ridge causing a ragged appearance of the ridge
      2) Immediately posterior to the ridge not always appearing to be connected with it
      3) Into the vitreous body perpendicular to the retinal plane
   d. Stage 4
      In addition to the findings of stage 3, retinal detachment has occurred.
4. "Plus" disease
   "Plus" is added to the ROP stage number when there are vascular changes such as dilation and tortuosity of the peripheral retinal vessels, iris vascular engorgement (rubeosis), pupillary rigidity, and viterous haze. The progression of ROP may be very rapid when it is located in zone I or II and "plus" disease is present.

D. Supportive Management

1. All premature infants less than 36 weeks or less than 2,000 gm who have received oxygen therapy should be examined for ROP. See Table 11–1 for time schedule for fundus examination. Dilate the pupils with 1% phenylephrine and 0.2% cyclopentolate. Complications include hypertension, tachycardia, abdominal distension, delayed gastric emptying, possible NEC, temperature instability, aerophagia, vagal stimulation, increased intracranial pressure, etc.
2. Findings of ROP should be recorded on an ophthalmic examination record (see Fig 11–4).
3. Approximately 20% of fullterm infants may have immature retinas. Therefore, some neonatologists feel that all infants below 44 weeks should have a fundal

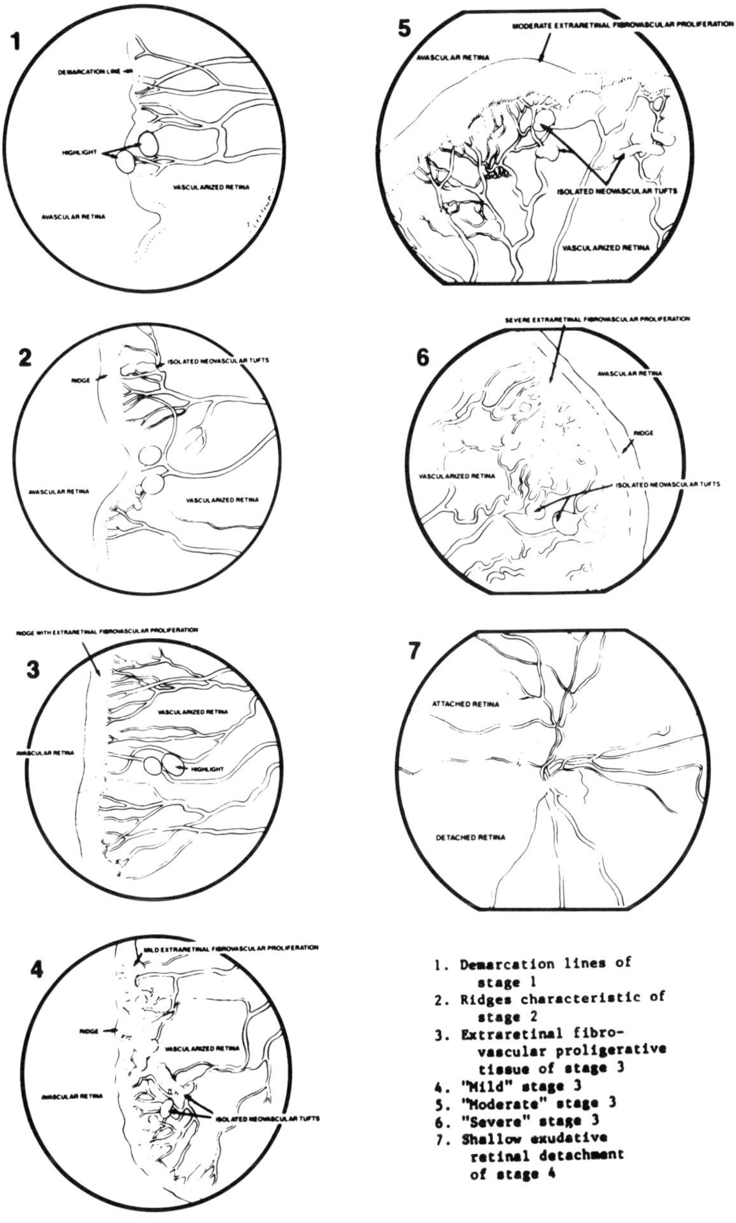

FIG 11–5.
ROP fundus findings. (From Garner A.: An international classification of retinopathy of prematurity. *Pediatrics* 74:127, 1984. Used by permission.)

TABLE 11–1.—TIME SCHEDULE FOR FUNDUS EXAMINATION*

GESTATIONAL AGE AT BIRTH	FIRST EXAM	FOLLOW-UP EXAM
Less than 30 wk	6–8 wk	If normal: Repeat every 3–4 wk, until mature retina, and again in 3–6 mo. If ROP present: Mild, re-examine every 2–3 wk until signs of resolution noted; severe (grade 3+), re-examine every 1–2 wk until disease is no longer progressing, then every 2–3 wk until signs of resolution noted. Resolving retrolental fibroplasia: every 2–4 weeks until resolved.
30–34 wk	6–7 wk	If normal: Repeat in 3–6 mo. If ROP present: Follow schedule as noted in less than 30 wk.
Greater than 34 wk	6 wk	If normal: No subsequent exam necessary. If ROP present: Follow schedule as noted in less than 30 wk.

If anterior chamber hyperemia occurs, immediate eye examination should be obtained.
For detection of late complications:
Infants with fully regressed ROP: Eye exam every 1 to 2 yr.
Infants with cicatricial retrolental fibroplasia: Eye exam every 6 to 12 mo.

*From Porat R.: Care of the infant with retinopathy of prematurity. *Clin. Perinatol.* 11:127, 1984. Used by permission.

examination before administration of general anesthesia and that air instead of oxygen should be used as the main anesthetic carrier if the retina is immature.

4. Inform and discuss the progress and prognosis of various modes of treatment of ROP and counsel parents concerning the possible residual visual defects.

E. Specific Therapy

1. Medical therapy with vitamin E (under investigation)
   Premature infants have low blood tocopherol levels due to inadequate tissue storage, dietary deficiency, transient malabsorption, and rapid growth. Vitamin E is reported to possibly prevent and modify ROP possibly due to prolonging plasma clotting time, reducing thrombosis by decreasing platelet aggregation, preventing irreversible endothelial damage by blocking free radicals, reducing cellular oxygen toxicity by preserving retinal superoxide dismutase, reducing fibrous scar formation as an anti-inflammatory agent, or suppressing gap junction formation allowing normal blood vessel growth.
   a. For prevention
      Oral vitamin E (Aquasol), 25 IU/day, for the first 2 months of life or until birth weight has been doubled (controversial).

b. For treatment
Increase vitamin E supplementation to maintain vitamin E level, 1.2 to 3.0 mg/dl, until the disease has regressed and retinal vascularization is almost mature.
c. Complications
Increased rates of infection, intraventricular hemorrhage, and NEC with high serum levels of vitamin E, 4 to 5 mg/dl, have been reported. The levels of 1.2 to 3.0 mg/dl were not associated with side effects.

2. Surgical Therapy
   a. Laser photocoagulation may be used. Technical problems are still present and this therapy is not applicable for advanced vitreal hemorrhage and retinal detachment at the present time.
   b. Cryotherapy to induce remission and obliterate neovascularization, thereby reducing traction on the retina and preventing further detachment, is used for extensive vitreal hemorrhage and retinal detachment. It is important to wait to determine if there is spontaneous regression, but not to wait so long that the lesions become inoperable. Cryotherapy complications include hemorrhage into the vitreous body, freezing the macula, scleral erosion, and occlusion of central retinal artery from buckling.
   c. Vitrectomy is limited to infants with bilateral traction, retinal detachment, and exudative elevation of the retina.
   d. Scleral buckling is used for retinal breaks and detachment. Cure rates are reported to be high.

F. Prognosis

1. Stages I and II of ROP usually show regression of all pathology with no scarring, but some small vessels growing from the shunt into the available area may remain. The resolution may occur as early as 11 to 16 weeks of postnatal age. Treatable ocular abnormalities, e.g., strabismus, amblyopia, and refractive errors, may occur.
2. Stages III and IV of ROP may show cicatricial changes that may occur proportional to the extent of active disease.
   a. Infants with cicatricial changes often develop retinal detachment as early as 5 months of age or as late as the first and second decades of life.
   b. Myopia occurs in almost 80% of children with cicatricial ROP as early as 6 months of age and may progress rapidly.
   c. Strabismus and pseudostrabismus may occur. Pseudostrabismus occurs when the macula is dragged by peripheral cicatricial changes.
   d. Amblyopia may be due to strabismus or anisometropia.
   e. Glaucoma may be due to angle closure from a shallow anterior chamber and forward displacement of the lens-iris diaphragm in severe cicatricial ROP, usually with blindness.
   f. Displacement of the retina and vitreous membranes (50% of chronic retrolental fibroplasia) and retinal breaks may occur (retinal detachment may occur at 2 to 14 years of age from retinal breaks).

3.

GRADE	ABNORMAL FUNDUS FINDINGS	OUTCOME FOR VISUAL ACUITY
0	None	
I	Minor peripheral pigmentation	I & II
	Vascular irregularities	
	Posterior pole vascular tortuosity	Myopia, strabismus, amblyopia, corrected acuity of 20/20 to 20/100
II	I + peripheral fibrosis	
III	II + dragged retina in the posterior pole	Acuity of 20/200 to 30/300
IV	III + retinal fold	Vision of hand motion
V	Retrolental mass	Vision of some light perception or total blindness
VI	V + anterior chamber compromise	Total blindness

The grade of ROP was based upon the international classification for retrolental fibroplasia, Washington, D.C., 1981.

Adapted from Porat R.: Care of the infant with retinopathy of prematurity. *Clin. Perinatol.* 11:134, 1984.

REFERENCES

Garner A.: An international classification of retinopathy of prematurity. *Pediatrics* 74:127, 1984.

Lucey J.F., Dangman B.: A re-examination of the role of oxygen in retrolental fibroplasia. *Pediatrics* 73:82, 1984.

Glass P., Avery G.B., Subramanian K.N.S., et al.: Effect of bright light in the hospital nursery on the incidence of retinopathy of prematurity. *N. Engl. J. Med.* 313: 401, 1985.

VI. ASSISTED VENTILATION

To support adequate alveolar ventilation and oxygenation and reduce the work of breathing, assisted ventilation is provided until the infant can breathe adequately and maintain normal Pa_{O_2} and Pa_{CO_2} independently. Types of assisted ventilation include the following: intermittent positive-pressure breathing (IPPB), intermittent negative-pressure breathing, continuous positive airway pressure (CPAP), and very high frequency oscillation. Indications for each type of ventilation may be modified depending upon pulmonary pathology. Each type of assisted ventilation can be administered in various ways. One such method for each type is presented here.

A. Intermittent Positive-Pressure Breathing

IPPB is a method of periodic administration of oxygen and removal of carbon dioxide by intermittent positive-pressure application via bag and mask.

1. Indications
   a. A Pa_{O_2} less than 50 mm Hg in 40% oxygen, or
   b. A Pa_{CO_2} greater than 55 mm Hg.
   c. During emergency situation and/or when equipment fails.

2. Procedures
   a. Place the infant supine with a roll under his or her shoulder to extend the neck slightly and open the airway. Do not hyperextend the infant's neck because the airway may be compromised.
   b. Suction the infant before beginning the procedure.
   c. Select an appropriately sized mask to fit over the lower half of the infant's nose and mouth. A size 1 mask usually fits an infant less than 1,000 gm, a size 2 mask usually fits an infant 1,001 to 1,750 gm, a size 3 mask usually fits an infant 1,751 to 2,500 gm, and a size 4 mask usually fits an infant greater than 2,501 gm.
   d. Attach the mask to a 250- to 500-ml bag equipped with a 40 cm H_2O pressure safety valve.
   e. Place the mask attached to the bag over the infant's nose and mouth and ventilate the infant by gently squeezing the bag synchronized with the infant's respiration.
   f. Judge the pulmonary compliance by the degree of resistance felt during application of positive pressure. When the resistance is high, a higher pressure is required to ventilate the infant. The incidence of pneumothorax rises as a higher pressure is applied to the stiff lung.
   g. Initially, ventilate the infant for 5 to 10 minutes every ½ to 1 hour to lower a high Pa_{CO_2}. Obtain a Pa_{CO_2} level before and after ventilation to determine the efficiency of the procedure. Ventilate as frequently as needed to keep the Pa_{CO_2} or $TcPCO_2$ at the desired level (see appendix A–8, A–9).
   h. Accomplish ventilation using the infant's resting ambient oxygen concentration (or lower) as the Pa_{O_2} level rises abruptly with the procedure.
   i. Signs of adequate ventilation
      1) Upper third of chest rises with each inspiration.
      2) The infant's skin, lips, finger tips, etc., become pinker.
      3) The blood gas studies improve.
   j. Complications
      Pulmonary air leak syndrome, skin abrasions, etc.

B. Continuous Positive Airway Pressure (CPAP)

CPAP is a method to provide continuous distending pressure (CDP)—positive pressure through the expiratory phase—when the infant is breathing spontaneously. Positive end expiratory pressure (PEEP) is a method to provide CDP to an infant receiving mechanical ventilation. CPAP may improve oxygenation by the following:

Preventing progressive alveolar collapse (atelectasis) by reducing progressive increase in intrapulmonary right to left shunt, effecting a higher effective alveolar ventilation due to decreased alveolar dead space ventilation, and conserving surfactant since atelectasis consumes surfactant due to reduced surface area

Decreasing work of breathing due to the constant gas flow and decreasing total airway resistance

Increasing alveolar ventilation and decreasing dead space ventilation by regularizing breathing patterns. CPAP shortens, but intensifies, inspiratory effort while prolonging expiratory time and decreasing respiratory rate.

Increasing functional residual capacity. However, lung and dynamic compliance are reduced due to overdistension of normal air spaces rather than distension of collapsed alveoli.

Maximum increase in Pa_{O_2} is noted with low to moderate CDP. A drop of Pa_{O_2} and an increase of Pa_{CO_2} may be noted with high CDP since overdistension with decreased lung compliance decreases alveolar ventilation, capillary flow, venous return, and cardiac output.

1. Indications
   a. A Pa_{O_2} less than 50 mm Hg in 40% ambient oxygen with the infant breathing unassisted in atelectatic disease (e.g., respiratory distress syndome)
   b. Recurrent apnea
   c. Patent ductus arteriosus with or without pulmonary edema
   d. Meconium aspiration syndrome
   e. Postsurgery (cardiac, omphalocele, gastroschisis, etc.)
   f. During weaning from mechanical ventilation, particularly to prevent postextubation atelectasis
2. Indications to be used with caution
   CDP, particularly PEEP, may not be used or should be used with caution in the following conditions:
   a. Persistent pulmonary hypertension of the newborn
      CDP, especially PEEP, may increase intrapulmonary vascular resistance, enhance extrapulmonary right to left shunt, and cause further hypoxia.
   b. Pulmonary edema
      PEEP enhances extravascular fluid accumulation in the lungs due to increased pulmonary arterial pressure with normal interstitial fluid pressure. In this situation, CPAP may still increase Pa_{O_2} possibly due to increasing functional residual capacity.
   c. Meconium aspiration syndrome
      Low to moderate CDP is shown to increase Pa_{O_2}, but should be used with caution in meconium aspiration syndrome because of frequent association of meconium aspiration syndrome with persistent pulmonary hypertension of the newborn and pulmonary air leak syndrome.
3. Procedure to place an infant on CPAP
   CPAP can be administered through an endotracheal tube, nasal prongs, face mask, or head chamber. An endotracheal tube and nasal prongs are commonly used.
   a. To institute CPAP
      1) Correct hypothermia, acidosis, anemia, hypovolemia, etc.
      2) Assemble the conventional CPAP set as shown in Figure 11–6 or set the ventilator on the CPAP mode since CPAP can be delivered via a CPAP set or a ventilator in a CPAP mode.
         All the technical methods by which CPAP is delivered include a

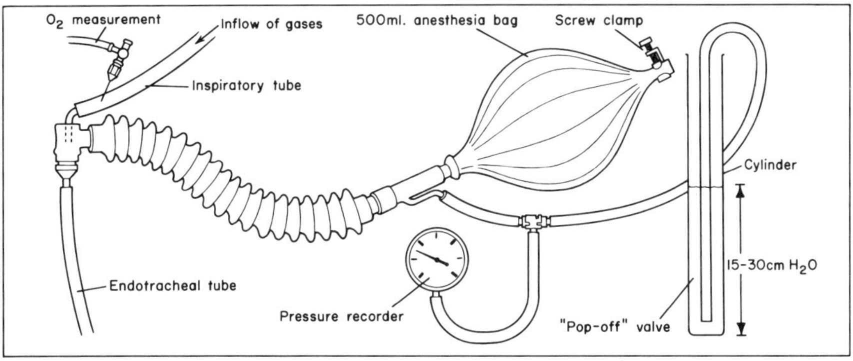

FIG 11–6.
Assembled equipment for administering conventional CPAP. (From Gregory G.: Continuous PPB therapy for neonatal respiratory distress. *Hosp. Pract.* 7:100, 1972. Used by permission.)

source of continuous gas flow, a reservoir bag, a humidifier, and a valve to produce pressures greater than ambient expiratory pressure. The amount of CPAP may be varied by changing the amount of gas flowing to the infant or the degree of obstruction to the gas outflow.

3) If the conventional CPAP set is used, set the bottom of the "pop-off" valve under 15 to 30 cm of water to prevent pneumothorax secondary to accidental occlusion of the anesthesia bag or system.
4) Apply nasal prongs or intubate the infant with an appropriately sized endotracheal tube. Try nasal prongs prior to endotracheal intubation since this method is less invasive.
5) Use warmed and humdified oxygen of the desired concentration. Measure and record the inspiratory oxygen concentration continuously with an in-line O_2 analyzer.
6) Set the flow rate at 5 to 10 L/minute with a minimum of 2 L/minute. Gas inflow should exceed two times the infant's respiratory minute volume in L/minute through the respiratory tubing: 2 × respiratory rate/minute × tidal volume (8 to 10 ml/kg). For example, for a 3-kg infant with 40 breaths/minute: 2 × 40/minute × 8 ml × 3 kg = 1.92 L/minute.
7) Prior to connecting the ventilator to the infant, if the ventilator is used, occlude nasal prongs or endotracheal tube connector and set the end expiratory pressure to 5 to 6 cm of water for nasal prongs and 3 to 4 cm of water for an endotracheal tube. If the conventional CPAP is used, adjust the screw clamp on the anesthesia bag to obtain desired pressure. Endotracheal tube CPAP can deliver the same CDP to the lungs with less flow rate and end expiratory pressure. For apnea, a CPAP of 2 to 3 cm of water may be started.
8) Attach nasal prongs or endotracheal tube connector to the infant and

re-adjust the settings. Antibiotic ointment may be applied outside the prongs.

9) Place an orogastric tube during CPAP therapy to decompress the stomach.

10) Obtain arterial blood gases within 10 to 15 minutes after the commencement of CPAP and after any change of CPAP or $F_{I_{O_2}}$.

b. When the infant's Pa_{O_2} is not improving

1) If the Pa_{O_2} is less than 50 mm Hg and Pa_{CO_2} is greater than 55 mm Hg:

a) Increase CDP pressure by 2-cm of water increments to a maximum of 12 cm of water via nasal prongs and 10 cm of water via an endotracheal tube, or

b) Increase oxygen concentrations by 5%- to 10%-increments to 60%.

2) If Pa_{O_2} is still less than 50 mm Hg with nasal CPAP, endotracheal CPAP may be employed.

3) When the Pa_{O_2} is decreasing and/or Pa_{CO_2} is increasing, reduce CDP by 2-cm of water decrements to reduce overdistension of alveoli and decreased compliance.

4) If Pa_{O_2} is still less than 50 mm Hg and Pa_{CO_2} is greater than 55 mm Hg, institute mechanical ventilation.

c. When the infant's Pa_{O_2} has improved, wean the infant from CPAP gradually.

1) Decrease oxygen concentrations by 3%- to 5%-decrements when the Pa_{O_2} is 70 mm Hg until O_2 concentration is 40%.

2) Then decrease CDP by 2-cm of water decrements gradually until CDP is 2–3 cm of water. Maintain the Pa_{O_2} between 50 and 70 mm Hg.

3) Then place the infant in an oxygen hood with 5% to 10% higher O_2 concentration when blood gases are normal on nasal CPAP of 2 to 3 cm of water for at least 4 to 6 hours and for a few days in infants with bronchopulmonary disease.

4) If apnea (of prematurity) occurs, re-institute CPAP or increase CPAP to the previous setting and decrease oxygen concentrations by 3% to 5%.

4. Complications

a. Obstruction of the endotracheal tube or nasal prongs with secretions

b. Pulmonary air leak, i.e., pneumothorax, pneumomediastinum, pulmonary interstitial emphysema. The incidence increases during recovery stage with better compliance.

c. Infection

d. Gastric dilatation and/or rupture

e. Hoarseness and/or stridor after endotracheal tube extubation, secondary subglottic edema/stenosis

f. Bronchopulmonary dysplasia

g. Aspiration during the procedure

h. Reduced cardiac output and renal blood flow and increased intracranial pressure. Secondary increase in central venous pressure (CVP) and right atrial pressure and decrease in venous return may result in reduced cardiac output.

C. Mechanical Ventilation

Mechanical ventilation is indicated to maintain normal arterial blood gases (pH, 7.30 to 7.40; Pa_{O_2}, 50 to 70 mm Hg; and Pa_{CO_2}, 35 to 45 mm Hg) when the following occur:

1. The Pa_{O_2} is less than 50 mm Hg while the infant is receiving CPAP of 10 to 12 cm of water and an ambient oxygen of greater than 60%.
2. The Pa_{CO_2} rises acutely beyond 50 to 55 mm Hg with a decrease in pH below 7.25.
3. Significant periods of apnea are present.

An infant should not be placed on a respirator unless adequately educated personnel and laboratory facilities are constantly available to maintain and support the infant's life functions. However, it must be remembered that the ventilator alone does not save infants. It is the diligence, knowledge, and skill of the physician and nursing team managing ventilatory care that facilitates the critically ill neonate's survival.

1. Types of ventilators

   Mechanical ventilation may be achieved by use of intermittent positive- or negative-pressure devices. Intermittent negative-pressure devices are rarely used and the majority of intermittent positive-pressure devices are volume or pressure limited (pressure or time cycled). In both types, compliance will change the pressure or volume.

   a. Positive-pressure ventilators

      Most of the positive-pressure ventilators available for the newborn have the following: (1) CPAP mode that can be applied to the spontaneously breathing infant, (2) IPPB mode with or without PEEP for the infant on a ventilator with or without continuous flow of gases through the circuit, and (3) intermittent mandatory ventilation (IMV) mode with continuous flow and PEEP in the circuit.

      1) Pressure-limited ventilators

         There are two types of pressure-limited ventilators: pressure cycled and time cycled.

         a) The pressure-cycled ventilator (Baby Bird, Bio-Med MVP-10) delivers a preset peak inspiratory pressure (PIP). Inspiration ends when the preset PIP is reached. To deliver the preset PIP, less tidal volume is delivered to the infant with poorer compliance in a shorter inspiratory time.
         b) The time-cycled ventilator (Int Med Bear Cub, Bourns-BP 200, Healthdyne, Sechrist) without pressure limit will end the inspiratory cycle when a preset time is reached. To deliver the preset time,

less volume is delivered, but higher pressure is generated in an infant with poor compliance.

2) The volume-limited ventilator

The volume-limited ventilator (Bourns-LS 104) delivers a preset tidal volume. Inspiration ends when the preset volume is reached. To deliver the preset volume, a higher PIP is generated to the infant with poor compliance. If there is uneven ventilation, normal areas with normal compliance will be ventilated, and areas of atelectasis may remain atelectatic.

b. Negative-pressure ventilators

Negative-pressure ventilators are rarely used today.

c. Very high frequency oscillation

Very high frequency (3 to 30 Hz, 180 to 1,800 cycles/minute) oscillation is in the research stage.

2. Establishing ventilatory settings
   a. Set up the ventilator with securely fit connectors.
   b. Turn power on.
   c. Check alarm systems.
      1) Check the power disconnect alarm. Use only grounded (three prong) plugs.
      2) Check the pressure alarm (50 PSI) of air and O_2 sources.
      3) Set the low PIP alarm to 10 cm of water.
      4) Set the high PIP limit to 30 cm of water to prevent pulmonary air leaks and reduced venous return unless the patient requires higher PIP (e.g., in infants with high Pa_{CO_2}).
      5) For the pressure-limited time cycled ventilator, set the insufficient expiratory time control usually at 0.2 seconds, which is determined by the preset inspiratory:expiratory (I:E) ratio and ventilator rate.
   d. Set the desired oxygen concentration.

      Select FI_{O_2} of the same percent as the infant has been receiving. Be certain the oxygen concentration will be monitored using continuous electronic sensors. Oxygen should be warmed and humidified.
   e. Set the mode of the ventilator.

      For either type of pressure-limited ventilator, set mode to IPPB/IMV.

      For the volume-limited ventilator, set mode to control, assist, or assist/control. The volume-limited ventilator is triggered to initiate the inspiratory cycle by the infant's respiratory effort (assist mode), by the ventilator (control mode), or by the infant's effort and the ventilator (assist/control mode) with predetermined frequency of IMV. If the infant's rate falls to 60% of the set breathing rate for 10 seconds in the assist mode, the apnea alarm will ring and the unit will remain in control for 5 seconds and then return to assist. The assist mode is not useful for the newborn since it is triggered by an inspired volume of 0.5 to 1.5 ml, which is too much for the small newborn's tidal volume, and its response time (80 msec) is too long for the infant's respiratory rate.

f. Set PIP or volume.
For either type of pressure-limited ventilator, set PIP by occluding the end of the tubing where the endotracheal tube will be connected. Dial PIP directly with the time-cycled ventilator and regulate PIP by flow rate, ventilator rate, and I:E ratio with the pressure-cycled ventilator. An initial PIP in moderate atelectatic disease (e.g., respiratory distress syndrome) would be 20–25 cm of water. Change PIP according to blood gases. Infants with severely decreased compliance and lung volume may require a high pressure. Pulmonary arterial resistance may be reduced in persistent pulmonary hypertension of the newborn with hyperventilation (increase PIP and/or increase ventilator rate). For the volume-limited ventilator, dial the volume directly. The volume to be set usually is 8 to 10 ml/kg for premature infant's tidal volume plus volume lost in the ventilator system (mainly in the tubings, usually 8 to 10 ml). Volume lost around an uncuffed endotracheal tube is proportional to alveolar pressure (with low compliance). The volume lost can be calculated as follows: (PIP − PEEP) × machine compliance. PIP and PEEP can be obtained when the machine is connected to the infant. Machine compliance is obtained when the infant is disconnected from the ventilator and the infant's connection is completely occluded and PIP is read. The machine compliance is then read on the sliding scale obtained from the ventilator company.

g. Set flow rate.
For both types of pressure-limited ventilators and volume-limited ventilators, set flow rate at approximately 5 L/minute. A minimum flow rate of at least 2L/minute (2 × minute ventilation) is required but most pressure ventilators operate at flow rates of 4 to 10 L/minute. With a low flow rate (0.5 to 3.0 L/minute), a slower inspiratory time and sine wave pressure curve are obtained (Fig 11–7). Low flow may be associated with lower mean airway pressure and hypercapnea. With high flow rates (4 to 10 L/minute), a square wave pressure curve will result and air leaks may occur (see Fig 11–7).

h. Set the ventilator rate.
For the pressure-limited pressure-cycled ventilator, set the ventilator rate by varying the I:E ratio and flow rate.
For the pressure-limited time-cycled ventilator or the volume-limited ventilator, dial directly the initial ventilator rate between 40 and 60/minute on the face of the ventilator.
Hyperventilation with a high ventilator rate (100 to 150/minute), low PIP, and low PEEP less than 5 cm of water to maintain a Pa_{CO_2} of 20 to 30 mm Hg may be required for persistent pulmonary hypertension of the newborn. Hyperventilation may be associated with air trapping and decreased compliance. A low ventilator rate less than 40/minute with or without square wave pressure curve and reverse I:E ratio will increase Pa_{O_2}, but may result in overdistension.
The pressure-limited time-cycled ventilator may be set for IMV. When the

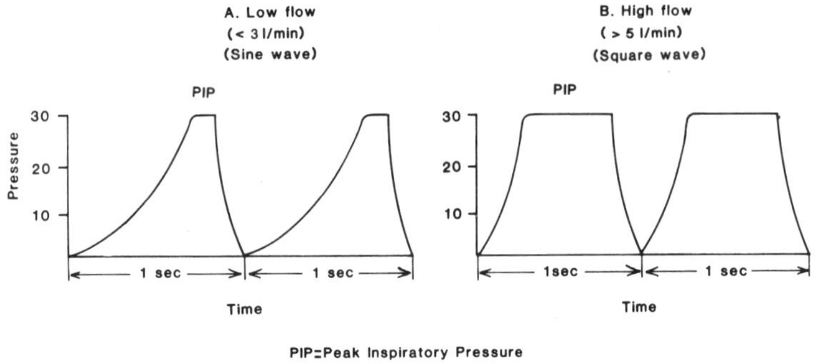

FIG 11–7.
Sine wave and square wave patterns of positive pressure ventilation. (From Fox W.W., Shutack J.G.: Positive pressure ventilation, in Goldsmith J.P., Karotkin E.H. (eds.): *Assisted Ventilation of the Neonate.* Philadelphia, W.B. Saunders Co., 1981, p. 103. Used by permission.)

infant is spontaneously breathing at his or her own rate, the machine will give the set rate in addition to the infant's own rate. The respirator provides a continuous gas flow and prevents the infant from rebreathing his or her exhaled gas in the ventilatory circuit. IMV is used for gradual withdrawal of ventilatory assist while the infant develops adequate spontaneous breathing.

i. Set the I:E ratio.

For the pressure-limited pressure-cycled ventilator, set the I:E ratio by adjusting both inspiratory and expiratory time. For the pressure-limited time-cycled ventilator, set the I:E ratio by direct dialing or adjusting the inspiratory time of the I:E ratio on the face of the ventilator.

For the volume-limited ventilator, calculation of the I:E ratio using tidal volume, ventilator rate and flow rate can be obtained from the calculator supplied by the company. At a given set of ventilator rate and tidal volume, the desired I:E ratio can be obtained by changing flow rate.

An I:E ratio of 1:1 is the most physiologic, and gas exchange takes place during the last two thirds of inspiratory time and the first one third of the expiratory cycle.

An I:E ratio of 3:1 or 2:1 (reverse) may improve distribution of ventilation in mild respiratory distress syndrome without asphyxia (studied only on the pressure-limited ventilator). A reverse I:E ratio (with high ventilator rate) is disadvantageous in severe respiratory distress syndrome particularly with asphyxia due to reduced venous return and insufficient expiratory time.

An I:E ratio of 1:2 or 3 may be used during the weaning process to avoid air trapping when oxygenation is not the problem.

j. Set PEEP.
For both types of pressure-limited and volume-limited ventilators, set PEEP by direct dialing.
For intubated infants, at least 2 to 3 cm of water PEEP is required to maintain normal end expiratory pressure and prevent atelectasis.
Moderate PEEP, 3 to 7 cm of water, is suggested for infants with atelectatic disease requiring 70% to 80% oxygen (e.g., respiratory distress syndrome). High PEEP, 8 to 10 cm of water, may be required for infants with markedly decreased compliance requiring 80% O_2. Greater than 8 cm of PEEP is often associated with pulmonary air leak syndrome.

3. Connecting the patient to the ventilator
Once the ventilator has been set to the starting settings, the physician is ready to connect the patient to the ventilator.
   a. Intubate the infant and stabilize the endotracheal tube as discussed in chapter 3.
   b. Minimize the endotracheal tube dead space. Cut the endotracheal tube approximately 1.5 cm longer than the level of the infant's lips or nares.
   c. Attach the endotracheal tube with a T-connector-adaptor to the ventilator tubings.
   d. Secure ventilator tubing to a resting (Christmas tree, Zee-Frame or Angel frame) device to prevent the tubing from pulling on the infant.
   e. Place rolls on both sides of the infant's head or a doughnut to prevent the infant's head from movement.
4. Medical management of the mechanically ventilated infant
   a. Maintain the infant's skin temperature at approximately 36.5° C.
   b. Monitor the infant's vital signs including blood pressure.
   c. Weigh the infant daily.
   d. Support the infant's fluid, electrolyte and caloric needs with appropriate intravenous and/or GI alimentation.
   e. Monitor and obtain electrolytes, BUN, blood glucose, and hematocrits as clinically indicated.
   f. Maintain the hematocrit above 40%–45% on acutely ill neonates on the ventilator.
   g. Pass a nasogastric tube and leave it in place to decompress the stomach.
   h. Be prepared with a bag and mask to administer IPPB by manual ventilation if the equipment fails.
   i. Have suction equipment readily available.
   j. Perform chest physiotherapy every 2 to 4 hours (see chapter 11–VII).
   k. Handle the infant as little as possible since handling may decrease the Pa_{O_2}.
   l. Paralyze or sedate the infant if the infant fights the ventilator or blood gases are labile. Paralysis (with pancuronium) is not usually required for newborn infants.
   m. Monitor the FI_{O_2} and follow arterial blood gases as clinically indicated. Obtain blood gases within 15 minutes of any setting change. Maintain the Pa_{O_2} between 50 and 70 mm Hg and the P_{CO_2} between 35 and 45 mm

Hg. Adjust the $F_{I_{O_2}}$, PIP, flow rate, ventilator rate, I:E ratio, and PEEP as required. Utilize $TcPO_2$ and Tc PCO_2.

n. Lower the $F_{I_{O_2}}$ as soon as clinically indicated to prevent complications of oxygen therapy.
o. Lower PIP, flow rate, ventilator rate, I:E ratio, and PEEP as soon as the infant can tolerate to prevent pulmonary air leak syndrome and reduced venous return.
p. Correct acidosis.
q. Correct hypotension with volume expander and/or dopamine (start 2 mcg/kg/minute and gradually increase to maximum dose of 20 mcg/kg/minute).
r. Change ventilator tubings every day.
s. Take cultures of endotracheal tube suction every other day and treat laryngeal-tracheal infection promptly.

5. Weaning process

As the infant is improving, decrease mechanical ventilatory support gradually. Do not decrease ventilatory settings rapidly as the "flip-flop phenomenon" may occur. This is a disproportionate drop in Pa_{O_2} in relation to the reduction of $F_{I_{O_2}}$ and failure to return to the prior Pa_{O_2} with increased $F_{I_{O_2}}$ to the previous level. There is no single well established method for weaning an infant from a ventilator. Each method must be tailored for the infant. Monitor $TcPO_2$ and $TcPo_2$ continuously and/or obtain arterial blood gas studies approximately 15 minutes after each change in ventilator setting. The following is a guideline for the pressure limited ventilator and must be modified for each individual infant depending upon pulmonary pathology and infant's size.

a. Gradually decrease PIP. Then obtain blood gases and/or monitor $TcPO_2$ and $TcPCO_2$ to ascertain that the blood gases are adequate. If so,
b. Gradually reduce $F_{I_{O_2}}$ by .05–.10. Again ascertain that blood gases are normal. If $F_{I_{O_2}}$ is high, you may reduce $F_{I_{O_2}}$ prior to reducing PIP if blood gases are adequate,
c. Reduce IMV rate gradually by 2–5 breaths per minute. If IMV rate is high, you may reduce the IMV rate prior to reducing $F_{I_{O_2}}$ or PIP.
d. When $F_{I_{O_2}}$ is .30–.40, the PIP is 15–20 cm H_2O, and IMV rate is 5/minute, gradually reduce PEEP to 2–3 cm H_2O.
e. When the PIP is 15–20 cm H_2O, $F_{I_{O_2}}$ is .40 or below and IMV rate is 5/minute, ET CPAP may be tried. Some neonatologists prefer to extubate the infant from IMV rate 5/minute and skip the ET CPAP process.
f. Extubate when the infant tolerates ET CPAP 2–3 cm H_2O for approximately 12 to 24 hours and for several days when the infant has chronic lung disease.
g. Theophylline 1–2 days prior to planning extubation may be helpful in weaning patient with respiratory distress syndrome and bronchopulmonary dysplasia because of either central stimulation and/or bronchodilatation.
h. Dexamethasone (Decadron), 0.5 to 1.0 mg IM or IV every 6 to 8 hours, may be used to reduce laryngeal edema in infants intubated longer than 72 hours (no proven benefit).
i. Suction nose and mouth and aspirate stomach contents. Prior to extuba-

tion, apply chest physiotherapy followed by re-inflation (see chapter 11–VII).

j. Send the tip of the endotracheal tube for culture.
k. Racemic epinephrine, 0.25 ml every 2 hours × 3, may be applied via micronebulizer to relieve laryngeal edema immediately after extubation.
l. After extubation, connect the infant to nasal CPAP with 5% higher O_2 and a PEEP of 4 to 6 cm of water.
m. Heart rate, blood pressure, $TcPO_2$, $TcPCO_2$ and arterial blood gases should be monitored after each change of ventilator settings.
n. Increase in retractions (work of breathing) may be caused by atelectasis, decreased compliance, or increased airway resistance.
o. Obtain a chest x-ray film 2 to 3 hours after extubation for evaluation of atelectasis.
p. Give nothing by mouth at least 8 hours after extubation or until audible cry is heard.

REFERENCES

Gregory G.A., Kitterman J.A., Phibbs R.H., et al.: Treatment of idiopathic respiratory distress syndrome with continuous positive airway pressure. *N. Engl. J. Med.* 284:1333, 1971.

Peabody J.L., Gregory G.A., Willis M.M.: Transcutaneous oxygen tension in sick infants. *Am. Rev. Resp. Dis.* 118:83, 1978.

VII. CHEST PHYSIOTHERAPY

Chest physiotherapy is necessary for infants on oxygen therapy with or without mechanical ventilator. The procedures include cupping, tapping, and vibration of the chest; suctioning; and postsuction hyperventilation. Chest physiotherapy is not without complications and is potentially dangerous since Pa_{O_2} may decrease significantly during chest physiotherapy, and bradycardia, decreased compliance, and possible CNS hemorrhage may occur after chest physiotherapy.

A. Indications

1. Infants on mechanical ventilator
2. Infants with potential and/or present atelectasis or increased volume of secretions

B. Procedures

1. Position the infant so that the area that requires suction can be aided by gravity and air flow. Position and duration should be modified for critically ill infants particularly when an endotracheal or chest tube is in place or the infant is postsurgery. Do not leave very small prematures in Trendelenburg's position (d,e,g, and h).

a. Upper lobe posterior seg: Lean forwards in sitting position.
b. Upper lobe anterior seg: Lie flat on back.
c. Upper lobe apical seg: Lean backwards in sitting position.
d. Right middle lobe, left upper lobe, left lingular seg: Elevate hips higher than head and roll backwards one-fourth turn right or left.
e. Lower lobe lateral basal seg: Place on right or left side with hips higher than head and roll forward one-fourth turn right or left.
f. Lower lobe superior seg: Lie flat on stomach.
g. Lower lobe posterior basal seg: Lie flat on stomach with hips higher than head.
h. Lower lobe anterior basal seg: Place on right or left side with hips higher than head.

2. Then cup by using neonatal palm cups (DHD medical products) or IPPB mask occluded with an adaptor to maintain the air pocket (black rubber from the piston of a 50-ml syringe occludes the mask well). Tap with fingers and/or vibrator during exhalation using a padded electric toothbrush to the infant's chest to loosen and drain secretions from the periphery of the lungs. Duration of chest physiotherapy is judged by the infant's tolerance and the frequency should depend upon the infant's need.
3. Set the vacuum pressure at about 60 to 100 mm Hg (44 to 74 cm of water: 0.736 cm H_2O/mm Hg). Higher pressure may be required for thick meconium.
4. Prepare a large-bore suction catheter to suction viscous secretions but not too large that the suction catheter exceeds more than two thirds of the endotracheal tube internal diameter as total airway obstruction will occur.

ENDOTRACHEAL TUBE SIZE (MM)	SUCTION CATHETER SIZE (FRENCH UNITS)
2.5	5
3.0	6½
3.5	6½
4.0	8

5. Maintain strict sterile techniques. It is best for two people to work together to suction an infant.
6. Instill 0.25–0.5 ml of normal saline into the endotracheal tube.
7. Give IPPB by bag via the endotracheal tube for 15 to 30 seconds with the same O_2 concentration.
8. Pass the appropriate suction catheter with a sterile, gloved hand with no suction until resistance is felt, then withdraw 0.5 to 1.0 cm.
9. Evaluate the infant's condition during the procedure as to the endotracheal tube position, color, heart rate, ventilator rate, etc.
10. Apply suction with pressure not more than 60 to 100 mm Hg (44 to 74 cm of water).
11. Do not suction longer than 30 seconds.

12. Withdraw the suction catheter with a twirling motion.
13. Apply IPPB by bag with pressure approximately 25% greater than the pressure received prior to the procedure.
14. Repeat steps 6 to 13 at different positions as the infant tolerates. Be careful not to overstress the infant as $TcPo_2$ falls during the procedure.
15. Give IPPB for 60 to 90 seconds prior to reconnection to the ventilator.
16. Monitor the infant's heart rate, color, or $TcPo_2$ during the procedure.
17. Blood-tinged secretions may be obtained from the local trauma that can lead to blockage due to blood clots, pulmonary hemorrhage, coagulopathy, necrotizing tracheobronchitis, and tracheal tears.
18. Re-evaluate the infant's condition after the procedure.

REFERENCE

Fox W.W., Schwatz J.G., Shaffer T.H.: Pulmonary physiology in neonates: Physiologic changes and respiratory management. *J. Pediatr.* 92:977, 1978.

VIII. RESPIRATORY DISTRESS SYNDROME (HYALINE MEMBRANE DISEASE)

Respiratory distress syndrome is a disease primarily of the premature infant in which pulmonary hyaline membranes and atelectasis are the principal findings at autopsy. Atelectasis is secondary to alveolar collapse from impaired or diminished surfactant production and/or release by type II alveolar cells. Diminished surfactant causes decreased lung complicance, alveolar hypoventilation, and ventilation/perfusion abnormalities. Diminished surfactant synthesis occurs in the presence of acidosis, hypothermia, hypovolemia, and hypoxia. Maternal diabetes, bleeding hypotension, and fetal/neonatal asphyxia increase the risk of occurrence. The spectrum of respiratory distress syndrome in premature infants includes not only respiratory failure (due to surfactant deficiency), but also pulmonary edema, cardiomegaly, pulmonary venous engorgement, left-to-right shunting via a patent ductus arteriosus, and others. The disease accounts for 30% of neonatal deaths and 50% of premature deaths.

A. Prevention

1. Ascertain gestational age and/or pulmonary maturity by the mother's last menstrual period, maternal pelvic examination at less than 16 weeks, ultrasonogram before the 30th week gestation, or evaluation of amniotic fluid lecithin/sphingomyelin (L/S) ratio before elective delivery. A false mature L/S ratio is seen in diabetic pregnancies and severe isoimmunization but the presence of phosphatidylglycerol (PG) indicates functionally mature lungs. The shake test may be helpful at the maternal bedside (see chapter 2 and Tables 2–2 and 2–3).

2. Delay spontaneous premature delivery with tocolytic agents if at all possible until lung maturity is assured. A decreased incidence of respiratory distress syndrome occurs in infants of mothers treated with isoxsuprine hydrochloride and ritodrine hydrochloride.
3. Avoid trauma during delivery, resuscitate promptly, avoid chilling, and correct hypoxia, hypercarbia, and acidosis quickly.
4. Various pharmacologic agents, including corticosteroids, aminophylline, thyroxine, and prolactin, have been reported to increase the quantity of surfactant. Prenatally administered glucorcorticoids to the mother in premature labor at 28 to 32 weeks' gestation when delivery is expected 24 to 72 hours later (but not later than 7 days after the dose) will lessen the incidence and severity of the disease. Routine administration of corticoids is not indicated because of possible side effects.
5. Administration of natural aerosolized surfactant for prevention and therapy is under investigation.

B. Who Is at Risk?

1. The disease occurs in 10% to 15% of less than 2,500-gm premature infants, and the incidence is inversely proportional to gestational age.
   Less than 28 weeks: 60% of infants
   32 to 36 weeks: 15% to 20% of infants
   Greater than 37 weeks: 5% of infants
2. Premature infants whose mothers bled or were hypotensive during pregnancy
3. Premature infants who developed perinatal asphyxia or who became hypoxic, acidotic, hypercapneic, or hypothermic at birth
4. Infants born by elective repeat cesarean section (possibly due to inaccurate dating of the gestational age of the infant and/or ? insufficient labor)
5. Infants with Rh incompatibility due to retardation of the development of surfactant
6. Infants of diabetic mothers, especially when the diabetes is poorly controlled
7. Males have a 1.5 times higher incidence.
8. Infants with decreased cord prolactin
9. A premature sibling of a premature infant who had respiratory distress syndrome
10. The second-born twin

C. Clinical Manifestations

Respiratory distress usually begins before 8 hours of age and may develop in the delivery room. If no signs of respiratory distress occur by 8 hours of age, the family may be assured that respiratory distress syndrome is unlikely. Uncomplicated cases are characterized by worsening of the disease for 2 to 3 days with recovery at 72 hours, and with severe disease, recovery may be delayed for days, weeks, or months. Chronic lung disease may develop.

The clinical signs of respiratory distress syndrome include the following:

1. Tachypnea, dyspnea, retractions, cyanosis in room air, and an expiratory grunt due to partial closure of the glottis on expiration to keep alveoli open
2. Apnea
3. Harsh bronchial breath sounds by auscultation
4. A tendency toward a fixed heart rate (100 to 120 beats/minute)
5. Edema
6. Systemic hypotension
7. Hypothermia despite an adequate environment temperature

D. Laboratory Findings

1. Surfactant deficiency
   a. L/S ratio less than 2 and/or absent phosphatidylglycerol in the amniotic fluid
   b. L/S ratio less than 2 and absence of phosphatidylglycerol in gastric, hypopharyngeal, or direct tracheal aspirate

   Surfactant deficiency is not specific for hyaline membrane disease as deficiency may occur with congenital pneumonia, transient tachypnea of the newborn, and other conditions.
2. Low Pa_{O_2} and/or high Pa_{CO_2} level
3. Respiratory acidosis early; respiratory and metabolic acidosis later
4. High serum bilirubin level as respiratory distress subsides
5. Nonspecific ECG findings of a tall T wave in V_1 and V_2 and prolonged PR and QRS intervals caused by increased potassium

E. Radiologic Features

1. There is a diffuse reticulogranular pattern throughout the lung fields with or without air bronchograms that is indistinguishable from (group B streptococcal) pneumonia. As the disease progresses, the lung fields may become completely opaque and obliterate the cardiac border ("white-out lung").
2. Lung volume is reduced in severe cases with normal heart size.
3. The thymic shadow may appear large at first but later becomes smaller.
4. The x-ray film appearance may clear simultaneously with clinical improvement.

F. Supportive Management

1. See chapter 11–IIIB for "general supportive management for infants with respiratory distress," 11–IV for "oxygen therapy," and 11–VI for "assisted ventilation."

2. Maintain a neutral thermal temperature.
3. Administer adequate fluids and electrolytes. Prevent fluid overload (see chapter 6–IID2).
4. Correct acid-base disturbances (see chapter 11–IIIB12).
5. Treat with penicillin and an aminoglycoside since the clinical and radiologic manifestations of (group B streptococcal) pneumonia mimic respiratory distress syndrome (see chapter 16–XV for "group B streptococcal infection").
6. Maintain venous hematocrit at 40% to 45% while on O_2 therapy.
7. Maintain effective gas exchange, systemic perfusion, and venous return.
8. Administer adequate continuous distending pressure throughout the respiratory cycle to increase Pa_{O_2} without compromising cardiovascular function.
9. High frequency positive-pressure ventilation (1 to 3 Hz, 60 to 180 cycles/minute) allows improved distribution of ventilation, lower peak inspiratory pressures, minimal interference with cardiac output, and inhibition of spontaneous ventilation.

G. Specific Therapy

Natural surfactant (homologous or heterologous, e.g., from the amniotic fluid or bovine lungs), and synthetic aerosolized phospholipids administered directly into the endotracheal tube have been shown to reduce the severity of respiratory distress syndrome and lessen the inspired O_2 and ventilatory pressure requirement. Abrupt improvements of gas exchange, ventilatory and cardiovascular changes may result in increased left to right shunt via the patent ductus arteriosus, CNS hemorrhage, necrotizing enterocolitis, air leak syndrome, and decreased endogenous surfactant secretion (no evidence yet). Serious chronic lung disease (bronchopulmonary dysplasia) associated with surfactant administration may be related to immunologic abnormality and autoantibodies. Because of possible serious complications and few long-term follow-up studies, surfactant administration is not recommended for routine respiratory distress syndrome therapy at this time.

H. Complications

Complications are frequently related to therapeutic intervention and include the following:

1. Pulmonary air leak syndrome
2. Tracheal erosions, stenosis, and metaplasia
3. Bronchopulmonary dysplasia
4. Intracranial hemorrhage
5. Patent ductus arteriosus
6. Left heart failure due to a patent ductus arteriosus and immature left ventricle
7. Hydrostatic pulmonary and alveolar edema due to low plasma oncotic pressure and retained fetal lung fluid
8. Infection

9. Retinopathy of prematurity
10. Surfactant deficiency

I. Prognosis

1. Developmental handicaps
   a. Infants greater than 1,500 gm have been reported to have a 15% incidence of severe handicaps.
   b. Infants less than 1,500 gm have been reported to have a 35% incidence of severe handicaps when requiring mechanical ventilation.

REFERENCES

Collaborative group on antenatal steroid therapy: Effect of antenatal dexamethasone administration on the prevention of respiratory distress syndrome. Sponsored by the Division of Lung Diseases, National Heart, Lung, and Blood Institute, NIH, Bethesda, Md. *Am. J. Obstet. Gynecol.* 141:276, 1981.

Fawcett W.A., Gluck L.: Respiratory distress syndrome in the tiny baby. *Clin. Perinatol.* 4:411, 1977.

Fujiwara T., Maeta H., Chida S., et al.: Artificial surfactant therapy in hyaline membrane disease. *Lancet* 1:55, 1980.

Hallman M., Gluck L.: Respiratory distress syndrome: Update 1982. *Ped. Clin. N. Am.* 29:1057, 1982.

IX. TRANSIENT TACHYPNEA OF THE NEWBORN

Transient tachypnea of the newborn (wet lung) is defined as respiratory distress due to a delay in the resorption of fetal lung fluid. The diagnosis is made by exclusion of other causes of respiratory distress.

A. Who Is at Risk?

1. Term infants or close-to-term premature infants
2. Infants born by cesarean section
3. Infants whose mothers were oversedated or received sodium-free solution
4. Infants with polycythemia or delayed cord clamp

B. Clinical Manifestations

1. Cyanosis, grunting, flaring, and tachypnea without dyspnea in a nonasphyxiated term or close-to-term premature infant
2. Respiratory and radiologic improvement occurs over 12 to 72 hours, and the disease is self-limiting.

C. Laboratory Findings

1. Laboratory findings are usually normal.
2. Some degree of hypoxia may be present.
3. Lung secretions on the first day may show decreased surfactant.

D. Radiologic Features

1. Chest x-ray film shows prominent perihilar streaking (sunburst pattern) with fluid in the minor fissure or costophrenic angles.

E. Supportive Management

1. Rule out other causes of respiratory distress, such as respiratory distress syndrome, group B streptococcal pneumonia, and cerebral hyperventilation.
2. See chapter 11–IIIB for "general supportive management for infants with respiratory distress."
3. Maintain adequate oxygenation. Infants may need oxygen therapy but a requirement for CPAP or assisted ventilation is unusual. If the infant requires more respiratory support than oxygen alone, be suspicious that another respiratory process may be present.

F. Specific Therapy

A specific therapy is unknown.

G. Prognosis

There is no known residual pulmonary dysfunction.

REFERENCES

James D.K., Chiswick M.L., Harkes A., et al.: Specificity of surfactant deficiency in neonatal respiratory disorders. *Br. Med. J.* 288:1635, 1984.

Sundell H., Garrott J., Blankenship W.J.,, et al.: Studies on infants with type II respiratory distress syndrome. *J. Pediatr.* 78:754, 1971.

X. APNEA

Apnea is defined as a cessation of breathing for more than 20 seconds and usually occurs in conjunction with periodic breathing (recurrent sequences of cessation of breathing of 5 to 10 seconds followed by 10 to 15 seconds of rapid respiration). Premature infants have reduced respiratory response to hypercarbia, biphasic respiratory response to hypoxia (increased respiration by stimulated chemoreceptor, followed by decreased respiration via respiratory center depression), and functional immaturity of pulmonary irritant receptor.

A. Prevention

1. Prevent oropharyngeal obstruction in small premature infants. Do not flex or hyperextend excessively the infant's head or neck.

2. Prevent hypoxia. See chapter 11–IIIB for "general supportive management for infants with respiratory distress."
3. Prevent metabolic derangements. Follow calcium, glucose, and electrolytes carefully and correct if necessary.
4. Minimize infant care procedures that may increase vagal tone, feed slowly, and remove indwelling nasogastric tube if apnea occurs frequently. Handling of small premature infants is often associated with falling $TcPo_2$.
5. Maintain neutral thermal temperature (36.5° C skin temperature).

B. Who Is at Risk?

1. The premature infant: At least 25% to 50% of premature infants experience apneic episodes. Classic (idiopathic) "apnea of prematurity" occurs at 72 hours of age (central apnea). The more immature the infant, the greater the incidence and severity.
2. Infants with tissue hypoxia: hypoxia, anemia, shock, patent ductus arteriosus, etc.
3. Infants with CNS dysfunction: CNS hemorrhage, seizure disorder, metabolic derangements (hypoglycemia, hypocalcemia, hyponatremia, hypernatremia, dehydration, hyperammonemia, etc.), or CNS infection can present as apnea.
4. Infants with increased vagal tone: stomach dilatation secondary to overfeeding, rapid feeding, indwelling nasogastric tube, gastroesophageal reflux, and rectal stimulation can present as apnea.
5. Infants with hypothermia or hyperthermia: this phenomenon is seen especially with rapid rewarming.
6. Infants with maternal and/or neonatal drug effects (see Table 2–5)

C. Clinical Manifestations

1. Apnea is usually associated with cyanosis and a decrease in heart rate and pH.
   a. Central apnea is defined as simultaneous cessation of both respiratory movements and airflow at the mouth or nose.
   b. Obstructive apnea is defined as absence of airflow while respiratory movements continue.

   Central apnea is frequently seen in immature newborns often during active (REM) sleep while obstructive apnea is frequently seen in infants beyond 1 month of age.

D. Laboratory Findings

1. Metabolic derangements (occasionally)
2. Positive bacterial cultures (occasionally)
3. Abnormal blood gases
4. Abnormal spinal fluid (occasionally)

5. Intraventricular, subependymal, subarachnoid, or subdural hemorrhage
6. Often no abnormal laboratory findings are present.

Be aware that the aforementioned findings are associations only. One may appropriately correct abnormal findings only to find that apnea continues.

E. Supportive Management

1. Maintain a clear airway. Aspirate oropharynx.
2. Maintain the infant at a neutral thermal temperature.
3. Study the infant appropriately (e.g., electrolytes, glucose, calcium, BUN, CBC, blood gases, cultures, liver function, chest x-ray film, ECG, barium swallow, pneumogram, cranial sonography, and EEG). Correct if abnormal. See appropriate chapters for methods of correction.
4. Correct positioning and avoid overfeeding.
5. Monitor respiratory and heart rate continuously.

F. Specific Therapy

1. Attempt to abolish apneic episodes in the following manner:
   a. Institute tactile or proprioceptive stimulation by flicking the sole of the infant's foot or rubbing the infant's chest.
   b. If bradycardia persists and infant is cyanotic, administer oxygen. Obtain Pa_{O_2} and avoid administering excessive oxygen.
   c. If the apneic episodes continue, institute IPPB by bag and mask. Intermittent tactile stimulation, apnea mattress, or water bed may be helpful.
2. If apnea appears intractable, consider nasal CPAP, xanthine derivatives, or mechanical ventilation.
   a. Nasal CPAP, 3 to 5 cm of water, will abolish apnea in the majority of prematures possibly due to increasing functional residual capacity, increasing oxygenation, influencing stretch reflexes, and stabilizing alveoli (see chapter 11–VIB).
   b. Xanthine derivatives (e.g., theophylline) may be effective in the treatment of neonatal apnea by modifying the respiratory center's activity, increasing the respiratory center sensitivity to CO_2, and improving cardiac contractibility and output.
      1) Theophylline (orally)
         Maintenance: 1.1 mg/kg/6 to 8 hours after loading with 5.5 mg/kg
      2) Aminophylline (IV) (contains 70% to 85% theophylline)
         Maintenance: 2 mg/kg/8 to 12 hours after loading with 7 mg/kg
      3) Caffeine
         Maintenance: 2.5 mg/kg/day single dose (orally or IV) after loading with 10 mg/kg

   Monitor blood levels carefully; keep xanthine level at 10 to 15 μg/ml. Observe for side effects (tachycardia, diuresis, jitteriness, seizures, hyperglycemia, abdominal distension, vomiting, and others).

If no further apnea is noted for 7 to 14 days, then theophylline can be slowly tapered in 3 to 7 days. Observe the infant for at least 1 week after discontinuation.

c. Mechanical ventilation may be required if the infant does not improve with xanthine therapy (see chapter 11–VI).

REFERENCES

Anderson J.V., Martin R.J., Fanaroff A.A.: Neonatal respiratory control and apnea of prematurity. *Perinatol. Neonatol.* 7:65, 1983.

Aranda J.V., Turmen T.: Methylxanthines in apnea of prematurity. *Clin. Perinatol* 6:87, 1979.

Kattwinkel J.: Neonatal apnea: Pathogenesis and therapy. *J. Pediatr.* 90:342, 1977.

Rigatto H., Brady J.P.: Periodic breathing and apnea in preterm infants: I. Evidence for hypoventilation possibly due to central respiratory depression. *Pediatrics* 50:202, 1972.

Rigatto H., Brady J.P.: Periodic breathing in preterm infants: II. Hypoxia as a primary event. *Pediatrics* 50:219, 1972.

XI. PNEUMONIA

Pneumonia is the most common serious infection occurring during the perinatal period, and may be acquired prenatally, perinatally, or postnatally. The mortality rate for bacterial pneumonia is quite high. Early recognition of infection in the newborn and prompt antibiotic therapy have reduced mortality.

A. Who Is at Risk

1. Congenital pneumonia via transplacental and/or ascending infection
   a. Infants with maternal history of urinary tract infection, prolonged rupture of membranes, prolonged labor, obstetric manipulation, etc.
   b. Premature, "sick," asphyxiated, or compromised newborns
   c. Infants with intrauterine infection (TORCH syndrome)

   Organisms involved are group B streptococci, *Escherichia coli, Klebsiella,* group D streptococci, *Listeria,* pneumococci, staphylococci, *Chlamydia trachomatis,* and TORCH (see chapter 16–III).
2. Infection (pneumonia) acquired in the nursery
   a. Infants may become infected through human contact (hands) or contaminated equipment, particularly infants on assisted ventilation.
   b. Infants with congenital anomalies, e.g., tracheoesophageal fistula, choanal atresia, diaphragmatic hernia, CNS malformations, or congenital heart disease, are at high risk.

   Those infections acquired in the newborn nursery are frequently caused by *Pseudomonas, Klebsiella, Staphylococcus,* and *Proteus.* Respiratory syncytial virus or *Candida* may occasionally cause pneumonia in the newborn.

B. Clinical Manifestations

1. Infants with congenital (or intrauterine) pneumonia often are stillborn or critically ill with asphyxia, apnea, and respiratory distress at birth. Infants may die within 24 hours.
2. Infants with pneumonia acquired postnatally have respiratory distress: cyanosis, tachypnea, retractions, grunting, apnea with rales or decreased breath sounds, or general signs of sepsis (temperature instability, weak cry, poor suck, decreased activity, weak Moro's reflex, lethargy, etc.).

C. Laboratory Findings

Laboratory findings are usually not significant, but if abnormal, aid in diagnosis.

1. Leukocytosis or leukopenia with shift to left
2. Thrombocytopenia
3. Positive gram's stain and/or cultures of tracheal aspirates
4. Lung biopsy should not be a routine procedure, but may be of help for the diagnosis of *Pneumocystis carinii.*
5. Increased cord blood IgM for intrauterine infection

D. Radiologic Features

1. Patchy densities in parenchyma with linear streaking toward the periphery
2. Confluent mottled opacities
3. Diffuse reticulogranular appearance with air bronchogram mimicking findings in respiratory distress syndrome, particularly with group B streptococci, pneumococci, *Hemophilus influenzae,* or others
4. "Snowstorm" appearance of meconium aspiration syndrome with severe pneumonia
5. Pleural effusion, abscess cavities, and pneumatoceles are frequently seen in staphylococcal pneumonia and less frequently in group A streptococcal, *E. coli,* or *Klebsiella* pneumonia.
6. Prominent perihilar streaking with fluid in the fissure

E. Supportive Management

See chapter 11–IIIB for "general supportive management for infants with respiratory distress," 11–IV for "oxygen therapy" and 11–VI for "assisted ventilation."

F. Specific Therapy

1. Administer antibiotics after blood, CSF, (endotracheal aspirates, if present), and urine cultures have been obtained.
   a. Ampicillin, 100 mg/kg/day IV in two divided doses (see Table 16–1)

b. Gentamicin, 3 to 5 mg/kg/day IM in two divided doses (see Table 16–1) or other aminoglycosides
2. Change or maintain the single most effective antibiotic depending upon sensitivities, and treat for at least 10 days.
3. Drainage of pleural effusion with or without intrapleural instillation of antibiotic has been recommended for staphylococcal effusion and abscess (e.g., penicillin G, 10,000 units; ampicillin, 10 mg; or nafcillin or methicillin, 10 mg, diluted with 5 to 10 ml of normal saline) for 1 hour with clamped chest tube three or four times daily.

REFERENCES

Harris H., Wirtschafter D., Cassady G.: Endotracheal intubation and its relationship to bacterial colonization and systemic infection of newborn infants. *Pediatrics* 58:816, 1976.
Sherman M.P., Goetzman B.W., Ahlfors C.E., et al.: Tracheal aspiration and its clinical correlates in the diagnosis of congenital pneumonia. *Pediatrics* 65:258, 1980.

XII. MECONIUM ASPIRATION SYNDROME

Normal fetal breathing movement is associated with movement of lung fluid from the airway into the amniotic fluid. Gasping induced by hypoxia and acidosis in utero is a forceful inspiration that may cause meconium-contaminated amniotic fluid to enter the lung. This occurs rarely in utero, but frequently the first respiratory efforts after birth force any fluid present in the nasopharynx or trachea into the smaller airways. Meconium fills the alveoli, impairs normal ventilation, obstructs the trachea and bronchi, and prevents expansion of the lungs. Rapid distal migration of meconium results in airway obstruction, areas of atelectasis from total small airway obstruction, and areas of overexpansion (emphysema) from gas trapping with partial obstruction. In 8% to 20% of all deliveries, meconium is passed in utero as a response to fetal asphyxia.

A. Prevention

1. Prevent perinatal asphyxia.
2. Suction meconium from the trachea and pharynx while the infant's head is on the perineum prior to the onset of respiration since severe pulmonary involvement can be almost completely prevented by this procedure.
3. Suction the trachea and pharynx under direct vision prior to the first breath. Meconium may remain in the trachea more than 20 minutes despite spontaneous respirations. In 1 hour, meconium may reach small airways.

B. Who Is at Risk?

1. All infants with meconium-stained amniotic fluid are considered to have had fetal distress and are at risk to develop meconium aspiration syndrome. See chapter 15–IV for "perinatal asphyxia."

a. Postmature infants
b. Infants who are small for gestational age, usually greater than 34 weeks' gestation
c. Infants with a maternal history of prolonged labor, hypertensive disease of pregnancy, prolapsed cord, breech extraction, maternal hemorrhage, hypotension, abruptio placentae, or other conditions

C. Clinical Manifestations

Many infants with meconium-stained amniotic fluid are not in any distress. Infants who aspirate meconium manifest respiratory distress within a few hours after birth, which may be mild or fulminating.

1. Depressed, irregular, or gasping respiration at birth that becomes labored tachypneic breathing later on
2. Increased anteroposterior diameter of the chest (barrel-shaped chest)
3. Coarse bronchial sounds, prolonged expiration, and rales may be audible.
4. Cyanosis. Occasionally severe cyanosis not improved by oxygen therapy may be present due to concurrent persistent pulmonary hypertension of the newborn.

D. Radiologic Features

1. Hyperinflation with flattened diaphragm
2. Unilateral or bilateral coarse; irregular, streaky densities (infiltration) with areas of atelectasis or hyperaeration. Massive aspiration is characterized by a "snowstorm" appearance with cardiomegaly.
3. Radiologic findings consistent with pulmonary air leaks: pneumothorax, pulmonary interstitial emphysema, and pneumomediastinum frequently develop
4. Pleural effusion may be present.

E. Laboratory Findings

1. Metabolic acidosis initially during the first few hours of life that reflects prenatal or perinatal hypoxia
2. Respiratory alkalosis in mild meconium aspiration syndrome and respiratory and metabolic acidosis in severe meconium aspiration syndrome
3. Hypoxia (decreased Pa_{O_2}) due to abnormal ventilation perfusion ratio (air trapping), intrapulmonary right-to-left shunt (atelectasis), and reduced diffusion and dynamic lung compliance (chemical pneumonitis)
4. Hypercarbia (CO_2 retension) due to alveolar hypoventilation and increased dead space ventilation in spite of increased minute ventilation

F. Supportive Management

1. See chapter 11–III B for "general supportive management for infants with respiratory distress," 11–IV for "oxygen therapy," and 11–VI for "assisted ventilation."
2. Continuous distending pressure (CPAP or PEEP) improves arterial oxygenation and occasionally decreases Pa_{CO_2} possibly due to a decrease in intrapulmonary shunt. However, CDP should be used with caution since it may reduce venous return and cardiac output and induce hypotension, acidosis, and pulmonary air leak syndrome.
3. Begin antibiotic therapy after cultures of blood, spinal fluid, and urine have been obtained since sepsis in utero may have been the precipitating cause of meconium aspiration (controversial).
   a. Ampicillin, 100 mg/day IV in two divided doses
   b. Gentamicin, 5 mg/kg/day IM in two divided doses, or other aminoglycosides
4. Observe closely for development of pulmonary air leaks.
5. Assess the infant's neurologic status closely since perinatal asphyxia with meconium aspiration may predispose the infant to convulsions and/or neurologic sequelae.
6. Steroids are not of value.
7. Meconium aspiration may be associated with persistent pulmonary hypertension of the newborn (see chapter 11–XIII).
8. Extracorporeal membrane oxygenation (ECMO) may be life-saving.

G. Specific Therapy

No specific therapy is known to remove meconium from the alveoli.

H. Complications

1. Pulmonary air leak syndrome
2. Persistent pulmonary hypertension of the newborn
3. Secondary bacterial infection
4. Subglottic stenosis if intubated
5. Pulmonary hemorrhage

I. Prognosis

Prognosis is dependent upon the initial asphyxial insult.

REFERENCES

Bancalari E., Berlin J.A.: Meconium aspiration and other asphyxial disorders. *Clin. Perinatol.* 5:317–334, 1978.

Carson B.S., Losey R.W., Bowes W.A. Jr., et al.: Combined obstetric and pediatric approach to prevent meconium aspiration syndrome. *Am. J. Obstet. Gynecol.* 126:712, 1976.
Fox W.W., Berman L.S., Downes J. Jr., et al.: The therapeutic application of end-expiratory pressure in the meconium aspiration syndrome. *Pediatrics* 56:214, 1975.

XIII. PERSISTENT PULMONARY HYPERTENSION OF THE NEWBORN (PERSISTENT FETAL CIRCULATION)

Persistent pulmonary hypertension of the newborn (PPHN) is a clinical entity wherein pulmonary hypertension, right-to-left shunting (via a patent ductus arteriosus and/or foramen ovale), and severe hypoxia occur with a structurally normal heart. PPHN may be primary or secondary to various conditions associated with pulmonary vasoconstriction (e.g., hypoxia or acidosis). Primary PPHN was first described as persistent fetal circulation with pulmonary hypertension and normal cardiac function without primary pulmonary pathology in term infants.

A. Who Is at Risk?

1. Term or preterm infants with pulmonary vasoconstriction secondary to asphyxia with or without severe pulmonary disease (e.g., meconium aspiration syndrome), group B streptococcal or E. coli (or other bacterial) sepsis, premature ductal closure, maternal ingestion of prostaglandin inhibitors (aspirin or indomethacin), and other conditions
2. Infants with functional obstruction of pulmonary vascular bed, e.g., hyperviscosity syndrome (polycythemia)
3. Infants with structural obstruction of pulmonary vascular bed, e.g., pulmonary hypoplasia, congenital or secondary (Potter's syndrome, diaphragmatic hernia, oligohydramnios syndrome)
4. Infants with left-sided heart failure (hypoplastic left heart syndrome, coarctation of aorta, endocardial fibroelastosis, etc.) or other coronary heart diseases, such as infradiaphragmatic total anomalous pulmonary venous return, mitral obstruction, or transient left ventricular dysfunction due to hypoxia
5. Infants with increased pulmonary blood flow, e.g., peripheral arteriovenous fistula, single ventricle without pulmonary stenosis, endocardial cushion defect.

B. Clinical Manifestations

Clinical manifestations are nonspecific.

1. Marked cyanosis in oxygen greater than 60% and/or sudden changes of color from pink to cyanotic in a matter of seconds (very sensitive to manipulation) at birth or as late as 24 hours of age. Early onset is seen in perinatal asphyxia and pulmonary hypoplasia; intermediate onset in meconium aspiration, group B streptococcal infection, and moderately severe pulmonary hypoplasia; and

late onset in idiopathic pulmonary disease and mild pulmonary hypoplasia. This condition is difficult to differentiate from cyanotic heart disease.
2. Increased anteroposterior diameter of chest
3. Retractions, tachypnea
4. Visible or easily palpable prominent right ventricular impulse at the lower left sternal border
5. Single, loud second heart sound or narrow, split second heart sound with loud pulmonic component
6. Pulmonary systolic ejection click due to dilated main pulmonary artery
7. Long, harsh systolic murmur at the lower left sternal border of tricuspid insufficiency or at the apex due to mitral insufficiency (in perinatal asphyxia)
8. Signs compatible with the underlying cause

C. Laboratory Findings

1. Low Pa_{O_2} with O_2 greater than 60% and very sensitive to handling
   a. When the infant has right-to-left shunting via a patent ductus arteriosus, simultaneously obtained preductal Pa_{O_2} from the right arm or right temporal artery is approximately 15 to 20 mm Hg higher than postductal Pa_{O_2} from the descending aorta. The absence of ductal shunt does not rule out PPHN. Similar pre- and postductal Pa_{O_2} may be seen with right-to-left shunting via both PDA and foramen ovale.
   b. Hyperoxia-hyperventilation test
   Hyperventilation with 100% O_2 and a high ventilatory rate of 100 to 150/minute, which decrease Pa_{CO_2} to less than 20 to 30 mm Hg, will reduce pulmonary artery pressure, reverse the right-to-left shunt, and increase Pa_{O_2} to greater than 100 mm Hg at least once. In cyanotic congenital heart disease, hyperventilation does not increase Pa_{O_2} significantly.
2. Acidosis
3. Right axis deviation and right ventricular hypertrophy and/or ST depression in the midprecordial leads and T-wave inversion in the left precordial leads on ECG
4. Echocardiogram findings
   a. Prolonged biventricular systolic time interval
      1) A prolonged right pre-ejection period (RPEP) and shortened right ventricular ejection time (RVET) (increased RPEP/RVET ratio) indicate increased pulmonary vascular resistance and pulmonary hypertension.
      2) A prolonged left pre-ejection period (LPEP) and a shortened left ventricular ejection time (LVET) (increased LPEP/LVET ratio) indicate left ventricular dysfunction.
   b. Contrast M mode may reveal the degree of right-to-left intra-atrial shunt.
   c. Decreased myocardial function due to ischemia
5. Increased total or alveolar ventilation and tidal volume and a large alveolar-arterial O_2 and CO_2 gradient because of many overventilated, underperfused alveoli

6. For secondary PPHN, findings consistent with primary problems are present. CBC, platelet count, blood sugar, serum calcium, and chest x-ray film are helpful in diagnosis.

D. Radiologic Features

1. Clear or hyperinflated pulmonary parenchyma; often with decreased pulmonary vascular markings secondary to pulmonary underperfusion
2. Findings consistent with primary pulmonary parenchymal disease
3. Prominent pulmonary artery segment
4. Cardiomegaly (cardiothoracic ratio greater than 0.60 on an anteroposterior projection)
5. Prominent right side of heart border suggesting tricuspid insufficiency

E. Supportive Management

1. See chapter 11–IIIB for "general supportive management of infants with respiratory distress," 11–IV for "oxygen therapy," and 11–VI for "assisted ventilation." Pharmacologic paralysis may be of value.
2. Extracorporeal membrane oxygenators (ECMO) may be attempted when hyperventilation and vasodilator do not increase Pa_{O_2} for term or near-term infants.

F. Specific Therapy

1. Treat the primary cause of the increased pulmonary vascular resistance. Correct hypoxia, acidosis, hypoglycemia, or other causes.
2. Decrease pulmonary artery pressure.
   a. Hyperventilate with mechanical ventilator. Maintain low Pa_{CO_2} less than 20 to 30 mm Hg with high ventilatory rate of 100 to 150/minute and adequate but lowest PIP possible. Ventilator-induced respiratory alkalosis often is effective in inducing pulmonary vasodilation. Infants with PPHN are very sensitive to changes of ventilator settings. Weaning process should be very slow with 1% O_2 or 1 cm of water PIP changes at a time. After 2 to 3 days of hyperventilation, when the infant no longer demonstrates P_{O_2} sensitivity, the Pa_{CO_2} may be increased to 35 to 45 mm Hg to prevent pulmonary air leak syndrome or chronic lung damage (bronchopulmonary dysplasia). Hyperventilation should be administered with extreme caution for premature infants with respiratory distress syndrome since pulmonary air leak syndrome is common.
   b. Administer tolazoline when hyperventilation fails to improve Pa_{O_2} through a peripheral scalp or arm vein to facilitate infusion into pulmonary vascular bed via the superior vena cava. Tolazoline increases Pa_{O_2} in approximately 60% of infants with PPHN possibly due to significant hemodynamic

alterations and decreases in pulmonary vascular resistance (more than systemic resistance). Correct hypotension prior to starting tolazoline.

1) Tolazoline dose
   Loading: 1 to 2 mg/kg over 10 minutes
   Maintenance: 0.28 mg/kg/hour IV
   Tolazoline is an adrenergic blocker and can cause systemic histamine release.
2) Side effects
   a) Histamine-like effect: from abdominal distension to severe GI hemorrhage
   b) Hyponatremia possibly due to oliguria and/or GI loss
   c) Hypotension
   d) Oliguria, hematuria
   e) Pulmonary hemorrhage (due to thrombocytopenia)
   f) Possible seizures

   If hypotension develops, discontinue tolazoline and correct with volume expanders and dopamine infusion, starting with a dose of 2 to 5 μg/kg/minute and increasing to a maximum of 15 to 20 μg/kg/minute. Avoid a high dopamine dose of greater than 4 μg/kg/minute if possible for infants with PPHN since sudden discontinuation of high dose may significantly increase pulmonary vascular resistance/systemic resistance, suddenly increase right-to-left shunt, and deteriorate the infant's condition.

G. Prognosis

High incidence of poor neurodevelopment with hearing loss has been reported.

REFERENCES

Drummond W.H., Gregory G.A., Heymann M.A., et al.: The independent effects of hyperventilation, tolazaline and dopamine on infants with persistent pulmonary hypertension. *J. Pediatr.* 98:603, 1981.

Gersony W.M., Duc G.V., Sinclair J.C.: "PFC" syndrome. *Circulation* (A) 40(suppl. 2): III–87, 1969.

Fox W.W., Duara S.: Persistent pulmonary hypertension in the neonate: Diagnosis and management. *J. Pediatr.* 103:505, 1983.

Philips J.B. III (ed.): Neonatal pulmonary hypertension. *Clin. Perinatol.* 11(3), 1984.

XIV. PULMONARY AIR LEAK SYNDROME

Pulmonary air leaks may occur as pneumothorax, pneumomediastinum, pulmonary interstitial emphysema, or pneumopericardium. The physician must be aware a pulmonary air leak may develop in those infants receiving assisted ventilation or spontaneously at any time. The overall incidence is reported to be approximately 1% of live births.

Pneumothorax is the most common type of pulmonary air leak syndrome and develops secondary to dissection of pulmonary interstitial emphysema into the mediastinal space and subsequent rupture of mediastinal air into the pleural space. A pneumothorax may progress to a tension pneumothorax, which will shift the mediastinum and compromise and compress the contralateral lung.

Pneumomediastinum develops secondary to interstitial air movement medially along the bronchi. Ultimately, the parenchymal air dissects into the mediastinal space.

Pulmonary interstitial emphysema (PIE) is usually the result of positive intra-alveolar pressure secondary to assisted ventilation (mechanical or manual) or spontaneous Valsalva's maneuvers associated with crying.

Pneumopericardium occurs secondary to dissection of pulmonary interstitial emphysema medially along vascular sheaths (great vessels, especially) and ultimate rupture into the pericardial space. Pneumopericardium usually occurs in association with the mechanically ventilated newborn who has other extra-alveolar air leaks.

A. Who Is at Risk?

1. Infants who have meconium aspiration syndrome (20% to 50%) or aspirated blood or gastric contents
2. Infants with atelectatic disease (e.g., respiratory distress syndrome or hypoplastic lungs). In infants with respiratory distress syndrome, pneumothorax usually occurs during the recovery stage with improvement of lung compliance.
3. Infants who have had vigorous resuscitation at birth or high positive mean airway pressure with assisted ventilation
4. Infants with renal malformations with pulmonary hypoplasia
5. Infants with pneumothorax rarely develop pneumoperitoneum through the diaphragmatic apertures
6. Infants <1500 gm requiring PIP > 25 cm H_2O (high mortality with PIE)

B. Clinical Manifestations

1. Often asymptomatic
2. Increasing respiratory distress: tachypnea, retractions, grunting, and cyanosis. When sudden deterioration occurs, pneumothorax should be considered.
   a. Pneumothorax
      Symptoms are decreased movement or distension of the thorax, a decrease in breath sounds, and an increase in resonance to percussion of the affected thorax in addition to shift of the mediastinum (cardiac apex, trachea, etc.) away from the affected side if unilateral. A sudden deterioration with persistent cyanosis, pallor, hypotension, and bradycardia may be present.
   b. Pneumomediastinum
      The infant is usually asymptomatic, but may have respiratory distress with a barrel chest (increased anteroposterior diameter).

c. Pulmonary interstitial emphysema
The usual presenting symptom is sudden deterioration of the infant's clinical condition often associated with pneumothorax or pneumopericardium. The high mortality has been reported particularly in the first 24 hours of life.

d. Pneumopericardium
Symptoms may be absent or occur secondary to cardiac tamponade with reduced stroke volume and venous return and include muffled heart sounds, hypotension, decreased pulse pressure, extreme cyanosis, and friction sound (rare).

C. Laboratory Findings

1. Pneumothorax
Transillumination of the chest with a transilluminating light (Chun Gun or Welch-Allyn fiberoptic transilluminator) has been extremely helpful as an immediate aid. Increased transillumination of the hemithorax ipsilateral to the pneumothorax supports the diagnosis. Increased vasopressin with syndrome of inappropriate antidiuretic hormone is often seen.
2. Pneumopericardium
Low voltage of R waves in the ECG.

D. Radiologic Features

1. Pneumothorax
   a. Free air outlines the partially collapsed lung.
   b. Pulmonary markings are absent beyond the border of the collapsed lung.
   c. A tension pneumothorax will be associated with a mediastinal shift, atelectasis of the contralateral lung, and downward displacement of the diaphragm. Because of poor compliance in respiratory distress syndrome, total lung collapse is rarely seen even with a tension pneumothorax.
2. Pneumomediastinum
   a. On anteroposterior view of the chest, areas of radiolucency are noted in the mediastinum.
   b. On the lateral and oblique chest x-ray films, the thymus is lifted upward by mediastinal air ("sail" sign on anteroposterior chest film).
3. Pulmonary interstitial emphysema
   a. A diffuse, rarely localized pattern of multiple linear and/or small cystlike radiolucent areas radiating to the lung periphery with radiologically increasing lung volume is visible. Pseudocysts, a localized pulmonary interstitial emphysema within the parenchyma beneath the visceral pleura or along fissure lines, appear as single or multiple circular areas of radiolucency that are well demarcated. This is seen occasionally for weeks in infants with respiratory distress syndrome or high mean airway pressure.
   b. The radiographic findings may resolve or may progress to pneumothorax, pneumomediastinum, pneumopericardium, or pneumoperitoneum. Pro-

gression to subcutaneous emphysema is uncommon during the neonatal period.

4. Pneumopericardium
   a. Air encircling the heart on both the anteroposterior and lateral views may be seen.
   b. The pericardial lining may be visualized with mediastinal air lying directly outside and around the pericardial sac.

E. Supportive Management

1. See chapter 11–IIIB for "general supportive management for infants with respiratory distress," 11–IV for "oxygen therapy," and 11–VI for "assisted ventilation."
2. If an infant develops spontaneous unexplained pneumothorax or pneumomediastinum, a thorough physical examination and appropriate laboratory studies for underlying renal malformations should be performed.

F. Specific Therapy

1. Asymptomatic infants with pneumothorax or pneumomediastinum require observation.
2. Symptomatic infants
   a. Pneumothorax
      1) Immediate relief of pneumothorax may be a life-saving procedure and may also prevent CNS hemorrhage.
         If the respiratory distress increases or the infant's clinical condition deteriorates, thoracentesis by needle (angiocath) aspiration is indicated. See chapter 19-IID for thoracentesis.
         If a tension pneumothorax is present or the pneumothorax extensive, closed intercostal drainage through an anteriorly placed chest tube (at the first to third intercostal space just lateral to the midclavicular line) should be instituted using a Pleur-evac drainage system with 10 to 20 cm of water suction pressure until no fluctuation of air in the tube and/or no air bubbling is present. Iatrogenic lung perforation is a common complication of chest tubes. Dramatic improvement in color and circulation follows the relief of tension pneumothorax, which may be confirmed by transillumination or chest x-ray film (see chapter 19–IIE).
      2) Administration of 100% oxygen will increase the nitrogen washout of gas in the pleural space. Do not give 100% O_2 to premature infants unless required to maintain normal Pa_{O_2}.
2. Pneumomediastinum
   Specific therapy is usually not indicated. With time, the pneumomediastinum will resolve spontaneously.
3. PIE: Pulmonary interstitial emphysema
   Adequate therapy to resolve pulmonary interstitial emphysema is unknown.

Suggestions include the following:

a. Decrease peak inspiratory pressure and distending pressure. (This is often impossible because arterial blood gases mandate the need for vigorous ventilatory support.) High frequency ventilation (or oscillation) may be of value.

b. If significant localized pulmonary interstitial emphysema is present, selective intubation of the uninvolved bronchus may be tried prior to surgical intervention (lobectomy).

4. Pneumopericardium
   a. Without evidence of cardiac tamponade
      Follow height of the R wave on the ECG and repeat the chest x-ray film. Administer high ambient FI_{O_2} to term infants.
   b. With evidence of cardiac tamponade
      1) Use repeated needle aspiration since recurrence is common. See chapter 19–IIC for pericardiocentesis.
      2) Place a pericardial tube for severe tension pneumopericardium.
      3) Surgically aspirate the pericardial sac.

REFERENCES

Allen R.W., Jung A.L., Lester P.D.: Effectiveness of chest tube evacuation of pneumothorax in neonates. *J. Pediatr.* 99:629, 1981.

Fletcher B.D., Outerbridge E.W., Dunbar J.S.: Pulmonary interstitial emphysema in the newborn. *J. Can. Assoc. Radiol.* 21:273, 1970.

Gaylord M.S., Thieme R.E., Woodall D.L., et al.: Predicting mortality in low-birth-weight infants with pulmonary interstitial emphysema. *Pediatrics* 76:219, 1985.

Kuhns L.R., Bednarek F.J., Wyman M.L., et al.: Diagnosis of pneumothorax or pneumomediastinum in the neonate by transillumination. *Pediatrics* 56:355, 1975.

Yeh T.F., Vidyasagar D., Pildes R.S.: Neonatal pneumopericardium. *Pediatrics* 54:429, 1974.

XV. PULMONARY HEMORRHAGE

Pulmonary hemorrhage may be alveolar, interstitial, or both. Since the hematocrit of the "hemorrhage" is usually significantly lower than the venous hematocrit, it has been postulated that pulmonary hemorrhage in most instances may be secondary to an acute rise in the pressure of the pulmonary capillary bed from advanced pulmonary edema. In some instances, pulmonary hemorrhage represents true hemorrhage from bleeding diasthesis or trauma, and the hematocrit of the pulmonary effluent will be similar to the venous hematocrit. The incidence of massive pulmonary hemorrhage is reported as 10% of neonatal autopsies.

A. Who Is at Risk?

1. Infants with perinatal asphyxia, low birth weight, hypoglycemia, respiratory distress syndrome, hypothermia, sepsis, pneumonia, oxygen therapy, breech

presentation, Rh immunization, kernicterus, bleeding disorders, and congenital heart disease with a large left-to-right shunt
2. Infants with erosion of the trachea or bronchi secondary to trauma

B. Clinical Manifestations

Symptoms include bloody froth from mouth or trachea, tachypnea, retractions, and cyanosis. Pallor, shock, apnea, bradycardia, and frank blood or red frothy liquid from the mouth with or without an endotracheal tube may occur. In 50% of the cases, blood will not be observed from the endotracheal tube.

C. Laboratory Findings

1. Reduced hematocrit
2. Reduced blood pressure
3. Worsening pulmonary function (e.g., acidosis, etc.)

D. Radiologic Features

Findings are nonspecific and variable. A reticulogranular appearance, nodular densities, and complete opacification have been described. Sudden radiographic changes and clinical deterioration should raise suspicion.

E. Supportive Management

1. Maintain as clear an airway as possible by suctioning.
2. Administer oxygen as required and assist ventilation (see chapter 11–IV and 11–VI).
3. Maintain the infant's temperature in the thermal neutral range (36.5° C skin or 37° C rectal temperature).
4. Administer vitamin K_1 (Aquamephyton or Konakion), 1 to 2 mg IV or IM, after obtaining coagulation studies.
5. Obtain coagulation studies.
   a. Obtain a peripheral blood smear and platelet count.
   b. Draw blood for prothrombin time, partial thromboplastin time, fibrinogen, and fibrin-split products.
   c. Obtain and follow the infant's hematocrit.
6. Obtain and follow blood pressure and/or central venous pressure.
7. Start an intravenous infusion to support intravascular pressure. Transfuse fresh whole blood if necessary (see chapter 14–III).
8. Exchange transfusion with fresh whole blood, high MAP, and intratracheal epinephrine may be of value.

F. Specific Therapy Prognosis

There is no specific therapy. There is a high mortality associated with this condition.

REFERENCE

Massive pulmonary hemorrhage in the newborn, editorial. *Br. Med. J.* 3:553, 1973.
Cole V.A., Normand I.C.S., Reynolds E.O.R., et al.: Pathogenesis of hemorrhagic pulmonary edema and massive pulmonary hemorrhage in the newborn. *Pediatrics* 51:175, 1973.

XVI. BRONCHOPULMONARY DYSPLASIA (BPD)

Bronchopulmonary dysplasia is a major form of chronic lung disease generally attributed to the direct toxic effects of prolonged high inspired oxygen concentrations upon the immature lung. The cytotoxicity and damage to the cell membranes have been reported to be related to the free radical (superoxide radical, hydrogen peroxide, hydroxyl radical, and singlet excited oxygen) reaction. Other proposed causative factors include the following: barotrauma secondary to positive-pressure ventilation, endotracheal intubation with secondary cilia dysfunction, immature lungs, left-to-right shunting through the patent ductus arteriosus, and lack of adequate humidity. The oxygen-induced lesions are ultimately expressed in all respiratory tissues: mucosal, bronchiolar, alveolar, and vascular.

A. Prevention

1. Administer minimum F_{IO_2} required and lowest mean airway pressure to maintain adequate blood gases. Wean the infant from the ventilator and extubate the infant as soon as possible.
2. The effect of bovine superoxide dismutase, pancuronium, fluid restriction and/or indometacin (to close PDA and prevent CHF), high frequency ventilation, surfactant replacement, and vitamin E is under investigation.

B. Who Is at Risk?

1. Premature infants who received O_2 therapy and positive-pressure assisted ventilation via an endotracheal tube. The more immature the infant, the higher the incidence.
2. Less commonly, term or postterm infants with meconium aspiration syndrome, high and prolonged ventilatory therapy, persistent pulmonary hypertension of the newborn, diaphragmatic hernia, pneumonia (viral, *candida, chlamydia,* etc.), cardiopulmonary disease, or other conditions.

C. Clinical Manifestations

1. As acute respiratory distress improves, chronic respiratory failure supervenes and manifests as continued need for oxygen therapy or assisted ventilation, tachypnea, dyspnea, or cyanosis.
2. Fine, diffuse rales may be heard throughout the lung. Expiratory wheezing may be audible with advanced BPD.

D. Laboratory Findings

1. Abnormal cytology of the tracheal aspirate (bronchial epithelial exfoliated cells, etc.)
2. Pulmonary function
   a. Marked maldistribution of ventilation
   b. Normal minute volume (with increased respiratory rate and decreased tidal volume)
   c. Hypercarbia with or without hypoxia
   d. Increased work of breathing
      1) Decreased dynamic compliance
      2) Increased airway resistance
   e. Decreased effective capillary blood flow
   f. Increased functional residual capacity
   g. Increased oxygen consumption
      (Remember $TcPo_2$ is decreased with handling up to 48 weeks postconceptual age and then decreases with sleep after that.)
3. Right ventricular hypertrophy on ECG or echocardiogram
   Pulmonary hypertension may be seen on catheterization.

E. Radiographic Findings

Radiographic findings may be classified according to Northway's staging.

1. Stage I (mild)
   Reticulogranular pattern with air bronchograms consistent with respiratory distress syndrome
2. Stage II (moderate)
   Confluent irregularly shaped densities throughout the lung parenchyma with perihilar small radiolucent areas. These findings are consistent with congestive heart failure from the patent ductus arteriosus, fluid overload, or pulmonary hemorrhage.
3. Stage III (severe)
   Mild radiolucent areas becoming cystic dense patches and developing hyperinflation

4. Stage IV (advanced)
   Chronic disease usually appearing at 20 to 30 days of age. Hyperinflation, nonhomogeneity, scattered translucent cysts, and multiple fine, lacy densities extending to the periphery.
   These findings are consistent with the Wilson-Mikity syndrome, which is a syndrome of chronic respiratory distress in premature (less than 36 weeks) infants who have an initial benign course, gradual insidious onset of cyanosis, hypercapnea, and retractions followed by severe respiratory distress requiring O_2 therapy and then gradual improvement within 6 to 24 months. One third of the patients die during the acute phase of Wilson-Mikity Syndrome.

F. Supportive Management

1. O_2 therapy and assisted ventilation are required for a prolonged period (1 month to 2 years). See chapter 11–IIIB for "general supportive management of the infant with respiratory distress," 11–IV for "oxygen therapy," and 11–VI for "assisted ventilation."
   Weaning from IMV and/or oxygen therapy must be cautious and gradual.
2. Control heart failure (see chapter 11–XXIX for "congestive heart failure").
3. Administer high caloric diet to meet high oxygen consumption, prevent frequent infection, and promote growth, new alveolar development, and the ventilatory weaning process.
4. Administer diuretics (e.g., furosemide) with close monitoring of intake and output, electrolytes, urine specific gravity, weight, etc., to prevent pulmonary edema from abnormal lymphatic drainage, right-sided heart failure, and/or cor pulmonale.
5. Administer adequate calcium and vitamin D to prevent rickets with chronic furosemide therapy.
6. Aggressively control infection. Pneumonia is a common complication and routine culture of tracheal aspirate may be helpful.
7. Administer theophylline 1.1 mg/kg/6–8 hour after loading dose of 5.5 mg/kg for bronchospasm possibly due to hypertrophy of peribronchiolar smooth muscle. Theophylline has been reported to increase dynamic compliance and decrease pulmonary resistance for infants less than 30 days old.
8. Promote infant stimulation for the infant to achieve maximum potential using a team of physical therapists, child developmentalists, medical and nursing counselors, social workers, etc.
9. Support parents and allow them to develop expertise by participating in daily infant care.

G. Specific Therapy

A specific therapy is not known.

H. Complications

1. Bronchiolitis
2. Bronchopneumonia
3. Recurrent atelectasis
4. Large airway obstruction
5. Pulmonary edema
6. Cor pulmonale
7. Congestive heart failure with or without right ventricular hypertrophy
8. Pulmonary hypertension
9. Systemic hypertension

I. Prognosis

1. Mortality is 10% to 40% in the first year of life.
2. Morbidity
   Complete healing is usually achieved if the infant survives.
   a. Delayed growth due to high O_2 consumption
   b. Delayed development in approximately 50% and severe developmental delay in 25% of infants with bronchopulmonary dysplasia
   c. Speech and hearing defects
   d. Visual impairment (amblyopia, blindness, myopia)
   e. Behavior and psychologic problems
   f. Surgery (often inguinal hernia, tubes for otitis media)
   g. Re-admission rate is approximately 50% in the first 1 to 2 years after discharge.
   h. Impaired pulmonary function over 2 years or more
   i. Obstructive airway disease as late as 8 years

REFERENCES

Hodgman J.E., Mikity V.G., Tatter D., et al.: Chronic respiratory distress in the premature infant. *Pediatrics* 44:179, 1969.
Koops B.L., Abman S.H., Accurso F.J.: Outpatient management and follow-up of bronchopulmonary dysplasia. *Clin. Perinatal.* 11:101, 1984.
Markestad T., Fitzhardinge P.M.: Growth and development in children recovering from bronchopulmonary dysplasia. *J. Pediatr.* 98:597, 1981.
Northway W.H., Rosan R.C., Porter D.Y.: Pulmonary disease following respirator therapy of hyaline-membrane disease. *N. Engl. J. Med.* 276:357, 1967.
Wilson M.G., Mikity V.G.: A new form of respiratory disease in premature infants. *Am. J. Dis. Child.* 99:489, 1960.

XVII. CONGENITAL LUNG CYST

A congenital lung cyst is a rare anomaly that is usually seen in the periphery of the lung, may communicate with the bronchi, may be solitary or multiple in other organs, and must be differentiated from other cysts, such as, cysts due to staphylococcal infections, bronchopulmonary dysplasia, or cystic adenomatoid malformation of the lung. Five types are recognized.

1. Small, almost microscopic cysts continuous with the epithelium of the bronchi.
2. Congenital cystic bronchiectasis. These cysts are visible grossly and appear to be widely dilated bronchi and bronchioles.
3. Cystic enlargement of the alveoli.
4. Solid mass of tissue with only occasional cysts.
5. The cysts appear to be widely dilated lymphatics and the disease is also known as pulmonary lymphangiectasis.

A. Who Is at Risk?

Infants from Yemen and Iraq are particularly at risk.

B. Clinical Manifestations

Symptoms are persistent episodes of respiratory distress, cough, wheezing, and stridor often aggravated by crying. Superimposed pneumonia is common. If air can enter the cyst, but not leave it, a tension pneumothorax may develop.

C. Radiologic Features

Chest x-ray films will delineate the cyst in the pulmonary parenchyma periphery. The size of the cyst may change on subsequent films. Displacement of the esophagus may be present. Complete obstruction of the bronchi will result in resorption atelectasis.

D. Laboratory Findings

Abnormal blood gas values depending on the extent and severity of the cyst.

E. Supportive Management

1. Asymptomatic infants
   Asymptomatic infants should be observed and given supportive therapy.
2. Symptomatic infants
   See chapter 11–IIIB for "general supportive management of the infant with respiratory distress," 11–IV for "oxygen therapy," and 11–VI for "assisted ventilation."

F. Specific Therapy/Prognosis

Acute compression of the lung requires immediate resection. If extensive, the disease may be incompatible with life.

REFERENCE

Stowens D.: *Pediatric Pathology,* ed 2. Baltimore, Williams & Wilkens Co., 1966, p. 454.

XVIII. TRACHEOESOPHAGEAL FISTULA

Esophageal atresia with tracheoesophageal fistula occurs in 1 out of 3,000 live births. Five varients exist.

1. Esophageal atresia with distal tracheoesophageal fistula (86%)
2. Esophageal atresia without tracheoesophageal fistula (8%)
3. Tracheoesophageal fistula without esophageal atresia (H type) (4%)
4. Esophageal atresia with proximal tracheoesophageal fistula (1%)
5. Esophageal atresia with both distal and proximal tracheoesophageal fistula (1%)

A. Who Is at Risk?

1. Infants born to mothers with a history of polyhydramnios
2. Infants of low birth weight especially those who are small for gestational age
3. Infants with excessive bubbly secretions

B. Clinical Manifestations

1. The infant usually has a good Apgar score.
2. Oral secretions are abundant and flow from the infant's mouth.
3. Various degrees of respiratory distress are present (e.g., tachypnea, labored respiratory effort, retractions).
4. Examination of the chest reveals rales, rhonchi, and abnormal breath sounds.
5. Feedings frequently result in gagging, aspiration, and choking.
6. Abdominal signs vary.
   a. Infants with a fistula between the trachea and the distal esophagus may have a distended abdomen.
   b. Infants with a fistula between the trachea and the proximal esophagus may have a scaphoid abdomen.
   c. Infants with an H-type fistula may appear normal except for choking with feedings.
7. The diagnosis is suggested when a nasogastric catheter cannot be passed into the infant's stomach. (Occasionally the length of the nasogastric tube appears to have passed to the stomach but simply has coiled in the esopha-

geal pouch. Use of a larger catheter, slowly passed, will avoid this error.)

8. T–E fistula may be part of the VATER syndrome (vertebral anomalies, anal atresia, T–E fistula, and renal anomalies). Twenty to 30% of the infants with a T–E fistula have associated congenital heart disease and 10% have imperforated anus.

C. Radiologic Features

1. Air in the blind pouch may be seen on chest x-ray film.
2. A radiopaque nasogastric catheter can be seen coiled in the pouch on chest x-ray film.
3. Barium can be instilled carefully and slowly through the nasogastric tube to define the outline of the pouch or any potential fistulous connections between the proximal esophagus and trachea, although this procedure is rarely necessary. The medium should be removed after the study.

D. Supportive Management

1. Withhold oral feedings to prevent aspiration pneumonia.
2. Suction the nasopharynx frequently. Leave a no. 8 catheter or Replogle tube in the pouch attached to continuous suction to facilitate drainage.
3. Keep the infant in a head-up position.
4. Consult the pediatric surgeon immediately.
5. Rule out associated cardiac, renal, vertebral, and anal malformations.
6. Administer total parenteral nutrition (TPN) for those infants with short-term delay or staged repair.
7. Some surgeons prefer the infant to be on antibiotics.
8. See chapter 11–IIIB for "general supportive management of infants with respiratory distress," 11–IV for "oxygen therapy," and 11–VI for "assisted ventilation."

E. Specific Therapy

1. Surgical correction is the treatment of choice.
   a. Provide surgical repair when the infant is of adequate weight, maturity, and stable condition.
   b. Short term delay and stabilize when the infant has pneumonia, cardiac disease, or is unstable. A gastrostomy may be placed and kept open to prevent aspiration pneumonia from regurgitation until surgery.
   c. Use staged repair for very sick, low birth weight, or severely malformed infants.

   Complications include leaks at the anastomotic site, recurrence of fistulae, esophageal dysmotility, strictures, hiatal hernias and gastroesophageal reflux.

F. Prognosis

1. Premature infant: 70% survival
2. Fullterm infant: greater than 85% survival

REFERENCES

Koop C.E.: Recent advances in the surgery of oesophageal atresia. *Progr. Pediatr. Surg.* 2:41, 1971.
Martin L.W., Alexander F.: Esophageal atresia. *Surg. Clin. North Am.* 65:1099. 1985.
Randolph J.G., Altman R.P., Anderson K.D.: Selective surgical management based upon clinical status in infants with esophageal atresia. *J. Thorac. Cardiovasc. Surg.* 74:335, 1977.

XIX. DIAPHRAGMATIC HERNIA

The abdominal viscera (stomach, large and small bowel, liver, spleen, kidney, and/or pancreas) may herniate into the thoracic cavity through a congenital diaphragmatic defect (70% to 85% are on the left posterolateral side, Bochdalek's type) and compress the lung. Incomplete rotation of the bowel without a true hernial sac is present in approximately 60% of cases. Hypoplasia of the ipsilateral lung and persistent pulmonary hypertension are associated findings. Coarctation of aorta, patent ductus arteriosus, or Meckel's diverticulum may be associated. If serious respiratory embarrassment is present, immediate surgical correction is indicated. The incidence is one in 2,000–5,000 live births.

A. Who Is at Risk?

1. Infants whose pleuroperitoneal canal failed to close and whose body cavity did not divide into abdominal and thoracic components (8 to 10 weeks of gestation) are at risk.
2. Infants with a history of polyhydramnios.

B. Clinical Manifestations

Clinical manifestations depend upon pulmonary vascular resistance, myocardial function, hypoplasia of the contralateral lung, and ductal status.

1. Severe respiratory distress and cyanosis may be present from birth and may become worse with assisted ventilation via bag and mask.
2. Mediastinal and PMI shift to the contralateral side.
3. Decreased or absent breath sounds and occasionally peristaltic sounds may be heard on the ipsilateral side.
4. The abdomen is scaphoid because the abdominal viscera are displaced into the chest cavity.
5. Occasionally, an asymptomatic infant may be diagnosed adventitiously by chest x-ray.
6. Respiratory distress may occur after a few days of life, particularly with right-sided hernia since the liver may prevent other viscera from herniating.

C. Laboratory Findings

1. Hypoxia, hypercarbia, and severe acidosis may become worse in spite of assisted ventilation from birth. Hypercarbia is due to inadequate ventilation. Hypoxia may be due to inadequate ventilation and right-to-left shunt at ductal level and/or atrial level due to persistent pulmonary hypertension.
2. ECG findings may be abnormal with peak P waves and ST, and/or T wave changes.

D. Radiologic Features

The diagnosis is established by x-ray film.

1. The air-filled bowel is seen occupying the hemithorax (left more frequent than right). Air-filled loops of bowel may appear as cysts above the diaphragm. Bowel gas patterns are usually diminished below the diaphragm.
2. The mediastinum is displaced toward the unaffected side. (Be certain the right and left side of the x-ray film are marked correctly!).

E. Supportive Management

See chapter 11–IIIB for "general supportive management for infants with respiratory distress," 11–IV for "oxygen therapy," and 11–VI for "assisted ventilation."

1. IPPB by bag and mask is contraindicated since it dilates the GI tract and further compresses the lung.
2. Decompress the GI tract with a nasogastric (Replogle) tube to low suction.
3. Ventilate the infant with the minimum amount of mean airway pressure necessary.
4. Correct acidosis and hypoxia, but do not delay surgery since it may not be possible to correct acidosis and hypoxia before surgery.

F. Specific Therapy

Emergency definitive surgical correction is indicated.

1. Do not attempt to expand the ipsilateral hypoplastic lung beyond its state of maturation since it may develop pulmonary air leak syndrome.
2. A ventral Silastic silo pouch may be necessary to prevent increased intra-abdominal pressure and compromised visceral blood supply.
3. Persistent pulmonary hypertension of the newborn with right-to-left shunt via the patent ductus arteriosus and/or foramen ovale may be difficult to manage and may require a vasodilator (tolazoline, see chapter 11–XIII).
4. Be aware that high Pa_{O_2} with functional closure of the patent ductus arteriosus after surgery increases pulmonary resistance further, which may result in right ventricular failure in addition to tissue hypoxia and acidosis. Extracorporeal

membrane oxygenation (ECMO) and prostaglandins therapy to keep ductus arteriosus patent may be life-saving.

G. Prognosis

1. The mortality rate varies from 30% to 50%.
   a. Asymptomatic infants have a better prognosis.
   b. Infants who become symptomatic and require surgery within 24 hours of life, and infants with Pa_{CO_2} greater than 50 mm Hg with adequate ventilation have poor prognosis.
   c. Infants requiring endotracheal intubation in the delivery room seldom survive.
2. If the infant survives, the ipsilateral lung will expand and become functional. The contralateral lung is able to maintain adequate ventilation. The size and number of alveoli of the ipsilateral lung increases, but the number of alveoli and airways never reach normal and the ipsilateral lung has decreased compliance.
3. Recurrent hernia in 10%–20% requires reoperation.

REFERENCES

Collins D.L., Pomerance J.J., Travis K.W., et al.: A new approach to congenital posterolateral diaphragmatic hernia. *J. Pediatr. Surg.* 12:149, 1977.

Cullen M.L., Klein M.D., Philipport A.I.: Congenital diaphragmatic hernia. *Surg. Clin. North Am.* 65:1115, 1985.

Dibbins A.W.: Congenital diaphragmatic hernia, hypoplastic lung and pulmonary vasoconstriction. *Clin. Perinatol.* 5:93, 1978.

Grmoljez P.F., Lewis J.E. Jr.: Congenital diaphragmatic hernia: Bochdalek's type. *Am. J. Surg.* 132:744, 1976.

XX. PULMONARY HYPOPLASIA

Pulmonary hypoplasia, a group of congenital anomalies varying from mild pulmonary parenchymal hypoplasia to complete pulmonary agenesis, may be unilateral or bilateral. Pulmonary hypoplasia includes a decreased number of alveoli, reduced peripheral bronchioles, and reduced arterioles. Decreased fetal respiratory movement, hypoxia, neuromuscular disease, reduction in thoracic size, and compression of the lung have all been postulated as causative agents. Complete pulmonary agenesis usually is unilateral and on the left side. The contralateral lung is usually hypertrophic.

A. Who Is at Risk?

1. Infants with a maternal history of oligohydramnios or chronic leakage of amniotic fluid for longer than four weeks' duration starting at less than 26 weeks of gestation

2. Infants with renal dysgenesis: renal agenesis (Potter's syndrome) or bilateral renal dysplasia with or without cysts
3. Infants with reduced thoracic size: Jeune's syndrome, (asphyxiating thoracic dystrophy), thanatophoric dysplasia syndrome, camptomelic dysplasia, or cleidocranial dysostosis syndrome
4. Infants with diaphragmatic hernia or eventration
5. Infants with nonimmune hydrops

B. Clinical Manifestations

Bilateral pulmonary hypoplasia presents as respiratory distress immediately after birth associated with abnormal blood gases. These infants frequently develop persistent pulmonary hypertension of the newborn and pneumothorax. In unilateral pulmonary agenesis/hypoplasia, decreased breath sounds and displacement of the mediastinum to the ipsilateral side are observed.

Clinical findings associated with renal dysgenesis (see chapter 18–IX), diaphragmatic hernia (see chapter 11–XIX), and reduced thoracic size (Jeune's syndrome, thanatophoric dysplasia syndrome, camptomelic dysplasia, and cleidocranial dysostosis syndrome, Tables 9–4 and 11–2) may be present. Those infants with Potter's syndrome have multiple nodules on the fetal surface of the placenta called amniom nodosum and a characteristic facies (see Potter's syndrome, Table 9–4).

C. Laboratory Findings

1. Abnormal blood gases, low pH, elevated Pa_{CO_2}, low Pa_{O_2}
2. Elevated BUN and creatinine in infants with renal anomalies

D. Radiologic Features

1. Unilateral pulmonary hypoplasia/agenesis presents as a radiopaque hemithorax with mediastinal shift to the affected side. Vertebral defects may be present.
2. Bilateral pulmonary hypoplasia presents as a small but clear lung field often associated with pneumothorax. (In contrast, lung fields are small but opaque in atelectasis.)
3. Other radiologic anomalies occur depending on the underlying disease, e.g., diaphragmatic hernia (see chapter 11–XIX).
4. Abnormal renal sonogram may be present.

E. Supportive Therapy

1. See chapter 11–IIIB for "general supportive management for infants with respiratory distress," 11–IV for "oxygen therapy," and 11–VI for "assisted ventilation."

TABLE 11–2.—Infants With Thoracic Cage Anomalies (see Table 9–4)

	CLINICAL FINDINGS	X-RAY FILM FINDINGS
Asphyxiating thoracic dystrophy Jeune syndrome	Narrow thorax Respiratory distress Short limbs Dwarfism Polydactyly Renal anomalies	Horizontal short ribs Low diaphragm Narrow thorax Trident iliac bones Double-notched acetabula
Thanatophoric dwarfism	Narrow thorax Micromelia with normal trunk Large head Prominent eyes Depressed nasal bridge	Short ribs Low diaphragm Narrow thorax Foreshortened long bones Flattened vertebral bodies Small iliac wings, flat acetabula Flaring of long bones
Hypophosphatasia	Multiple fractures Vomiting, failure to thrive	Poor skull mineralization Fractures
Achondrogenesis	Large head, short neck Narrow thorax	Short limbs, poor ossification Low diaphragm

Spondyloepiphyseal dysplasia congenita	Growth retardation Normal face Short trunk	Short ribs Flaring shapes of long bones Scoliosis, short spine Fragmentation of the epiphysis
Achondroplasia	Large head with bulging forehead Narrow chest Short, broad hands Short stature	Short ribs Short, broad long bone Short, broad pelvis Small sacrosciatic notch
Osteogenesis imperfecta	Blue sclerae Multiple fractures Skeletal deformities	Multiple wormian bones in skull Poorly ossified bones Multiple fractures of ribs and long bones
Ellis-van Creveld syndrome	Narrow chest Congenital heart disease Polydactyly Distal shortening of extremities	Normal skull x-ray films Short, thick long bones Progressive shortening of long bones, greatest at extremities

REFERENCE

Smith D.W.: *Recognizable Patterns in Human Malformation,* Philadelphia, W.B. Saunders Co., 1982.

2. Look for associated congenital anomalies.
   a. Examine the infant carefully. Palpate the abdomen to define renal size and configuration.
   b. Obtain an abdominal/renal sonogram to elucidate renal structure and presence of urinary bladder.
   c. Evaluate the chest x-ray film to assess thoracic skeletal configuration, lung volumes, and placement of GI tract.
3. Obtain electrolytes, glucose, calcium, and baseline BUN. (Remember, BUN reflects mother's renal status the first 24 to 48 hours.)
4. Extracorporeal membrane oxygenation (ECMO) may yield time for the lungs to develop (controversial).

F. Specific Therapy

No specific therapy is known.

REFERENCES

Langston C.: Normal and abnormal structural development of the human lung. *Prog. Clin. Biol. Res.* 140:75, 1983.
Nimrod C., Gitting F.V., Machin G., et atl.: The effect of very prolonged membrane rupture of fetal development. *Am. J. Obstet. Gynecol.* 148:540, 1984.
Swischuk L.E., Richardson C.J., Nichols M.M., et al.: Primary pulmonary hypoplasia in the neonate. *J. Pediatr.* 95:573, 1979.
Thibeault D.W., Beatty E.C., Hall R.T., et al: Neonatal pulmonary hypoplasia with premature rupture of fetal membranes and oligohydroamnios. *J. Pediatr.* 107:273, 1985.

XXI. ATELECTASIS

Lobar atelectasis, the segmental or subsegmental collapse of a portion of the lung, occurs secondary to increased bronchial secretions, ciliary dysfunction and/or endotracheal tube misplacement. Diffuse atelectasis, collapse of alveoli due to surfactant deficiency, usually occurs secondary to respiratory distress syndrome.

A. Prevention

1. For the infant on a ventilator or postextubation: application of 2 to 3 cm of continuous distending pressure (CPAP or PEEP) and chest physiotherapy with postural drainage (see chapter 11–VIB and 11–VII).
2. For the infant off a ventilator: administration of chest physiotherapy with postural drainage (see chapter 11–VII) for the infant with surfactant deficiency (e.g., respiratory distress syndrome, bronchopulmonary dysplasia or pneumonia).

B. Who Is at Risk?

1. Lobar atelectasis
   a. Approximately 40% to 50% of infants postextubation (right upper, right middle, and left lower lobes)
   b. Infants with bronchopulmonary dysplasia (frequently recurrent atelectasis)
   c. Infants with phrenic nerve palsy
   d. Infants with misplaced endotracheal tube.
2. Diffuse atelectasis
   Infants with respiratory distress syndrome

C. Clinical Manifestations

1. Lobar atelectasis
   A sudden increase in respiratory distress and ventilatory requirements
2. Diffuse atelectasis
   See respiratory distress syndrome (see chapter 11–VIII)

D. Radiologic Features

1. Lobar atelectasis
   a. Radiopacification of the involved area
   b. A change in the position of the fissures
   c. A shift of the mediastinum toward the side of the collapse
   d. Narrowing of the intercostal spaces over the affected area
   e. Compensatory hyperinflation of the uninvolved portion of the lung
   f. Endotracheal tube, if present, in the right or rarely left main bronchus.
2. Diffuse atelectasis
   a. A diffuse reticulogranular pattern due to microatelectasis interspersed with dilated air space
   b. A "white out" lung may occur in severe cases.

E. Laboratory Findings

Abnormal blood gases, e.g., increased Pa_{CO_2}, decreased Pa_{O_2}

F. Supportive Therapy

See chapter 11–IIIB for "general supportive management for infants with respiratory distress," 11–IV for "oxygen therapy," 11–VI for "assisted ventilation," and 11–VII for "chest physiotherapy."

G. Specific Therapy

Bronchoscopy utilizing a flexible, fiberoptic bronchoscope to remove mucous plugs and casts

REFERENCES

Nussbaum E.: Pediatric flexible bronchoscopy and its application in infantile atelectasis. *Clin. Pediatr.* 24(7):379, 1985.

Wyman M.L., Kuhns L.R.: Lobar opacification of the lung after tracheal extubation in neonates. *J. Pediatr.* 91:109, 1977.

XXII. UPPER AIRWAY OBSTRUCTION

A. Choanal Atresia

Choanal atresia, a membranous (10%) or bony (90%) obstruction between the anterior nasal airway and the nasopharynx, causes respiratory distress in the newborn infant because most newborns are obligatory nasal breathers up to the third to sixth week of life. The incidence is 0.02% to 0.04% of live births. Some infants survive as mouth breathers; others develop periods of respiratory distress, apnea, and inability to feed.

1. Who Is at Risk?
   a. Infants with a family history of "mouth breathers"
   b. Infants with the following congenital malformations:
      1) Treacher Collins syndrome, Apert's syndrome
      2) Palatal abnormalities
      3) Colobomas
      4) Hypoplastic nipples
      5) Tracheoesophageal fistula
      6) Congenital heart disease
   c. Females more than males
2. Clinical Manifestations
   Acute respiratory distress and cyanosis occur in the delivery room if bilateral choanal atresia is present; frequently, the infant holds his or her head in hyperextension and breathes rapidly until exhaustion ensues. The infant becomes pink while crying. Respiratory distress may be mild but worsens with feedings. The physician will be unable to pass a catheter through one or both nasal passages.
3. Radiographic Features
   Radiopaque dye will not pass from the nasal cavity into the nasopharynx.
4. Supportive Management
   Establish a satisfactory oral airway by inserting an infant oropharyngeal air-

way or an endotracheal tube if necessary. A rubber nipple with a large hole strapped by tape over the ears is a useful aid. Subsequently, many infants learn to breathe through their mouths. Feed with a large-hole nipple until the ability to breathe through the mouth occurs. Tube feedings may be required at first, but within a month many infants learn to breathe through their mouths and feed.

Rule out other congenital anomalies, e.g., congenital heart disease, palatal abnormality, or tracheoesophageal fistula.

5. Specific Therapy

   Surgical therapy should be used to relieve the obstruction, i.e., transnasal perforation of membrane obstructions via a transnasal or transpalatal approach. Carbon dioxide laser therapy has recently been advocated.

REFERENCES

Hall B.D.: Choanal atresia and associated multiple anomalies. *J. Pediatr.* 95:395, 1979.

Healy G.B., McGill T., Strong M.S.: Surgical advances in the treatment of lesions of the pediatric airway: The role of the carbon dioxide laser. *Pediatrics* 61:380, 1978.

B. Subglottic Stenosis

Intrinsic narrowing of the trachea and subglottic region secondary to intubation is the most frequent cause of laryngeal obstruction in infancy and has been noted in approximately 1% of less than 1.5-kg survivors of mechanical ventilation.

1. Prevention
   a. Avoid prolonged intubation.
   b. Ensure space surrounding the endotracheal tube.
   c. Avoid extreme hyperextension of the neck.
   d. Secure the endotracheal tube carefully.
   e. Treat superficial infection promptly.
2. Who Is at Risk?

   Infants who have been intubated for more than 3 to 4 weeks
3. Clinical Manifestations

   Increased respiratory distress, apnea, stridor, cyanosis, and inability to maintain adequate ventilation after extubation
4. Laboratory Findings

   Increased Pa_{CO_2} and decreased Pa_{O_2} after extubation

   Bronchoscopy reveals narrowing of the airway.
5. Radiologic Features

   Narrowing of airway on magnified films
6. Supportive Therapy

   Tracheostomy may be necessary.

   See chapter 11–IIIB for "general supportive management for infants with respiratory distress," 11–IV for "oxygen therapy," and 11–VI for "assisted ventilation."

7. Specific Therapy
   Serial endoscopic resection (or laser therapy) of scar tissue, dilation, and intralesional steroids have proven to be effective therapy.

REFERENCE

O'Nelll J.A.: Experience with iatrogenic laryngeal and tracheal stenoses. *J. Pediatr. Surg.* 19:235, 1984.

C. Laryngeal Web

Laryngeal web, a membranous obstruction above or below the true vocal cords, is a rare congenital anomaly.

1. Who Is at Risk?
   Infants with ventricular septal defects
2. Clinical Manifestations
   The infant may have upper airway obstruction with gasping, retractions, and cyanosis or the infant may have stridor and a hoarse cry. Direct laryngoscopy usually reveals a thin, transparent web. Occasionally, the web is thick and fibrous.
3. Laboratory Findings
   Abnormal arterial blood gases
4. Supportive Therapy
   See chapter 11–IIIB for "general supportive management for infants with respiratory distress," 11–IV for "oxygen therapy," and 11–VI for "assisted ventilation."
5. Specific Therapy
   a. For thin, transparent web: intubation and perforation of the web
   b. For thick and fibrous web: do not force endotracheal tube through the web. Tracheostomy is the treatment of choice, with later surgical repair or laser therapy. Bronchoscope to rule out the possibility of associated anomalies.

REFERENCE

Shearer W.T., Biller H.F., Agura J.H., et al.: Congenital laryngeal web with intraventricular septal defect. *Am. J. Dis. Child.* 123:605, 1972.

XXIII. CONGENITAL LOBAR EMPHYSEMA

Congenital lobar emphysema is an uncommon, but potentially life-threatening, cause of respiratory distress in the newborn. It is characterized by overdistension and air trapping in the affected lobe, compression atelectasis of the ipsilateral lung, and displacement of the mediastinum. The left upper lobe is the most frequently affected area. The disease almost always involves a single lobe.

A. Who Is at Risk?

1. Infants with partial intraluminal bronchial obstruction (e.g., congenital deficiency of bronchial cartilage in greater than 50% of patients)
2. Infants with extrabronchial compression often by pulmonary artery or mediastinal mass
3. Infants with partial airway collapse
4. Twice as many males affected as females, usually white and fullterm

B. Clinical Manifestations

Approximately one half of patients develop symptoms in the first few days of life and one half of patients between 1 and 4 months of age. Rarely, infants develop fulminating symptoms and die within several hours of age. Once symptoms develop, the course is progressive with emphysema and compression of normal lobes.

1. Dyspnea, cyanosis (in one half of patients, worse with cry or feeding), wheezing, cough, tachypnea, or intercostal retractions
2. Prominent chest of the involved side with shift of PMI away from the involved side
3. Hyperresonant and decreased breath sounds of the involved side
4. No signs of inflammation

C. Radiologic Features

1. Chest x-ray film demonstrates hyperinflation of a lobe with bronchovascular markings in the hyperlucent area in contrast to pneumothorax, pneumatocele, and congenital lung cysts where bronchovascular markings are not seen. Mediastinal shift away from the affected lobe may be seen.
2. Atelectasis of adjacent lung tissue
3. Little movement of the flattened diaphragm on the affected side
4. Bowing of the sternum and herniation across the anterior mediastinum on the lateral view
5. An enlarged opaque lobe, due to retention of fluid within the lobe, may be seen at birth, which clears and becomes hyperlucent within a few days.

D. Supportive Management

1. Bronchoscopy will rule out associated cause of airway obstruction when the newborn has respiratory distress and radiologic features of radiolucent emphysema.
2. See chapter 11–IIIB for "general supportive management for infants with respiratory distress," 11–IV for "oxygen therapy," and 11–VI for "assisted ventilation."

E. Specific Therapy

1. Lobectomy is curative when severe respiratory distress is present due to emphysematous lobe and atelectatic uninvolved lobe(s) and decreased venous return. Infants with symptoms in the first few days of life usually require surgery.
2. Asymptomatic infants or infants with the onset of symptoms between 1 and 4 months of age usually do not require surgical treatment.

REFERENCES

Buckner D.M.: Congenital lobar emphysema. *Clin. Perinatol.* 5:105, 1978.
DeLuca F.G., Wesselhoeft C.W.: Surgically treatable causes of neonatal respiratory distress. *Clin. Perinatol.* 5:377, 1978.
Ryckman F.C., Rosenkrantz J.C.: Thoracic surgical problems in infancy and childhood. *Surg. Clin. North Am.* 65:1423, 1985.

XXIV. CONGENITAL CYSTIC ADENOMATOID MALFORMATION OF THE LUNG

Congenital cystic adenomatoid malformation is a form of hamartomas formed from uncontrolled overgrowth of bronchioles. This rare form of congenital cystic lung disease is classified as follows:

Type I: Multiple large cysts that mimic lobar emphysema (50% of cases)
Type II: Multiple even-spaced cysts not greater than 1.2 cm in diameter (40% of cases)
Type III: Firm mass with even-spaced small cysts

A. Who is at Risk?

1. Infants with a maternal history of polyhydramnios
2. Infants with nonimmune hydrops fetalis

B. Clinical Manifestations

Progressive respiratory distress is usually noted at birth or in the first week of life. Anasarca (hydrops fetalis) is noted in 50% of infants, especially those who are stillborn. Associated congenital anomalies are present in one fifth of the infants. Some infants are asymptomatic or exhibit recurrent infection due to poor bronchopulmonary drainage.

C. Radiologic Features

Chest x-ray film reveals an extensive multicytic pattern with mediastinal shift. When cysts are fluid filled, a homogeneous opaque mass may be seen. Diaphragmatic hernia should be differentiated.

D. Supportive Therapy

See chapter 11–IIIB for "general supportive therapy for infants with respiratory distress" and 18–XII for "hydrops fetalis."

E. Specific Therapy

Resection of the affected lobe to prevent further compression of normal lung tissue is indicated if respiratory distress or infection is present.

REFERENCES

Ryckman F.C., Rosenkrantz J.G.: Thoracic surgical problems in infancy and childhood. *Surg. Clin. North Am.* 65:1423, 1985.

Stocker J.T., Drake R.M., Madewell J.E.: Cystic and congenital lung disease in the newborn. *Perspect. Pediatr. Pathol.* 4:93, 1978.

XXV. PLEURAL EFFUSION

Collection of fluid in the plural space is a rare but occasional cause of respiratory distress in the newborn.

A. Who Is at Risk?

Infants with the following diagnoses are at risk for plural effusion:

1. Pneumonia
2. Hydrops fetalis
3. Turner's syndrome
4. Congestive heart failure
5. Trauma to the lymphatic ducts (inadvertent complication of surgical closure of a patent ductus arteriosus)
6. Viral infection
7. Transient tachypnea of the newborn
8. Meconium aspiration syndrome
9. TPN solution inadvertently placed in the chest due to misplaced catheter

B. Clinical Manifestations

Infants usually have tachypnea, retractions, and cyanosis. When the effusion is unilateral, there are decreased breath sounds and dullness to percussion on the affected side and a shift of the mediastinum to the contralateral side.

C. Radiologic Features

Fluid is seen as a characteristic opacity in the pleural space.

D. Laboratory Findings

Thoracentesis will reveal the following:

1. In chylothorax: clear fluid at first; fluid becomes opalescent with visible fat globules after feeding; greater than 90% of cells are lymphocytes. Protein concentration is half of the plasma protein while cholesterol and triglyceride levels exceed the plasma level.
2. In hemothorax: a high hematocrit in the pleural fluid
3. In hydrothorax due to pneumonia: positive smear and culture for responsible organism; increased polymorphonuclear neutrophils in pleural fluid

E. Supportive Therapy

1. See Chapter 11–IIIB for "general supportive management for infants with respiratory distress," 11–IV for "oxygen therapy," and 11–VI for "assisted ventilation."
2. Perform thoracentesis with chest tube placement. Replacement of protein loss may be necessary.
3. Feeding a medium-chain triglyceride formula to lessen chyle formation in chylothorax may be of value.

F. Specific Therapy

Treat specific disease if known.

G. Prognosis

Most infants recover after single or multiple thoracentesis.

REFERENCES

Randolph J.G., Gross R.E.: Congenital chylothorax. *Arch. Surg.* 74:405, 1957.

Ryckman F.C., Rosenkrantz J.G.: Thoracic surgical problems in infancy and childhood. *Surg. Clin. North Am.* 65:1423, 1985.

XXVI. PULMONARY LYMPHANGIECTASIS

Congenital dilatation of the lymphatics may be localized to the lungs or may be associated with generalized lymphedema in multiple organs. Pulmonary lymphangiectasis is frequently associated with congenital heart disease.

A. Who Is at Risk?

Infants with Turner's syndrome, Noonan's syndrome, and congenital heart disease are at risk.

B. Clinical Manifestations

Term infants have respiratory distress and cyanosis at birth or shortly afterwards. Death frequently occurs in the neonatal period or early infancy.

C. Radiologic Features

Chest x-ray film reveals hyperaerated lungs with a fine, diffuse, ground-glass appearance representing dilated lymphatics.

D. Supportive Therapy

See chapter 11–IIIB for "general supportive management of infants with respiratory distress," 11–IV for "oxygen therapy," and 11–VI for "assisted ventilation."

E. Specific Therapy

No specific therapy is known.

F. Prognosis

The prognosis is poor.

REFERENCE

Noonan J.A., Walters L.R., and Reeves J.T.: Congenital pulmonary lymphangiectasis. *Am. J. Dis. Child.* 120:314, 1970.

XXVII. PHRENIC NERVE PALSY

Injury to the phrenic nerve sustained during birth may produce respiratory distress from unilateral paralysis of the diaphragm. Paralysis of the phrenic nerve, usually on the right, is frequently associated with a brachial plexus palsy and occasionally with Horner's syndrome.

A. Prevention

Avoid trauma to the infant during delivery.

B. Who Is at Risk?

1. Infant delivered by difficult breech extraction
2. Infants delivered by mothers experiencing dystocia, especially large infants
3. Infants receiving negative-pressure ventilation therapy

C. Clinical Manifestations

1. An infant may be asymptomatic.
2. With severe injury: recurrent episodes of cyanosis, paradoxic respirations, labored respirations, apnea, tachypnea, or feeble cry
3. On physical examination of affected side: diminished breath sounds, dullness to percussion, and absence of the downward thrust of diaphragm

D. Radiographic Features

1. Elevation of affected diaphragm on chest x-ray film
2. Mediastinal shift away from the affected side
3. Fluoroscopic evaluation reveals paradoxic movement of the diaphragm during respiration (during inspiration, ascent of the diaphragm on the affected side and descent on the normal side)

E. Supportive Management

1. See chapter 11–IIIB for "general supportive management for infants with respiratory distress," 11–IV for oxygen therapy," and 11–VI for "assisted ventilation."
2. Observe for signs of infection, especially pneumonia.
3. Feed carefully to prevent aspiration pneumonia.
4. Plication of the diaphragm may be life saving in severely symptomatic infants.

F. Specific Therapy

There is no known specific therapy.

G. Prognosis

Remission may occur in a few days or several weeks. Most infants have a return of function by 3 to 4 months of age. If the newborn is severely symptomatic or if by 3 to 4 months of age the infant is mildly symptomatic but radiologically unchanged, surgical plication is indicated.

REFERENCE

Smith B.T.: Isolated phrenic nerve palsy in the newborn. *Pediatrics* 49:449, 1972.

XXVIII. CONGENITAL HEART DISEASE

Cardiovascular malformations are recognized in the neonatal period in 8 in 1,000 births. Congenital heart disease (CHD) accounts for approximately 50% of deaths due to congenital defects during the first year of life. During the neonatal period, the congenital heart defects usually causing critical illness are the hypoplastic left heart syndrome, complicated coarctation of the aorta, transposition of the great vessels, and right ventricular outflow obstruction (severe tetralogy of Fallot and hypoplastic right heart syndrome). Patients with isolated ventricular septal defects, patent ductus arteriosus, and atrial septal defects comprise about 50% of all infants and children with congenital malformations and rarely do these patients have serious difficulties in the neonatal period. During the neonatal period, it is sometimes difficult to differentiate infants with parenchymal lung disease or persistent pulmonary hypertension from infants with heart disease. Careful evaluation of history, physical examination, laboratory data (Pa_{O_2} in 100% oxygen), radiologic findings, ECG, echocardiogram and catheterization are often helpful.

A. Normal Newborn Infants

The normal newborn may mimic the infant with CHD. Transient heart murmurs, tachypnea, and cyanosis during cry may all be seen in the normal newborn infant, especially in the first few hours after birth. Tachypnea, cyanosis, and a heart murmur, however, should resolve by the end of the first few postnatal days. See appendix A1 to A9 and Figs A–1 and A–2 for normal cardiorespiratory data.

B. Who Is at Risk?

The following infants are at risk for CHD:

1. Infants of diabetic mothers (D-transposition of great vessels, hypoplastic left-heart syndrome)
2. Infants with congenital rubella (congenital infection with cytomegalovirus, coxsackievirus B, or herpes virus has a low correlation with CHD)
3. Infants whose mothers ingested teratogenic drugs during the first trimester of pregnancy, i.e., thalidomide, diphenylhydantoin, trimethadone, or alcohol
4. Infants with chromosomal abnormalities, i.e., trisomy 21, 13, or 18 or Turner's syndrome (XO)
5. Infants with family history of CHD especially with a sibling as a proband for CHD
6. Infants born of incest (consanguinity of parents)

C. Clinical Manifestations (Table 11–3)

1. The newborn with CHD usually has a good Apgar score and often initially appears well with or without cyanosis for the first 24 hours of life.
2. Central cyanosis may be the initial presenting symptom of cyanotic CHD with intracardiac right-to-left shunting. Cyanosis often fails to disappear with 100% oxygen administration for 5 to 10 minutes (hyperoxia test). Central cyanosis may be present in infants with primary pulmonary disease, sepsis, hypogly-

TABLE 11–3.—CONGENITAL HEART DISEASE (CHD) IN THE NEWBORN (NB)

GROUP (INCIDENCE IN NB) TYPE	ONSET OF SYMPTOMS (AGE)	PRESENTING SYMPTOMS	MURMUR/ PULSE	ECHOCARDIOGRAM	ECG	CHEST X-RAY FILM	INITIAL MANAGEMENT FOR SX
L → R shunt (15%)							
VSD (large)	>4 weeks, earlier in prematures	Tachypnea CHF No cyanosis	syst. ⓜ	LV overload ↑ LA size LV size	LVH RVH c̄ ↑ pul. resist. or nl	Cardiomegaly ↑ pul. flow	Digoxin Diuretics
A-V canal (endocardial cushion defect)	<2 weeks	CHF No cyanosis Trisomy-21 in ⅓	syst. ⓜ (holo syst.)	Abnl mitral valve c̄ paradoxical septum	Indeterminate axis LVH and RVH ↑ PR interval	Cardiomegaly ↑ pul. flow	Digoxin Diuretics
Single ventricle (common ventricle)	early	CHF s̄ ps cyanosis	syst. ⓜ	No ventricular septum	NS or LVH qRS in all pre-cordial	Variable cardiomegaly ↑ pul. flow	Digoxin Diuretics, pul. artery banding
Mixture (25%)							
TOGV	<3 days	Tachypnea Cyanosis-marked CHF Abnormal hyperoxia test (Usually large infant)	NS unless VSD or PS present	no aortic-mitral valve continuity, nl or RVH, abnl STI, aorta ant. to pul. art.	nl or RVH Upright T in R precordial	"Egg-shaped" heart-narrow base ↑ pul. flow	Digoxin Diuretics PGE$_1$, septostomy
Truncus arteriosus	1st few days	CHF Cyanosis-variable	Syst. or diast. ⓜ at base	Two ventricles c̄ VSD Truncal root overiding	LVH and/or RVH	R. aortic arch, ↓ or ↑ pul. flow, nl or ↑ heart size	Digoxin Diuretics Pul. artery banding
TAPVR (Subdiaphragmatic) c̄ pul. venous obst	<3 days	Tachypnea CHF Severe cyanosis	Ejection or continuous syst. ⓜ	Large RV, occ paradoxical septal motion, small LA	RAD RVH or nl	↑ pul. flow Curley B lines, nl heart size, pulmonary edema like RDS	Digoxin Diuretics Cardiac cath Surgery

LV obstruction (25%)							
Hypoplastic left heart syn.	1st few days	Ashen gray, sudden CHF, shock as PDA closes, ↓ pH, sudden deterioration	NS/weak pulses	Large RV, small or no aortic valve & LV	normal or RVH RAD	Variable cardiomegaly ↑ pul. flow	Digoxin Diuretics O_2, PGE_1
Coarctation of the aorta	Usually >1st month	CHF, shock, palor, arm BP > leg BP, ↓ femoral pulses, edema, tachypnea	syst. ⓜ, LLSB and/or back	Two ventricles, aortic-mitral valve continuity, ↓ aortic diameter	RVH LVH BVH	Cardiomegaly ↑ pul. flow, pul. edema	Digoxin Diuretics O_2, PGE_1, catheterization
Aortic stenosis	1st month if CHF	CHF, palor, cyanosis-pul. edema, ↓ BP	Stenotic syst. ⓜ URSB, poor pulse	Small deformed aortic valve	LVH	Cardiomegaly ↑ pul. flow	Digoxin Diuretics O_2, PGE_1, catheterization
RV obstruction (15%)							
Pulmonic atresia or stenosis s̄ VSD	1st few days	CHF, cyanosis-marked	ejection syst. ⓜ xULSB	↑ or rarely ↓ RV size small or no pul. artery	RAD, RVH RAE, rarely LAD	RAE, RVE ↓ pul. flow	PGE_1, O_2 Inotropic agents Digoxin (?)
Ebstein's anomaly	1st hours	CHF, cyanosis-marked, tachypnea	long syst. ⓜ xLLSB	↓ RV size tricuspid valve-abnl	RAE, rsr' in V_1 ↓ RV force (c̄ WPW or PAT) RBBB	"Box-car" cardiomegaly ↓ pul. flow	PGE_1, O_2 Inotropic agents Digoxin (?)

(continued)

TABLE 11–3.—*(continued)*

INCIDENCE IN NEWBORN	ONSET OF SYMPTOMS (AGE)	PRESENTING SYMPTOMS	MURMUR/ PULSE	ECHOCARDIOGRAM	ECG	CHEST X-RAY FILM	INITIAL MANAGEMENT
R-L shunt (20%)							
Tetralogy of Fallot	usually >1 week, may be several months	Cyanosis, tachypnea	ejection syst. ⓜ U-MLSB	Two ventricles c̄ aortic root overriding interventricular septum.	RAD RVH RAH	"Boot-shaped" heart, ↓ pul. flow, R aortic arch	PGE_1, O_2
Tricuspid atresia (hypoplastic R. heart syn)	usually first day	Cyanosis-marked, tachypnea	syst. ⓜ × LLSB, continuous ⓜ in ¼	Small or no RV, large LV, absent tricuspid	LAD LVH RAH ↓ RV force	Cardiomegaly Large RA ↓ pul. flow	PGE_1

Abbreviations: L = left; R = right; V = ventricle; A = atrium; H = hypertrophy; E = enlargement; VSD = ventricular septal defect; PDA = patent ductus arteriosus; TOGV = transposition of great vessels; TAPVR = total anomalous pulmonary venous return; Sx = symptoms; CHF = congestive heart failure; BP = blood pressure; NS = not significant; STI = systolic time interval; AD = axis deviation; ↑ = increased; ↓ = decreased; Pul. = pulmonary; Syst. = systolic; Diast. = diastolic; ⓜ = murmur; LLSB = lower left sternal border; ULSB = upper left sternal border; URSB = upper right sternal border; s̄ = without; nl = normal; c̄ = with; PGE_1 = prostaglandin E_1; RBBB = right bundle branch block.

REFERENCES

Rudolph A.M.: *Congenital Diseases of the Heart*. Chicago, Year Book Medical Publishers, Inc., 1974.

King T.D.: Cardiovascular aspects, in Goldsmith J.P., Karatkin E.H. (eds.): *Assisted Ventilation of the Neonate*. Philadelphia, W.B. Saunders Co. 1981.

cemia, polycythemia, methemoglobinemia, seizures, or cyanotic CHD. When cyanosis occurs without dyspnea or metabolic abnormalities, consider the following:

a. Right ventricular obstruction
   Severe pulmonic stenosis with intact septum, Ebstein's anomaly
b. Right-to-left shunt (intracardiac)
   Tricuspid atresia, tetralogy of Fallot
c. Mixtures
   Transposition of great vessels, total anomalous pulmonary venous return, truncus arteriosus
d. Cyanosis due to congestive heart failure (CHF)
   Hypoplastic left heart syndrome, coarctation of aorta, myocarditis, arteriovenous fistula
e. Persistent pulmonary hypertension of the newborn
   Since the newborn with cyanotic CHD has many features similar to infants with persistent pulmonary hypertension, a hyperoxia-hyperventilation test should be performed to differentiate cyanotic CHD from persistent pulmonary hypertension (see chapter 11–XIII).
f. Methemoglobinemia
   Infants with methemoglobinemia have cyanosis, but normal Pa_{O_2}.

3. CHF is often the first recognized sign of CHD, but term newborns with left-to-right shunts usually do not develop CHF until 4 weeks of age. CHF presents in infants as tachypnea without dyspnea, tachycardia, occasionally hepatomegaly, pallor, poor perfusion, active precordium, gallop, and full or bounding pulse.
   a. If CHF with shock is present, consider left ventricular obstruction (hypoplastic left heart syndrome, coarctation of aorta, aortic stenosis).
   b. If CHF is present after 2 weeks of life, consider left-to-right shunt (ventricular septal defect, patent ductus arteriosus, atrioventricular canal).
   c. If CHF is present without murmur, consider systemic arteriovenous fistula or thyrotoxicosis.
   d. If CHF is present without murmur, but with cardiomegaly, consider myocarditis, endocardial fibroelastosis, anomalous left coronary artery, glycogen storage disease, severe aortic or pulmonary stenosis (murmur appears when CHF is controlled), or median calcinosis of the coronary artery.
   e. If CHF with marked cyanosis is present, consider right ventricular obstruction (pulmonic stenosis with intact septum or Ebstein's anomaly) or mixtures (transposition of great vessels, total anomalous pulmonary venous return, truncus arteriosus).
4. Heart murmurs are not common in the newborn with CHD and not as helpful as in older children.
   A loud systolic murmur in the first 2 to 3 days of life suggests valvular stenosis or insufficiency murmur while a loud systolic murmur after 2 weeks of life suggests left-to-right shunt (ventricular septal defect, patent ductus arteriosus, etc.). Murmurs due to a patent ductus arteriosus sound similar to those of a ventricular septal defect. In prematures, murmurs due to left-to-right shunt are heard in the first week of life.

5. Shock, pale and ashen gray color, and feeble pulses develop suddenly after the patent ductus arteriosus closes in infants with left ventricular obstruction, e.g., hypoplastic left heart syndrome.

D. Laboratory Findings

1. See Table 11–3 for chest x-ray film, echocardiogram, and ECG findings.
2. A normal glucose and hematocrit are seen. Low blood glucose is possible with CHF.
3. A normal ECG is seen in most infants with CHD within a few days of age.
4. A chest x-ray film can not only rule out pulmonary pathology, but also evaluate heart size and shape and pulmonary blood flow. If Curley B lines are present, consider subdiaphragmatic total anomalous pulmonary venous return or left ventricular obstruction.
5. An echocardiogram (two-dimensional real time) is a very useful diagnostic test in infants with transposition of great vessels, tetralogy of Fallot, atrioventricular canal, single ventricle, and total anomalous pulmonary venous return, but less helpful in ventricular septal defect, patent ductus arteriosus, or coarctation of the aorta.
6. Cardiac catheterization should be reserved for infants who need surgery. Complications of catheterization include hypertonicity, blood loss, fluid overload, and hemopericardium due to cardiac perforation.

E. Supportive Management and Specific Therapy

1. See chapter 11–III B for "general supportive management of the infant with respiratory distress," 11–IV for "oxygen therapy," and 11–VI for "assisted Ventilation."
2. For infants with cyanotic heart disease
   a. Maintain Pa_{O_2} greater than 25 mm Hg since lactic acidosis may develop. However, additional O_2 therapy is not indicated unless pulmonary edema, severe shock, and/or pulmonary disease coexist.
   b. Maintain a hematocrit greater than 40% to assure O_2 carrying capacity and tissue oxygenation.
   c. Keep the hematocrit less than 60% to prevent cerebrovascular accidents. Prevent dehydration.
   d. Prostaglandin E_1 to keep ductus arteriosus patent is necessary to maintain life in infants with cyanotic heart disease with decreased pulmonary flow and may improve the hemodynamics of infants with transposition of the great vessels and interrupted aortic arch until surgery.
      1) Obtain CBC, platelet count, coagulation studies, electrolytes, calcium, glucose, BUN/creatinine, arterial blood gases, liver function, and urinalysis before infusion.
      2) Administer prostaglandin E_1, 0.05 to 0.10 μg/kg/minute, via an umbilical catheter at T-4 or a peripheral venous catheter. During infusion, obtain

vital signs every 15 minutes and arterial blood gases every 30 minutes. Pa_{O_2} should increase from about 20 to 40 mm Hg when ductus arteriosus opens in 15 minutes after infusion. Repeat electrolytes, calcium, and glucose every 4 hours.

3) Consider side effects: flushing, apnea, jitteriness, hypotension, and necrotizing enterocolitis.
4) After surgery, decrease prostaglandin E_1 dosage.
5) After discontinuation, repeat aforementioned laboratory tests.

3. For infants with CHF, see chapter 11–XXIX.
4. Surgical procedures for infants with CHD
   a. Total anomalous pulmonary venous return
      Cardiopulmonary bypass in the first few months of life
   b. Transposition of great vessels
      1) Balloon atrial septostomy followed by baffle procedure, then pulmonary artery banding procedure, or
      2) Early total correction by Jatene's procedure
   c. Truncus arteriosus
      1) Pulmonary artery banding
      2) Corrective Rastelli's operation with a weight greater than 10 kg
   d. Hypoplastic left heart syndrome
      1) Balloon atrial septostomy
      2) Surgical palliation (poor prognosis)
   e. Coarctation of the aorta
      1) Prostaglandin E_1 into the pulmonary artery or peripheral vein
      2) Subclavian patch angioplasty
      3) Propranolol for postoperative residual hypertension with CHF
   f. Aortic stenosis
      1) Prostaglandin E_1
      2) Valved conduit to bypass the obstruction
      3) Aortic valvotomy
   g. Single ventricle
      1) Pulmonary artery banding in the newborn
      2) Later:Fontan conduit procedure
   h. Ventricular septal defect
      1) Defects become smaller with age.
      2) Pulmonary banding in the newborn, then total repair to prevent pulmonary vascular obliterative disease if large or multiple ventricular septal defects are present
   i. Pulmonic stenosis with intact septum
      1) Prostaglandin E_1
      2) Pulmonary valvotomy or a right pulmonary artery to aorta shunt (Waterston's procedure)
   j. Ebstein's anomaly
      Tricuspid valvuloplasty
5. Postoperative complications
   a. postpericardiodectomy syndrome

Postpericardiodectomy syndrome has a possible viral or immunologic origin.

1) Who is at risk?
   Infants who received the following are at risk:
   a) Open heart procedures
   b) Central and Waterston shunts
   c) Pulmonary artery banding
2) Clinical manifestations
   a) Onset: several days to a month postoperatively
   b) Polyserositis (pericardial friction rub, pericardial and/or pleural effusions, hepatomegaly, ascites, fever, weight gain, increased white blood cells and erythrocyte sedimentation rate)
3) Treatment
   a) Drainage of effusions
   b) Diuretics
   c) Anti-inflammatory agent (aspirin or prednisone) for 2 to 4 weeks

b. Postoperative fever
   Postoperative fever may be due to sepsis, wound infection, UTI, pneumonia, otitis media, meningitis, gastroenteritis, or bacterial endocarditis.

REFERENCE

Adams F.H., Emmanouilides G.C.: *Heart Disease in Infants, Children and Adolescents,* ed. 3. Baltimore, Williams & Wilkins Co., 1983.

XXIX. CONGESTIVE HEART FAILURE

Congestive heart failure (CHF) is defined as decreased cardiac output associated with inadequate systemic perfusion. In the newborn, right heart failure is uncommon and is a poor prognostic sign when present.

A. Who Is at Risk?

Infants with the following diseases are at risk:

1. Within first postnatal week
   a. Hypoplastic left heart syndrome
   b. Severe tricuspid and pulmonic regurgitation
   c. Patent ductus arteriosus in extremely immature infant
   d. Critical aortic stenosis
   e. Coarctation of aorta
   f. Endocardial fibroelastosis
   g. Neonatal myocarditis
   h. Rhythm disturbances: premature atrial tachycardia, atrial flutter, complete atrioventricular block

  i. Severe anemia and/or shock secondary to hemolytic disease in utero or chronic fetomaternal transfusion or fetofetal transfusion
  j. Sepsis
2. After first week of life
  a. Transposition of great vessels
  b. Coarctation of aorta
  c. Ventricular septal defect and/or patent ductus arteriosus
  d. Endocardial cushion defect, i.e., atrioventricular communis
  e. Total anomalous pulmonary venous return
  f. Tricuspid atresia
  g. Hypervolemia secondary to iatrogenic overload
  h. Sepsis
  i. Shock

B. Clinical Manifestations

1. Tachypnea without dyspnea
2. Tachycardia: a diastolic gallop rhythm and/or pulsus alternans is suggestive of left-sided heart failure or myocarditis.
3. Hepatomegaly: palpable liver 3 to 5 cm below the costal margin at the right midclavicular line
4. Pulmonary rales
5. Poor feeding and easy fatigability
6. Peripheral edema with or without ascites
7. Poor peripheral perfusion and/or mild perioral cyanosis
8. Poor weight gain
9. Diaphoresis

C. Laboratory Findings

1. Abnormal arterial blood gases: metabolic and/or respiratory acidosis, hypoxia due to pulmonary edema, cyanotic heart disease, or other primary problems causing CHF
2. Increase in systemic venous pressure
3. Poor ventricular contractility on echocardiogram
4. Dilutional anemia and/or hyponatremia

D. Radiologic Features

Chest x-ray film may reveal cardiomegaly and increased or decreased pulmonary flow.

E. General Supportive Management and Specific Therapy

Medical management depends on the cause of the CHF. The etiology of CHF in the neonate can be divided into two general categories: hypervolemia and hypovolemia.

1. CHF with hypervolemia
   a. Administer oxygen if necessary to maintain Pa_{O_2} greater than 50 mm Hg.
   b. Position the infant at a 10- to 30-degree head-up incline.
   c. Withhold oral feedings until CHF is under control.
   d. Restrict intravenous fluids (usually less than 130 ml/kg/day) or oral intake. Oral intake should consist of maintenance fluids (insensible water loss plus urinary loss plus stool output minus planned weight loss if edematous).
   e. Monitor electrolytes since hyponatremia (sodium less than 130 mEq/L) and hypokalemia (potassium less than 3.5 mEq/L) are common due to dilutional effects and/or wasting from diuretics.
      1) Restrict fluid to correct hyponatremia.
      2) Provide adequate potassium in the diet if glomerular filtration rate and serum potassium are normal because of secondary hyperaldosteronism and increased potassium loss in the urine.
   f. Administer diuretics for respiratory distress and/or hepatomegaly: furosemide, 1 mg/kg/dose, one to four times daily with potassium supplements (spironolactone, 1 mg/kg/dose, three to four times daily may be added for potassium sparing).
   g. Correct anemia (a frequent association due to dilution).
      1) Transfuse with packed red blood cells, 5 to 10 ml/kg, over 2 to 4 hours with additional dose of diuretic only when necessary to maintain hematocrit greater than 40%. If CHF is due to severe anemia from in utero chronic blood loss or hemolysis, administer a *slow* transfusion or exchange transfusion with packed red blood cells (see chapter 13–VI for "exchange transfusion" and 14–IIID for in utero hemorrhage).
      2) Correct a dilutional effect by diuretic therapy.
      3) Correct hypochromic microcytic iron deficient anemia with iron supplementation.
   h. Consider digitalization after consultation with the pediatric cardiologist.
      1) Total digitalizing dose (TDD) over 24 hours for digoxin (IV)
         a) Preterm infants: 0.015 to 0.020 mg (15 to 20 mcg)/kg IV
         b) Term infants: 0.025 to 0.035 mg (25 to 35 mcg)/kg IV
      2) Give one half of TDD immediately; then give the remainder in two divided doses over the next 18 to 24 hours. The daily maintenance dose is one fourth the TDD; it is given as one eighth of the TDD every 12 hours.
      3) Check the written dosage carefully; *a decimal point overdose error can cause death.*
      4) Perform an ECG before each digoxin dose to screen for digitalis toxicity for approximately 2 weeks of therapy.
      5) The digoxin level should be obtained 6 to 8 hours after a dose following

the first weeks of digitalization, and the therapeutic level should be 1 to 2 ng/ml. Adjustment in dosage should be made according to weight gain. A level greater than 2 ng/ml may be associated with toxic effects, such as vomiting or arrhythmia (premature atrial tachycardia with block, ventricular ectopy, nodal rhythm, and atrioventricular block).

6) Digoxin toxicity is exacerbated by hypokalemia (less than 3.5 mEq/L), hypercalcemia, and hypoxia.

7) Treatment of digoxin toxicity includes cessation of digoxin, correction of hypokalemia, phenytoin for malignant tachyarrhythmias, and atropine or temporary pacing for bradyarrhythmias.

i. When the infant can tolerate oral feeding, administer breast milk or PM 60/40 or Lonalac (formula with reduced sodium). Polycose (Ross Labs, 30 calories tablespoon; Mead Johnson, 30 calories tablespoon), Moducal, and medium-chain triglyceride oil (115 calories tablespoon) may be added to breast milk, and Similac PM 60/40. Do not restrict feeding, but increase of diuretics may be necessary for an excess weight gain of greater than 30 gm/day.

2. CHF with hypovolemia due to acute hemorrhage/shock/sepsis (see chapter 14–IIID)
   a. Initially support intravascular volume/blood pressure with volume expanders (fresh frozen plasma, 5% albumin, or normal saline).
   b. If there is acute hemorrhage (e.g., fetomaternal transfusion or fetoplacental transfusion), replace estimated blood losses. Consider a partial exchange transfusion if volume overloaded.
   c. If shock is secondary to sepsis:
      1) Support intravascular volume.
      2) Start appropriate antibiotics after sepsis workup.
      3) Administer hydrocortisone, 25 mg IV, and start dopamine infusion, 2 to 20 mcg/kg/minute, if patient is still hypotensive after appropriate volume replacement and antibiotics.

REFERENCE

Adams F.H., Emmanouilides G.C.: *Heart Disease in Infants, Children and Adolescents,* ed. 3. Baltimore, Williams & Wilkins Co., 1983.

XXX. PATENT DUCTUS ARTERIOSUS

The ductus arteriosus is patent during fetal life and closes functionally between 10 and 15 hours of age in response to an increased oxygen environment and to bradykinin, acetylcholine, prostaglandin inhibitors, and prostaglandin F. The anatomic closure may take anywhere from 5 to 7 days in fullterm infants and 20 days (as long as 3 months) in preterm infants. In the fetus, the elevated pulmonary vascular resistance causes a significant shunt (90%) of right ventricular output across the ductus arteriosus to the aorta.

A. Prevention

1. Conservatively administer fluids to sick premature infants as increased fluids greater than 150 ml/kg/day have been associated with an increased incidence of patent ductus anteriosus.
2. Prevent or promptly treat hypoxia, acidosis, or hypocalcemia as these are associated with opening of the ductus arteriosus.

B. Who Is at Risk?

1. Premature infants with the following:
   a. Respiratory distress syndrome
   b. Hypoxia
   c. Acidosis
   d. Fluid overload
   e. Hypocalcemia
   The incidence of failure to close is inversely related to the gestational age (over 80% in infants less than 1,000 gm and 10% to 15% in infants 1,500 to 2,000 gm). Spontaneous closure occurs more frequently in larger and healthier infants than smaller and sicker infants.

C. Clinical Manifestations

Clinical manifestations of left-to-right shunting and congestive heart failure in prematures occur earlier (5 to 8 days) than in term infants (6 to 8 weeks) because in prematures, the ductus arteriosus is less muscular, pulmonary vascular resistance is lower, the incidence of hypoxia and acidosis is higher, and myocardial contractibility is depressed. Clinical manifestations include the following:

1. Apnea
2. Persisting tachypnea and tachycardia
3. Mild intercostal and subcostal retractions due to decreased lung compliance
4. Hyperactive precordium
5. Heart murmur: systolic only or intermittent systolic murmur along left sternal border or under left clavicle may continue into early diastole. The most typical patent ductus arteriosus murmur, a harsh, continuous one, is rarely heard in premature infants. A patent ductus arteriosus may produce no murmur in infants with severe cardiac failure.
6. Full or bounding peripheral pulses
7. Widening of the pulse pressure
8. Deterioration of the general condition due to pulmonary venous congestion and high pulmonary artery pressure
   a. Requirement of higher concentration of oxygen
   b. CO_2 retention

9. Congestive heart failure
10. Difficulty in weaning off ventilator

D. Radiologic Features

1. Findings consistent with respiratory distress syndrome only
2. Enlarged heart (increased cardiothoracic ratio)
3. Increased pulmonary vascular markings and/or patterns of pulmonary edema
4. Left aortic arch

E. ECG

The ECG is normal or has suggestions of left arterial enlargement.

F. Echocardiographic Features (M-mode, two dimensional, and/or contrast)

1. Heart structurally normal.
2. Increased left atrium/aortic ratio greater than 1.3 (greater than 1 in prematures). The left atrium/aortic ratio may be normal in large patent ductus arteriosus of the premature infant due to fluid restriction or cardiac compression by severe sternal retractions.
3. Increased left atrial size
4. Increased left ventricular end-diastolic dimensions
5. Decreased left pre-ejection period/left ventricular ejection time ratio; a short left pre-ejection period may differentiate a patent ductus arteriosus from a ventricular septal defect
6. Middiastolic or holodiastolic pulmonary valve flutter
7. Direct visualization of the patency of the ductus arteriosus by two-dimensional (real-time) echocardiogram.

G. Supportive Management

1. See chapter 11–IIIB for "general supportive management for infants with respiratory distress."
   a. Continue ventilatory support to keep Pa_{CO_2} less than 40 mm Hg.
   b. Promptly treat hypoxia, acidosis, and hypocalcemia.
   c. Keep the hematocrit at greater than 40%.
   d. Administer positive airway pressure by CPAP or PEEP.
2. Restrict fluids to 80 to 100 ml/kg/day and add 20 ml/kg/day if phototherapy is used.
3. Administer diuretics, furosemide (Lasix) 1 to 2 mg/kg/dose IV or IM, to reduce left ventricular end-diastolic and pulmonary venous pressure.
4. Consider digitalis if no. 2 and no. 3 are not successful and indomethacin can

not be used because of contraindications. Digitalis is not usually effective and it gives frequent toxicity in premature infants.

H. Specific Therapy

No treatment is required for premature infants without CHF or other clinical manifestations of a patent ductus arteriosus except heart murmur since spontaneous closure usually occurs by 40 weeks of conceptual age.

1. Medical therapy for symptomatic infants
   Administer indomethacin (prostaglandin synthetase inhibitor), 0.2 mg/kg every 12 hours for 3 doses orally. Recommended IV dosage according to age is as follows:

AGE AT FIRST DOSE	DOSE (mg/kg) 1st	2nd	3rd
$<$48 hours	0.2	0.1	0.1
2–7 days	0.2	0.2	0.2
$>$7 days	0.2	0.25	0.25

   Infants should have normal platelet counts, BUN, and creatinine. If the ductus arteriosus closes or infant develops complications from indomethacin, discontinue the medication. This regimen may be repeated after 48 hours if the ductus arteriosus does not close or reopens provided the infant does not have any complications from indomethacin.
   A high failure rate has been reported in infants less than 1,000 gm and infants more than 2 weeks of age when indomethacin was given orally.
   a. Indications for indomethacin
      Premature infants (preferably less than 2 weeks of age) with left-to-right shunting through a patent ductus arteriosus, inability to be weaned from the ventilator, and/or minimal evidence of CHF
   b. Contraindications to the use of indomethacin
      1) Necrotizing enterocolitis
      2) Hyperbilirubinemia greater than 10 to 12 mg/dl
      3) Renal failure or serum creatinine greater than 1.8 mg/dl
      4) Bleeding diasthesis, thrombocytopenia
      5) Dehydration
      6) Hepatic dysfunction
   c. Complications
      1) Transient renal dysfunction: oliguria due to vasopressin release, elevated BUN and creatinine, elevated potassium
      2) Hyponatremia due to potentiating antidiuretic hormone and decreased urinary sodium excretion; hypoglycemia
      3) Reduced platelet aggregation greater than 1 week
      4) Displace bilirubin from binding sites only with high doses.

2. Surgical management
   If the ductus arteriosus stays open in spite of the three courses of indomethacin, the infant may require surgical ligation of the ductus arteriosus.

REFERENCES

Bhat R., Fisher E., Raju T.N.K., et al.: Patent ductus arteriosus: Recent advances in diagnosis and management. *Ped. Clin. N. Am.* 29:1117, 1982.

Friedman W.F., Hirschklau M.J., Printz M.P., et al.: Pharmacologic closure of patent ductus arteriosus in the premature infant. *N. Engl. J. Med.* 95:526, 1976.

Friedman W.F., Kurlinski J., Jacob J., et al.: The inhibition of prostaglandin and prostacyclin synthesis in the clinical management of patent ductus arteriosus. *Sem. Perinatol.* 4:125, 1980.

XXXI. ARRHYTHMIAS (DYSRHYTHMIAS)

Healthy normal fullterm and premature infants have heart rates usually between 100 and 180 beats/minute and occasionally 90 to 195 beats/minute. Transient periods of sinus bradycardia may be seen during straining, micturition, crying, and compression of the anterior fontanelle and are more frequent in premature infants. Sinus tachycardia may occur with increased activity, crying, fever, and hyperthyroidism. Maternal medications (reserpine or propranolol) may result in bradycardia.

Premature supraventricular and ventricular beats, brief periods of sinus arrest, ectopic atrial rhythm, and wandering atrial pacemaker may be observed on ECG monitoring of asymptomatic newborns.

Arrhythmia may be seen in infants with cardiac pathology or extracardiac disease and may be potentially dangerous; therefore, it is important to differentiate.

Congenital atrioventricular block is often diagnosed in utero.

(See Table 11–4.)

TABLE 11–4.—Common Arrhythmias Seen in the Newborn Infant

ARRHYTHMIAS	CAUSE AND/OR ASSOCIATIONS	CLINICAL MANIFESTATIONS	ECG	MANAGEMENT
Tachycardia				
Supraventricular tachycardia (most common tachycardia)	Transposition of great vessels; Ebstein's anomaly, cardiomyopathy	Severe congestive heart failure or shock in utero, first hour or later; pale, ashen color; tachycardia >210–300/min; poor feeding; irritability	Heart rate >210/min, fixed RR interval; no change with cry, absent or abnormal P wave shape, Wolff-Parkinson-White Syndrome (short PR interval and slow upstroke of QRS "delta" wave tachycardia.)	IV digitalization and maintain ½–1 year (20% recurrence in 1 year). Direct current synchronized cardioversion of ¼ watt-second/pound is usually effective; increased recurrence with Wolff-Parkinson-White Syndrome; propranolol, 0.05–0.1 mg/kg IV, if not corrected; maternal propranolol may convert intrauterine SVT
Atrial flutter	Stretched atria, mitral valve disease, endocardial fibroelastosis, tricuspid atresia, Ebstein's anomaly, ventricular septal defect, etc.; normal newborns	May be diagnosed in utero; signs of congestive heart failure, regular tachycardia not influenced by effort or position	Atrial rate 250–400/min, regular atrial beats, characteristic "sawtooth" pattern, some degree of atrioventricular block	Direct current cardioversion, digitalization after conversion and maintain for 1 yr; propranolol if not converted

Bradycardia				
Atrioventricular block (most common bradycardia)	Congenital heart block, transposition of great vessels, ASD, Ebstein's anomaly, postsurgery infection (viral), fibrous degeneration, digitalis administration (1%), maternal connective tissue disease, no evidence of heart disease	Usually asymptomatic, syncope, easy fatigability, ventricular rate $<$55/min, atrial rate $>$140/min, often die in the first yr, congestive heart failure common, ⅓ recognized in utero	Heart rate 90/min; first degree: prolonged PR interval, second degree: not all atrial beats conduct to the ventricle, third degree: atrial depolarizations not related to QRS complexes; no increase in heart rate with exercise	Atrial sensing ventricular-inhibited pacemaker implantation for third-degree atrioventricular block with congestive heart failure, neonatal stress (e.g., respiratory distress syndrome), syncope, wide QRS escape rhythms, ventricular rhythm $<$55/min or $<$65–70/min with congenital heart defects or ventricular arrhythmia Pacemaker implantation when bradycardia becomes life-threatening
Sinus bradycardia	Severe systemic disease, hypoxia, acidosis, fetal distress, hydrops fetalis, increased intracranial pressure, electrolyte imbalance; other arrhythmias, premature atrial tachycardia, premature ventricular contraction	May be intermittent bradycardia with intermittent sinus arrest and paroxysmal tachycardia	Heart rate $<$90/min, no increase in heart rate with stimulation	Correct primary causes

REFERENCE

Adams F.H., Emmanouilides G.C.: Heart Disease in Infants, Children and Adolescents, ed. 3. Baltimore, Williams & Wilkins Co., 1983.

Chapter 12

Cyanosis

Cyanosis, a blue or dusky hue, may indicate a trivial or life-threatening condition. Cyanosis is usually perceived when O_2 saturation is reduced to less than 85%, but some physicians perceive cyanosis at a higher O_2 saturation and some at a lower saturation. The degree of cyanosis depends upon the arterial oxygen saturation (Sa_{O_2}), hemoglobin concentration, pH, peripheral circulation, and temperature of the infant.

It is important to obtain an arterial blood gas as soon as cyanosis is noted to establish if a process impairing oxygenation exists. The old axiom is true that once an infant is noted to be persistently cyanotic during the first day or two of life, only one thing generally happens: the infant gets worse. Rapid evaluation to establish the diagnosis is therefore mandatory.

I. CLINICAL EVALUATION

A. Factors Affecting the Degree of Cyanosis

1. Hemoglobin concentration
   Cyanosis is apparent when the reduced hemoglobin concentration of arterial blood is beyond 3 to 5 gm/dl. In infants with 20 gm/dl hemoglobin, cyanosis is apparent with an Sa_{O_2} of 75% to 85%. Sa_{O_2} = [actual hemoglobin (20 gm/dl) − reduced hemoglobin (3 to 5 gm/dl)] ÷ actual hemoglobin (20 gm/dl) × 100 = 85% to 75%. In infants with anemia (e.g., 8 gm/dl hemoglobin), cyanosis is not apparent until Sa_{O_2} is decreased to 37.5% to 62.5%.
2. Peripheral perfusion
   Even when Sa_{O_2} is normal, the infant may appear cyanotic if there is poor peripheral perfusion (due to hypothermia, acidosis, etc.) because relatively slow peripheral blood flow results in a large arteriovenous difference. Therefore, it is important to observe central cyanosis of the lips and/or mucous membranes.
3. Experience
   Skilled attendants may observe cyanosis with 3 gm/dl of reduced hemoglobin

while neophytes may only observe cyanosis with 5 gm/dl of reduced hemoglobin.

4. Illumination
   Infants in a dark blue painted room, under a blue phototherapy light, or in blue clothing may look cyanotic with normal Sa_{O_2}.

B. Types of Cyanosis

1. Peripheral cyanosis (acrocyanosis)
   Peripheral cyanosis, a blue discoloration or duskiness confined to the skin of the extremities, is usually ascribed to "vasomotor instability"; is frequently seen in normal infants; may be due to a cold environment, a high hematocrit, or local obstruction; and may persist for days or weeks.
2. Central cyanosis
   Central cyanosis, a blue discoloration of the mucous membranes and periphery due to the presence of 3 gm/dl or more of reduced hemoglobin in arterial blood may be considered pathologic. Persistent central cyanosis always requires immediate evaluation.

II. COMMON CAUSES OF CYANOSIS IN THE NEWBORN

A. Alveolar Hypoventilation

Decreased $P_{A_{O_2}}$, increased $P_{A_{CO_2}}$, decreased Sa_{O_2}, decreased Pa_{O_2}, increased Pa_{CO_2}, e.g.:

1. CNS abnormalities
   Narcotics, CNS hemorrhage or malformation, infection, apnea of prematurity
2. Airway obstructions
   Choanal atresia, laryngeal webs, tracheal stenosis, vascular ring
3. Space-occupying lesions of the chest
   Congenital lobar emphysema, air leak syndrome (pneumothorax, pulmonary interstitial emphysema, etc.), diaphragmatic hernia, pleural effusion, abdominal distention (ascites, etc.)
4. Decreased pulmonary parenchyma
   Hypoplastic lung
5. Decreased pulmonary compliance
   Respiratory distress syndrome, pulmonary edema, TTNB, congestive heart failure
6. Interference with neuromuscular control of breathing
   Diaphragmatic paralysis
7. Metabolic
   Hypoglycemia, Hypocalcemia

B. Right-to-left Shunt

Normal PA_{O_2}, normal or decreased PA_{CO_2}, decreased Sa_{O_2}, decreased Pa_{O_2}, normal or decreased Pa_{O_2}, e.g.:

1. Intracardiac
   a. With increased pulmonary blood flow
      Transposition of great vessels, truncus arteriosus, etc.
   b. With decreased pulmonary blood flow
      Tetralogy of Fallot, tricuspid atresia, pulmonary atresia, etc.
2. Extracardiac
   Patent ductus arteriosus with high pulmonary resistance
3. Intrapulmonary
   Atelectatic disease (respiratory distress syndrome, atelectasis, etc.)
4. Persistent pulmonary hypertension of the newborn

C. Uneven Ventilation/Perfusion Ratio

Variable PA_{O_2}, PA_{CO_2}, Pa_{CO_2}, decreased Sa_{O_2} and Pa_{O_2}, e.g., meconium aspiration syndrome, respiratory distress syndrome, polycythemia, pneumonia, pulmonary hemorrhage, regional atelectasis, etc.

D. Diffusion Interference

Normal PA_{O_2}, PA_{CO_2}, and Pa_{CO_2}; decreased Sa_{O_2} and Pa_{O_2}, e.g., meconium aspiration syndrome, pulmonary edema

E. Decreased Affinity of Hemoglobin for O_2

Normal PA_{O_2}, PA_{CO_2}, Pa_{O_2} and Pa_{CO_2}; decreased Sa_{O_2}, e.g., methemoglobinemia

III. WHAT THE PHYSICIAN SHOULD DO WHEN CONFRONTED WITH AN INFANT WITH CYANOSIS

The following table shows the diagnostic workup for the infant with cyanosis.

WORKUP	FINDINGS	RISKS
1. Review maternal or family history	a. Maternal diabetes	a. Hypoglycemia, hypocalcemia, polycythemia, respiratory distress syndrome
	b. Maternal medications (narcotics for labor pain)	b. Respiratory depression
	c. Prolonged rupture of the membranes	c. Infection

WORKUP	FINDINGS	RISKS
	d. Family history of methemoglobinemia	d. Methemoglobinemia
2. Review prenatal and/or delivery history	a. Oligohydramnios	a. Hypoplastic lungs
	b. Polyhydramnios	b. Esophageal atresia
	c. Fetal distress	c. Congestive heart failure and pulmonary edema, persistent pulmonary hypertension of the newborn
	d. Difficult, traumatic delivery	d. CNS hemorrhage, diaphragmatic paralysis
	e. Cesarean section	e. Respiratory distress syndrome, TTNB
3. Review of cyanosis history	a. Intermittent cyanosis	a. CNS abnormalities
	b. Cyanosis with first feeding	b. Esophageal atresia
	c. Cyanosis at birth and pink during crying	c. Choanal atresia
4. Physical examination	a. Low blood pressure	a. Shock
	b. Tachypnea with dyspnea Tachypnea without dyspnea	b. Pulmonary pathology Cyanotic congenital heart disease, methemoglobinemia
	c. Apnea or depressed breathing	c. CNS or metabolic disease
	d. Premature infants	d. Respiratory distress syndrome
	e. Postmature infants	e. Meconium aspiration syndrome, polycythemia
	f. Large- or small-for-gestational-age	f. Polycythemia, hypoglycemia
	g. Scaphoid abdomen	g. Diaphragmatic hernia
	h. Abdominal distention	h. Ascites
	i. Plethora	i. Polycythemia
	j. Poor perfusion	j. Polycythemia, sepsis with shock, hypoplastic left heart syndrome, hypothermia
	k. Decreased tone and activity	k. Shock, sepsis, CNS disease, acidosis
	l. Unable to pass a nasogastric tube or nasal catheter	l. Esophageal atresia or choanal atresia
	m. Increased precordial activity loud murmur	m. Congenital heart disease, congestive heart failure
5. Obtain chest x-ray film	a. Abnormal pulmonary parenchyma	a. Primary pulmonary disease (respiratory distress syndrome, pneumonia, meconium aspiration syndrome, pulmonary air leak syndrome, diaphragmatic hernia, etc.)
	b. Enlarged heart	b. Congestive heart failure
	c. Fluid in the minor fissure and costophrenic angles	c. Polycythemia, TTNB

(continued)

WORKUP	FINDINGS	RISKS
5. Obtain chest x-ray film–*(continued)*	d. Normal chest x-ray film	d. Choanal atresia, CNS disease, metabolic disease, methemoglobinemia
6. Obtain appropriate laboratory tests	a. Hematocrit (venous or arterial), increased or decreased	a. Polycythemia, anemia
	b. Low serum glucose	b. Hypoglycemia
	c. Low serum calcium	c. Hypocalcemia
	d. Arterial blood gases: increased Pa_{CO_2}	d. Alveolar hypoventilation
	1) Hyperoxia test with 100% O_2 Pa_{O_2} of $\geq$150 mm Hg	Uneven ventilation/perfusion ratio, diffusion interference, decreased hemoglobin affinity for O_2 (but cyanotic in methemoglobinemia)
	Little effect on Pa_{O_2}	Right-to-left shunt (congenital heart disease, persistent pulmonary hypertension of the newborn)
	2) Hyperoxia-hyperventilation test Increased Pa_{O_2}	Persistent pulmonary hypertension of the newborn
	Little effect on Pa_{O_2}	Cyanotic congenital heart disease
	3) Differential Pa_{O_2}, Sa_{O_2} between right arm and lower body (taken simultaneously)	Right-to-left shunt via patent ductus arteriosus
	e. CBC, platelet count, and culture of CSF, blood, and urine	e. Infection
	f. Increased CSF protein and red blood cells	f. Infection, CNS hemorrhage
	g. A drop of blood on a glass slide remains brown with air blown on it	g. Methemoglobinemia
7. Administer vasodilator, 100% O_2, and hyperventilate	a. Pa_{O_2} increment of $>$15 mm Hg with tolazoline 1–2 mg/kg/$>$10 min	a. Persistent pulmonary hypertension of the newborn
	b. No Pa_{O_2} increase with tolazoline	b. Persistent pulmonary hypertension of the newborn, congenital heart disease
8. Obtain echocardiogram (rarely cardiac catheterization)	Diagnose or rule out cyanotic heart disease	

IV. GENERAL SUPPORTIVE MANAGEMENT

1. Position the infant in the supine position with a roll under his or her shoulders to extend the neck and keep the airway patent. Place an oropharyngeal airway if necessary.
2. Suction the infant as frequently as necessary.
3. Maintain the infant's abdominal skin temperature at approximately 36.5° C. Work within a warmed environment to avoid precipitous drops in body temperature associated with procedures, e.g., performing an ECG, inserting a catheter, and drawing a blood specimen.
4. Administer oxygen to keep the arterial oxygen tension between 50 and 70 mm Hg. Ventilate as required.
5. Consider withholding oral fluids to prevent aspiration or bradycardia.
6. Start IV fluids to maintain fluid and electrolyte status and to have an IV route for emergency and therapeutic IV medications.
7. If a right-to-left shunt with decreased pulmonary blood flow is present (ductus-dependent congenital heart disease: tetrology of Fallot, pulmonary stenosis or atresia, or tricuspid atresia), initiate therapy with prostaglandin E_1 to maintain a patent ductus. Surgical correction is then indicated. See chapter 11-XXVIII.
8. Diuretics and digitalization are required for congestive heart failure (see chapter 11–XXIX).
9. If a pulmonary process is present, see chapter 11.
10. If hypoglycemia and/or hypocalcemia is present, see chapter 15–IX and 15–X.
11. If infection is present, see chapter 16.
12. If intracranial hemorrhage is present, see chapter 15–VI to 15–VIII.
13. If apnea is present, see chapter 11–X.
14. If seizures are present, see chapter 15–III.

REFERENCES

Goldman H.I., Maralit A., Sun S. et al.: Neonatal cyanosis and arterial oxygen saturation. *J. Pediatr.* 82:319–324, 1973.

Kitterman J.A.: Cyanosis in the newborn infant. *Pediatr. Rev.* 4:13, 1982.

Lees M.H.: Cyanosis of the newborn infant. *J. Pediatr.* 77:484, 1970.

Readinger R., Norton J.B., Dungan W.T.: Pediatric review: An approach to cyanosis in the newborn. *J. Arkansas Med. Soc.* 76:365, 1980.

V. POLYCYTHEMIA AND HYPERVISCOSITY

Polycythemia, a marked increase in red blood cell mass associated with an increase in blood viscosity, is noted in 1.8% to 6% of newborns (venous hematocrit greater than 65% or cord hematocrit greater than 56%). The increased blood viscosity interferes with tissue perfusion as well as cardiopulmonary and metabolic adaptation.

A. Who Is at Risk?

1. Infants who have had excessive placental transfusion
   a. Delayed cord clamping (more than 2.5 minutes after birth)
   b. Maternal fetal transfusion
   c. Twin-to-twin transfusion (recipient)
2. Infants who are small for gestational age
   a. Postmature infants
   b. Fullterm or premature infants
3. Infants whose mothers had a complicated pregnancy
   a. Toxemia of pregnancy
   b. Placenta previa
4. Infants who have had, or infants whose mothers have had, endocrine disorders
   a. Congenital adrenal hyperplasia
   b. Neonatal thyrotoxicosis
   c. Maternal diabetes
5. Infants with Down's syndrome
6. Infants with Beckwith's syndrome

B. Clinical Manifestations

Clinical manifestations are often related to poor perfusion within the cardiopulmonary system, CNS, GI tract, kidney, and muscle.

1. Tachypnea, cyanosis, persistent pulmonary hypertension of the newborn
2. Poor feeding, vomiting, NEC
3. Convulsions, irritability, hypertonia, tremors
4. Priapism
5. Jaundice
6. Congestive heart failure
7. Renal vein thrombosis
8. Gangrene of fingers and toes

C. Laboratory Findings

1. Venous hemoglobin greater than 21 gm/dl and hematocrit greater than 65%, cord hematocrit greater than 56%
2. Increase in blood viscosity greater than 7.5 cps at a shear rate of 115/second^{-1} (cord viscosity greater than 5.6 at 115/second^{-1})
3. Transient thrombocytopenia
4. Increased number of circulating nucleated red blood cells

5. Hyperbilirubinemia (secondary to breakdown of increased hemoglobin)
6. Hypocalcemia
7. Hypoglycemia (secondary to glucolytic activity of red blood cells)
8. Proteinuria, hemoglobinuria
9. Decreased cerebral blood flow
10. Decreased cardiac output and increased ductal right-to-left shunting

D. Supportive Management

See chapter 12–IV for "general supportive management" of the infant with cyanosis.

E. Specific/Supportive Therapy

1. Monitor the levels of venous blood hematocrit, glucose, calcium, and bilirubin and correct as required.
2. Obtain a urinalysis to determine the presence of red blood cells in the urine (renal vein thrombosis).
3. Obtain a platelet and a nucleated red blood cell count.
4. Monitor the infant for respiratory, cardiac, and CNS symptoms.
5. Perform a partial exchange transfusion using fresh frozen plasma, Plasmanate, or 5% albumin if the infant develops any symptoms or Hct is greater than 65%.

   $$\text{Volume of exchange (ml)} = \text{Blood volume (80–100 ml/kg)} \times \frac{\text{Observed} - \text{Desired Hct (55\%)}}{\text{Observed Hct}}$$

   Since volume of exchange is usually less than 60 ml, complications from umbilical catheterization can be prevented by using a peripheral arterial catheter (radial arterial catheter) for drawing blood and a peripheral venous catheter for infusing Plasmanate, etc.
6. Monitor vital signs during exchange transfusion.
7. Obtain a hematocrit before and 1 hour, 8 hours, and 24 hours after exchange transfusion.
8. Measure central venous pressure immediately before and after exchange transfusion if possible.
9. Obtain a chest x-ray film and ECG as necessary.

F. Prognosis

Twenty-five percent of infants with symptoms have significant neurologic and developmental abnormalities. Neurologic abnormalities are more common in the nonexchanged group (especially with hypoglycemia) than in the exchanged group.

REFERENCES

Black V.D., Lubchenco L.O.: Neonatal polycythemia and hyperviscosity. *Ped. Clin. N. Am.,* 29:1137, 1982.

Goldberg K., Wirth F.H., Hathaway W.E., et al.: Neonatal hyperviscosity: II. Effects of partial plasma exchange. *Pediatrics* 69:419, 1982.

Shohat M., Merlob P., Reisner S.H.: Neonatal polycythemia: 1. Early diagnosis and incidence relating to time of sampling. *Pediatrics* 73:7, 1984.

VI. METHEMOGLOBINEMIA

Methemoglobin is an otherwise normal hemoglobin in which the iron is oxidized from the ferrous to the ferric state. Iron in the ferric state is not able to form a complex with oxygen for transport. Normally less than 2% of hemoglobin is present as methemoglobin.

A. Who Is at Risk?

1. Infants with increased methemoglobin production by oxidizing agents, e.g., aniline dyes, bismuth subnitrate, sodium nitrate, well water (nitrates), nitrate food additives, benzocaine, partially cooked spinach, home-prepared carrot juice.
2. Infants with impaired reduction of methemoglobin
   a. Infants with transient deficiency of $NADH_2$-dependent methemoglobin diaphorase reductase (e.g., prematures)
   b. Infants with congenital deficiency of NADH-dependent diaphorase. (In the Navajo Indians, this is an autosomal recessive trait.)
   c. Newborns less than 4 months of age since those infants have a high level of hemoglobin F, and the γ chain of hemoglobin F is more susceptible to methemoglobin formation than hemoglobin A
3. Infants with abnormal hemoglobin, e.g., hemoglobin M (five hemoglobin M variants have been described, but this hemoglobinopathy is rare)

B. Clinical Manifestations

1. Slate gray, lavender, or deep generalized cyanosis
2. Absence of respiratory distress, pulmonary rales, and cardiac murmurs
3. With greater than 30% methemoglobin, infants may be tachypneic and tachycardic.

C. Laboratory Findings

1. With methemoglobin greater than 10%, drops of capillary blood do not turn red on shaking with air or oxygen but remain chocolate brown.

2. Normal chest x-ray film and ECG
3. Methemoglobin is detected spectroscopically with absorption peak at 634 mμ that disappears on addition of cyanide.
4. Hemoglobin electrophoresis detects hemoglobin M.
5. Enzyme studies for methemoglobin reductase show a decrease in activity.
6. Hemolytic anemia and jaundice in methemoglobinemia due to toxins (e.g., aniline dye)

The diagnosis depends on a high degree of clinical suspicion. Enzyme studies and electrophoresis are rarely obtained in an emergent clinical situation.

D. Supportive Management

See chapter 12–IV for "general supportive management" of the infant with cyanosis.

E. Specific Therapy

1. Identify the potential oxidant-toxin and remove the infant's exposure to the toxin.
2. Administer methylene blue, 1 to 2 mg/kg of a 1% solution in normal saline IV. Persisting methemoglobinemia in spite of methylene blue suggests methemoglobin M. Otherwise the infant becomes pink within 1 to 2 hours. Recurrence suggests hereditary methemoglobinemia due to enzyme deficiency.
3. Continuous therapy can be maintained with oral methylene blue for enzyme deficiency. Large dose of oral ascorbic acid, 300 to 400 mg/24 hours may be tried. Observe for hemolytic anemia from excessive dose of methylene blue.

REFERENCES

Balsamo P., Hardy W.R., Scott E.M.: Hereditary methemoglobinemia due to diaphorase deficiency in Navajo Indians. *J. Pediatr.* 65:928, 1964.

Bartos H.R., Desforges J.F.: Erythrocyte DPNH dependent diaphorase levels in infants. *Pediatrics* 37:991, 1966.

Chapter 13

Jaundice

Jaundice (bilirubin greater than 2 mg/dl) is one of the most common abnormal physical signs noted in the newborn. It is known that hyperbilirubinemia greater than 20 mg/dl due to hemolysis is often associated with severe neurologic damage or death due to bilirubin toxicity (kernicterus) and that very low birth weight infants with bilirubin levels as low as 6 mg/dl can also develop kernicterus. Therefore, every physician who cares for the newborn should be thoroughly acquainted with the causes and problems associated with neonatal jaundice.

I. NORMAL DATA

A. Bilirubin Metabolism

Bilirubin, a tetrapyrol, is derived from the catabolism of heme proteins, mainly hemoglobin of erythrocytes, and partly myoglobin and heme-containing enzymes. Bilirubin, under physiologic conditions, is insoluble in the serum and is bound tightly to albumin at primary and secondary binding sites for transport. Bilirubin is transferred from the circulation to the liver, bound by Y and Z proteins, conjugated by glucuronyl transferase (UDPG-T), converted to the water-soluble conjugated direct-reacting bilirubin, and excreted into the bile. Conjugated bilirubin enters the intestine and is reduced to stercobilin by bacteria. Some conjugated bilirubin is hydrolyzed to unconjugated bilirubin by the enzyme β-glucuronidase in the absence of bacteria and reabsorbed from the gut into the circulation, and the reabsorbed bilirubin requires repeat liver metabolism. This phenomenon is called the enterohepatic circulation.

B. Physiologic Jaundice

Almost every newborn infant develops some degree of jaundice. Jaundice is considered physiologic if the serum indirect bilirubin does not exceed 5 mg/dl in the first 24 hours; 12 mg/dl in fullterm infants or 15 mg/dl in premature infants at 2 to 6 days of age; and 10 mg/dl after the first week of life. In low birth weight infants, the increased levels of bilirubin and prolonged jaundice are noted as long as 2 weeks after birth due to immaturity of the liver and increased enterohepatic reabsorption. Serum direct bilirubin levels should not exceed 1 mg/dl.

The causes of physiologic jaundice are considered to be as follows:

1. An increased bilirubin load on liver cells due to the following:
   a. Increased red blood cell volume in the newborn period
   b. Decreased fetal red blood cell survival time (90 days)
   c. Increased enterohepatic circulation of bilirubin
2. A defective uptake of bilirubin from the plasma, because of decreased transport and a deficient caloric intake in the first 48 to 72 hours of life
3. A decreased ability of the liver to conjugate bilirubin caused by a decrease in glucuronyl transferase.
4. A decreased ability of the liver to excrete bilirubin
5. An altered hepatic circulation through the ductus venosus after birth

II. COMMON CAUSES OF JAUNDICE IN THE NEWBORN INFANT

A. Indirect Hyperbilirubinemia

1. Presenting during the first day of life
   a. Blood-group incompatiblity: Rh, ABO, other minor blood groups (Kell, c,E, Duffy, Kidd, etc.)
   b. Intrauterine infection: rubella, cytomegalovirus, toxoplasmosis, syphilis, occasionally other bacteria (*Escherichia coli, Staphylococcus, Pseudomonas, Klebsiella, Proteus, Streptococcus,* etc.)
   c. Erythropoietic porphyria
2. Presenting during second or third day of life
   a. Physiologic jaundice
   b. Blood-group incompatibility
   c. Infection, often caused by gram-negative or gram-positive organisms (*E. coli* or streptococci, etc.)
   d. Polycythemia (hyperviscosity syndrome) or hyponatremia
   e. Extravascular blood: skin bruises, subdural hematoma, subcapsular liver hemorrhage, bone fracture, pulmonary or CNS hemorrhage, swallowed maternal blood during parturition, etc.
   f. Increased enterohepatic circulation: mechanical intestinal obstruction or reduced peristalsis
   g. Abnormal red blood cell morphology: spherocytosis, elliptocytosis, stomatocytosis, infantile pyknocytosis, etc.
   h. Red blood cell enzyme deficiencies: glucose-6-phosphate dehydrogenase (G-6-PD), 6-phosphogluconate dehydrogenase, pyruvate kinase, hexokinase, phosphoglucose isomerase, glutathione perioxidase, etc.

i. Respiratory distress syndrome
j. Heinz body anemia caused by drugs and toxins: vitamin K_3, naphthalene, menadione, phenylhydrazine, naphthoguinone, sodium nitrite, and phenolic disinfectant
k. Transient familial neonatal hyperbilirubinemia

3. Presenting during the fourth and fifth days of life
   a. Breast feeding
   b. Respiratory distress syndrome
   c. Maternal diabetes
   d. Crigler-Najjar syndrome
   e. Gilbert's syndrome
4. Presenting after one week of life
   a. Herpes simplex
   b. Pyloric stenosis
   c. Hypothyroidism
   d. Neonatal giant cell hepatitis
   e. Infection, usually acquired infection in the neonatal period
   f. Galactosemia

B. Direct Hyperbilirubinemia

Direct hyperbilirubinemia usually occurs after 1 week of life. It may be caused by hepatocellular disturbances in bilirubin excretion.

1. Primary hepatitis
   a. Neonatal idiopathic hepatitis (giant cell hepatitis)
   b. Hepatitis caused by identified infectious agents
   Hepatitis B (HB_sAg), rubella, cytomegalovirus, *Toxoplasma* organisms, coxsackievirus, syphilis, herpes simplex, varicella-zoster, *Listeria* organisms, tubercle bacillus
2. Toxic hepatitis caused by systemic infectious diseases, etc.
   E. coli (sepsis or urinary tract), pneumococci, *Proteus* organisms, *Salmonella* organisms, idiopathic diarrhea, intestinal obstruction, parenteral alimentation, ischemic necrosis
3. Hematologic disorders
   Erythroblastosis fetalis (severe forms), congenital erythropoietic porphyria
4. Metabolic and heredofamilial disorders
   α-1-Antitrypsin deficiency, galactosemia, tyrosinemia, fructosemia, glycogen storage disease type IV, lipid storage diseases (Niemann-Pick disease, Gaucher's disease, Wolman's disease), cerebrohepatorenal syndrome (Zellweger's syndrome), trisomy 18, cystic fibrosis, familial idiopathic cholestasis (Byler's disease).
5. Ductal disturbances in bilirubin excretion
   Extrahepatic biliary atresia (without associated malformations, associated with trisomy 18, or associated with polysplenia-heterotaxia syndrome), intrahepatic atresia associated with lymphedema, extrahepatic stenosis and choledochal

cyst, bile plug syndrome, cystic fibrosis, tumors of the liver and biliary tract, periductal lymphadenopathy

6. Parenteral nutrition

C. Combined Indirect and Direct Hyperbilirubinemia

Combined indirect and direct hyperbilirubinemia can occur at any time.

1. Intrauterine or perinatal infections (rubella, cytomegalovirus, toxoplasmosis, herpes simplex, syphilis, hepatitis, etc.), postnatal infections
2. Severe hemolytic disease

III. WHAT THE PHYSICIAN SHOULD DO WHEN CONFRONTED WITH AN INFANT WITH JAUNDICE

A. Diagnostic Workup for Indirect Hyperbilirubinemia

1. Obtain baseline hematocrit and bilirubin levels (direct and indirect) and follow as necessary.
2. Obtain the blood group and Rh factor of the mother and the infant. Subgroup, if necessary, and repeat, if necessary.
3. Perform a direct Coombs' test. If positive, the antibody should be eluted from the infant's red blood cells.
4. Review the infant's family history to determine a history of the following:
   a. Blood-group incompatibility
   b. Jaundice or exchange transfusion in other siblings
   c. Red blood cell enzyme deficiency
   d. Abnormality in red blood cell morphology
5. Review the prenatal history to determine the presence of possible intrauterine infection, maternal drug ingestion, difficult delivery, or other conditions.
6. Review the infant's feeding history, frequency and quantity of meconium, and type and quantity of drugs ingested.
7. Examine the infant carefully considering the causes of neonatal jaundice, such as intrauterine infection, polycythemia (hyperviscosity syndrome), hydrops fetalis, subcapsular hemorrhage with hepatomegaly, or extravasated blood (see chapter 13–II for "common causes of jaundice in the newborn infant").
8. Make a smear of the infant's peripheral blood to determine the following:
   a. The red blood cell morphology (spherocytosis, elliptocytosis, stomatocytosis, infantile pyknocytosis, etc.). These are best seen on an unstained blood smear. Examine the parent's red blood cells if spherocytosis or another disorder is suspected. The presence of spherocytosis, polychromatophilia, acanthocytes, and/or anisocytosis is suggestive of hemolysis.
   b. The presence of increased numbers of reticulocytes and nucleated red blood cells

9. Obtain a complete blood count (CBC) for leukopenia, leukocytosis, or increased immature cells and cultures of the urine, blood, and CSF if infection is suspected.
10. Obtain total protein, albumin levels, and electrolytes.
11. Check the mother's serologic test for syphilis (STS). Obtain the infant's STS if mother's test is positive.
12. Analyze a urine specimen for the presence of reducing substances and signs of infection (white blood cells, protein, etc.).
13. If red blood cell enzyme deficiency is suspected, perform screening tests.
14. Obtain serum thyroxine, triiodothyronine, and thyroid-stimulating hormone if indirect hyperbilirubinemia is prolonged.

B. Diagnostic Workup for Direct Hyperbilirubinemia

1. Review history of duration and quantity of parenteral nutrition. Direct hyperbilirubinemia often occurs after 2 weeks of total parenteral nutrition.
2. Obtain direct and indirect bilirubin levels and follow as necessary.
3. Obtain liver function tests: total protein, serum glutamic oxaloacetic transaminase (SGOT), serum glutamic pyruvic transaminase (SGPT), alkaline phosphatase, 5′ nucleotidase, γ-glutamyl transpeptidase (GGTP), prothrombin time, partial thromboplastin time, α-1-antitrypsin, cholesterol, and α-fetoprotein.
4. Obtain appropriate tests for bacterial and viral infection: IgM, TORCH (complement fixation) titers, HB_sAg (in both mother and infant), viral cultures of blood, nose, throat, stool, and CSF.
5. Obtain urine for protein, glucose, reducing substances, amino acids, bilirubin, and urobilinogen.
6. Obtain 24-hour collection of duodenal fluid for bile pigment if necessary.
7. Obtain iodine 131-labelled rose bengal excretion test or ^{99m}TcPIPIDA scan.
8. Obtain inborn-error metabolic disease screening test.
9. If laboratory tests for evaluation of direct hyperbilirubinemia indicate, consult a pediatric gastroenterologist for a liver biopsy.

C. General Supportive Management for the Infant With Indirect Hyperbilirubinemia

1. Handle the infant gently (as always).
2. Maintain the infant's abdominal skin temperature at approximately 36.5° C (97.7° F) and rectal temperature at approximately 37.0° C (98.6° F).
3. Eliminate the "possible" predisposing factors of kernicterus (hypothermia, hyperthermia, hypoxia, acidosis, dehydration, competing drugs).
4. Administer oral feedings if the infant can tolerate feeding by mouth. If not, give parenteral fluids.
5. Draw blood to check bilirubin and hematocrit levels every 4 hours and plot results against the infant's age on a bilirubin chart.

6. Administer phototherapy, and exchange transfusion, as indicated (see chapter 13–V and 13–VI).

REFERENCE

Cashore W.J., Stern L.: Neonatal hyperbilirubinemia. *Ped. Clin. N. Am.* 29:1191, 1982.

IV. KERNICTERUS: BILIRUBIN ENCEPHALOPATHY

Kernicterus refers to yellow staining of nuclear areas of the brain seen on gross postmortem examination. The yellow staining is often associated with irreversible neuronal damage and frequently is in the same areas as those affected by hypoxia. The basal ganglia and hippocampus are the most frequently affected areas. Severe hyperbilirubinemia due to hemolytic disease may result in kernicterus, functional impairment, or death; lower levels of bilirubin associated with an open blood-brain barrier may have a similar result in low birth weight or impaired infants. The pathogenesis of kernicterus is not fully understood and it is not known whether bilirubin is a primary or secondary cause of CNS injury.

A. Who Is at Risk?

Infants with conditions in which bilirubin crosses the blood-brain barrier and deposits in the neuron are reported to be at risk.

1. Fullterm infants with serum bilirubin greater than 20 mg/dl due to hemolytic disease. Several factors predispose the infant:
   a. Hypoalbuminemia
   b. Conditions competing with the primary binding site
      1) Increased nonesterified fatty acids due to total parenteral nutrition, hypothermia, fasting, septicemia, etc.
      2) Hematin arising from hemolysis or other causes
   c. Drugs competing with the secondary binding site
      salicylate, sulfonamide, sodium benzoate, diazepam (Valium), novobiocin, oxacillin sodium, cephalothin, furosemide
2. Infants with decreased albumin binding sites for bilirubin
3. Sick, premature low birth weight infants with serum bilirubin as low as 6 mg/dl. The mechanism of kernicterus in low birth weight infants is not known and may be different from that of hemolytic disease.

B. Clinical Manifestations

1. Kernicterus with severe hemolytic disease: indirect bilirubin greater than 20 mg/dl in fullterm infants
   a. Decreased activity, lethargy, hypotonia, diminished Moro's reflex, poor feeding
   b. Irritability, hypertonia, high-pitched cry, rigid extension of all four extremi-

ties, opisthotonos with marked rigid arching of the back, seizures, gastric or pulmonary hemorrhage, hyperthermia, and death

c. If the infant survives, hypotonia and poor feeding followed by spastic chorioathetoid cerebral palsy with tremors, fine motor clumsiness, paralysis of upward gaze, high-frequency hearing loss, and mental retardation

2. Bilirubin encephalopathy in low birth weight infants
   a. No symptoms, only mild neurologic manifestations, hearing loss, or subtle developmental problems have been reported in low birth weight infants with bilirubin levels of 10 to 20 mg/dl who survive.

C. Laboratory Findings

Both diffusion of unbound bilirubin at high bilirubin levels and entry of albumin-bound bilirubin due to reversible opening of the blood-brain barrier as a result of injury to the CNS or to the cerebral circulation may be responsible for the development of kernicterus. Factors other than unbound bilirubin such as degree of transfer of albumin-bound bilirubin across the blood-brain barrier and cellular uptake can not be measured. Therefore, no specific test can predict infants at risk.

The following methods have been proposed to assist identifying infants at risk:

1. Sephadex G-25 or peroxidase method measuring unbound or loosely bound bilirubin
2. HBABA binding capacity test measuring reserve binding sites
3. Salicylate saturation index measuring percent of bilirubin displaced
   Infants with hyperbilirubinemia have reversible abnormal auditory brain stem response in relation to the level of unbound bilirubin.

D. Specific Therapy

No known therapy is available. It is not clear if early exchange transfusion reverses the pathologic process once kernicterus has occurred.

E. Supportive Management

See chapter 13–IIIC for "general supportive management for the infant with indirect hyperbilirubinemia."

F. Prevention

See chapter 13–V for "phototherapy" and 13–VI for "exchange transfusion."

REFERENCES

Cashore W.J., Stern L.: Neonatal hyperbilirubinemia. *Ped. Clin. N. Am.* 29:1191, 1982.

Kim M.H., Yoon J.J., Sher J. et al.: Lack of predictive indices in kernicterus: A comparison of clinical and pathologic factors in infants with or without kernicterus. *Pediatrics* 66:852, 1980.

Lucey J.F.: Bilirubin and brain damage: A real mess. *Pediatrics* 69:381, 1982.

V. PHOTOTHERAPY

Phototherapy, the photoisomerization (80%) and photooxidation (20%) of bilirubin, has been shown to be an efficient method of preventing hyperbilirubinemia and lowering serum bilirubin. During phototherapy, bilirubin IXα(ZZ) is photoisomerized in the skin and subcutaneous tissues into photobilirubin. Photobilirubin is carried to the liver and secreted into the bile without conjugation. During phototherapy, bilirubin is also oxidized and these photodegradation products are excreted in the urine. Phototherapy is not without hazard and should not be used unless the physician is aware of the possible dangers and contraindications.

A. Guidelines for the Use of Phototherapy

There is no clear guideline as to when to start phototherapy at present since the safe level of bilirubin, the mechanism of bilirubin toxicity, and the efficacy of phototherapy to prevent bilirubin toxicity are not known. No test predicts with 100% accuracy the need for phototherapy.

In general, the following indications to start phototherapy are practiced by many physicians:

1. In fullterm infants with nonhemolytic jaundice and an indirect bilirubin level above 15 mg/dl (e.g., hyperbilirubinemia caused by Crigler-Najjar syndrome, polycythemia, and extravasation of blood from cephalohematoma, ecchymosis, and fracture)
2. In sick, less than 1,500-gm premature infants with nonhemolytic jaundice and an indirect bilirubin level above 6 to 8 mg/dl
3. In infants with Rh hemolytic jaundice without rapid hemolysis e.g., bilirubin rising less than 0.5 mg/dl/hour or less than 10 mg/dl during first day of life or a cord bilirubin level of less than 5 mg/dl
4. In term infants with ABO hemolytic disease, phototherapy may be started at total serum bilirubin levels of $\geq$10 mg/dl $<$12 hours of life, $\geq$12 at 18 hours, $\geq$14 at 24 hours, and $\geq$15 over 24 hours of life, and may be continued until $\geq$20 mg/dl, when exchange transfusion may be indicated.
5. In infants with erythroblastosis after the first exchange transfusion

B. Contraindications for the Use of Phototherapy

Phototherapy is not indicated

1. Until the physician has tried to determine the cause of the infant's jaundice (see chapter 13–III for "what the physician should do when confronted with an infant with jaundice")
2. As a substitute for exchange transfusion
3. In infants with copious eye discharge whose eyes cannot be covered
4. In infants with hepatocellular liver disease. Infants with impaired biliary excretion develop a complication of phototherapy, the bronze baby syndrome.

These infants have an increased level of photoproducts of dark brown-black (bronze) pigment. It is not clear if this affects the CNS or not. If direct bilirubin is elevated, phototherapy should not be started or should be discontinued.

C. Practical Considerations of Administering Phototherapy

1. Mechanical techniques
   a. Specify the type of light to be used: blue, green, or daylight. Although blue light is a more effective reducer of bilirubin levels than daylight, daylight lamps are used in the most nurseries because blue light obscures cyanosis and makes the staff nauseous. The standard phototherapy unit is fitted with eight 20-watt daylight fluorescent lamps with a 400- to 500-nm wavelength and will provide an irradiation of 5 to 6 μW/sq cm/nm at a standard distance of 42 to 45 cm below the lamp. Phototherapy often decreases bilirubin levels approximately 2 to 3 mg/dl in 24 hours for infants with nonhemolytic hyperbilirubinemia. The greatest reduction is seen in the first day of exposure in the smallest infant.
   b. Order the light to be administered either continuously or intermittently. Substantial data as to which is preferable are lacking. Lights should be turned off during feeding and blood sampling.
   c. Position the light source between 42 to 45 cm to the top surface of the infant. The irradiance diminishes as the square of the distance is increased.
   d. Record the light-use hours of the phototherapy unit. The bulbs can be used 1,000 hours or more.
2. Procedures for the infant
   a. Specify whether the infant is to receive phototherapy in the incubator or warmer. The phototherapy unit must have a 0.25-inch thick thermoplastic cover with approximately 2 inches of space between the thermoplastic incubator hood and the cover of the lamp to minimize overheating of the incubator.
   b. Undress the infant with the exception of a small diaper before placing the infant under phototherapy.
   c. Order the infant to be turned every 2 to 4 hours.
   d. Monitor the infant's temperature hourly to avoid chilling or overheating.
   e. Cover the infant's eyes securely with an opaque eye shield to prevent retinal and optic nerve damage. Be sure to have the eye shield removed at least once every 4 hours to ascertain that the infant has not developed conjunctivitis or an eye discharge and to enhance visual contact.
   f. Weigh the infant every 8 to 24 hours and provide 10 to 25 ml/kg/day of extra fluid to compensate for increased insensible water loss especially in low birth weight infants.
   g. Monitor the infant's serum bilirubin level every 6 to 12 hours during phototherapy and for at least 24 hours after discontinuation of phototherapy; this is necessary as a rebound phenomenon may occur. Do not rely on the infant's skin color as a sign of jaundice because phototherapy

"bleaches" the skin while the bilirubin level may still be elevated. The usual methods for plasma bilirubin measurement do not distinguish bilirubin from photobilirubins.

h. Monitor the infant's hematocrit level during and for several months after discontinuation of phototherapy since phototherapy does not stop the hemolytic process and severe anemia may occur.

i. To avoid exposure of nearby unprotected infants, those receiving phototherapy should be placed at a sufficient distance from unshielded infants so that the eyes of the latter are not exposed to the phototherapy light source.

j. Discontinue phototherapy as soon as possible. In general, phototherapy may be discontinued when the indirect bilirubin level is less than 10 mg/dl and has been falling for 24 hours.

k. A rebound of 1 to 2 mg/dl of bilirubin is common particularly in low birth weight infants when phototherapy is discontinued.

3. Procedures for the family

Discontinue phototherapy and uncover the infant's eyes periodically to allow the family to see and touch their infant. Explain the phototherapy procedure to the family. They may be frightened when they see their infant under the light and wearing eye shields.

D. Complications of Phototherapy

1. Human infants
   a. Increased insensible and GI water loss with dehydration
   b. Loose, greenish stools
   c. Skin rash
   d. Jaundice or cyanosis masked by light
   e. Overheating or chilling
   f. Mild reduction of platelet counts
   g. Hypocalcemia
   h. Stimulation of the synthesis of melanin and vitamin D.
   i. Alteration of circadian rhythm (theoretical)
   j. Photosensitization
   k. Bronze baby syndrome, in the presence of direct hyperbilirubinemia
   l. Damaging effect of ultraviolet spectral emissions
   m. Nasal obstruction due to improper placement of eye shields
2. Animals
   a. Eye damage in piglets, rats, hamsters, mice, and monkeys
   b. Darkness-delayed pineal development in rabbits
   c. Retarded gonadal growth in rats
   d. Increased liver glycogen values in rats
3. In vitro data
   a. Decreased bilirubin-binding capacity of photooxidized albumin
   b. Increased hemolysis
   c. Transient G-6-PD deficiency

REFERENCES

Brown A.K., McDonagh A.F.: Phototherapy for neonatal hyperbilirubinemia: Efficacy, mechanism and toxicity. *Adv. Pediatr.* 27:341, 1980.

McDonagh A.F.: Phototherapy: A new twist to bilirubin. *J. Pediatr.* 99:909, 1981.

Osborn L.M., Lenarsky C., Oakes, R.C., et al.: Phototherapy in fullterm infants with hemolytic disease secondary to ABO incompatibility. *Pediatrics* 74:371, 1984.

VI. EXCHANGE TRANSFUSION

Exchange transfusion is a method for slowly exchanging the infant's blood for fresh adult blood.

A. Purposes

1. In infants with hyperbilirubinemia
   a. To remove Rh or ABO sensitized (antibody-coated) red blood cells and circulating antibodies
   b. To prevent kernicterus by reducing excessive hyperbilirubinemia
   c. To correct anemia
2. In infants exposed to toxic substances such as magnesium, either transplacentally or neonatally, to remove the toxic substances
3. In infants with hyperviscosity syndrome (polycythemia) or hyperkalemia to reduce intravascular red blood cell mass and correct electrolyte imbalance

B. Preparation Before Delivery in Case of Rh Incompatibility

When the obstetrician reports that the maternal Rh-antibody titer is greater than 1:64 and the ΔOD of the amniotic fluid is in Liley's zone 3 (see Fig 13–2), when the mother has lost a previous infant because of Rh incompatibility, or the fetus is hydropic, preparations for exchange transfusion should be completed before delivery.

1. Obtain 500 ml of group O, Rh-negative, low-titer blood compatible with maternal serum.
2. Prepare the exchange transfusion set.
3. Prepare for cardiorespiratory support. In cases of severe hydrops fetalis, the infant may need simultaneous paracentesis and thoracentesis.
4. Prepare to obtain the cord-hematocrit and bilirubin levels, blood group, and Coombs' test.
5. Prepare to obtain fetal scalp pH.

C. Criteria for Exchange Transfusion in Case of Rh Incompatibility

The level of indirect serum bilirubin continues to be the most widely used criterion for exchange transfusion. The criteria for exchange transfusion vary with the age and clinical condition of the newborn. No satisfactory validated criteria exist that can be relied on in all circumstances to prevent kernicterus.

1. Indications at birth (with hemolysis)
   A cord hemoglobin level of 13.5 gm/dl or less, a cord indirect bilirubin level of more than 5 mg/dl, and/or the clinical findings of hydrops fetalis
2. Indications in the first 24 hours of life and thereafter
   A rise in indirect bilirubin of 1 mg/dl/hour or more, or indirect bilirubin level greater than 20 mg/dl at any age due to severe hemolysis.
   Many neonatologists feel that exchange transfusion is indicated at an indirect bilirubin level below 20 mg/dl in septic, hypothermic, acidotic, hypoalbuminemic, asphyxiated, hypoglycemic, meconium-stained, and premature infants. The serum indirect bilirubin levels of 15 mg/dl or more for high-risk, less than 1,500-gm infants and 10 mg/dl or higher for less than 1,000-gm infants have been recommended to be indications for exchange transfusion since kernicterus has been reported in these situations. Lethargy, irritability, poor muscle tone, and hyporeflexia may also indicate the need for exchange transfusion (e.g., sepsis).
3. Indications for repeat exchange transfusion
   Use the same serum indirect bilirubin concentration level as used for the first exchange transfusion. A number of infants require repeated exchange transfusions due to continued hemolysis and early and late bilirubin rebound as a result of re-equilibration of bilirubin between tissue and blood.

D. Selection of Blood for Exchange Transfusion

1. Type
   If the blood is selected before birth, obtain group O, Rh-negative, low-titer blood compatible with maternal serum. When a minor group incompatibility involves a "public" antigen, washed red blood cells of the antigen-negative mother or a relative may be prepared before delivery if possible.
   If the blood is selected after birth, obtain blood that is of the same major group as the infant's red blood cells and compatible with maternal serum. Obtain ABO-compatible, Rh-negative blood for Rh incompatibility and group O, Rh-specific blood with low anti-A and anti-B or resuspend the group O, Rh-specific red blood cells in AB plasma for ABO incompatibility.
2. Age
   The blood should be as fresh as possible to minimize the loss of coagulation factors and platelets as well as to prevent excessive potassium from accumulating as a result of leakage. When possible, the blood should be drawn less than 4 days before the exchange.
   To prevent sudden death due to hyperkalemia in the sick or low birth weight

infant, use blood less than 2 days old, measure potassium prior to the procedure, and use centrifuged and saline-washed packed cells reconstituted with fresh frozen plasma just prior to the procedure.

3. Type of anticoagulant.
   Citrate phosphate dextrose (CPD) or CPD adenine is the most commonly used anticoagulant at present and has replaced acidcitrate dextrose (ACD). CPD blood has less acid load than the ACD blood. Heparin-treated blood is preferable for infants with acidosis or hypocalcemia but impractical because it must be used within 24 hours after being drawn, may aggravate hypocoagulability, and may compete with bilirubin for albumin-binding sites due to the presence of nonesterified fatty acids.
4. Concentration of red blood cells
   Whole-blood exchange transfusion is preferable when treatment is primarily for bilirubin withdrawal or removal of other toxic substances. Packed-cell single volume exchange transfusion is preferred when the initial treatment is for congestive heart failure or impending heart failure caused by severe anemia, e.g., infants with severe hydrops fetalis. It should be followed by an exchange transfusion with whole blood.
5. Amount
   Estimate double the infant's blood volume for an exchange transfusion, i.e., 160 to 200 ml of blood/kg of the infant's body weight (serum bilirubin concentration usually will be reduced by 50%).

E. Procedure

1. Order 160 to 200 ml/kg of whole blood or 80 to 100 ml/kg of packed cells of the appropriate type. Whole blood should be used for removing bilirubin.
2. Slowly warm refrigerated blood to the infant's body temperature to prevent cold stress. Allow the refrigerated blood to warm to room temperature for approximately 30 minutes to 1 hour. Take care to prevent excessive heating or fast warming of the red blood cells, which will result in hemolysis and potassium release. Sudden death may occur.
3. Albumin priming is controversial. It may be of value when the bilirubin binding capacity is already compromised and exchange transfusion is delayed.
   One to two hours before the exchange transfusion, administer 1 gm/kg IV of 5 or 25% salt-poor human albumin. (Be sure to plan to exchange transfuse the infant before the administration of albumin.) Albumin increases the movement of bilirubin from the extravascular space into the vascular compartment and thereby improves the efficiency of the exchange transfusion. Do not give albumin if the infant is hydropic, severely anemic, or has a high central venous pressure (CVP) with or without congestive heart failure or anemia.
4. Place the infant in a warmed environment under a radiant warmer. Be careful not to lower the infant's oxygen concentration and/or temperature. Transcutaneous Po_2 monitoring will be helpful if the infant requires oxygen therapy.

5. Monitor the infant's cardiac and respiratory status before and throughout the procedure. Stabilize cardiorespiratory status before starting the procedure.
6. Correct asphyxia and acidosis promptly if present and maintain normal intravascular volume. If CVP is greater than 10 cm of water, remove 10 to 15 ml/kg of blood; if CVP is less than 3 cm of water or blood pressure is low, infuse 10 ml/kg of blood or blood volume expander until CVP and/or blood pressure is in the normal range.
7. Restrain the infant by strapping the upper and lower extremities to padded splints.
8. Aspirate the stomach contents.
9. An assistant is required to record the quantity of blood given and withdrawn.
10. Wash hands thoroughly.
11. Using surgical aseptic technique, prepare the umbilicus with antiseptic solution such as Betadine and isolate the area with sterile towels.
12. Cut the umbilical cord to a length of 1.0 cm to permit cannulation with a sterile umbilical vessel catheter if the infant is less than 1 week of age and there is no omphalitis. Traction with a mouse-toothed forcep on the umbilical cord will facilitate the catheter entry. The catheter should be filled with saline before cannulating the umbilical vessel (see chapter 3–IIIC3). If the umbilical vessels can not be used, supraumbilical cutdown or saphenous cutdown may be performed. Percutaneous central venous line may be performed instead of cutdown (see chapter 19–IE). The commercially available exchange transfusion set (Pharmaseal, Pharmaseal Laboratories, Glendale, Calif.) may be used.
13. Obtain chest and abdominal x-ray films to ascertain the level of the umbilical or central vein catheter in the inferior or superior vena cava, if possible.
14. When a free flow of blood is obtained from the umbilical or central vein, measure the infant's CVP by the pressure monitor or by holding the venous catheter upright at a right angle to the infant's body. Raise the catheter cautiously and slowly, as the fluid filling the catheter will run into the infant and air will be introduced into the circulation if the CVP is below 1 cm. Then measure the height of the column of blood from the level of the heart.
15. If the pressure is between 3 to 10 cm (normal CVP), connect the catheter to a three-way stopcock and attach the stopcock to the banked blood and a disposal unit.
16. If the pressure is above 10 cm, reposition the catheter (check the x-ray films) as pressure can be erroneously high when the catheter is in the liver. If the pressure is still above 10 cm, withdraw 10 ml of blood and redetermine the pressure. Do not use whole blood to exchange transfuse an infant when the infant has an elevated (greater than 10 cm) venous pressure. Use packed cells to start the exchange on this infant.
17. Method
    a. The Diamond single-site "push-pull" method
       Withdraw 15–20 ml of blood if the infant weighs more than 2,500 gm, 10 ml if between 1,500 and 2,500 gm, 5 ml if between 1,000 and 1,500 gm or if severely anemic or hydropic, and 3 ml if less than 1,000 gm. After

withdrawal, transfuse the same amount as was withdrawn via the same vessel. Repeat withdrawal and transfusion ("push-pull") procedure until double the infant's blood volume is exchanged.

b. The automated two-site method
Withdraw blood via the umbilical artery or a peripheral arterial catheter (e.g., radial) and transfuse through the umbilical vein or peripheral vein by using a modified volumetric infusion pump at the same rate as the withdrawal. This method may be a more effective exchange and may avoid many of the potential problems associated with the single-site "push-pull" exchange procedure with sudden changes in pressure predisposing infants to necrotizing enterocolitis, CNS hemorrhage, and other complications.

18. Send the initial withdrawn blood specimen to be analyzed (direct and indirect bilirubin, hematocrit, glucose, calcium, electrolytes, total protein and albumin). If needed, send blood for IgM, viral and protozoan studies, liver function, and coagulation profile tests. Keep the rest of the initially withdrawn plasma in the freezer for further evaluation if necessary.
19. Monitor blood pressure and intracranial pressure (if possible) continuously as blood pressure and intracranial pressure are seen to rise during infusion and decrease during blood withdrawal. Slow exchange (5 ml/kg/3 minutes) minimizes the hemodynamic changes.
20. Monitor pH in hypoxic or sick infants througout the procedure every 30 minutes. Give 2 mEq $NaHCO_3$ or tromethamine (Tham) per 100 ml of exchanged blood to buffer the acid load to infants with acidosis. $NaHCO_3$ cannot be given directly after calcium gluconate is given without flushing the catheter. Monitor calcium and correct hypocalcemia as required.
21. Measure the venous pressure during and at the end of the procedure and adjust the venous pressure by adding or withdrawing blood to maintain a venous pressure of 3 to 10 cm H_2O. Measure the venous pressure after each 50 ml of blood exchanged in hydropic infants since a shift of edema fluid into the intravascular space may occur and result in cardiac failure.
22. Mix (slowly agitate) the donor blood during the procedure as the red blood cells sediment at the bottom.
23. Save the last specimen withdrawn to be analyzed (hematocrit, bilirubin, glucose, pH, calcium, and electrolytes). The postexchange serum bilirubin is usually half the pre-exchange value after the double volume exchange.
24. Remove the umbilical catheter and clamp the cord with a cord tie. Suture with 000 silk if necessary. Apply pressure until hemostasis is certain.
25. Occasionally, abdominal distension occurs after the exchange transfusion and probably is caused by increased portal venous pressure resulting in passive ischemia of the bowel if an umbilical venous catheter was utilized.
26. Consider antibiotic therapy if signs of sepsis occur after the exchange transfusion.
27. Readminister medications except digoxin if exchange procedure is done soon after the last dose.
28. After exchange, monitor vital signs every 15 to 30 minutes for the first 3 to 6 hours.

29. Resume feedings by 4 hours after the exchange transfusion if the infant's condition is stable.
30. Check pH after a few hours to determine the presence of alkalosis resulting from the metabolism of citrate to bicarbonate.
31. During the 4 to 6 hours postexchange transfusion period, check serum calcium for hypocalcemia, potassium for hypokalemia, and glucose for rebound hypoglycemia.
32. Check CBC and platelet count for a few days after exchange since leukopenia and thrombocytopenia are observed especially in prematures because of smaller granulocyte reserves and bone marrow depression.
33. Since Rh antibody is still present after exchange transfusion, hemolysis can continue and the infant may develop severe anemia requiring packed cell transfusion at 2 to 5 weeks of age.

F. Complications of Exchange Transfusion

1. Vascular
   a. Embolization with air or clots
   b. Thrombosis
   c. Necrotizing enterocolitis with or without perforation
   d. False abdominal aortic aneurysm
   e. Sickling (donor blood)
2. Cardiac
   a. Arrhythmia, arrest
   b. Volume overload
   c. Decreased blood pressure with fast exchange
   d. Fluctuation of cerebral blood flow
3. Electrolytes
   a. Hyperkalemia
   b. Hypernatremia
   c. Hypocalcemia
   d. Hypomagnesemia
   e. Acidosis during or immediately after exchange due to acid load (less often with CPD blood)
   f. Alkalosis 2 to 3 hours after exchange transfusion
   g. Hypoglycemia
4. Bleeding
   a. Overheparinization when heparinized blood is used
   b. Thrombocytopenia
5. Infection
   a. Bacteremia
   b. Viral infections: hepatitis, cytomegalovirus, and acquired immune deficiency syndrome
   c. Malaria
6. Miscellaneous
   a. Mechanical injury to donor cells
   b. Hypothermia

c. Perforation of umbilical vein
d. ROP (RLF)
7. Mortality
The mortality rate is usually reported as less than 1% (reported to be as high as 5% in the past).

G. Complications of Heparin-Treated Blood Versus ACD or CPD Blood

1. Heparin-treated blood
Hypoglycemia, bleeding tendency, marked increase in nonesterified fatty acids that compete with bilirubin for albumin-binding sites
2. ACD or CPD blood
Acidosis, hypernatremia, hyperkalemia, thrombocytopenia, hypocalcemia, hypomagnesemia, postexchange hypoglycemia

REFERENCES

Diamond L.K., Allen F.H. Jr., Thomas W.O. Jr.: Erythroblastosis fetalis:VII. Treatment with exchange transfusion. *N. Engl. J. Med.* 244:39, 1951.

Goldman S.L., Tu H.C.: Automated method for exchange transfusion: A new modification. *J. Pediatr.* 102:119, 1983.

Oski F., Naiman J.L.: Hematologic problems in the newborn, in *Major Problems in Clinical Pediatrics,* vol. IV, 1982, p. 308.

Wennberg R.P., Depp R., Heinrichs W.L.: Indications for early exchange transfusion in patients with erythroblastosis fetalis. *J. Pediatr.* 92:789, 1978.

VII. Rh INCOMPATIBILITY

Hemolytic disease caused by maternal anti-Rh(D) antibody against the corresponding Rh-positive red blood cells of the infant is one of the most serious hemolytic processes in the newborn. An Rh-negative pregnant woman carrying an Rh-positive fetus develops Rh antibodies (both 19S and 7S) against Rh-positive red blood cells that crossed the placenta during pregnancy or at parturition. The maternal 7S anti-Rh antibodies return to the Rh-positive fetal circulation and coat fetal red blood cells, which are then destroyed in the fetal liver and spleen with resultant anemia.

A. Prevention

1. Management of the Rh-negative pregnant woman before delivery
   a. If anti-Rh antibodies are not present during the first trimester, repeat the test at approximately 28 weeks.
      1) If negative, repeat the test at 34 weeks. Rh immunoglobulin, 300 μg, may be administered at 28 weeks. Although the safety of both infant and mother has been well documented, antenatal prophylaxis is contro-

versial since it is unnecessary in about 40% of pregnancies where the fetus is Rh-negative.

2) If positive, repeat the test at 2- to 4-week intervals until 34 weeks and 1- to 2-week intervals from 34 weeks.
3) If the maternal anti-D titers (indirect Coombs' titers) have reached 1:16 or 1:32, obtain at least two ΔOD readings at 450 mμ of amniotic fluid at 1- to 2-week intervals and interpret the results according to the zone (see Figs 13–1 and 13–2) the bilirubin falls into. Depending on the zone, early delivery may be undertaken to prevent further deterioration in utero. A high reading that remains flat or rises is often associated with intrauterine or neonatal death.

b. If sensitization occurred before the present pregnancy, no known measures are available to prevent the Rh-positive fetus from being immunized.

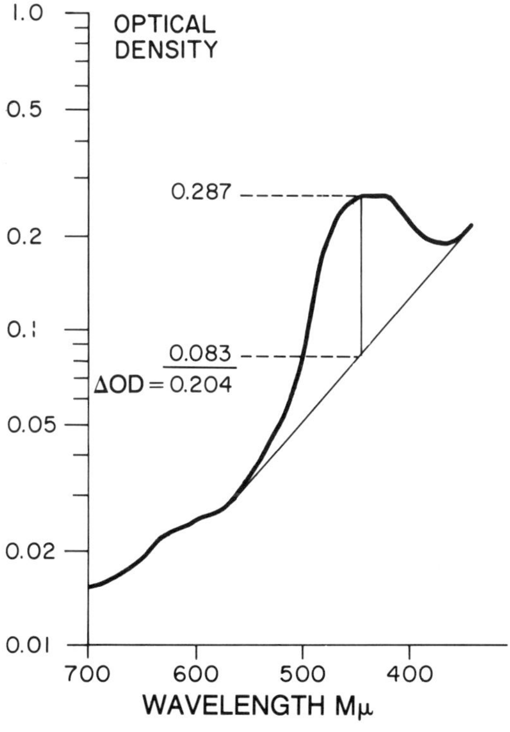

FIG 13–1.
Spectral absorption curve of amniotic fluid in hemolytic disease. In the presence of bilirubin, the absorbance at 450 mμ will be increased. The *ΔOD* at 450 represents the difference in optical density (OD) between the reading at 450 mμ and a tangential line drawn between 375 mμ and 525 mμ. (From Liley A.W.: Liquor amnii analysis in management of pregnancy complicated by Rh sensitization. *Am. J. Obstet. Gynecol.* 82:1359, 1961. Used by permission.)

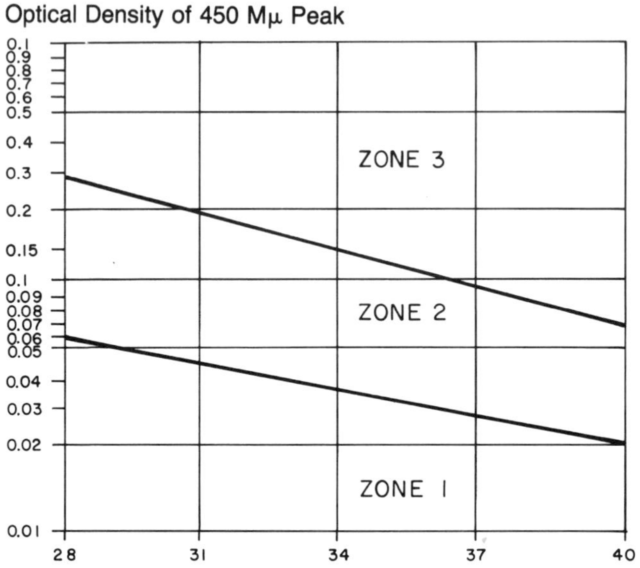

FIG 13–2.
Fetal involvement reflected by spectrophotometric analysis of amniotic fluid. From Liley A.W.: Liquor amnii analysis in management of pregnancy complicated by Rh sensitization. *Am. J. Obstet. Gynecol.* 82:1359, 1961. Used by permission.)

Obtain the anti Rh antibody titer at 6 to 8 weeks of gestation as a baseline. Then obtain amniotic fluid and determine the ΔOD when the titers rise or 10 weeks before the gestation when the previous pregnancy ended with stillbirth or severely affected infant. Intrauterine transfusion may be helpful for 30% of fetuses that would die at 25–32 weeks' gestation.

2. Management of the Rh-negative woman after delivery
   a. If the Rh-negative woman is not sensitized and the fetus/infant is Rh negative, nothing further is required.
   b. If the Rh-negative woman is not sensitized and the fetus/infant is Rh positive, injection of anti-D (Rh) immune globulin leads to rapid clearance of circulating Rh-positive red blood cells (mainly to the spleen) and prevents sensitization.
      1) After abortion, ruptured ectopic pregnancy, or manual version, administer 50 mcg anti-D immune globulin if pregnancy is before 12 weeks' gestation and 100 mcg after 12 weeks.
      2) After amniocentesis, administer 50 mcg.
      3) After delivery, determine the amount of fetomaternal transfusion that often occurs at the time of labor and delivery. Then administer 300 μg of anti-D immune globulin within 72 hours after exposure to Rh positive red blood cells. If exposure exceeds 30 ml, administer an additional dose of anti-D immune globulin. The protection rate is approximately

90%. Failures are largely due to sensitization by massive fetomaternal transfusions prior to delivery or failure to administer anti-D globulin following abortion or delivery of a previous Rh-positive infant.

3. Management of the nonpregnant Rh-negative woman
   a. When a transfusion of blood components (e.g. platelets, granulocytes, or plasma) contains a small amount of Rh-positive red blood cells, administer 300 mcg of Rh-immunoglobulin. Most components contain some red blood cells.
   b. When a blood transfusion is mismatched, administer Rh-immunoglobulin 10 to 15 μg/ml of whole blood or 25 to 35 μg/ml of red blood cells.

B. Who Is at Risk?

1. Rh-positive infants born to sensitized Rh-negative mothers are at risk. Mothers are frequently sensitized by transplacental hemorrhage of greater than 0.5 ml, which occurs often during active labor and obstetric complications such as breech delivery, twin pregnancy, transverse lie, adherent placenta, placenta previa, abruptio placenta, normal removal of placenta, amniocentesis, or abortion (particularly therapeutic). The greater the number of previously affected siblings, the greater the risk.
2. Mothers who are hyperresponders can be sensitized during their first pregnancies.
3. Males are more seriously affected since their Rh-positive erythrocytes are more antigenic.
4. Whites have a higher incidence: 15% of the population have the Rh-negative genotype versus 5% to 6% in blacks and 0% in Orientals.
5. Rarely, Rh-negative mothers of Rh-positive grandmothers may be sensitized in utero from maternofetal transfusion.
6. Conditions decreasing the incidence of severity or maternal sensitizations
   a. Rh heterozygosity of the father
   b. Associated ABO incompatibility
   c. Avoidance of obstetric factors that might injure the placental barrier
   d. Maternal corticosteroid administration to enhance fetal lung maturation, which is associated with a sharp fall in the optical density rise at 450 mμ wavelength and has a beneficial effect on hemolytic disease

C. Clinical Manifestations

1. Unaffected infants
   Fifteen percent to 20% of Rh-positive infants born to Rh-negative sensitized mothers show no clinical signs of illness.
2. Mildly affected infants
   a. Jaundice appears within 24 to 36 hours of life and becomes moderately intense.
   b. Hepatosplenomegaly of mild-to-moderate degree occurs.

c. As the jaundice and hepatosplenomegaly begin to lessen, pallor becomes noticeable and persists for a few months.

3. Moderately affected infants
   a. Jaundice appears within a few hours of life (rarely at birth) and rapidly becomes more intense until the third or fourth day of life.
   b. Edema, especially of the extremities
   c. Hepatosplenomegaly
   d. Poor feeding, regurgitation
   e. Pallor
   f. Rapid and labored respiration
   g. Irritability and lethargy
   h. Progressive decrease in hemoglobin concentration (late anemia) may occur with or without exchange transfusion(s) after 1 to 2 weeks of life.
   i. Kernicterus may develop (see Chapter 13–IV).
4. Severely affected infants
   a. Jaundice appears within a few hours of life, occasionally at birth, and quickly becomes more and more intense.
   b. Infants may be born with hydrops fetalis
      1) Severe pallor
      2) Generalized edema, pleural effusion, and ascites, which may be due to hypoalbuminemia as a consequence of reduced hepatic synthesis
      3) Abdominal distension with dullness to percussion
      4) Severe hepatosplenomegaly. Rarely, splenic rupture may occur.
      5) Infant appears critically ill: poor suck, rapid and labored respiration, etc.
      6) Petechiae and purpuric spots with severe anemia. Intracranial and pulmonary hemorrhages are common.

      These infants are often stillborn or die within a few hours of age.
   c. Kernicterus may occur (see chapter 13–IV).
   d. Maternal history of polyhydramnios and pre-eclampsia.

D. Laboratory Findings

1. Serologic abnormalities (in the infant)
   a. Direct Coombs' test

      Anti-Rh antibodies to Rh-positive red blood cells are present. Saline-reacting anti-Rh antibodies are IgM (19S) and do not cross the placenta while albumin-reacting incomplete anti-Rh antibodies are usually detectable by the indirect Coombs' test or by the Autoanalyzer and are able to cross the placenta. The incidence of stillbirth or hydrops fetalis is high when albumin-reacting titers are greater than 1:64. A positive direct Coombs' test occurs as a result of the anti-Rh antibody coating the infant's Rh-positive cells.
   b. False-negative direct Coombs' test caused by low titers of anti-Rh antibody of the mother or by atypical antibodies (uncertain)
   c. False Rh typing of the infant

      An Rh-positive infant occasionally is typed as Rh-negative because the anti-Rh antibody coats the infant's Rh-positive cells so heavily that it blocks the Rh antigenic sites, causing a false-negative Rh typing ("blocked D").

These infants have a strongly positive direct reaction to Coombs' test. It can be presumed that the infant is Rh-positive if the direct Coombs' test is strongly positive.

2. Hematologic abnormalities (see chapter 14-I for normal values)
   a. Decreased hemoglobin concentration less than 14 gm/dl
   b. Increased reticulocyte count greater than 6%
   c. Increased nucleated red blood cell count greater than 10/100 white blood cells
   d. Decreased platelet count less than 100,000/cu mm
   e. Marked polychromasia and anisocytosis on the peripheral smear
3. Increased serum bilirubin level
   a. Increased bilirubin in amniotic fluid (see Fig 13–1 and 13–2)
   b. Indirect-reacting serum bilirubin is usually increased.
      1) The cord bilirubin level is rarely more than 4 mg/dl since fetal bilirubin crosses the placenta and is conjugated by the maternal liver; cord bilirubin greater than 4 mg/dl suggests severe hemolytic disease.
      2) The rate of increase (mg/hour) in serum bilirubin reflects both the kinetic equilibrium between the rate of production from hemolysis and the rate of excretion of bilirubin. An increase of 1 mg/dl/hour represents severe hemolytic disease. Under 0.3 mg/dl/hour represents mild hemolysis. Peak bilirubin levels are usually reached by the third day of life.
   c. Elevated direct-reacting serum bilirubin is observed in the severely affected infant possibly due to impaired hepatic excretion.
   d. Increased unbound (free) bilirubin or decreased bilirubin binding capacity
4. Hypoglycemia
   a. Hypoglycemia before exchange transfusion, attributed to compensatory hyperplasia of the pancreatic islets
   b. Hypoglycemia after exchange transfusion, probably secondary to pancreatic β-cell stimulation from high-glucose level of the ACD or CPD donor's blood
5. Intravascular hemolysis and hemoglobinuria are rare because complement is not activated during extravascular destruction.
6. Deficiencies of the vitamin-K-dependent coagulation factors due to hepatic dysfunction are seen.

E. Supportive Management

1. See chapter 13–IIIC for "general supportive management for the infant with indirect hyperbilirubinemia."
2. The degree of anemia, hypoxia, and acidosis can be evaluated in labor from fetal scalp sampling.

F. Specific Therapy

1. Specific management of the fetus affected by Rh hemolytic disease.
   Intrauterine intraperitoneal or intravascular transfusion is limited to only those

who are certain to die due to hydrops fetalis in utero and to immaturity if delivered.

Consider early delivery if the fetus is severely affected (ΔOD in Liley's zone 3) and 33 weeks or more with the lecithin-sphingomyelin ratio greater than 1.5 (Fig 13–1 and 13–2).

2. Specific management of the infant affected by Rh-hemolytic disease
   a. Exchange transfusion (see chapter 13–VI for indications, procedure, and complications)
   b. Phototherapy (see chapter 13–V)
   c. Transfusion with or without exchange transfusion for anemia. Hemoglobin and hematocrit should be followed every week for the first 1 to 2 months of age.

REFERENCES

Frigoletto F.D. Jr., Umansky I.: Erythroblastosis fetalis: Identification, management and prevention. *Clin. Perinatol.* 6:321, 1979.

Peddle L.J.: The antenatal management of the Rh sensitized woman. *Clin. Perinatol.* 11:251, 1984.

Zipursky A.: Rh hemolytic disease of the newborn: The disease eradicated by immunology. *Clin. Obstet. Gynecol.* 20:759, 1977.

VIII. ABO INCOMPATIBILITY

Hemolytic disease caused by maternal anti-A and anti-B antibodies against the corresponding A or B erythrocytes of the infant is more common but generally milder than hemolytic disease caused by Rh incompatibility.

A. Who Is at Risk?

1. Group A (mostly A) or B infants of group O mothers. Virtually all infants have ABO incompatibilities since the "natural" anti-A and anti-B of group O mothers are of the IgG type that cross the placenta while those of group A and B mothers are mainly IgM that cannot cross the placenta. Increased anti-A and anti-B were reported after vaccines and possibly intestinal parasite infestation. Group OA (mother O, baby A) incompatibility is more common but OB incompatibility is more severe.
2. Group B or AB infant of group A mother
3. Group A or AB infant of group B mother
4. First-born infants frequently affected

B. Clinical Manifestations

1. Jaundice

   Jaundice occurs in 10% to 20% of ABO incompatible infants, usually appears within the first 24 to 48 hours of life (slightly later than Rh disease), and disappears in 3 to 7 days. Rarely, it may be severe enough to cause kernicterus and death.

2. Pallor
   Pallor is usually mild or absent.
3. Hepatosplenomegaly
   Hepatosplenomegaly is usually mild or absent.

C. Laboratory Findings

1. Hematologic findings
   a. Anemia
      Anemia is uncommon, as is delayed anemia.
   b. Polychromasia, reticulocytosis (10% to 30%); increased number of nucleated red blood cells
   c. Spherocytosis (3% to 40%)
      Spherocytosis is usually present in clinically significant cases. Autohemolysis cannot be corrected by the addition of glucose. This differentiates spherocytosis caused by ABO incompatibility from hereditary spherocytosis.
2. Elevated serum bilirubin levels
   Mainly indirect-reacting bilirubin levels are increased.
3. Serologic findings
   a. Demonstration of incompatible blood groups

MOTHER	INFANT
O	A or B
A	B or AB
B	A or AB

   b. Results of a direct Coombs' test of the infant's red blood cells may be negative; but, using a newer method, autoanalysis, results are usually mildly to moderately positive.
      ABO-incompatible infants with positive direct Coombs' test have a greater chance of developing significant hyperbilirubinemia than those with a negative Coombs' test.
   c. The indirect Coombs' test demonstrating anti-A or anti-B using adult red blood cells of the same group as the infant's is almost always positive when hemolytic disease is present.
   d. The antibody titers in maternal serum have limited value since titers are the highest in late pregnancy and fall after delivery and false positive tests are common.

D. Supportive Management

See chapter 13–IIIC for "general supportive management for infants with indirect hyperbilirubinemia."

E. Specific Therapy

1. Exchange transfusion for hyperbilirubinemia (see chapter 13–VI)
   Group O low-titer blood of the same Rh type as that of the infant should be used. Replacement of the donor plasma with AB plasma offers no additional advantage.
2. Phototherapy (see chapter 13–V)
   Hyperbilirubinemia can be controlled by phototherapy in most infants with ABO hemolytic disease. The majority do not even require phototherapy.
3. Transfusion for anemia
   Packed-cell transfusion is indicated if the central venous pressure is high or if there is late onset of anemia from continuous hemolysis while maternal antibodies are present.

REFERENCES

Dufour D.R., Monaghan W.P.: ABO hemolytic disease of the newborn. *Am. J. Clin. Pathol.* 73:369, 1980.

Levine, D.H., Meyer H.B.P.: Newborn screening for ABO hemolytic disease. *Clin. Pediatr.* 24(7):391, 1985.

Zipursky A., Chintu C., Brown E., et al.: The quantitation of spherocytes in ABO hemolytic disease. *J. Pediatr.* 94:965, 1979.

IX. MINOR GROUP INCOMPATIBILITY

Less than 2% of the infants with hemolytic disease have isoimmunization caused by minor group antibodies: anti-c, anti-Kell, anti-E, anti-Duffy, and anti-Kidd antibodies. Anti-Le^a, Le^b, E, M, and P are "natural" antibodies of IgM class that do not cross the placenta and are of no consequence to the fetus.

A. Prevention

Screen the serum of all pregnant women for atypical antibodies early in pregnancy. If present, serial antibody titers should be obtained. The management in pregnancy is similar to that of Rh sensitization (see chapter 13–VII).

B. Who Is at Risk?

1. Infants with a positive Coombs' test that can not be explained by Rh(D) or ABO incompatibility are at risk.
   (Remember, however, that many drugs (e.g., Keflex) may also be associated with a positive reaction to a direct Coombs' test.)
2. Infants whose mothers have anti-Kell mainly following transfusion and whose fathers are Kell-positive (10% of the population and all are heterozygous) have a 5% chance of developing hemolytic disease.

Fifty percent of infants whose mothers develop anti-Kell following pregnancy and whose fathers are carriers of the Kell antigen are at risk of developing hemolytic disease.

3. The c-positive infant born to a c-negative mother with anti-c antibody from a previous pregnancy and a c-heterozygous father (70% of population) has an approximately 50% chance of developing hemolytic disease.

C. Clinical Manifestations

Clinical manifestations are the same as those seen in Rh incompatibility (see chapter 13–VIIC).

D. Laboratory Findings

1. The direct Coombs' test is positive in the absence of Rh or ABO incompatibility.
2. The identity of the antibody is determined by testing maternal serum, an eluate of the infant's cells, and the father's cells against a panel of standard test cells.

E. Supportive Management and Specific Therapy

See chapter 13–IIIC for "general supportive management for infants with indirect hyperbilirubinemia," 13–VI for "exchange transfusion," and 13–V for "phototherapy."

REFERENCES

Astrup J., Kornstad L.: Presence of anti-c in the serum of 42 women giving birth to c-positive babies: Serological and clinical findings. *Acta Obstet. Gynecol. Scand.* 56:185, 1977.

Frigoletto F.D. Jr., Davies I.J.: Erythroblastosis fetalis with hydrops from anti-Kell isoimmune disease. *Am. J. Obstet. Gynecol.* 127:887, 1976.

X. GLUCOSE-6-PHOSPHATE DEHYDROGENASE DEFICIENCY

G-6-PD deficiency is a sex-linked, recessive trait that may be associated with hemolytic anemia and jaundice even in the absence of a recognized "trigger agent" or event in the newborn period. The incidence and severity of the disease and the agents capable of initiating hemolysis differ in the racial groups. The incidence is high among whites (mainly-B type) residing in the Mediterranean areas and Sardinia (30% of males), Sephardic Jews, Greeks (0.7% to 3%), Iranians, Mongolians, Chinese (5.5% of males), Malayans, Filipinos (13%), Indonesians, and American blacks (9% to 10% of A type in males and 2% to 3% in females) and in some areas of Africa (25%). Jaundice with kernicterus has been observed in whites, blacks, and Mongolians.

Transient nongenetic G-6-PD deficiency has also been observed in premature infants.

A. Prevention

1. Potential hemolytic agents should not be given to the pregnant mother or newborn with G-6-PD deficiency (see Table 13–1). Routine administration of Vitamin K_1 (AquaMEPHYTON or Konakion) does not produce hemolysis in G-6-PD-deficient blacks.
2. Potential hemolytic agents should not be given to the mother if the infant is to be breast fed.
3. Consider phenobarbital administration for a male infant or pregnant women carrying a male fetus if there is a family history of severe hyperbilirubinemia due to G-6-PD deficiency.

B. Who Is at Risk?

1. Infants who develop neonatal jaundice without evidence of isoimmunization, especially those with histories of exposure to certain drugs (see Table 13–1) and/or evidence of infection, hypoxia, or acidosis
2. Male infants
3. Infants with a family history of neonatal jaundice. Recurrence of severe neonatal jaundice with G-6-PD deficiency is observed in certain families and this may be due to an independent genetic icterogenic factor.
4. Premature infants who have transient nongenetically determined G-6-PD deficiency that lasts 3 to 5 days

C. Clinical Manifestations

1. Jaundice
   Approximately 5% of infants with G-6-PD deficiency develop clinically significant jaundice, and jaundice usually appears after 24 hours of life and after the infant is exposed to a trigger agent or circumstance. Maximum bilirubin concentration is reached usually between the third and fifth days of life, as in normal physiologic jaundice, or between the third and fifth days after exposure to a precipitating factor. If the mother ingested a triggering agent, e.g., ascorbic acid during the last month of pregnancy, the infant may develop jaundice at birth or in the first day of life.
2. Pallor
3. Signs of kernicterus (Lethargy, hypotonia, poor feeding, opisthotonos, convulsions, and irregular respirations)

TABLE 13–1.—SOME AGENTS REPORTED TO PRODUCE HEMOLYSIS IN PATIENTS WITH G-6-PD DEFICIENCY*

Antimalarials
- Primaquine
- Pamaquine
- Pentaquine
- Plasmoquine
- Quinocide
- Quinacrine (Atabrine)
- Quinine (C)

Sulfonamides
- Sulfanilamide
- N^2-Acetylsulfanilamide
- Sulfacetamide (Sulamyd)
- Sulfamethoxypyridazine (Kynex, medicel)
- Salicylazosulfapyridine (Azulfidine)
- Sulfisoxazole (Gantrisin) (in large doses)
- Sulfapyridine
- Sulphamethoxazole (Gantanol)
- Trisulphapyrimidine (Sultrin)

Nitrofurans
- Nitrofurantoin (Furadantin)
- Furazolidone (Furoxone)
- Furaltadone (Altafur)
- Nitrofurazone (Furacin)

Antipyretics and Analgesics
- Acetylsalicylic acid (in large doses)
- Acetanilid
- Acetophenetidin (Phenacetin) (in large doses)
- Antipyrine (C)†
- Aminopyrine (C)†
- *p*-Aminosalicylic acid

Sulfones
- Thiazolesulfone

Others
- Aniline dyes
- Ascorbic acid
- Dimercaprol (BAL)
- Methylene blue (in large doses)
- Naphthalene
- Phenylhydrazine
- Acetylphenylhydrazine
- Probenecid
- Vitamin K (large doses of water-soluble analogues)
- Chloramphenicol (C) (in massive doses)
- Quinidine (C)
- Fava beans (C)
- Chloroquine
- Nalidixic acid (Negram)
- Sulfoxone (in large doses)
- Tolbutamide (Orinase)
- Toluidine blue
- Trinitrotoluene (TNT)

Infections
- Respiratory viruses
- Infectious hepatitis
- Infectious mononucleosis
- Bacterial pneumonias

Diabetic Acidosis

*From Oski F.A., Naiman, J.L.: *Hematologic Problems in the Newborn,* ed. 2. Philadelphia, W.B. Saunders Co., 1972. Used by permission.
†(C) To date, only in Caucasians.

D. Laboratory Findings

1. Hyperbilirubinemia
   Occasionally, hyperbilirubinemia exceeds 20 mg/dl on the third to fifth day of life. The serum bilirubin level may be as high as 50 mg/dl.
2. Anemia
   Hemoglobin may be as low as 7 to 8 gm/dl during first week of life.
3. Elevated reticulocyte count

4. Elevated nucleated red blood cells
5. Peripheral blood smear showing spherocytes, poikilocytes, and crenated and fragmented red blood cells, blister cells, and red blood cells containing Heinz bodies.
6. Reduced levels of G-6-PD activity determined by direct assay of the enzyme (spectrophotometric technique) or by screening tests such as the decolorization test and the methemoglobin reduction test. However, the screening tests are not reliable during the hemolytic episode.

E. Supportive Management

1. Eliminate predisposing factors (see Table 13–1).
2. Careful instruction should be given to the parent on discharge particularly with respect to exposure to naphthalene (moth balls, flakes, or vaporizer containing naphthalene or its derivatives) and to the importance of immediate medical attention if pallor, jaundice, or dark urine is noted.
3. See chapter 13–IIIC for "general supportive management for the infant with indirect hyperbilirubinemia."

F. Specific Therapy

A specific therapy is not known.

REFERENCES

Piomelli S., Vora S.: G-6-PD deficiency and related disorders of the pentose phosphate pathway, in Nathan D.G., Oski F.A. (eds.): *Hematology of Infancy and Childhood,* Philadelphia, W.B. Saunders Co., 1981, p. 608.

Valaes T.: Bilirubin and red cell metabolism in relation to neonatal jaundice. *Postgrad. Med. J.* 45:86, 1969.

XI. HEREDITARY SPHEROCYTOSIS

Hereditary spherocytosis is characterized by spherocytic erythrocytes that are abnormally fragile under osmotic stress. The disease is inherited as a Mendelian dominant trait.

A. Who Is at Risk?

Infants with family histories of neonatal jaundice caused by hereditary spherocytosis are at risk. Neither parent may have spherocytosis in 10% to 25% of cases.

B. Clinical Manifestations

Fifty percent of infants with spherocytosis develop neonatal jaundice, which is usually misdiagnosed as physiologic jaundice. Occasionally, the infant develops severe hyperbilirubinemia resulting in pallor, splenomegaly, and kernicterus.

C. Laboratory Findings

1. Mild anemia
2. Mild reticulocytosis
3. Hyperbilirubinemia, usually
4. Spherocytosis: small, thick, and more intensely stained spherical red blood cells on peripheral blood smear
5. Positive reaction to osmotic fragility test of freshly drawn blood (80% to 90%) or of blood cells incubated under sterile conditions for 24 hours (100%). The increased autohemolysis of hereditary spherocytosis is reduced by the addition of glucose to the incubated blood. But, glucose has no beneficial effect on infants with spherocytic cells in hemolytic disease as a result of ABO incompatability.

D. Supportive Management

See chapter 13–IIIC for "general supportive management for infants with indirect hyperbilirubinemia."

E. Specific Therapy

These infants eventually require splenectomy to cure hemolysis due to spherocytosis, but splenectomy should be delayed until 4 to 6 years of age because of the increased risk of infection.

REFERENCES

Robinson G.C.: Hereditary spherocytosis in infancy. *J. Pediatr.* 50:446, 1957.

Kostinas J.E., Cantow E.F., Wetzel R.A.: Autohemolysis of cord blood in congenital spherocytosis and ABO incompatibility. *J. Pediatr.* 70:273, 1967.

XII. BREAST MILK JAUNDICE

Jaundice caused by breast feeding usually starts at 4 to 5 days of life and can continue after 5 to 7 days of life. Cessation of breast feeding leads to a prompt decline in serum bilirubin, which reaches normal in 4 to 6 days. Breast feeding can be resumed safely after 2 to 3 days, but jaundice may continue for weeks or months if due to an inhibitor.

A. Early Onset Breast Milk Jaundice

An exaggerated indirect hyperbilirubinemia within 3 to 5 days of life in breast-fed babies has been reported to be related to underfeeding.

B. Late Onset Breast Milk Jaundice

A few otherwise normal, usually fullterm infants develop indirect hyperbilirubinemia (10 to 27 mg/dl) at the end of the first week of life due to a glucuronyl transferase inhibitor. This entity originally was reported to be related to 3α20β-pregnanediol but more recently has been associated with high concentrations of nonesterified long-chain fatty acids.

REFERENCES

Gartner L.M., Arias I.M.: Studies of prolonged neonatal jaundice in the breast-fed infant. *J. Pediatr.* 68:54, 1966.

Osborn L.M., Reiff M.I., Bolus R.: Jaundice in the full term neonate. *Pediatrics* 73:520, 1984.

XIII. HEINZ BODY ANEMIA

Heinz bodies are multiple small, round inclusions that are composed of precipitated, membrane-bound denatured hemoglobin, usually seen in the periphery of the red blood cell. A defect in the detoxification of hydrogen peroxide has been postulated to be the cause.

A. Who Is at Risk?

1. Premature infants
   In the normal adult, naturally occurring Heinz bodies are removed by the spleen and are not seen in the peripheral blood, but in the premature infant, Heinz bodies may be seen even in the absence of oxidant drugs possibly due to inability of the premature spleen to remove Heinz bodies from the circulation.
2. Infants who are exposed to a toxic drug
   A progressive oxidating injury to hemoglobin occurs normally as an aging process, but is accelerated by certain oxidant drugs such as phenylhydrazine, naphthoquinone and its derivatives (menadione, naphthalene), sodium nitrite, and phenolic disinfectant.
3. Infants with a defect of red blood cell metabolism such as G-6-PD deficiency, methemoglobin reductase deficiency, and the presence of hemoglobinM or hemoglobinH who are exposed to a normal dosage of oxidant drugs
4. Congenital Heinz body anemia does not usually appear until child or adulthood.

B. Clinical Manifestations

1. Pallor, which is usually progressive during the second to third week
2. Jaundice, which usually begins after the first day

C. Laboratory Findings

1. Anemia, hyperbilirubinemia
2. Heinz bodies, which are not visible on Wright-stained blood smears but can be demonstrated in wet preparations by phase microscopy or by supravital stains such as brilliant cresyl blue

D. Supportive Management

See chapter 13–IIIC for "general supportive management for infants with indirect hyperbilirubinemia."

E. Specific Therapy

Remove the toxic agent.

REFERENCES

Acevedo G., Mauer A.M.: The capacity for removal of erythrocytes containing Heinz bodies in premature infants and patients following splenectomy. *J. Pediatr.* 63:61, 1963.

Cohen G., Hochstein P.: Glucose-6-phosphate dehydrogenase and detoxification of hydrogen peroxide in human erythrocytes. *Science* 134:1756, 1961.

Varadi S., Hurworth E.: Heinz-body anemia in the newborn. *Br. Med. J.* 1:315, 1957.

XIV. FAMILIAL NONHEMOLYTIC UNCONJUGATED HYPERBILIRUBINEMIA: CRIGLER-NAJJAR SYNDROME, TYPES I AND II

A. Type I

This rare familial nonhemolytic unconjugated hyperbilirubinemia has been attributed to a structural defect in glucuronyl transferase and is transmitted in an autosomal recessive pattern. Unconjugated hyperbilirubinemia greater than 25 to 35 mg/dl during the first week of life persists thereafter and fails to respond to phenobarbital therapy. All type I patients to date have developed kernicterus, either in the neonatal period or later despite therapy with phenobarbital, exchange transfusions, or phototherapy.

B. Type II

Type II is similar to type I but less severe (indirect bilirubin usually is 10 to 15 mg/dl). Inheritance is as an autosomal dominant trait with variable penetrance. Infants respond readily to phenobarbital, 5 mg/kg/day.

REFERENCE

Arias I.M., Gartner L.M., Cohen M., et al.: Chronic non-hemolytic unconjugated hyperbilirubinemia with glucuronyl transferase deficiency: Clinical, biochemical, pharmacologic and genetic evidence of heterogeneity. *Am. J. Med.* 47:395, 1969.

XV. HEPATOCELLULAR CHOLESTATIC JAUNDICE

Hepatocellular cholestatic jaundice represents persistent liver dysfunction in the early months of life with liver cell necrosis, bile stasis, fibroblast proliferation, variable inflammatory cell infiltration, extramedullary hematopoiesis, and multinucleated giant cell transformation.

A. Who Is at Risk?

1. Infants with infection (viral, syphilis, bacterial, etc.)
2. Infants with α_1-antitrypsin deficiency
3. Infants with galactosemia
4. Infants with severe hemolytic disease (Rh or ABO)
5. Infants with shock, multiple transfusions, congestive heart failure
6. Premature infants
7. Infants with parenteral alimentation
8. Infants with cystic fibrosis

B. Clinical Manifestations

1. Poor feeding, failure to thrive
2. Jaundice, which may occur at any time after birth
3. Hepatomegaly

C. Laboratory Findings (see Table 13–2)

1. Total and direct hyperbilirubinemia
2. Abnormal liver function tests
   Low albumin, prolonged prothrombin time, elevated serum glutamic oxaloacetic transaminase and serum glutamic pyruvic transaminase
3. Percutaneous liver biopsy reveals cholestasis, fibroblast, proliferation of inflammatory cells and multinucleated giant cells

TABLE 13–2.—LABORATORY TESTS DIFFERENTIATING BILIARY ATRESIA FROM HEPATOCELLULAR CHOLESTASIS*

TESTS	BILIARY ATRESIA	HEPATOCELLULAR CHOLESTASIS
Serum glutamic oxaloacetic transaminase (IU)	<500	>500
^{131}I rose bengal excretion in stool after cholestyramine and phenobarbital for 72 hours	<10%	>10%
Serum 5′ nucleotidase (average IU/L)	>25	<14
Serum lipoprotein-X (with cholestyramine)	>300	<200
Serum α-fetoprotein (μg/ml)	<10	>40
Serum γ-glutamyl transpeptidase (IU/L)	760 ± 492	183 ± 54

*Adapted from Sunaryo F.P., Watkins J.B.: Evaluation of diagnostic techniques, in Daum F. (ed.): *Extrahepatic Biliary Atresia in Extrahepatic Biliary Atresia.* New York, Marcel Dekker, Inc., 1983.

4. ^{131}I rose bengal excretion test
   Fecal excretion greater than 10% of injected dose rules out biliary atresia.
5. Depending on the cause, the infant may have one of the following:
   a. Positive culture for bacteria or virus
   b. Positive serology for rubella, cytomegalovirus, toxoplasmosis, herpes simplex, syphilis, or hepatitis A and B virus
   c. Increased cord serum IgM
   d. Decreased α_1-antitrypsin by serum protein electrophoresis
   e. The presence of nonglucose reducing substances or organic acids in the urine
   f. Laboratory findings of Rh or ABO incompatibility
   g. Positive sweat test in cystic fibrosis

D. Supportive Management

1. See chapter 13–IIIC for "general supportive management for infants with indirect hyperbilirubinemia."
2. Medium-chain triglycerides supplement to compensate for malabsorption
3. Supplement fat-soluble vitamins (A,D,E,K) with greater than twice the recommended daily doses, e.g., 2,000 IU of vitamin D and 2.5 to 5.0 mg of vitamin K.
4. Cholestyramine (240 mg/kg/day divided into 3–4 doses) to relieve pruritus and phenobarbital (3 to 5 mg/kg/day) to improve bile flow
5. 1,25-hydroxycholecalciferol, 0.20 μg/kg/day orally to prevent rickets

E. Specific Therapy

No known specific treatment is available.

F. Prognosis

1. Severe and prolonged hepatocellular cholestasis with early onset of portal fibrosis, coexistence of systemic disease, and family history of cholestasis in a sibling are associated with poor prognosis.
2. Surgery has an adverse effect on infants with hepatocellular cholestasis. Progressive liver failure (30%) or death may occur.

REFERENCES

Kaplinsky C., Sternlieb I., Javitt N., et al.: Familial cholestatic cirrhosis associated with Kayser-Fleischer rings. *Pediatrics* 65:782, 1980.

Thaler M.M., Gellis S.S.: Studies on neonatal hepatitis and biliary atresia: II. The effect of diagnostic laparotomy on long term prognosis of neonatal hepatitis. *Am. J. Dis. Child.* 116:262, 1968.

XVI. CHOLESTATIC JAUNDICE DUE TO BILIARY ATRESIA

Biliary atresia refers to a group of diseases in which there is luminal obliteration or apparent absence of all or segments of the biliary duct system. The occurrence has been reported as 1 in 8,000 to 20,000 live births. Previously, biliary atresia was thought to represent a congenital developmental anomaly. At the present time, biliary atresia is considered to be an acquired hepatocellular disease associated with toxins, viruses, and developmental malformations.

A. Who Is at Risk?

1. Infants with antibodies to rubella, hepatitis, rotavirus type 3, cytomegalovirus, herpes, and toxoplasmosis
2. Infants with the fetal alcohol syndrome, polysplenia-heterotaxia syndrome or extra chromosomes (trisomy 18)
3. Infants born to families with Alagille's syndrome (cholestasis, paucity of intrahepatic bile ducts, unusual facies, vertebral malformations, cardiac disease, and retardation) or other familial diseases with paucity of the bile ducts

B. Clinical Manifestations

1. The infant is well until a few weeks of life.
2. Jaundice persists beyond the first week of life, gradually increases, rarely fluctuates, and usually becomes apparent between the second and third week.
3. Meconium and early stools are normal in color, but gradually become acholic. The stools may intermittently have color.

4. The urine appears dark yellow.
5. Hepatomegaly, splenomegaly, ascites, and portal hypertension develop and may progress over the first month of life.
6. Malabsorption leads to malnutrition and deficiencies of vitamins (especially vitamin E), zinc, magnesium, and other minerals.
7. Pruritus occurs at approximately 3 months of age.

C. Laboratory Findings (See Table 13–2)

1. Elevated direct and, to a lesser extent, indirect bilirubin
2. Abnormal liver function test. An abnormal serum glutamic oxaloacetic transaminase (but usually not over 300 units) suggests biliary atresia rather than hepatitis. A γ-glutamyl transpeptidase greater than 300 units suggests biliary atresia.
3. ^{131}I rose bengal excretion test. Excretion of less than 5% of the injected dye after 72 hours indicates complete obstruction. (Normally, 90% of injected dye is recovered.)
4. Abdominal scanning techniques may reveal inadequate (less than 10%) radioactivity in the intestine.
5. Elevated alkaline phosphatase, 5′ nucleotidase, cholesterol, α_1-antitrypsin, bile acid, lipoprotein, and/or α-fetoprotein may be present.
6. Tests for infectious diseases may be positive, e.g., cord IgM, HBs antigen, STS.
7. Percutaneous liver biopsy may reveal periportal bile duct proliferation, inflammatory exudate, dilation of lymphatic channels, thick-walled arterioles, and cholestasis.

D. Supportive Management

1. See chapter 13–IIIC for "general supportive management for infants with indirect hyperbilirubinemia."
2. Cholestyramine, 240 mg/kg/day divided into 4 doses, relieves pruritus.
3. Administer fat-soluble vitamins (A: 10,000–15,000 IU/day; D: 5,000–8,000 IU/day; E: 50–400 IU/day; K: 2.5–5.0 mg/2 days) water-soluble vitamins with twice recommended daily allowance, and medium-chain triglycerides for nutritional support.

E. Specific Therapy

Kasai portoenterostomy requires the presence of portohepatic bile ducts and should be performed before 3 months of age to maximize bile drainage and minimize liver damage. In spite of adequate bile drainage after surgery, recurrent cholangitis and progressive cirrhosis with portal hypertension may develop. Liver transplantation may be performed in infants with end-stage liver disease.

F. Prognosis

Infants with untreated biliary atresia usually survive 16 to 19 months. With surgery, bile drainage is reported in 90% of patients (Japan), and the 5-year survival rate is as high as 36%. Over 50% of infants with a successful portoenterostomy develop postoperative cholangitis and progressively deteriorating liver function.

REFERENCES

Altman R.P.: Biliary atresia. *Pediatrics,* 68:896, 1981.

Balistreri W.F., Suchy F.J., Farrell M.K., et al.: Pathologic versus physiologic cholestasis: Elevated serum concentration of a secondary bile acid in the presence of hepatobiliary disease. *J. Pediatr.* 98:399, 1981.

Barkin R.M., Lilly J.R.: Biliary atresia and Kasai operation: Continuing care. *J. Pediatr.* 96:1015, 1980.

Balistreri W.F.: Neonatal cholestasis. *J. Pediatr.* 106:171, 1985.

XVII. INHERITED CONJUGATED HYPERBILIRUBINEMIA: DUBIN-JOHNSON SYNDROME, ROTOR'S SYNDROME

Inherited conjugated hyperbilirubinemia is inherited as an autosomal recessive or an autosomal dominant trait with variable expression and is due to the inability of the hepatocyte to transport certain organic anions (e.g., conjugated bilirubin, rose bengal, methylene blue, indocyanine green, cholecystographic dye) into the bile. Bile salt excretion is normal. There are no abnormalities in production, hepatic uptake, or conjugation of bilirubin or in the extrahepatic biliary tract.

A. Who Is at Risk?

1. Infants with a family history of inherited conjugated hyperbilirubinemia
2. Infants born to parents who are consanguinous

B. Clinical Manifestations

1. Jaundice may be noted at birth or later in life but the onset is usually later.
2. Mild, occasionally tender, hepatomegaly may occur.
3. Nonspecific generalized symptoms such as poor feeding, nausea, vomiting, and weakness may be present.
4. Occasionally, a bleeding tendency due to decreased factor VII may be present.

C. Laboratory Findings

1. Direct hyperbilirubinemia 2 to 5 mg/dl
2. Prolonged bromsulphalein (BSP) retention and nonvisualized gallbladder

3. Pale stool
4. Dark urine
5. Normal serum uroporphyrinogen, increased urinary coproporhyrin I, and decreased urinary coproporhyrin III
6. Abnormal granular, brown pigment in the cytoplasm of the centrilobar hepatocytes in Dubin-Johnson syndrome.

D. Supportive Management

1. See chapter 13–IIIC for "general supportive management for infants with indirect hyperbilirubinemia."
2. Avoid estrogen and anabolic steroids since conjugated bilirubin excretion is inhibited.

E. Specific Therapy

No treatment is necessary.

REFERENCES

Schimizu Y., Kondo T., Kuchiba K., et al.: Uroporphyrinogen III cosynthetase in liver and blood in Dubin-Johnson syndrome. *J. Lab. Clin. Med.* 89:517, 1977.

Swartz H.M., Sarna T., Varma R.R.: On the nature and excretion of the hepatic pigment in the Dubin-Johnson syndrome. *Gastroenterology* 76:958, 1979.

Chapter 14

Anemia and Hemorrhage

Neonatal anemia can result from hemorrhage, hemolysis, or decreased red blood cell (RBC) production. The clinical manifestations of neonatal anemia depend upon the severity and duration of the anemia. Rapid diagnosis and therapy are essential since acute loss of approximately 20% to 25% of blood volume will result in shock.

I. NORMAL DATA (SEE APPENDIX A–10 to A–22)

A. General

Hematologic values at birth are influenced by gestational age, method of delivery, time of umbilical cord clamping, and site and time of sampling.

B. Blood Volume

Term infants have a blood volume of 80 to 110 ml/kg. Those with early umbilical cord clamp average 78 ml/kg of whole blood, while those with late clamp (greater than 30 seconds) average 98 ml/kg. Infants held below the level of the placenta will continue to gain blood; infants held above the placenta may bleed into the placenta. Asphyxiated infants tend to have a higher blood volume than normal infants. Premature infants have a blood volume of 90 to 115 ml/kg, which is somewhat higher than term infants (see Appendix A–4).

C. Hemoglobin/Hematocrit

The hemoglobin (Hb) level rises from approximately 10 gm/dl at 16 weeks to 15 gm/dl at 32 weeks. Normal mean cord Hb at birth is 16.8 gm/dl (13.7 to 20.1 gm/dl). Cord Hb values less than 13.5 gm/dl should be considered as anemia and Hb greater than 21 gm/dl as polycythemia. Cord Hb values from the umbilical artery tend to be 0.5 gm/dl higher than those from the umbilical vein. The mean Hb value the first day is 18.7 ± 3.4 gm/dl in term infants and 15.6 ± 1.0 gm/dl in premature infants. There is a Hb increase in the first several hours after birth; Hb then slowly declines and stays stable during the first 2 weeks of age. Capillary blood Hb levels may be 3.5 gm/dl higher than venous Hb levels, and venous levels are higher than arterial levels. Capillary Hb should be checked by venous specimens since capillary values may be unreliable due to the site being cold, edematous, or poorly perfused.

D. Reticulocytes

The mean cord reticulocyte count in blood of normal term infants is 2.8% ± 1.7%. Premature infants have higher reticulocyte counts at birth. The reticulocyte count increases slightly during the first 2 to 3 days after birth then drops abruptly to about 1% by the seventh day. Small-for-gestational-age infants have a more rapid decrease. Persistent reticulocytosis suggests the presence of a hemolytic process, blood loss, or hypoxia.

E. Nucleated Red Blood Cells (NRBCs)

Term infants have approximately 7.3 (range, 0 to 24) NRBCs/100 white blood cells (500 NRBCs/cu mm), and preterm infants have 21 NRBCs/100 white blood cells. By 12 hours, the NRBC count is decreased by approximately 50% and by the fourth day is decreased to 0%.

F. White Blood Cells (WBCs)

In term and premature infants, the total WBC count ranges from 5,000 to 25,000/cu mm during the first 2 weeks of life (see appendix A–12).

The total neutrophil count as well as band count rises during the first 12 hours of life, then slowly declines to reach a plateau by the fourth day. Prematures have a slightly lower total WBC count and higher percentage of young cells than term infants during the first 3 days. Polymorphonuclear cells predominate in the first days of life. Between the fourth and seventh day of life, lymphocytes predominate.

Both sample site and physical activity can produce alterations in WBC count. The capillary WBC count is higher than the venous count, which is higher than the arterial count. A vigorous cry increases WBC count with a shift to the left. Decreased WBCs may result from infection, asphyxia, or maternal hypertension. Neutropenia persists for the first 3 days in infants with history of asphyxia or maternal hypertension while neutropenia may not persist after 36 hours in infants with sepsis. Increased WBCs may result from intraventricular hemorrhage, hemolytic disease, infection, and other conditions. Increased young cells may result from conditions such as infection, asphyxia, meconium aspiration, and hypoglycemia.

G. Platelets

Both fullterm and preterm infants have platelet counts in the same range as normal older children and adults. Platelet counts of less than 150,000/cu mm should raise the suspicion of thrombocytopenia, and counts less than 100,000/cu mm indicate thrombocytopenia regardless of gestational age.

H. Coagulation Factors

A reduction in the activity of many clotting factors has been reported in the newborn. There is a deficiency of vitamin K, which is necessary for the normal function of factors II (prothrombin) VII, IX, and X. Even with the administration of vitamin K_1, factors II, VII, IX, and X are lower than normal adult values. Clotting factors I and V produced by the liver, which are not vitamin K dependent, are within the normal adult range. The range for the prothrombin time (PT) is 13–21 seconds and partial thromboplastin time (PTT) is 45–65 seconds in term and 45-75 seconds in preterm infants.

I. Physiologic Anemia

The Hb concentration of normal healthy newborns declines progressively to the minimum level of 11.4 ± 0.9 gm/dl by 8 to 12 weeks of age in full term infants and 7 to 10 gm/dl by 6 weeks of age in premature infants. This physiologic change in Hb concentrations (anemia) is most likely due to diminished erythropoiesis from high Hb and reticulocyte values at birth, shortened RBC survival (80 to 100 days in term infants and 60 to 80 days in premature infants), and rapid increase in blood volume. When the Hb concentration falls to a level low enough to limit tissue oxygen delivery, erythropoiesis occurs. Premature infants and infants with a low Hb concentration at birth have an earlier and more profound drop.

Rapid weight gain associated with increased total circulating volume may result in a static or falling peripheral Hb concentration despite active erythropoiesis.

J. Blood Pressure (See Appendix A–1 and Figs A–1 and A–2)

1. Normal blood pressure in the first 12 hours of life
   67/41 mm Hg for greater than 3,000-gm infants
   60/34 mm Hg for 2,001- to 3,000-gm infants
   51/30 mm Hg for 1,001- to 2,000-gm infants
   Systolic blood pressure during the awake state is approximately 5 to 7 mm Hg higher than during sleep.
2. Blood pressure in hypertension in the first 6 weeks of life
   Greater than 90/65 mm Hg for term infants
   Greater than 80/45 mm Hg for premature infants

3. Systolic blood pressure in shock (hypotension)
   Less than 50 mm Hg for term (3,000-gm) infants
   Less than 40 mm Hg for 1,000-gm infants

II. COMMON CAUSES OF ANEMIA AND/OR HEMORRHAGE

A. Hemorrhage Before and During Delivery

1. Occult hemorrhage before birth
   a. Fetomaternal transfusion
   b. Twin-to-twin transfusion
   c. Placental transfusion (e.g., nuchal cord)
   d. Traumatic amniocentesis
2. Bleeding from the placenta
   a. Placenta previa
   b. Marginal sinus rupture
   c. Abruptio placentae (usually associated with anoxia rather than hemorrhage)
   d. Incision of the placenta during cesarean section
3. Bleeding from the cord
   a. Rupture of a normal umbilical cord
   b. Hematoma of the cord or placenta
   c. Rupture of an abnormal umbilical cord
   d. Inability to control bleeding during insertion of an in-utero catheter
   e. Aberrant vessels
   f. Velamentous insertion of the cord with hemorrhage
4. Internal hemorrhage
   a. Intracranial hemorrhage
   b. Retroperitoneal hemorrhage
   c. Intra-abdominal hemorrhage
   d. Subperiosteal (cephalohematoma) or subgaleal hemorrhage
   e. Pulmonary hemorrhage

B. Hemorrhage in the Neonatal Period

1. Hemorrhagic disease of the newborn
2. Disseminated intravascular coagulation
3. Inherited deficiencies of the coagulation factors, e.g., factor VIII and IX
4. Platelet abnormalities
5. Vascular abnormalities
6. Rupture of a hollow viscus or umbilical vessel

C. Hemolysis Prenatally or Postnatally (See Chapter 13)

1. Isoimmune hemolytic disease
   Rh, ABO, minor blood group (Duffy, etc.) incompatibilities
2. Immune hemolytic disease due to maternal disease
   Connective tissue disorders (lupus erythematosus, rheumatoid arthritis, etc.)
3. Drug-induced immune hemolysis (penicillin)
4. Infections (bacterial, viral, treponemal, protozoal)
5. Vitamin E deficiency
6. Hereditary RBC membrane disorders (spherocytosis, elliptocytosis, pyknocytosis, stomatocytosis, etc.)
7. RBC enzyme (glucose-6-phosphate dehydrogenase, pyruvate kinase, hexokinase, etc.) deficiency
8. Abnormal hemoglobins (Bart's, β-thalassemia, etc.)

D. Failure of RBC Production

1. Physiologic anemia
2. Congenital hypoplastic anemia (Diamond-Blackfan syndrome)
3. Fanconi's anemia
4. Leukemia
5. Transcobalamin II deficiency
6. Refractory sideroblastic anemia
7. Congenital leukemia
8. Infection
9. Nutritional deficiencies (iron, folate, etc.)

III. WHAT THE PHYSICIAN SHOULD DO WHEN CONFRONTED WITH AN INFANT WITH ANEMIA AND/OR HEMORRHAGE

A. Diagnostic Workup for the Infant with Anemia and/or Hemorrhage Before or During Delivery or Recognized in the First 2 Days of Life

If severe anemia is first recognized at birth, consider hemorrhage or severe isoimmunization. If the anemia is recognized during the first 2 days of life, consider internal or external hemorrhage.

1. Review the prenatal and delivery history of the infant to determine the maternal and obstetric events that may predispose the infant to anemia or hemorrhage (see Tables 5–3 and 14–1 and chapter 15–IV). Was there any history of maternal vaginal bleeding in the last trimester? Placenta previa? Abruptio placentae? Traumatic amniocentesis? Ruptured umbilical cord? Incision of the placenta during cesarean section? Difficult, traumatic, or precipitous delivery? Fetal distress or low Apgar score? Maternal drug ingestion, especially barbiturates, phenytoin (Dilantin), or aspirin? Maternal infection?

TABLE 14–1.—Maternal Events Associated With Neonatal Hematologic Abnormalities*

	MATERNAL EVENT	NEONATAL HEMATOLOGIC ABNORMALITIES
Infection	Cytomegalovirus Toxoplasmosis Syphilis Rubella Coxsackie B Herpes simplex Malaria Echovirus Epstein-Barr virus	Hyperbilirubinemia, hemolytic anemia, thrombocytopenia, or disseminated intravascular coagulopathy
Illness	Lupus erythematosus	Thrombocytopenia, leukopenia, anemia
Systemic	Hyperthyroidism	Thrombocytopenia, hyperbilirubinemia, polycythemia
	Idiopathic thrombocytopenic purpura	Thrombocytopenia
	Eclampsia, maternal hypertension	Disseminated intravascular coagulation, leukopenia
	Autoimmune hemolytic anemia	Hemolytic anemia, thrombocytopenia
	Diabetus mellitus	Polycythemia, hyperbilirubinemia, hypercoagulable platelets, elevated HbA_{1c}
Malignancies	Malignant melanoma	Anemia, agranulocytosis, thrombocytopenia, normoblastemia
	Hodgkin's disease	Hodgkin's disease in infant
	Leukemia	Leukemia in late infancy (rare)
Sensitization in infants	Erythrocytes	Hemolytic anemia
	Leukocytes	Leukopenia
	Platelets	Thrombocytopenia
Drug ingestion	Thiazides	Thrombocytopenia, leukopenia, hemolytic anemia
	Hydralazine	Thrombocytopenia, leukopenia
	Tolbutamide	Thrombocytopenia
	Quinine	Thrombocytopenia
	Moth balls, antimalarials, sulfonamides, fava beans, nitrofurantoins, menadione	Hemolytic anemia if infant has G-6-PD deficiency, hyperbilirubinemia
	Dicumarol (Coumarin)	Hemorrhage
	Barbiturates	Prolongation of PT
	Salicylates	Prolongation of bleeding, platelet dysfunction
	Hydantoins	Aplastic anemia, abnormal PT, abnormal factor V, abnormal factor X
	Penicillin	Coombs' positive hemolytic anemia
	Epidural analgesics (prilocaine)	Methemoglobinemia
	Aspirin, glyceryl guaiacolate, dipyridamole, antihistamines	Impaired platelet aggregation, prolonged bleeding time
	Methylene blue	Heinz body hemolytic anemia
	Methadone	Thrombocytosis

*From Oski F.A., Naiman J.L.: *Hematologic Problems in the Newborn,* ed. 3. Philadelphia, W.B. Saunders Co., 1982. Used by permission.

2. Review family history of the infant. Is there a history of a hemolytic process? Does the mother have a history of isoimmune disease or Rh incompatibility? Is there a family history of RBC membrane disorder (e.g., spherocytosis or elliptocytosis)? Does the mother have a connective tissue disorder? Is there a family history of anemia?
3. Examine the infant noting the general physical condition: presence or absence of tachycardia, bradycardia, respiratory distress (including tachypnea), hepatosplenomegaly, abnormal blood pressure, and the quality of the peripheral pulses. Pay particular attention to the stigmata of intrauterine infection and congenital anomalies. Look carefully for bruises, scalp hemorrhage, petechiae, ecchymosis, blood from the gastrointestinal (GI) tract or trachea, and other signs of internal hemorrhage. (Table 14–2). Remember that infants who are asphyxiated appear pale, bradycardic, apneic, and cyanotic, but respond to oxygen therapy and have stable Hb.
4. Examine the placenta noting hematomas of the cord, incision of the placenta, etc.
5. For shock or severe anemia, insert umbilical arterial and venous lines (see chapter 3–IIIC3). Obtain the central venous pressure. The most effective indicator of blood loss is the central venous pressure.
6. Obtain appropriate laboratory studies.
   a. Obtain a complete blood count (CBC). The hematocrit value does not immediately fall after an acute bleed; therefore, the hematocrit value may be normal while the infant is in hypovolemic shock from blood loss.
   b. Obtain a reticulocyte count. Is it elevated or reduced?
   c. Examine the infant's peripheral smear to determine the RBC morphology.
   d. Obtain a Coombs' test to consider hemolysis.
7. Differentiate acute from chronic hemorrhage (Table 14–3).
8. If the infant is a twin, obtain Hb value for each twin to rule out the possibility of twin-to-twin transfusion. When the Hb difference is greater than 5 gm/dl and/or the weight difference exceeds 20% of the larger twin's weight, examine the vascular communication between the two placentae by injecting milk to determine if a twin-to-twin transfusion occurred.
9. If occult blood loss is suspected from fetomaternal transfusion, obtain a specimen of the mother's blood within 24 hours of the infant's birth to determine if fetal cells are present in the mother's blood by the acid elution method (Kleihauer-Betke test).
10. If no evidence of hemorrhage or hemolysis before or during delivery can be found, consider the possibility that the infant is bleeding at present.

B. Diagnostic Workup for the Infant With Neonatal Hemorrhage

1. Perform a rapid and careful physical examination to determine the infant's clinical condition and the site and extent of bleeding. If the infant is bleeding profusely or if the infant's vital signs are unstable, request a second physician to assist since multiple tests and support measures are frequently required simultaneously.

TABLE 14–2.—COMMON CLINICAL MANIFESTATIONS OF NEONATAL INTERNAL HEMORRHAGE

SITE OF HEMORRHAGE	CLINICAL MANIFESTATIONS
Adrenal glands	Commonly associated with macrosomia, difficult delivery, sepsis and/or breech presentation. Hemorrhage usually occurs at 24–72 hr of age. Clinical manifestations include sudden collapse, cyanosis, limpness, jaundice, irregular respiration, elevated or subnormal temperature, and the presence of a flank mass with bluish discoloration of the overlying skin. Blood in the adrenals can be confirmed by sonography. Calcification may be seen on x-ray film after 2–6 wk. A salt-losing syndrome may ensue.
Liver	
Subcapsular hematoma Rupture of the liver	Infant usually appears well first 24–48 hr. Commonly associated with a difficult delivery. Shock frequently occurs. Abdominal distention with a mass contiguous with the liver is noted. Shifting dullness may be present. Free fluid will be seen in the upright and supine films of the abdomen; blood may be obtained from paracentesis. Confirm the diagnosis by sonogram. Prompt surgical repair of the laceration is indicated.
Spleen Rupture of the spleen	Rare except in infants with history of difficult delivery, severe erythroblastosis fetalis, syphilis, or congenital leukemia (massive splenic enlargement). Pallor, abdominal distention, free fluid on the upright and supine films of the abdomen; blood will be obtained from paracentesis. Occasionally splenic rupture can occur in healthy macrosomic newborns.
CNS hemorrhage	See chapter 15–VI, 15–VII, 15–VIII.
GI tract	Associated with necrotizing enterocolitis and decreased platelets (see chapter 17–XVI), stress ulcers, maternal ingestion of drugs (e.g., aspirin), hemorrhagic disease of the newborn, platelet dysfunction, hemangiomas of the GI tract, etc. Infants with volvulus may show only minimal amounts of bleeding.
Skin	Ecchymoses and petechiae are commonly secondary to obstetric manipulation during delivery and/or sepsis. Ecchymosis of the legs is common with breech delivery; ecchymosis of the neck and face is frequent with a cord around the neck or maternal cervical clamping with the head delivered.
Pulmonary hemorrhage	See chapter 11–XV.
Cavernous hemangioma	Smaller hemangioma may regress spontaneously with growth of the infant; larger ones may predispose to a hemorrhagic diathesis associated with disseminated intravascular coagulation, thrombocytopenia; monitor clotting factors carefully.
Cephlohematoma	Subperiosteal or subgaleal bleeding may result in anemia.

Ref. Faix R.G., Donn S.M.: *Clin. Perinatol* 10:487, 1983.

TABLE 14–3.—CLINICAL AND LABORATORY MANIFESTATIONS OF ACUTE AND CHRONIC HEMORRHAGE*

	ACUTE HEMORRHAGE	CHRONIC HEMORRHAGE
Clinical manifestations	Acute distress Pale, dusky, occasionally pink in the delivery room Shallow, rapid and often irregular respirations Tachycardia, weak or absent peripheral pulses. Low or absent blood pressure. No hepatosplenomegaly	Marked pallor disproportionate to the evidence of distress Occasionally, signs of congestive heart failure (taychycardia, tachypnea, hepatomegaly, cardiomegaly, etc.)
Venous pressure	Low	Normal or elevated
Laboratory findings		
Hemoglobin/Hct	May be normal initially, then drops quickly during first 24 hr of life. Can be misleadingly high in infants with shock or acute hemorrhage	Low at birth
RBC morphology	Normochromic and macrocytic	Hypochromic and microcytic Anisocytosis and poikilocytosis.
Serum iron	Normal at birth	Low at birth
Course	Prompt treatment of anemia and shock necessary to prevent death (see chapter 14–IIID)	Generally uneventful
Treatment	Administer whole blood, plasma, or other blood-volume expander, 20 ml/kg and more for shock. Iron therapy later.	Packed RBC transfusion may be necessary Iron therapy

*From Oski F.A., Naiman J.L.: *Hematologic Problems in the Newborn,* ed. 3. Philadelphia, W.B. Saunders Co., 1982, p. 62. Used by permission.

2. Obtain and follow the infant's blood pressure, central venous pressure, heart rate, and respiratory rate.
3. Review the infant's familial, prenatal, and delivery history to determine if there is a family history of excessive bleeding or a maternal history of hematologic disorders. Determine if there has been a maternal history of infection during pregnancy or a complicated labor and/or delivery, evidence of birth trauma, prolonged anoxia, fetal distress, prematurity, breech presentation, or other problems. Note if there were drugs administered to the mother that might adversely affect the infant's hematologic status (see Table 14–1).
4. Review the infant's clinical status prior to the bleeding episode to determine if there were clinical abnormalities (e.g., sepsis, asphyxia, breech presentation) predisposing to platelet and/or clotting factor disorders.
5. Ascertain if Vitamin K_1, 1 mg, was administered to the infant at birth.
6. Obtain appropriate coagulation studies to judge whether the infant has disseminated intravascular coagulopathy, platelet insufficiency, hemorrhagic disease of the newborn, or other coagulation disorders (Table 14–4).

TABLE 14–4.—COAGULATION STUDIES*

TEST	STATUS IN DEFICIENCY	COAGULATION STAGES INVOLVED	FACTORS INVOLVED
Thromboplastin generation test	Prolonged and corrected by adding normal plasma	First phase (generation of thromboplastin)	Platelet thromboplastin factor, calcium and factors V, VIII, IX, X, XI, and XII
Prothrombin consumption test	More than 25% of its original plasma prothrombin concentration	First phase (generation of thromboplastin)	Platelet thromboplastin factor, calcium and factors V, VIII, IX, X, XI, and XII. Thrombocytopenia or qualitative defects of platelet function
Partial thromboplastin time (PTT)	Prolonged	First phase (generation of thromboplastin)	Platelet thromboplastin factor, calcium and factors V, VIII, IX, X, XI, and XII
Assay of factors	Decreased or absent	First phase (generation of thromboplastin)	Platelet thromboplastin factor, calcium and factors V, VIII, IX, X, XI, and XII
One-stage prothrombin time (PT)	Prolonged	Second stage (conversion of prothrombin to thrombin)	Thromboplastin, calcium and factors I (fibrinogen), II (prothrombin), V, VII, and X
Thrombin (TT) clotting time	Prolonged	Third phase (conversion of fibrinogen to fibrin clot)	Thrombin, fibrinogen, presence of coagulation inhibitor (Heparin or fibrin-split products)
Fibrinogen determination	Decreased	Third phase (conversion of fibrinogen to fibrin clot)	Fibrinogen
Fibrin-split products	Increased	Fibrinolytic system	Disseminated intravascular coagulation
Euglobulin lysis time	Shortened	Fibrinolytic system	Plasminogen activator

*Modified from Harper R.G., Yoon J.J.: *Handbook of Neonatology* ed. 1. Chicago, Year Book Medical Publishers, Inc., 1974, p. 187.

   a. Obtain a CBC, platelet count, and peripheral smear.
   b. Draw blood for PT, PTT, fibrinogen, and fibrin degradation products.
7. Obtain coagulation factor levels if PTT is prolonged (factors VIII, IX, etc.).
8. Obtain chest x-ray films and blood gas studies if blood is aspirated by nasotracheal suction and pulmonary hemorrhage is suspected.
9. If the infant has blood-stained gastric aspirate/vomitus or stool in the first few hours of life:
   a. Perform an APT test on the specimen. This test determines if the blood is from the mother or the newborn.
      APT test: Mix one part blood-stained vomitus or stool with 5 to 10 parts tap water. The mixture is centrifuged for several minutes at approximately 2,000 rpm to separate the debris. The pink supernatant is decanted or filtered. About 1 ml of 0.25 N(1%) sodium hydroxide is mixed with 5 ml of supernatant. The color change is read in 2 minutes. Blood containing adult hemoglobin changes from pink to brownish yellow, while blood containing predominantly fetal Hb remains pink. It is helpful to run two control tubes, one containing the peripheral blood of the infant being studied and the other adult blood.
   b. If the APT test indicates fetal blood, obtain a flat plate of the abdomen to determine the presence of necrotizing enterocolitis, volvulus, GI perforation, etc.
10. If the infant has anemia and flank mass with bluish discoloration over the skin, consider adrenal hemorrhage (see Table 14–2).
11. If the infant has anemia and abdominal distension with a mass contiguous with liver, consider subcapsular hematoma or rupture of the liver (see Table 14–2).
12. If the infant has anemia and abdominal distension with history of erythroblastosis or syphilis, consider rupture of the spleen (see Table 14–2).
13. If the infant has anemia, apnea, seizures, etc., consider intracranial hemorrhage (see chapter 15–VI, 15-VII, and 15-VIII).
14. If the infant has hemoglobinuria and/or hematuria, consider disseminated intravascular coagulation, transfusion reaction, acute renal cortical necrosis, nephrotoxic drugs, renal vascular accident, obstructive uropathy, etc. (see chapter 18).

C. Diagnostic Workup for the Infant With Anemia Recognized After the First 48 Hours of Life

1. If the anemia is first recognized:
   a. After 48 hours of age, consider hemolysis often associated with jaundice or iatrogenic loss due to blood drawing.
   b. After the first 2 to 4 weeks of life, consider physiologic anemia and nutritional deficiency.
2. Obtain a family history of abnormal RBC morphology or RBC enzyme deficiency, maternal history of drug ingestion, etc.

3. Obtain an initial investigation, e.g., Hb, reticulocyte count, peripheral smear, mean corpuscular volume, Coombs' test, etc.
4. If reticulocytopenia is present, consider congenital hypoplastic anemia or leukemia. Bone marrow examination is required. Late reticulocytopenia is associated with anemia due to iron, folic acid, and copper deficiency.
5. If reticulocytosis is present, consider hemorrhage or hemolysis.
   a. Obtain a direct Coombs' test. If positive, consider Rh, ABO, or minor group incompatibility. Rule out a Coomb's positive autoimmune hemolytic disease in the mother. See chapter 13 for jaundice.
      If negative, consider occult hemorrhage or hemolytic disease other than isoimmunization.
6. If reticulocytosis is present and the Coombs' test is negative, obtain a peripheral blood smear for RBC morphology.
   a. Spherocytosis, elliptocytosis, and pyknocytosis can be identified.
   b. If hypochromic microcytic anemia is present, consider iron deficiency anemia from chronic fetomaternal transfusion, twin-to-twin transfusion, fetoplacental bleeding, infection, or other causes.
   c. If the mean corpuscular volume is less than 95 fl, consider α-thalassemia trait.
   d. If RBCs are normocytic and normochromic, consider acute blood loss, congenital RBC enzyme defect, or systemic disease.

D. General Supportive Management for the Infant With Anemia, Hemorrhage, and/or Shock

1. Handle the infant gently (as always).
2. Support the infant's ventilatory status. Resuscitate the infant as required.
3. Apply pressure to an overt bleeding site. Apply topical thrombin or an absorbable gauze (Gelfoam or Oxycel) to bleeding wounds, circumcision sites, and other superficial bleeding areas.
4. Request a second physician to help if artificial ventilation and/or umbilical vessel catheterization is required simultaneously with multiple diagnostic tests (see chapter 3).
5. Maintain the infant's neutrothermal environment.
6. Monitor the infant's heart rate, respiratory rate, blood pressure, and central venous pressure frequently.
7. If the infant is pale and has delayed capillary filling (normally it takes only 4 seconds for pink color to return after blanching) with hypotension, systolic blood pressure less than 40 mm Hg for a 1,000-gm infant and less than 50 mm Hg for a 3,000-gm infant, consider the infant to be in shock (see appendix A–1, Figs A–1 and A–2). Note that occasionally infants can vasoconstrict so efficiently that blood pressure will not fall although the infant is hypovolemic until 20% to 25% of the blood volume is lost. Marked peripheral vasoconstriction, low tissue oxygenation, and increasing metabolic acidosis may be present before blood pressure falls. Other findings such as tachypnea, dyspnea, bradycardia, and hypothermia may also be present.

a. Insert an arterial and venous umbilical line if at all possible to have access for central arterial and central venous monitoring, and blood gas monitoring. If umbilical catheterization cannot be performed, insert a peripheral venous line with at least a 23-gauge needle or catheter as a route for administration of blood volume expanders.
b. Obtain a CBC and send a blood specimen for type and crossmatch. Replace blood loss with whole blood.
c. When shock is due to blood loss, rapidly administer 20 ml/kg of group O Rh-negative fresh whole blood (not greater than 72 hours since drawing) or 10 ml/kg of packed RBCs followed by 10 ml/kg of fresh frozen plasma. If neither whole blood nor fresh frozen plasma is available, administer Plasmanate, 5% albumin (or 25% salt-poor albumin diluted to 5%), or Ringer's lactate 20 ml/kg. Monitor the infant's heart rate during infusion to avoid overload. Do not use dextran prior to obtaining blood to be typed and crossmatched as dextran interferes with typing. *Do not wait for blood to arrive. Support intravascular pressure with other agents immediately if the infant is in shock.*
d. Monitor acidosis and hypoglycemia; both frequently occur concurrently with shock. Severe metabolic acidosis and/or hypoglycemia require immediate therapy.
e. Reassess management. Infants with acute blood loss will improve immediately after transfusion. If shock persists (small heart on x-ray film, central venous pressure below 3 cm of water, small liver), give another 10 to 20 ml/kg of whole blood or blood volume expander.
f. If hypotension persists despite the administration of adequate volume, consider the administration of inotropic agents such as dopamine at 2 to 20 μg/kg/minute. Usually the lower dose is adequate in those infants who benefit.
    1) For low cardiac output, normal or increased blood pressure, vasoconstriction, and tachycardia, administer either isoproterenol (1:5,000, 0.2 mg/ml), 0.05 to 0.50 μg/kg/minute diluted with D5W to a concentration of 1.0 mg/dl (10 μg/ml), or nitroprusside, 0.5 to 8.0 μg/kg/minute.
    Isoproterenol affects β-receptors and bronchodilation, and vasodilation (skeletal muscle, kidneys, and gut) and cardiac stimulation (cardiac output and maintenance of systemic atrial pressure) occur. In hypovolemia, isoproterenol may induce hypotension. Arrhythmia occurs frequently.
    2) For low cardiac output, normotension, and tachycardia, administer dobutamine, 2 to 20 μg/kg/minute.
    Dobutamine increases cardiac contractility directly without α-adrenergic effect.
    3) For low cardiac output, hypotension, and low urine output, administer dopamine, 2 to 20 μg/kg/minute diluted with D5W to a concentration of 10 mg/dl (100 μg/ml).
    Dopamine is a naturally occurring catecholamine. Low doses (2 to 4

μg/kg/minute) activate dopamine receptors and mediate renal, mesenteric, coronary, and cerebral vasodilation. It improves renal function and increases urine output, creatinine clearance, and fractional sodium excretion. It may decrease systemic atrial pressure. High doses may stimulate α- and/or β-receptors and increase systemic more than pulmonary resistance. However, sudden cessation of high-dose infusion increases pulmonary vascular resistance.

Inotropic action depends upon endogenous myocardial norepinephrine stores and left ventricular afterload. Therefore, a sick neonatal heart may not be able to respond to dopamine.

4) For bradycardia and/or asystole, administer epinephrine, 1:10,000 dilution (0.1 mg/ml), 100–200 μg/kg bolus.

g. If shock persists and endotoxemia is suspected, administer the following:
   1) Hydrocortisone IV, 35 to 50 mg/kg over 10 to 15 minutes, and if necessary repeat at not less than 30-minute intervals and not more than four times. Hydrocortisone may interrupt the vasodilatation effects of kallikrein released by granulocytes and vascular endothelial cells due to endotoxin.
   2) Naloxone, 0.01 mg/kg IV, in conjunction with hydrocortizone. Naloxone inhibits the hypotensive effect of the pituitary β-endorphin stimulated by endotoxin.

h. Follow the blood pressure and hematocrit and keep the hematocrit between 40% and 45% within the first week of life or if the infant is on a ventilator. Transfuse with 5 to 10 ml/kg of packed cells when the hematocrit is below 40% even if the central venous pressure and blood pressure are within normal limits during the first week of life. (The administration of 1 ml/kg of packed cells will raise the hematocrit approximately 1% or 3 ml/kg of packed cells will raise the Hb by 1 gm/dl.)

8. Administer vitamin K_1, 2 mg IV, if vitamin K_1 was not given and the infant is bleeding after obtaining coagulation studies. If vitamin K_1 was given, repeat the dose of vitamin K_1, 1 mg IV.
9. For those anemic infants in congestive heart failure with increased central venous pressure, administer furosemide, 1.0 mg/kg IV, prior to the transfusion.
10. If the infant looks pale but is not in distress, anemia may be due to chronic blood loss and blood transfusion is not required, but iron therapy should be started; ferrous sulfate, 2 mg of elemental iron/kg orally, three times a day for 3 months.
11. For those infants who had multiple blood drawings for diagnostic purposes, the quantity of blood removed should be recorded. When 10% of the blood volume has been removed in less than 48 hours it should be replaced.
12. If the infant is hemorrhaging from the stomach, attempt to stop the bleeding.
    a. Obtain an immediate plane and crosstable lateral abdominal x-ray film to determine if perforation has occurred.
    b. If there is no perforation, pass a nasogastric tube to the stomach and

wash the stomach with cool saline. The addition of 1 ml of aqueous epinephrine (1:1,000) to 1,000 ml of saline will help induce vasoconstriction.

c. If the infant continues to bleed from the GI tract, consult the pediatric surgeon. Loss of twice the infant's blood volume is the usual indication for surgical intervention. Most infants stop bleeding before surgical intervention is necessary, however.

13. If the infant has a cephalohematoma or subgaleal hemorrhage follow infant's hematocrit, bilirubin, and platelet levels. These infants occasionally have thrombocytopenia secondary to platelet consumption in the hematoma.
14. If the infant has disseminated intravascular coagulation, eliminate the causative factors and give exchange transfusion for severe disseminated intravascular coagulation with fresh whole blood or fresh packed RBCs reconstituted with fresh frozen plasma followed by platelet transfusion. In milder cases, give repeated fresh frozen plasma transfusions with platelet transfusions (see chapter 14–XII).
15. See chapters 15–VI, 15–VII, 15–VIII for intracranial hemorrhage, 11–XV for pulmonary hemorrhage, 17–XVI for necrotizing enterocolitis, 17–X for volvulus, etc.
16. For those infants with physiologic anemia with signs of decompensation, such as tachypnea (respiratory rate greater than 50/minute), tachycardia (heart rate greater than 160/minute), poor weight gain, easy fatigability with feeding, and central venous oxygen tension less than 25 mm Hg at 3 to 8 weeks of age, transfuse the infant with 5 to 10 ml/kg of packed RBCs.
17. Complications of transfusion should be considered.
    a. Hemolytic transfusion reaction
    True hemolytic transfusion reaction is rare in the newborn, but pseudohemolytic transfusion reaction may occur when the donor's RBCs are injured.
    b. Transmission of infection
    Cytomegalovirus, hepatitis, bacterial infection (more common with platelet transfusion since it is stored at 22° C), Epstein-Barr virus, acquired immune deficiency syndrome, and others
    c. Metabolic complications
    Hypoglycemia, acidosis, hypocalcemia, hyperkalemia, etc. (especially with exchange transfusion)
    d. Cardiac and vascular complications
    Volume overload (may be associated with CNS hemorrhage in premature infants)
    e. Sensitization to plasma and HLA antigen
    Sensitization is rare, but HLA alloimmunization may result from sensitization to maternal leukocytes as a result of maternofetal transfusion.
    f. Possible graft versus host disease
    Graft versus host disease is rare.

    To reduce transfusion complications, quadruple or triple packs of single donor for repeat transfusion may be used.

REFERENCES

Blajchman M.A., Sheridan D., Rawls W.E.: Risks associated with blood transfusion in newborn infants. *Clin. Perinatol.* 11:403, 1984.

Blanchette V.S., Zipursky A.: Assessment of anemia in newborn infants. *Clin. Perinatal.* 11:489, 1984.

Furman W.L., Menke J.A., Barson W.J., et al.: Continuous naloxone infusion in two neonates with septic shock. *J. Pediatr.* 105:649, 1984.

IV. FETOMATERNAL TRANSFUSION

Fetomaternal transfusions occur in approximately 50% of all pregnancies but only in 1% is blood loss severe enough to cause significant anemia in the newborn. Bleeding can occur acutely as well as chronically during labor or during pregnancy as early as the fourth to eighth week of gestation.

A. Who Is at Risk?

1. Infants whose mothers had a transabdominal amniocentesis, especially when the amniocentesis was traumatic
2. Infants who underwent external cephalic version prior to delivery or fundal pressure during delivery
3. Infants whose mothers received oxytocin during labor
4. Infants whose placenta was malformed (placental chorioangioma)
5. Fetomaternal transfusion can occur in infants without perinatal complications.

B. Clinical Manifestations (See Table 14–3)

Fetomaternal transfusion can be acute, chronic, or acute and chronic.

1. In the infant with acute hemorrhage
   a. Pale, dusky, occasionally pink in the delivery room
   b. Rapid and often irregular respirations without marked retractions, tachycardia, weak, feeble peripheral pulses, low blood pressure
2. In the infant with chronic hemorrhage
   a. Marked pallor disproportionate to the distress
   b. May have signs of congestive heart failure (tachycardia, tachypnea, hepatomegaly, cardiomegaly, etc.); hydrops fetalis in severe cases
3. In the mother with severe fetomaternal hemorrhage
   a. Shaking chills and fever may develop as a consequence of incompatible fetal blood entering the mother's circulation.
   b. Likewise, acute renal failure may ensue as a result of hemolytic transfusion reaction.

C. Laboratory Findings (See Table 14–3)

1. In the infant with acute hemorrhage
   a. Low hematocrit and Hb levels. Initial Hb and hematocrit levels can be misleadingly high if hemorrhage occurred recently. Hb and hematocrit drop quickly during the next several hours.
   b. Peripheral blood smear: normocytic and normochromic. Increased NRBCs may be seen.
   c. Jaundice is usually absent; the Coombs' test is negative unless erythroblastosis is present.
   d. Demonstration of fetal cells in the maternal circulation. As little as 0.1 ml of fetal RBCs may be demonstrated in the maternal circulation by several techniques. The tests are reliable only when the mother does not have conditions associated with increased maternal fetal Hb levels, e.g., sickle cell anemia. The mother normally may have an increase in her own fetal Hb during pregnancy from 1.5% to 5.7%, and this fetal Hb stains faintly. Dark-stained fetal Hb from the fetus should be differentiated from light-stained fetal Hb originated from the mother.
      1) The acid elution technique (Kleihauer-Betke test)
         The acid-elution technique is the simplest and most commonly used. It is based on the property of fetal Hb to resist elution from the intact RBCs in an acid medium. Unstained smears are fixed and then incubated in an acid buffer that elutes adult Hb from the erythrocytes. Fetal Hb resists elution and stains darkly, while maternal cells appear ghost-like.
         If there is ABO incompatibility, the mother's blood should be tested for the presence of fetal cells within several hours of birth since the infant's A or B cells are rapidly cleared from the maternal circulation by the mother's anti-A or anti-B antibodies.
      2) Direct differential agglutination
      3) Mixed agglutination and fluorescent antibody techniques
2. In the infant with chronic hemorrhage
   a. Low hematocrit and Hb as low as 3 to 6 gm/dl.
   b. Hypochromic and microcytic RBCs with anisocytosis and poikilocytosis on peripheral blood smear
   c. Increased NRBC and reticulocyte counts
   d. High central venous pressure (if the infant has congestive heart failure)
   e. Absent hyperbilirubinemia
   f. Low serum iron level or no stainable iron in the bone marrow
   g. Demonstration of fetal cells in maternal circulation

D. Supportive Management

See chapter 14–IIID for "general supportive management for the infant with anemia, hemorrhage, and/or shock."

E. Specific Therapy

1. Therapy for shock
   Rapidly administer whole blood, plasma, or other blood-volume expander (normal saline, Plasmanate, albumin, etc.), 20 ml/kg (see chapter 14–IIID7).
2. Therapy for anemia
   Transfuse with 10 ml/kg of packed cells if hematocrit is below 40% in the first week of life. Transfuse packed cells slowly if CHF is present (see chapter 11–XXIXE).
   Administer ferrous sulfate, 2 mg of elemental iron/kg orally, three times a day for three months to infants who have acute blood loss and have received blood transfusions or to infants who have mild blood loss but do not require blood transfusions. Iron therapy may be started after the first 2 weeks of life.

REFERENCES

Keith L., Berger G.S., Edelman D.A.: Evaluation of fetaldex: A new screening test for fetal erythrocytes in maternal circulation. *J. Repro. Med.* 20:109, 1978.

Pembrey M.E., Weatherall D.J., Clegg J.B.: Maternal synthesis of hemoglobin F in pregnancy. *Lancet* 1:1350, 1973.

Woo Wang M., McCutcheon E., Desforges J.F.: Fetomaternal hemorrhage from diagnostic transabdominal amniocentesis. *Am. J. Obstet. Gynecol.* 97:1123, 1967.

V. TWIN-TO-TWIN (FETO-FETAL) TRANSFUSION

Arteriovenous connections do not occur in dichorionic placentas, whether joined or separated, but do occur in monochorionic twins' placentas. In 33% of monochorionic twin placentas, there is significant blood loss from one twin to the other. Twin-to-twin anastomosis can be demonstrated by injecting milk into the vessels on one side of the placental vascular equator and demonstrating its emergence from the other side. Twin-to-twin transfusions should be suspected when the Hb difference is greater than 5 gm/dl between monochorionic twins. Hemorrhage may be acute or chronic.

A. Who Is at Risk?

Monochorionic twins are at risk (approximately 70% of monozygous twins).

B. Clinical Manifestations

When the weight difference exceeds 20% of the weight of the larger twin, the transfusion is chronic and the smaller twin is the donor.

1. Donor twin
   Clinical manifestations include pallor, low blood pressure, congestive heart failure, rapid and irregular gasping respirations, weak, feeble peripheral pulses, and a history of maternal oligohydramnios.
2. Recipient twin
   Clinical manifestations include recipient usually larger than donor; ruddy, plethoric, cyanotic, tachypneic, and tachycardiac; hepatomegaly and cardiomegaly as signs of congestive heart failure; cerebral vascular accidents caused by thrombosis; convulsions; priapism; renal vein thrombosis; and a history of maternal polyhydramnios. See chapter 12–V for polycythemia.

C. Laboratory Findings

1. Donor twin
   a. Anemia
   b. Low blood pressure
   c. Thrombocytopenia
   d. Elevated reticulocytes
   e. Elevated number of NRBCs
   f. Absence of hyperbilirubinemia
2. Recipient twin
   a. Polycythemia (hematocrit above 65%) and/or hyperviscosity
   b. Elevated blood pressure
   c. X-ray film evidence of pulmonary edema
   d. Hyperbilirubinemia
   e. Hypoglycemia
   f. Transient thrombocytopenia

D. General Supportive Management

1. Donor twin
   See chapter 14–IIID for "general supportive management for the infant with anemia, hemorrhage, and/or shock."
2. Recipient twin
   See chapter 11–IIIB for "general supportive management for infants with respiratory distress" and chapter 12–VE for "specific therapy" for infants with polycythemia, and 11–XXIXE for "general supportive management and specific therapy" for infants with congestive heart failure.

E. Specific Therapy

1. Donor twin
   Transfuse as required if the donor twin is in distress.
   See chapter 14–IIID7 for specific therapy of the infant with shock. Oral administration of iron at a later date may be necessary.

Administer ferrous sulfate, 2 mg of elemental iron/kg, three times daily for 3 months if the donor is anemic, but not in distress.

2. Recipient twin

   Partial exchange transfusion with plasma should be performed if the plethoric recipient twin is in respiratory distress with circulatory overload.

   See chapter 12–VE for specific therapy of the infant with polycythemia and hyperviscosity.

REFERENCES

Pochedly C., Musiker S.: Twin-to-twin transfusion syndrome. *Postgrad. Med.* 47:172, 1970.

Sacks M.O.: Occurrence of anemia and polycythemia in phenotypically dissimilar single ovum human twins. *Pediatrics* 24:604, 1959.

Tan K.L., Tan R., Tan S.H., et al.: The twin transfusion syndrome: Clinical observations on 35 affected pairs. *Clin. Pediatr.* 18:111, 1979.

VI. FETOPLACENTAL HEMORRHAGE

Infants with tight nuchal cords (where pressure on the cord obstructs the umbilical vein earlier than the artery) or infants who are held above the placenta prior to clamping the cord during delivery may lose blood into the placenta.

A. Who Is at Risk?

1. Infants born by cesarean section
2. Infants with tight nuchal cords
3. Infants held higher than the placenta prior to cord clamp
4. Infants born to mothers with acute hypotension

B. Clinical Manifestations

Clinical findings of acute hemorrhage such as pallor, duskiness, and rapid and often irregular respiration are seen (see Table 14–3).

C. Laboratory Findings

See Table 14–3.

D. Supportive Management

See chapter 14–IIID for "general supportive management for the infant with anemia, hemorrhage, and/or shock."

E. Specific Therapy

There is no known specific therapy.

REFERENCE

Lubin B.: Neonatal anemia secondary to blood loss. *Clin. Hematol.* 7:19, 1978.

VII. TRAUMATIC AMNIOCENTESIS

Amniocentesis is relatively safe; however, even in the most experienced hands placental trauma, transplacental hemorrhage, increased maternal antibody titer, and increased severity of erythroblastosis can occur. Exsanguination from massive transplacental hemorrhage is a potential but very unlikely hazard of amniocentesis. Ultrasound should be utilized to properly identify and locate fetus, placenta, and umbilical cord.

A. Who Is at Risk?

Any fetus subjected to amniocentesis through anteriorly placed placenta is at risk.

B. Clinical Manifestations

1. Lacerations due to misjudgement of position of placenta or fetus may result in trauma to any part of the fetus and/or anemia. Fetal risks include bleeding, needle puncture, gangrene, and death.
2. See Table 14–3.

C. Laboratory Findings

See Table 14–3.

D. General Supportive Management and Specific Therapy

1. See chapter 14–IIID for "general supportive management for infants with anemia, hemorrhage, and/or shock."
2. If puncture wounds are present, give appropriate therapy.

REFERENCE

Simpson J.L.: Diagnosing fetal chromosomal abnormalities, in Queenan J.T. (ed.): *Management of High Risk Pregnancy.* Oradell, N.J., Medical Economics Co., 1980, p. 35.

VIII. PLACENTA PREVIA

Placenta previa, the low implantation of the placenta, may be suspected whenever there is vaginal bleeding or when the fetus is breech or transverse. The incidence is 1 in 200 live births. Placentas that appear to be low-lying in early or middle pregnancy frequently migrate away from the lower uterine segment as pregnancy progresses. Placenta previa tends to be associated with fetal developmental defects and twins. In the majority of cases, the fetus can be carried to gestational maturity. Significant hemorrhage prior to maturity may necessitate delivery of a premature infant.

The types of placenta previa are as follows:

Central placenta previa: The implantation site entirely covers the internal os of the cervix; this is the most dangerous type.

Partial placenta previa: Only part of the internal os is covered by the placenta; the rest of the cervix is covered by fetal membranes.

Marginal placenta previa: The lowermost edge of the placenta reaches the edge of the internal os of the cervix.

Lateral placenta previa: The placenta is implanted on the lower section of the uterus but is distant from the internal os.

A. Who Is at Risk?

Mothers with the following conditions are at risk to have placenta previa:

1. Previous spontaneous or induced abortions or cesarean sections
2. Twin pregnancy
3. Heavy smoking
4. Advanced maternal age

B. Clinical Manifestations

The infant may be term or preterm. There is an increased incidence of prematurity and anemia in the newborn (see Table 14–3).

C. Laboratory Findings

See Table 14–3.

D. Supportive Management and Specific Therapy

See chapter 14–IIID for "general supportive management for the infant with anemia, hemorrhage, and/or shock."

E. Specific Therapy

There is no known specific therapy.

REFERENCE

Lubin B.: Neonatal anaemia secondary to blood loss. *Clin. Hematol.* 7:19, 1978.

IX. ABRUPTIO PLACENTAE

Abruptio placentae, the premature separation of the placenta from the uterine wall, occurs in 1% to 4.5% of all births. The placenta contains blood clots on the maternal side that may detach the placenta either partially or completely, progressively or abruptly, and result in perinatal asphyxia and disseminated intravascular coagulation if the mother is in shock or fetal side of the placenta is torn.

A. Who Is at Risk?

Mothers with the following conditions are at risk to develop abruptio placentae:
1. Diabetes mellitus
2. Hypertensive disease of pregnancy
3. Abdominal trauma (including coitus)
4. Uterine malformations
5. Vena cava compression
6. Heavy smoking
7. Twin pregnancy
8. Polyhydramnios
9. Premature labor

B. Clinical Manifestations

1. Central and paracentral hematomas present a considerable danger and predispose to fetal demise if they exceed 10% of total placental volume.
2. Fetal distress
3. Perinatal asphyxia
4. Signs of disseminated intravascular coagulation
5. Anemia (see Table 14–3)

C. Laboratory Findings

1. Consistent with findings of perinatal asphyxia (see chapter 15–IV)
2. Consistent with findings of anemia and/or shock (see Table 14–3)

3. Consistent with findings of disseminated intravascular coagulation (see chapter 14–XII)

D. General Supportive and Specific Therapy

See chapter 14–IIID for "general supportive management for infants with anemia, hemorrhage, and/or shock," 14–XII for "disseminated intravascular coagulation," and 15–IV for "perinatal asphyxia."

REFERENCE

Philippe E., Sauvage J.: The placenta and its membranes, in Iffy L., Kaminetzky H.A. (eds.): *Principles and Practice of Obstetrics and Perinatology.* New York, John Wiley & Sons, 1981, p. 181.

X. INTERNAL HEMORRHAGE

Anemia that appears in the first 24 to 72 hours of life and is not associated with jaundice is commonly due to internal hemorrhage. However, internal hemorrhage is often associated with hyperbilirubinemia 24 hours after bleeding.

A. Who Is at Risk?

1. Infants born after difficult delivery, vacuum extraction or asphyxia, or who are less than 32 weeks' gestation or who have rapid infusion of hyperosmolar solutions are at risk for periventricular-intraventricular hemorrhage (see chapter 15–VI).
2. Infants whose mothers have cephalopelvic disproportion, prolonged labor or who are born by difficult forceps extraction are at risk for subdural hematoma (see chapter 15–VII).
3. Premature, hypoxic, or fullterm infants born after a traumatic delivery are at risk for subarachnoid hemorrhage (see chapter 15–VIII).
4. Infants born by breech delivery are at risk for hemorrhage into the adrenals, kidney, spleen, or retroperitoneal area (see Table 14–2).
5. Large infants born by breech delivery are at risk for rupture of the liver or spleen (see Table 14–2).
6. Premature infants who have sustained stress or hypoxia or who have a sudden increment of feedings are at risk for necrotizing enterocolitis (see chapter 17–XVI).
7. Infants with malrotation and other GI anomalies are at risk for GI bleeding secondary to volvulus (see chapter 17–X).
8. Infants born with vitamin K_1 deficiency, platelet aberrations, coagulation factor deficiency, or sepsis are at risk for hemorrhage.

B. Clinical Manifestations

Clinical manifestations are related to the quantity, duration, time, and site of the hemorrhage (see Tables 14–2 and 14–3, chapter 11–XV for pulmonary hemorrhage, 15–VI, 15–VII, 15–VIII for CNS hemorrhage, and other relevant sections).

C. Laboratory Findings

1. Anemia, thrombocytopenia, and hyperbilirubinemia are the most consistent findings. Findings of disseminated intravascular coagulation may be seen.
2. See Table 14–3 for laboratory findings of acute and chronic hemorrhage.
3. Sonogram may be helpful to locate the site of the hemorrhage.

D. General Supportive Management and Specific Therapy

1. See chapter 14–IIID for "general supportive management for the infant with anemia, hemorrhage, and/or shock," 14–XII for "disseminated intravascular coagulation," and other relevant sections.
2. Multiple blood transfusions and prompt surgical repair of lacerations of the liver or spleen may be life-saving.

REFERENCES

Khuri F.J., Alton D.J., Hardy B.E., et al.: Adrenal hemorrhage in neonates: Report of 5 cases and review of the literature. *J. Urol.* 124:684, 1980.

Robinson R.J., Rossiter M.A.: Massive subaponeuretic hemorrhage in babies of African origin. *Arch. Dis. Child.* 43:684, 1968.

Schwartz O., Cohen B.D.: Rupture of the normal spleen in the newborn with survival. *Surgery* 59:1124, 1966.

XI. VITAMIN K DEFICIENCY (HEMORRHAGIC DISEASE OF THE NEWBORN)

Hemorrhagic disease of the newborn occurs during the first days of life and is caused by vitamin K deficiency and characterized by deficiency of factors II (prothrombin), VII, IX, and X.

A. Prevention

Vitamin K is required for the hepatic synthesis of factors II, VII, IX, and X. Administration of vitamin K_1, 1 mg IM, to the healthy term infant prevents a decrease in prothrombin activity and the prolongation of the prothrombin time that are normally observed during the first few days of life, although normal adult values for factors II, VII, IX, and X may not be reached for many weeks. The response to vitamin K_1 in prematures is less predictable.

B. Who Is at Risk?

1. Infants who did not receive vitamin K_1, 1 mg, after delivery
2. Infants with fat malabsorption due to chronic diarrhea, biliary atresia, neonatal hepatitis, cystic fibrosis, or other causes
3. Breast-fed infants
4. Infants receiving antibiotics
5. Infants whose mothers have taken drugs in pregnancy that impair vitamin K activity, e.g., phenobarbital or coumarin
6. Infants receiving parenteral nutrition without adequate vitamin K (200 μg/day or 1 mg/week)

C. Clinical Manifestations

Bleeding is noted most commonly on the second and third day of life.

1. Bleeding from multiple sites (GI tract, umbilical cord, circumcision site, nose, etc.) as well as generalized ecchymosis
2. Prolonged oozing from deep puncture wounds
3. Internal hemorrhage

D. Laboratory Findings

1. Prolonged clotting time
2. Prolonged prothrombin time
3. Decreased factors II, VII, IX, and X

E. Supportive Management

1. See chapter 14–IIID for "general supportive management for the infant with anemia, hemorrhage, and/or shock."
2. Administer fresh blood or fresh frozen plasma if hemorrhage is severe.

F. Specific Therapy

Administer vitamin K_1, 1 to 2 mg IV. In 2 to 4 hours, clotting factors rise.

REFERENCES

Aballi A.J., Banus V.L., deLamerens S., et al.: Coagulation studies in the newborn period: I. Alternation of thromboplastin generation and effects of vitamin K_1 in full term and premature infants. *Am. J. Dis. Child.* 94:589, 1957.

Van Doorm J.M., Hemker H.C.: Vitamin K deficiency in the newborn. *Lancet* 2:708, 1977.

XII. DISSEMINATED INTRAVASCULAR COAGULATION

Disseminated intravascular coagulation (DIC) is an acquired pathologic process characterized by the intravascular deposition of fibrin thrombi and consumption of platelets and plasma clotting factors (Factors I, II, V, VIII, and XIII), which results in inadequate factor levels to maintain hemostasis. Accumulation of fibrin in the microcirculation produces mechanical injury to the RBCs (fragmentation) and microangiopathic anemia.

A. Prevention

1. Close observation of the fetus before and at delivery to prevent compromise of the fetus and infant
2. Prevention or prompt correction of hypothermia, hypoxia, shock, dehydration, acidosis, sepsis, or other conditions

B. Who Is at Risk?

Infants with the following conditions are at risk for disseminated intravascular coagulation:

1. Obstetric complications, e.g., abruptio placentae, preeclampsia, eclampsia, dead-twin fetus, fetal distress, amniotic fluid embolism, or breech delivery
2. Severe hypoxia, hypotension, and acidosis
3. Asphyxia at or after birth
4. Sepsis (bacterial, viral, intrauterine, or postnatal)
5. Necrotizing enterocolitis
6. Severe respiratory distress syndrome or erythroblastosis fetalis
7. Thrombosis (giant hemangioma, renal vein thrombosis)
8. Polycythemia

C. Clinical Manifestations

1. Oozing at puncture sites
2. Petechiae, purpura, ecchymoses
3. Pulmonary or CNS hemorrhage
4. Bleeding from umbilical stump, melena, and/or hematemesis
5. Thrombosis of peripheral or central vessels with tissue necrosis and gangrene

D. Laboratory Findings

1. Hemolytic anemia with fragmented RBCs in the peripheral blood smear
2. Thrombocytopenia
3. Prolonged PT, PTT, and thrombin time
4. Decreased factor V and, occasionally, VIII and I (fibrinogen) levels
5. Elevated levels of fibrin degradation (split) products may be seen.

E. Supportive Management

See chapter 14–IIID for "general supportive management for infants with anemia, hemorrhage, and/or shock."

F. Specific Therapy

1. The best therapy is vigorous treatment/correction of the underlying disease, e.g., prompt treatment of sepsis, correction of hypoxia, or hypotension.
2. Those infants who have laboratory evidence of disseminated intravascular coagulation but no evidence of hemorrhage require no specific therapy unless the coagulation abnormalities are severe, e.g., platelet count less than 25,000/cu mm, fibrinogen less than 100 mg/dl, or PT and PTT more than twice their normal values after vitamin K therapy.
3. For those infants with abnormal laboratory study results and bleeding, therapy should be instituted.
   a. Administer vitamin K_1, 1 to 2 mg IV.
   b. Administer replacement therapy. Give 10 to 15 ml/kg of platelets and 10 to 15 ml/kg of fresh frozen plasma. Dose may be repeated every 8 to 12 hours.
   c. Exchange transfusion may be of value with fresh whole blood every 8 to 12 hours until coagulation becomes normal.
   d. The role of heparin remains controversial. Heparin, 50 units/kg loading dose followed by 10 to 20 units/kg/hour as a continuous infusion to maintain the whole blood clotting time in the range of 20 to 30 minutes, or activated PTT at about 1.5 to 2.0 times the normal for age should be reserved only for those infants who have overwhelming hemorrhage after replacement or exchange transfusion has been administered. The platelet count should be kept greater than 25,000 to 30,000/cu mm during the heparin therapy.
4. Follow laboratory parameters every 6 to 8 hours and replace as required.

REFERENCES

Buchanan G.R.: Neonatal coagulation: Normal physiology and pathophysiology. *Clin. Hematol.* 7:85, 1978.

Hathaway W.E., Bonnar J.: *Perinatal Coagulation.* New York, Grune & Stratton, 1978.

Woods W.G., Corman-Luban N.L., Hilgartner M.W., et al.: Disseminated intravascular coagulation in the newborn. *Am. J. Dis. Child.* 133:44, 1979.

XIII. INHERITED CLOTTING FACTOR DISORDERS

Hemorrhage due to a congenital clotting factor deficiency is rare in the neonatal period despite the fact that maternal clotting factors do not cross the placenta. If excessive bleeding is noted in a healthy fullterm infant after circumcision or from the umbilical stump, a congenital clotting factor deficiency should be considered. The majority of such infants have factor VIII (classic hemophilia) or IX (Christmas disease) deficiency. These two disorders together occur in approximately 1 in 5,000 male births.

A. Who Is at Risk?

1. Infants with a family history of "bleeding problems." Fifty percent to 75% of hemophiliacs have such a family history and almost all are male.
2. Infants with hematomas at injection sites; those with excessive spontaneous bleeding or bruising; those with excessive bleeding after circumcision or from the umbilical stump
3. See Table 14–5 for the mode of inheritance.

B. Clinical Manifestations

1. Spontaneous hemorrhage is rare.
2. Bleeding after circumcision may occur but is rare even with moderate hemophilia (factor VIII or IX over 1% to 2% of normal).
3. Only a few cases of intracranial hemorrhage have been reported.
4. Prolonged oozing from the umbilical stump may occur.

C. Laboratory Findings

See Table 14–4 and Appendix A–14 for coagulation factors.

1. Obtain screening tests.

TABLE 14–5.—Coagulation Factors and Mode of Inheritance

DEFICIENT FACTOR	MODE OF INHERITANCE
Factor V	Autosomal recessive
Factor VII	Autosomal recessive (incomplete)
Factor VIII (classic hemophilia)	X-linked recessive
Factor IX	X-linked recessive
Factor X	Autosomal recessive
Factor XI	Autosomal dominant
Factor XII	Autosomal recessive
Factor XIII	Autosomal recessive
Fletcher factor	Autosomal recessive
Von Willebrand's disease	
Classic	Autosomal dominant
Homozygous	Autosomal recessive
Factor II (prothrombin)	Autosomal recessive
Factor I (afibrinogenemia)	Autosomal recessive
Dysfibrinogenemia	Autosomal recessive or autosomal dominant

TABLE 14–6.—REPLACEMENT THERAPY FOR HEMOSTATIC DEFECTS*

FACTOR	AVAILABLE PREPARATIONS	INCREASE IN PLASMA AFTER 1 UNIT/KG†	50% DISAPPEARANCE TIME††	BIOLOGIC HALF-LIFE	HEMOSTATIC LEVELS, MINOR BLEED	HEMOSTATIC LEVELS, MAJOR BLEED
Fibrinogen	Fresh frozen plasma, cryoprecipitate	1.0–1.5 mg/dl	48 hr	4–6 days	150 mg/dl	200 mg/dl
Prothrombin	Fresh frozen plasma, commercial concentrate	2%		2–4 days	10%	25%
V	Fresh frozen plasma, less than 1 month old	1.5%		15–24 hr	10%	25%
VII	Fresh frozen plasma, commercial concentrate	1%		4–6 hr	5%–10%	10%
VIII	Fresh frozen plasma, cryoprecipitate, commercial concentrate	2%	5–8 hr	12–18 hr	20%–30%	40%–50%
XI	Fresh frozen plasma, commercial concentrate	1.0–1.5%	4–6 hr	30–32 hr	20%–30%	40%–50%
X	Fresh frozen plasma, commercial concentrate	1%	10 hr(?)	2–3 days	10%	15%
XI	Fresh frozen plasma	2%		2–3 days	10%–15%	20%–30%
XIII	Fresh frozen plasma	2%–3%		6 days	2%–3%	2%–3%
Von Willebrand's disease	Fresh frozen plasma, cryoprecipitate					

*From Abildgaard C.F.: Diseases of coagulation: The fluid phase, in Nathan D.G., Oski F.A. (eds.): *Hematology of Infancy and Childhood,* ed. 2. Philadelphia, W.B. Saunders Co., 1981, p. 1199. Used by permission.

†Expressed in 1 mg/kg for fibrinogen.

††Values listed for factors known to have an accelerated initial disappearance rate from the circulation.

TABLE 14–7.—BLOOD PRODUCTS AND OTHER FORMS OF THERAPY FOR COAGULATION DISORDERS*†

	USE	DOSE
Fresh whole blood (<4 hr old)	To replace acute hemorrhage from any cause; hemoglobin and volume deficits; unknown type hemophilia	As required to replace loss
	Exchange transfusion for DIC	
Fresh frozen plasma	Depletion of clotting factors in liver disease, DIC, congenital coagulation factor deficiencies	10–15 ml/kg/8–24 hr
Factor concentrates		Depends on severity of bleeding
Factor VIII cryoprecipitate	Factor VIII deficiency	
Prothrombin complex concentrate	Factor IX deficiency	
Vitamin K_1 oxide (AquaMEPHYTON)	Vitamin K deficiency	0.5–1.0 mg IV
Heparin	DIC	50 units/kg as a loading dose, then 10–20 units/kg/hr as a continuous infusion
Platelets		
Random donor	Thrombocytopenia with bleeding, DIC	1–2 units
Maternal	Isoimmune neonatal thrombocytopenia	1–2 units

*From Buchanan G.R.: *Clin. Haematol* 7:85, 1978. Used by permission.
†DIC, disseminated intravascular coagulation.

a. PTT and thrombin time are prolonged in factor I, II, V, VII, VIII, IX, X, XI (hemophilia C), and XII deficiency.
b. PTT and thrombin time are normal in factor XIII deficiency.
c. PT is normal in factor VIII, IX, XI, and XIII deficiency.
d. PT is prolonged in factor I, II, V, VII, and X deficiency.
e. Platelet counts are normal.
f. Prolonged PT and PTT after vitamin K administration are associated with factor I, V, or X deficiency.

2. If screening tests are abnormal obtain specific coagulation factor assay to determine which factor is deficient.

D. Supportive Management

See chapter 14–IIID for "general supportive management for the infant with anemia, hemorrhage, and/or shock."

E. Specific Therapy

See Table 14–6 for replacement therapy and 14–7 for blood products and other forms of therapy for the management of neonatal coagulation disorders. For mild or moderate bleeding secondary to factor VIII and IX deficiency, local measures with or without fresh plasma are usually adequate. Specific cryoprecipitate of factor VIII or IX is not indicated unless bleeding is severe. Infants with Christmas disease should be treated with 10 ml/kg of fresh frozen plasma for bleeding.

REFERENCES

Buchanan G.R.: Neonatal coagulation: Normal physiology and pathophysiology. *Clin. Hematol.* 7:85, 1978

Johnson C.A., Chung K.S., McGrath K.M., et al.: Characterization of a variant prothrombin in a patient congenitally deficient in factors II, VII, IX and X. *Br. J. Haematol.* 44:461, 1980.

Oski F.A., Naiman J.L.: *Hematologic Problems in the Newborn,* ed. 3. Philadelphia, W.B. Saunders Co., 1982, p. 137.

XIV. HEMORRHAGE DUE TO PLATELET ABNORMALITIES

Hemorrhage caused by a quantitative deficiency in platelet number or a qualitative impairment of platelet function is characterized by generalized and recurrent petechiae and purpura and is often associated with underlying pathology.

A. Who Is at Risk?

1. Infants at risk for thrombocytopenia
   a. Due to megakaryocytic hypoplasia
      1) TAR syndrome (thrombocytopenia, absent radii and ulnae, hand and heart defects)
      2) Fanconi's syndrome (constitutional aplastic anemia, hypoplastic thumb, multiple chromatid breaks)
      3) Isolated thrombocytopenia with megakaryocytic hypoplasia
      4) Congenital leukemia (usually acute myelogenous: ecchymoses and hepatosplenomegaly)
      5) Down's syndrome (possibly with thrombocytopenia, anemia, nodular skin infiltration, and acute granulocytic leukemia)
      6) Congenital Letterer-Siwe disease (systemic histiocytosis)
      7) Wiskott-Aldrich syndrome (thrombocytopenia, eczema, and immune deficiency)
      8) Inborn errors of metabolism (methylmalonic acidemia, ketotic glycinemia, isovaleric acidemia, holocarboxylase synthetase deficiency)
   b. Due to increased peripheral destruction of platelets
      1) Autoimmune thrombocytopenia (antiplatelet antibodies cross the placenta from the mother with idiopathic thrombocytopenic purpura, systemic lupus erythematosus, or hyperthyroidism)
      2) Alloimmune (isoimmune) thrombocytopenia (maternal antiplatelet antibodies cross the placenta and destroy fetal platelets; incidence is 1 to 2 in 10,000 live births)
      3) Maternal drugs (sulfonamides, quinine, quinidine, thiazides, etc.)
      4) Giant hemangioma (Kasabach-Merritt syndrome or disseminated intravascular coagulation)
      5) Platelet consumption (necrotizing enterocolitis, renal vein thrombosis, polycythemia, indwelling vascular catheter thrombi, perinatal aspiration syndrome in association with persistent pulmonary hypertension and chorionic vessel thrombosis)
   c. Due to both decreased production and increased destruction of platelets
      1) Bacterial sepsis or nonbacterial intrauterine infections
      2) Osteopetrosis (obliteration of the bone marrow space with anemia and thrombocytopenia, teardrop erythrocytes and leukocytosis)
2. Infants at risk for platelet dysfunction
   a. Due to maternal drugs that impair platelet aggregation (taken less than a week before delivery)
      Aspirin, promethazine hydrochloride, chlordiazepoxide hydrochloride (Librium), chlorpromazine hydrochloride (Thorazine), prochlorperazine maleate (Compazine), diazepam (Valium), alphaprodine (Nisentil), imipramine hydrochloride (Tofranil), phenothiazines, dextran, ethyl alcohol, glyceryl quaiacolate, and heparin
   b. Due to medications given to the infant
      Indomethacin

c. Due to hereditary thrombasthenia (Glanzmann's disease)
d. Due to severe hyperbilirubinemia with increased free bilirubin and severe acidosis

B. Clinical Manifestations

1. Generalized and recurrent cutaneous petechiae and/or purpura. Large cephalohematoma and bruising on the presenting part are common in infants delivered vaginally. Epistaxis or oozing from the umbilical cord or needle puncture site may be present. Hemorrhagic manifestations may be fulminating with CNS hemorrhage, melena, hematemesis, and hematuria.
2. Hepatosplenomegaly may be present in infection or congenital leukemia.
3. Early jaundice in infection and severe hemolytic disease and jaundice in 2 to 3 days of age in enclosed hemorrhage may be present.

C. Laboratory Findings

1. Thrombocytopenia
   a. Platelet count less than 100,000/cu mm. Capillary platelet count or difficult venipuncture may give falsely reduced platelet count.
   b. Platelet numbers are reduced, sparse, and single in peripheral smear. The presence of a larger number of platelets, particularly clumps of platelets, excludes thrombocytopenia.
   c. Both infant's and mother's platelet count is decreased in idiopathic thrombocytopenic purpura, systemic lupus erythematosus, and maternal drug-induced thrombocytopenia (thiazides). The infant's platelet count is not predictable from the maternal count. The infant's platelet counts continue to fall in the first few days of life then gradually improve and returns to normal within a few weeks to 2 months of age.
   d. In idiopathic thrombocytopenic purpura, a platelet agglutinin in both mother and infant may be demonstrated. The maternal level of platelet-associated IgG (unbound antiplatelet antibody) may predict the presence and severity of neonatal thrombocytopenia.
   e. In thrombocytopenia associated with maternal systemic lupus erythematosus, a transient positive lupus erythematosus factor, anti ANA, and platelet agglutinin may be demonstrated.
   f. In drug-induced thrombocytopenia, a platelet agglutinin in both mother and infant may be demonstrated by complement-fixing technique. Thrombocytopenia is not dose related.
   g. In alloimmune (isoimmune) thrombocytopenia, complement-fixing platelet isoantibody may be demonstrated and thrombocytopenia is more serious than autoimmune thrombocytopenia.
   h. In thrombocytopenia due to megakaryocytic hypoplasia, a bone marrow aspirate will show decreased or small, immature megakaryocytes or decreased cytoplasm.

2. Platelet dysfunction
   Decreased adenosine diphosphate-induced platelet aggregation may be present.

D. Supportive Management

1. See chapter 14–IIID for "general supportive management for the infant with anemia, hemorrhage, and/or shock."
2. If an offending drug is the causative agent, discontinue administration of the drug.

E. Specific Therapy

Transfusion with freshly prepared platelets or stored platelets at 20 to 22° C less than 48 hours may be needed for infants with a platelet count of less than 20,000/cu mm or with a platelet count of less than 50,000/cu mm with acute bleeding. Spontaneous bleeding does not generally occur with a platelet count greater than 20,000 to 30,000/cu mm. One unit of platelet transfusion will increase the platelet count by approximately 50,000/cu mm/5 kg (1 hour after). In the absence of increased platelet destruction, the recipient's platelet count falls by about 10% each day, reaching pretransfusion level in 5 to 7 days.

1. Infants with thrombocytopenia due to megakaryocytic hypoplasia are usually treated with transfusion of a platelet concentrate.
2. Infants with thrombocytopenia due to increased peripheral destruction are usually treated with exchange transfusion and/or corticosteroid therapy (prednisone, 1 to 3 mg/kg/day) for 1 to 2 weeks. Platelet transfusion may be used only for an emergency because of their short survival. Splenectomy is contraindicated. Breast feeding is not contraindicated.
   a. For those infants with autoimmune thrombocytopenia due to maternal idiopathic thrombocytopenic or systemic lupus erythematosus, increased platelet-associated IgG, and a reduced fetal scalp platelet count of less than 50,000/cu mm, maternal corticoid therapy (prednisone, 10 to 20 mg/day for 2 weeks before delivery) and cesarean section may prevent complications, e.g., CNS hemorrhage (controversial).
   b. For those infants with alloimmune thrombocytopenia, transfusion of platelets in utero followed by cesarean section may prevent CNS hemorrhage (controversial). Washed platelet concentrate prepared from the mother's blood should be employed and may be prepared just before delivery if the previous infant was affected.
   c. For those infants with giant hemangiomas, replacement therapy, steroids, and compression with a bandage may hasten involution of the tumor.
   d. For those infants with disseminated intravascular coagulation, correcting the underlying cause is the most important therapeutic measure. Replacement therapy with platelet concentrate plus clotting factors may be of value (see chapter 14–XII).

e. See chapters 17–XVI, 12–V, 11–XIII, and 16–VI, 16–IV, 16–VII for infants with necrotizing enterocolitis, polycythemia, persistent pulmonary hypertension, toxoplasmosis, rubella, and herpes simplex.

REFERENCES

Andrew M., Kelton J.: Neonatal thrombocytopenia. *Clin. Perinatol.* 11:359, 1984.

Corby D.G., Schulman I.: The effects of antenatal drug administration on aggregation of platelets of newborn infants. *J. Pediatr.* 79:307, 1971.

XV. ANEMIA OF PREMATURITY

The Hb concentration in premature infants is affected by erythropoietin, oxygen requirements, dilutional factors associated with weight gain, nutritional factors, and blood drawing (samples). Suppressed bone marrow erythropoiesis with decreased erythropoietin levels and reticulocytes (to 1% by 5 to 7 days), short RBC survival, and increased blood volume as a result of weight gain without any known nutritional deficiency causes physiologic anemia with the lowest Hb of 6.5 to 9.0 gm/dl reached by 8 to 12 weeks of age. Then a gradual increase in the Hb value occurs secondary to increased production. Premature infants develop an earlier and more profound physiologic anemia at a falling rate of Hb approximately 1 gm/dl/week during 2 to 8 weeks of age. The Hb level becomes similar to those of term infants by 5 months of age. Prematures have lower cord Hb at birth, since term Hb levels (16.8 gm/dl) are reached by 32 weeks' gestation in males and 38 weeks in females. Delayed erythropoiesis at lower Hb concentrations is seen in prematures possibly due to a shift to the right in the Hb oxygen dissociation curve and shorter RBC survival.

A. Who Is at Risk?

1. The smaller the infant at birth, the lower the lowest Hb level at approximately 6 to 8 weeks of age. However, small-for-gestational-age infants have a higher Hb concentration than appropriate-for-gestational-age infants at the same gestation.
2. Infants with early cord clamping, blood loss, or Hb destruction (from any cause) may have a more profound physiologic anemia.
3. Infants who received an exchange transfusion or numerous replacement transfusions for a significant blood loss (10% of blood volume) from multiple blood samples start to increase erythropoiesis at a 2 to 3 gm/dl lower Hb value than infants without transfusions because of high adult Hb concentrations and better tissue oxygen delivery.

4. Infants with nutritional deficiency may have an accentuated physiologic anemia.
   a. Iron
      In nonanemic infants, about 75% of iron endowment is present as Hb, and infants with low Hb will have a decreased iron endowment. Infants with low birth weight, low initial Hb, and subsequent blood removal (drawing) develop early iron-deficient anemia that accentuates physiologic anemia. Infants with normal Hb values at birth and infants who are fed milk without supplemental iron will generally deplete their iron reserves by the time they have doubled their birth weight.
   b. Vitamin E
      Newborns, particularly prematures, have low plasma and tissue vitamin E levels and their RBCs are susceptible to hemolysis by peroxide and other oxidative agents (e.g., lipid, iron) since vitamin E inactivates and inhibits lipid peroxides. Vitamin E deficiency is reported to contribute to hemolytic anemia and accentuate physiologic anemia in premature infants, and vitamin E administration ameliorates hemolytic anemia.
      1) The smaller the infant, the greater the degree of vitamin E deficiency. Most premature and very low-birth-weight infants are at increased risk of persistent postnatal vitamin E deficiency possibly due to decreased intestinal absorption of this lipid soluble vitamin.
      2) The higher the polyunsaturated fatty acid intake, the greater the vitamin E requirement. Dietary polyunsaturated fatty acids provide the substrate for peroxidation in the membrane and vitamin E as an antioxidant prevents continued membrane lipid peroxidation.
      3) Iron supplement to vitamin E-deficient infants produces a more severe anemia than no iron supplement because iron inhibits vitamin E absorption and enhances hemolysis.
   c. Folic Acid
      Serum and RBC folate levels are higher in both premature and term infants at birth than in normal adults and drop rapidly after birth in all infants; the fall is more rapid and severe in low-birth-weight infants. The deficiency of folic acid manifests as megaloblastic anemia.
      The following infants are at risk for folate deficiency:
      1) Premature infants
      2) Infants with chronic diarrhea or chronic infections
      3) Infants receiving diphenylhydantoin (Dilantin)
      4) Infants receiving goat's milk
   d. Copper
      The plasma copper levels in prematures are the same as in term infants. However, a microcytic hypochromic anemia due to copper deficiency has been reported in premature infants with inadequate intake, infants with protracted diarrhea, and infants with inadequate supplementation for total parenteral nutrition.

e. Zinc
The following infants are at risk for zinc deficiency:
1) Premature infants
2) Infants who have been on prolonged parenteral nutrition without adequate supplementation

B. Clinical Manifestations

1. The infant may appear pale but otherwise is clinically well.
2. Some infants may have persistent tachycardia (heart rate greater than 160/minute), tachypnea (respiratory rate greater than 50/minute), lethargy, poor weight gain, or easy fatigability with feeding. Occasionally, congestive heart failure secondary to severe anemia may occur.
3. Infants with vitamin E deficiency often have edema of legs and scrotum and rhinorrhea.
4. Infants with folic acid anemia often have chronic diarrhea.
5. Infants with zinc deficiency often are edematous and have acrodermatitis enteropathica.

C. Laboratory Findings

1. After 1 month of age, the lowest Hb concentration is 11.4 $\pm$ 0.9 gm/dl in fullterm infants and 6.5 to 9.0 gm/dl in premature infants when the erythropoiesis is stimulated (see appendix A–10 and A–11). Infants who received exchange transfusion or frequent transfusions have a 2 to 3 gm/dl lower Hb level before the erythropoietic stimulation occurs.
2. The reticulocyte count provides a good measure of bone marrow activity. Decreased reticulocytes are seen in physiologic anemia, exchange transfusion or replacement transfusion, and anemia due to iron, folic acid, and copper deficiency. Reticulocytosis is seen in blood loss and hemolysis (e.g., vitamin E deficiency or the recovery phase of physiologic anemia).
3. The following conditions accentuate physiologic anemia at approximately 4 weeks of age and should be ruled out.
   a. Iron deficiency
   Microcytic hypochromic anemia with decreased reticulocytes, serum ferritin level less than 10 ng/ml, elevated serum transferrin, and decreased saturation of transferrin
   b. Vitamin E deficiency
   Hemolytic anemia (anisocytosis, poikilocytosis, RBC fragmentation) associated with reticulocytosis and thrombocytosis with serum values less than 0.5 mg/dl (normal, 0.3 to 1.7 mg/dl) usually occurs at 4 to 6 weeks of age.
   c. Folic acid deficiency
   Megaloblastic anemia with decreased reticulocytes

d. Copper deficiency
   Microcytic hypochromic anemia with decreased reticulocytes and a serum copper level less than 40 μg/dl
e. Zinc deficiency
   Microcytic hypochromic anemia with plasma zinc levels less than 75 mcg/dl

D. Supportive and Specific Management

1. Physiologic anemia requires no therapy, especially if the infant is feeding well and growing normally.
2. The Hb and hematocrit of all premature infants should be obtained several times in the first week and at least weekly thereafter for the first 3 to 4 months until the Hb level starts to increase.
3. For those infants who are receiving multiple blood drawings for diagnostic purposes, the quantity of blood removed should be recorded. When 10% of the blood volume has been removed in less than 48 hours, it should be replaced.
4. In low-birth-weight infants, if the anemia is extensive and/or accompanied by tachycardia greater than 160/minute and tachypnea greater than 50/minute, lethargy, poor weight gain, easy fatigability with feeding, and central venous oxygen tension less than 25 mm Hg or an "available oxygen" value less than 7 ml/dl at 3 to 8 weeks of age, transfuse the infant with 5 to 10 ml/kg of packed RBCs. The "available oxygen" (ml/dl blood) $= [0.54 + 0.005 \times$ total age in weeks$] \times$ (Hb [gm/dl]). Infants with congenital heart disease or bronchopulmonary dysplasia may require transfusion at higher Hb levels.
5. In all infants whose Hb falls below 13 gm/dl in the first week of life or in excess of 1.0 to 1.5 gm/dl/week or who have unexplained reticulocytosis, further investigation should be instituted to rule out hemolysis or occult blood loss.
6. Infants who do not become symptomatic at 4 to 8 weeks of age are at risk for developing a late anemia at 8 to 12 weeks of age, mostly from nutritional (iron, vitamin E, folic acid, copper, etc.) deficiency.
   a. Iron
      1) For prevention:
         2 mg/kg/day for term infants at 3 to 4 months of age
         2 to 3 mg/kg/day for prematures less than 2,000 gm
         4 mg/kg/day for prematures less than 1,000 gm as early as 2 weeks of age or at the time that their weight is double the birth weight
      2) For therapy: 6 mg/kg/day
   b. Vitamin E
      1) For prevention:
         Formula should contain vitamin E/polyunsaturated fatty acid (PUFA) ratio greater than 0.6 mg vitamin E/gm PUFA
         5 IU/day for term infants
         25 IU/day for premature infants

2) For therapy: 50 to 200 IU/day orally according to the need for 2 weeks

c. Folic acids
   1) For prevention:
      30–50 μg/day for term infants
      65 μg/day for premature infants
   2) For therapy: 50 μg/day

d. Copper
   1) For prevention:
      80 μg/day with oral feeding
      63 μg/kg/day for parenteral nutrition for premature infants
   2) For therapy: 500 μg/day or 2 to 3 mg of 1% copper sulfate solution daily

e. Zinc
   1) For prevention:
      438 μg/kg/day for parenteral nutrition for prematures
   2) For therapy:
      1 mg/kg/day with oral feeding

REFERENCES

Barness L.A.: Nutrition in the tiny baby: Update and problems. *Clin. Perinatol.* 4:377, 1977.

O'Brien R.T., Pearson H.A.: Physiologic anemia of the newborn infant. *J. Pediatr.* 79:132, 1971.

Sabio H.: Anemia in the high risk infant. *Clin. Perinatol.* 11:59, 1984.

XVI. CONGENITAL HYPOPLASTIC ANEMIA

The major congenital hypoplastic anemias are Fanconi's anemia, Diamond-Blackfan syndrome, and Shwachman-Diamond syndrome. Table 14–8 describes clinical findings, laboratory features, and therapy.

TABLE 14–8.—Congenital Failure of RBC Production (Aplastic Anemia)

DISEASE ENTITY	CLINICAL FINDINGS	LABORATORY FEATURES	THERAPY
Fanconi's anemia	Abnormal skin pigmentation, anomalies of the radius, low birth weight, small stature, microcephaly, renal anomalies, thumb abnormalities	Chromosomal abnormalities, reduced stem cells, increased serum and urinary erythropoietin, increased incidence of acute nonlymphocytic leukemia and liver tumors	Bone marrow transplantation
Diamond-Blackfan syndrome (congenital hypoplastic anemia)	Maternal history usually includes previous stillbirths, abortions, abruptio placentae, or hypertensive disease of pregnancy. Infant has nonspecific anomalies: small for gestational age, high arched palate, eye anomalies, short neck, etc.	Normochromic macrocytic anemia, decreased or absent reticulocytes, decreased or absent NRBCs in bone marrow, normal chromosomes, anemia at birth or present by 6 mo. of age, increased serum and urinary erythropoietin levels	Corticosteroids; 60%–80% of patients will respond to this therapy. Transfuse as required.
Shwachman-Diamond syndrome	Exocrine pancreatic insufficiency, skeletal abnormalities, diarrhea, steatorrhea, weight loss, failure to thrive, recurrent infection, delayed skeletal maturation	Absent trypsin and lipase in duodenal aspirate, neutropenia, anemia (50%), thrombocytopenia (70%)	Pancreatic replacement therapy. Treat for infection as required

REFERENCE

Freedman M.H.: Congenital failure of hematopoiesis in the newborn. *Clin. Perinatol.* 11:417, 1984

Chapter 15

Tremors and Convulsions

Clinical manifestations of CNS irritability are variable because the cerebral cortex of the newborn is morphologically and physiologically immature. It is frequently difficult for the pediatric house officer to recognize convulsions in the newborn because manifestations differ from older children and adults. Hypoxic-ischemic encephalopathy, intracranial hemorrhage, intracranial infection, developmental defects, and metabolic disorders account for the largest proportion of infants with tremors and/or convulsions. The house officer must be able to recognize the various types of seizures, delineate the cause, and promptly treat because seizures may indicate significant underlying pathology, interfere with life functions, or cause additional brain injury.

I. CLINICAL EVALUATION

A. Normal Data

Neurologic assessment must be considered in relation to gestational age, sleep state, state of consciousness, degree of illness, time of feeding, and local comfort (temperature, position, etc.) as well as exogenous and endogenous insults, e.g., hypoxia-ischemia, hemorrhage, infection, or developmental defects.

1. Normal level of consciousness
   Evaluate in a quiet, alert state. While infant is in the appropriate flexion state per gestational age (see Figs 6–1 and 6–2), the infant exhibits symmetric, spontaneous, nonstereotyped activity.
2. Normal posture, tone, strength
   See Figures 6–1 and 6–2 for normal values per gestational age. Strength is evaluated in upper extremities, e.g., grasp reflex, and in lower extremities by the infant's ability to support weight per gestational age.
3. Sensation
   Perception of pain is evaluated in response to painful stimuli, such as crying, grimacing, change in respiratory pattern, or level of consciousness.

4. Cranial nerves

   Nerve II: Infant fixes and follows red ball or human face held 10 to 12 inches from infant's face through 60-degree arc.

   Nerve III: Pupils respond to light.

   Nerve III, IV: Infant has conjugate eye movements to the side of cold water injected into the ear canal (cold water test).

   Nerve V: Infant displays positive grimacing movements with pin prick of face (sensory function of V). Infant is able to close mouth adequately (motor function of V).

   Nerve VI: Infant has ability to abduct eye on the observed side.

   Nerve VII: Infant's facies and mouth remain symmetric while infant is crying and eyes are closed.

   Nerve VIII: Must be tested by auditory-evoked potential.

   Nerve IX, X, XII: Effective swallowing occurs.

B. Seizure Types

1. Subtle seizures
   Episodes of horizontal deviation of the eyes, staring, eye-rolling, lip-smacking, "swimming," "rowing," "pedaling," or apneic spells
2. Tonic seizures
   Tonic extension of upper and lower limbs or tonic flexion of upper limbs and extension of lower limbs. Usually seen in premature infants.
3. Multifocal clonic seizures
   Rhythmic jerking at a rate of 1 to 3/second. Movements may migrate from one part of the body to another.
4. Focal clonic seizures
   Localized clonic jerking, usually with the infant awake
5. Myoclonic seizures
   Single or multiple flexion jerks of upper or lower extremities

C. Tremors and Jitteriness

Episodes of tremulousness with occasional clonus may occur without external stimulation and are not accompanied by abnormal ocular movements. The dominant movement, tremors, can usually be stopped by flexion of the affected limb. (Convulsive movements will not be stopped by flexion.) Tremors and jitteriness are not seizures.

II. COMMON CAUSES OF TREMORS OR CONVULSIONS IN THE NEWBORN

A. Hypoxic Insults

Perinatal asphyxia, hypoxic-ischemic encephalopathy

B. Intracranial Hemorrhage

1. Periventricular-intraventricular
2. Subdural
3. Subarachnoid
4. Cortical vein thrombosis

C. Metabolic Aberrations

1. Hypocalcemia
2. Hypoglycemia
3. Hyperglycemia
4. Hypomagnesemia
5. Hyponatremia
6. Hypernatremia
7. Hyperammonemia
8. Pyridoxine deficiency/dependency

D. Drug Withdrawal or Intoxication

1. Drug withdrawal: heroin, methadone, cocaine, or other drugs
2. Fetal alcohol syndrome, alcohol-related birth defects, and neonatal alcohol withdrawal
3. Phenobarbital withdrawal
4. Intoxication with local anesthesia

E. Cerebral Infections

1. Meningitis with or without sepsis (group B β-hemolytic streptococcus, *Escherichia coli,* etc.)
2. Meningoencephalitis (herpes simplex, toxoplasmosis, cytomegalovirus, rubella, coxsackie B, etc.)

F. Developmental Anomalies (see Table 15–2)

1. Disorders of neuronal proliferation
   Macrencephaly, Beckwith-Wiedemann syndrome, achondroplasia, tuberous sclerosis, neurofibromatosis, Sturge-Weber syndrome, Klippel-Trenaunay-Weber syndrome, unilateral macrencephaly
2. Disorders of migration
   Schizencephaly, lissencephaly, pachygyria, polymicrogyria, heterotopia, agenesis of the corpus callosum
3. Disorders of organization
   Mental retardation, trisomy 21, congenital rubella, phenylketonuria, Rubinstein-Taybi syndrome, trisomy 13–15, perinatal insults

4. Disorders of myelination
   Cerebral white matter hypoplasia, Alexander's disease, Canavan's disease, Krabbe's Disease, Pelizaeus-Merzbacher disease, metachromatic leukodystrophy, amino and organic acidopathies, perinatal insults

G. Miscellaneous

1. Kernicterus
2. Inborn errors of metabolism (see Table 15–3)
   Maple syrup urine disease, nonketotic hyperglycinemia, methionine malabsorption, hyper-beta-alaninemia, carnosinemia, congenital hyperammonemia type I and II, argininosuccinic acid synthetase deficiency, argininosuccinase deficiency, pyruvate dehydrogenase deficiency, hereditary fructose intolerance, Von Gierke's disease, galactose-l-phosphate uridyl transferase deficiency, congenital lysine intolerance, propionic acidemia, methylmalonic acidemia, etc.
3. Disease associated with metabolic acidosis in the newborn (chapter 15–V)
4. Congenital hyperthyroidism (neonatal Grave's disease)
5. Adrenal hemorrhage (see Table 14–2)

III. WHAT THE PHYSICIAN SHOULD DO WHEN CONFRONTED WITH AN INFANT WITH TREMORS AND/OR CONVULSIONS

A. Diagnostic Workup

1. Review the perinatal history to determine if fetal distress, meconium-stained amniotic fluid, perinatal asphyxia, birth trauma, or other conditions occurred.
2. Review the maternal history to determine if the mother was diabetic; addicted to heroin, methadone, phenobarbital, alcohol, or other substances; ingested isoniazid (INH) or other vitamin B_6 antagonists, received sodium-free fluids IV; was infected with agents such as herpes simplex or rubella; was on medication for hyperthyroidism, etc.
3. Review the family history to consider inborn errors of metabolism associated with neonatal seizures, e.g., maple syrup urine disease or galactosemia, developmental anomalies, hyperthyroidism (with increased thyroid stimulating immunoglobulins), etc.
4. Examine the infant carefully, considering the physical abnormalities relating to tremors or convulsions. Are there signs of birth trauma, e.g., fracture? Is there a bulging or tense anterior fontanelle? Peculiar facies? Hemangioma over the distribution of first branch of the fifth nerve? Petechiae, vesicles, or other sign of infection? Hepatosplenomegaly? A peculiar smell? Jaundice? What is the state of consciousness? Posture? Tone? Strength? What type of movement is the infant exhibiting?

5. Send a blood specimen to the laboratory to determine the infant's blood sugar, calcium, magnesium, electrolytes, bilirubin, ammonia, arterial blood gases, IgM, serum amino, and organic acids if indicated. In addition, another specimen should be sent for bacterial (and viral) cultures, complete blood count (CBC), and differential and platelet measurements.
6. Perform a spinal tap to determine the presence of meningitis and/or CNS hemorrhage. Note the spinal fluid values (cells, protein, sugar) of the newborn in relation to age (see appendix A–39). Send bacterial and viral cultures.
7. Send a urine specimen for metabolic and drug screen if indicated.
8. Obtain a skull x-ray film for signs of calcification and fracture, chest x-ray film for signs of pneumothorax, long bone x-ray films for signs of intrauterine infection, etc., if indicated.
9. Obtain cranial ultrasonography and/or computerized tomography (CT) scan to identify CNS developmental defects, intracranial hemorrhage, etc.
10. Obtain an EEG.
11. Perform a subdural tap if indicated.

B. General Supportive Management for the Infant With Seizures

1. Handle the infant gently (as always).
2. Place the infant in the supine position with a roll under the shoulders to hyperextend the neck and open the airway.
3. Suction the infant as frequently as necessary.
4. Support cardiorespiratory status. Prevent hypoventilation, hypercapnia, hypoxemia, and apnea. Maintain adequate blood pressure.
5. Maintain the infant's abdominal skin temperature at approximately 36.5° C (97.7° F) and rectal temperature at approximately 37° C (98.6° F). Work within a warmed environment to avoid precipitous drops in body temperature associated with procedures such as inserting a catheter or drawing a blood specimen.
6. Establish an intravascular route for infusions.
7. If a blood glucose level is not immediately available, measure the infant's glucose level by a screening test, e.g., Glucoscan, Dextrostix, or Chemstrip BG.
8. If the infant is seizing and if the blood glucose level is 30 mg/dl or lower in a fullterm infant, 20 mg/dl or lower in a premature or small-for-gestational-age infant during the first 72 hours of life, or less than 40 mg/dl thereafter in a premature or fullterm infant, slowly inject 0.5 to 1.0 gm/kg of glucose in a 10% to 20% dextrose in water solution (not more than 25%) over 10 minutes. Then infuse 6 to 8 mg/kg/minute of glucose. Monitor the serum glucose level every 15 to 30 minutes to ascertain that the level is being maintained. See chapter 15–X for asymptomatic and symptomatic hypoglycemia.
9. If immediate blood calcium determinations are not available, record the in-

fant's ECG and indirectly determine the QT_c or QoT_c (see chapter 15–IX). A prolonged QT_c greater than 0.425 seconds or QoT_c greater than 0.18 seconds in term infants and greater than 0.20 seconds in premature infants is suggestive of hypocalcemia and low ionized calcium except in the presence of hypokalemia. If the QT_c or QoT_c is prolonged, slowly inject 1 to 5 ml/kg of 10% calcium gluconate solution IV. (Be certain the injection is IV and not subcutaneous, as local necrosis and sloughing occur with leaks.) Infants with convulsions secondary to hypocalcemia usually do not respond immediately to injected calcium. There is a lag period of 5 to 10 minutes (see chapter 15–IX for maintenance therapy for the infant with hypocalcemia). Hypomagnesemia should be ruled out when seizures associated with hypocalcemia are persistent.

10. If the trial of glucose and calcium do not result in relief of symptoms, administer pyridoxine hydrochloride, 50 mg IM or IV. Convulsions caused by pyridoxine deficiency or dependency will abate immediately.
11. If tremors and/or convulsions continue, control convulsions with anticonvulsant drugs, as repeated seizures may produce hypoxia, cerebral edema, or damage.
    a. Phenobarbital (IV)
    Administer 15 to 20 mg/kg IV stat as the loading anticonvulsant dose over 5 to 10 minutes. If an IV route is not available, give IM with 10% to 15% greater dose than IV dose. If respiratory depression ensues, place the infant on a ventilator. Then maintain the infant on phenobarbital, 3 to 5 mg/kg/day, in two divided doses to maintain a therapeutic blood level of 20 to 40 mcg/ml.
    b. Phenytoin (Dilantin)
    If the patient continues to exhibit active seizures after 20 mg/kg of phenobarbital, phenytoin may be given IV in a loading dose of 15 to 20 mg/kg. Monitor cardiac rate and rhythm during infusion. The maintenance dose is 4 to 5 mg/kg/day in two divided doses to maintain therapeutic blood level, 15 (10 to 20) mcg/ml.
    c. Diazepam (Valium)
    Administer 0.1 to 1.0 mg/kg IM or IV. When used with barbiturates, diazepam carries an increased risk of circulatory collapse and respiratory failure. This drug is not recommended for use in the newborn with hyperbilirubinemia since benzoate, with which diazepam is preserved, has been reported to compete with bilirubin for albumin-binding sites, predisposing the infant to kernicterus. Diazepam is a poor drug for maintenance as clearance from brain is very rapid.
12. Obtain a pediatric neurology consult.
13. Start antibiotic therapy if meningitis/sepsis is suspected (chapter 16–XIX, 16–XX).
14. Measure intracranial pressure/cerebral blood flow velocity if indicated and if appropriate equipment is available.
15. If cerebral edema is suspected:
    a. Limit fluid intake to 50 ml/kg/24 hours for 72 hours.

b. Dexamethasone, 2 mg/kg/day IV is controversial.

High-dose barbiturates have been shown to reduce cerebral edema due to ischemia.

16. If the infant is hyponatremic or hyperammonemic, has metabolic acidosis, has abnormal serum amino acids, is withdrawing, or has asphyxia, see the appropriate sections of chapter 15.
17. Discuss with the family the meaning of the seizure activity. Remember the underlying disease process, in general, determines the prognosis for seizures. Late-onset hypocalcemic seizures, for example, have a 80% to 100% normal outcome while intracranial infection has a 20% to 65% normal outcome.

    An abnormal EEG in a term infant is associated with an 86% chance of normal development at age 4. A "flat or periodic" or multifocal pattern is associated with a 12% chance of normal development. A "burst suppression" pattern is associated with a grave prognosis. In a preterm infant, EEG is not of prognostic value.

REFERENCES

Freeman J.M.: Neonatal seizures: Diagnosis and management. *J. Pediatr.* 77:701, 1970.

Hill A., Volpe J.J.: Seizures, hypoxic-ischemic brain injury, and intraventricular hemorrhage in the newborn. *Ann. Neurol.* 10:109, 1981.

Rose A.L., Lombroso C.T.: Neonatal seizure states: A study of clinical, pathological, and electroencephalographic features in 137 full-term babies with a long-term follow-up. *Pediatrics* 45:404, 1970.

Volpe J.J.: Neonatal seizures. *Clin. Perinatol.* 4:43, 1977.

IV. PERINATAL ASPHYXIA: HYPOXIC-ISCHEMIC ENCEPHALOPATHY

Hypoxic-ischemic encephalopathy caused by perinatal asphyxia is the most common cause of nonprogressive neurologic defects in older children.

Clinically, hypoxemia, a diminution in the quantity of oxygen, and ischemia, a diminution in the quantity of blood perfusing an area, occur together. Major causes of hypoxemia are (1) perinatal asphyxia, (2) postnatal respiratory insufficiency, and (3) severe right-to-left shunt due to cardiac disease or persistent pulmonary hypertension of the newborn. The major cause of ischemia is cardiovascular collapse due to (1) perinatal asphyxia, (2) postnatal cardiac disease, (3) sepsis or (4) hemorrhage.

Perinatal asphyxia is defined as an impairment in the exchange of oxygen and carbon dioxide. Perinatal asphyxia occurs in utero 90% of the time and post delivery 10% of the time.

Labor, the rhythmic contractions of the uterus, impedes the normal blood supply to the fetus. Animal studies have shown that any insult that causes the oxygen content to fall from a normal of 11 to 12 volume % to less than 4 to 5 volume

% will result in fetal heart rate and pattern changes. With a drop of oxygen content below 3 volume %, changes in CNS blood supply occur, and with a drop below 0.5 to 1.0 volume %, fetal death ensues.

Changes in oxygen supply can result in anoxia, the total cessation of oxygen supply, or hypoxia, a diminution of the oxygen supplied. Animal studies have shown that with 2.5 minutes of anoxia, pH decreases, P_{CO_2} increases, and P_{O_2} and base excess fall. Mean arterial blood pressure declines gradually and bradycardia is marked after 4 minutes. Blood is shunted from the muscles, gut, kidneys, and lungs to the heart, adrenals, brain, and placenta. The EEG shows a rapid reduction in amplitude and frequency and by 2.5 minutes the EEG is isoelectric. CNS glucose declines rapidly, lactate concentrate rises, and CNS phosphocreatine levels decrease markedly. The rise in CO_2 with asphyxia augments CNS blood flow and decreases the CNS metabolic rate. This first phase of asphyxia is termed primary apnea. If the infant is not resuscitated and if anoxia does not abate, the infant will commence rhythmic gasping with continued fall in heart rate and muscle tone. All activity will cease at approximately 12 minutes after the start of anoxia.

If the infant is hypoxic, as opposed to anoxic, the process can continue for considerably longer periods of time. Those infants with anoxia, if resuscitated, usually do not develop seizures. Those with hypoxia usually do seize. Pathologic examination of the CNS of infants with anoxia shows necrosis in the brain stem, thalamus, and spinal cord, while those with hypoxia show edema and necrosis in the basal ganglia, thalamus, and cerebral cortex.

For those infants who suffer asphyxia, multiple changes may occur in other organs due to hypoxia and ischemia, both local and central.

Gastrointestinal (GI) system: ulcers, hemorrhage, necrotizing enterocolitis, glucose and feeding intolerance, and vomiting

Cardiovascular system: cardiomegaly, congestive heart failure, papillary muscle necrosis, patent ductus arteriosus

Renal system: acute cortical necrosis, acute renal tubular necrosis, renal vein thrombosis, syndrome of inappropriate antidiuretic hormone

Pulmonary system: meconium aspiration, respiratory distress syndrome, persistent pulmonary hypertension of the newborn, "shock lung," pulmonary hemorrhage, edema

Hematopoietic system: disseminated intravascular coagulation, leukopenia

Metabolic disturbances: hypoglycemia, hyperkalemia, hypocalcemia, acidosis, hyperglycemia, hyperammonemia

Hepatic system: hepatocellular damage

A. Prevention

1. Prevent intrauterine asphyxia; recognize and carefully follow the "high-risk" mother; and carefully monitor the fetus throughout labor and delivery.
2. Avoid depressant drugs during labor (narcotics, barbiturates, local anesthesia, magnesium, etc.) if at all possible

3. Be prepared to resuscitate infants promptly and efficiently. Support infants with respiratory or cardiac disease or hypotension.
4. Treat seizures promptly.

B. Who Is at Risk?

1. Infants who are asphyxiated
2. Infants who have had a traumatic labor or delivery (only one fourth of the in utero asphyxiated infants are due to traumatic delivery)
3. Infants who develop postnatal asphyxic insults, e.g., severe pulmonary disease, recurrent apneic spells, congenital heart disease, vascular collapse, persistent pulmonary hypertension of the newborn

C. Clinical Manifestations

1. In utero
   Meconium-stained amniotic fluid, abnormal fetal heart rate patterns, low scalp pH, and decreased or increased fetal movements, etc. (see Table 2–2).
2. Postnatal manifestations
   a. Need for endotracheal intubation and assisted ventilation at birth, Apgar score of less than 3 at 1 minute and less than 5 at 5 minutes.
   b. Clinical course of serious intrauterine asphyxia
      1) In the first 12 hours after birth, clinical features include deep coma or stupor, periodic breathing, intact pupillary response, intact ocular motor response, hypotonia, and seizures.
      2) From 12 to 24 hours after birth, there is an apparent increase in the level of alertness. More seizures, apneic spells, jitteriness, and weakness may occur (weakness is more common in the upper limbs in fullterm infants and in the lower limbs in premature infants).
      3) Between 24 and 72 hours after the insult, the infant's level of consciousness deteriorates to stupor or coma. Respiratory arrest may occur. There is loss of responsiveness to cold water test. Premature infants frequently develop intraventricular hemorrhage.
      4) After 72 hours post insult, there may be persistent though diminished stupor. Abnormal suck, swallow, gag, and tongue movements are common. Hypotonia is seen more frequenty than hypertonia. Weakness is seen in the lower limbs in prematures, and hemiparesis and upper limb weakness are seen in fullterm infants.
   c. Feeding difficulties, apnea, seizures, and hypotonia are common.
   d. For the clinical manifestations of other organs previously listed, see the appropriate chapters.

D. Laboratory Findings in Asphyxiated Infants

1. In utero findings (see Table 2–2)
   a. Abnormalities of fetal heart rate patterns; a heart rate below 120 or above

160 beats/minute; loss of beat-to-beat variability, late decelerations, etc.
   b. Fetal blood pH less than 7.2 on two occasions or more
   c. Meconium-stained amniotic fluid
   d. Decreased fetal movements
2. Postnatal abnormalities
   a. Neurologic derangements
      1) Abnormalities in the cerebrospinal fluid (CSF) including increased pressure, increased cell count, high protein, low glucose, and high lactate levels
      2) EEG results
         a) Low amplitude or frequency
         b) Periodic pattern with multifocal or sharp focal activity
         c) Periodic pattern with voltage suppression
         d) Isoelectric pattern
      3) Technetium-99m brain scan may show increased uptake on the delayed image.
      4) CT scan of the brain may show periventricular leukomalacia in the premature infant. In the fullterm infant, periventricular leukomalacia, focal and multifocal ischemic changes, necrosis, and infarction in the distribution of the middle cerebral artery may be seen.
      5) Cortical-evoked stimulation and/or auditory-evoked stimulation may show increase in latency and abnormalities of the response pattern that can be quantified with the degree of asphyxia.
      6) Continuous monitoring of intracranial pressure (Ladd pressure transducer) may reveal brain edema.
   b. Metabolic derangements
      Metabolic acidosis, hypoglycemia, hyperkalemia, hypocalcemia, hyperammonemia, hyperglycemia, hyperinsulinemia, etc.
   c. Renal abnormalities
      1) Acute cortical necrosis: a rise in blood pressure, red and/or white blood cells in the urine, urine osmolarity greater than or equal to 300 mOsm/L, a rise in blood urea nitrogen (BUN) and creatinine, and an increase in the fractional excretion of sodium (see Chapter 18–V)
      2) Syndrome of inappropriate antidiuretic hormone; a rise in antidiuretic hormone, hyponatremia with an increase intravascular volume and an increase in plasma arginine vasopressin (see Chapter 18–XV)
   d. GI abnormalities
      Necrotizing enterocolitis with guaiac-positive stools with ileus pattern or pneumatosis intestinalis on x-ray film
   e. Liver abnormalities
      Abnormal liver function test results with hyperammonemia
   f. Pulmonary abnormalities
      Hypoxemia, acidosis, hypercarbia
   g. Cardiac abnormalities
      ECG evidence of myocardial ischemia or necrosis (ST-, T-wave changes)
   h. Hematologic abnormalities

Abnormal prothrombin time, partial thromboplastin time, fibrinogen, platelets (see chapter 14–XII for disseminated intravascular coagulation)

E. General Supportive Management

1. See chapter 15–IIIB for "general supportive management for the infant with seizures."
2. See appropriate sections for general supportive management for infants with associated problems, e.g., chapters 17–XVI for necrotizing enterocolitis, 11–XXIX for congestive heart failure, 18–IV for acute renal failure, 18–XV for syndrome of inappropriate antidiuretic hormone, 11–XIII for persistent pulmonary hypertension of the newborn, 14–XII for disseminated intravascular coagulation, etc.

F. Prognosis

When the infant with hypoxic-ischemic insult has a normal neurologic examination by 1 week of age, sequelae are minimal. Those who continue to have abnormal neurologic examination by 3 weeks of age are at risk to develop mental retardation, microcephaly, cortical blindness, hydrocephalus and/or cerebral palsy, primarily involving upper extremities in fullterm infants and lower extremities in premature infants.

REFERENCE

Hill A., Volpe J.J.: Seizures, hypoxic-ischemic brain injury and ventricular hemorrhage in the newborn. *Ann. Neurol.* 10:109, 1981.

V. METABOLIC ACIDOSIS IN THE NEWBORN

Metabolic acidosis may be caused by cellular hypoxia, hypothermia, cellular starvation (hypoglycemia), maternal factors, inborn errors of metabolism, renal disease, congenital malformations, and goat's milk ingestion. Specific therapy requires that the cause be identified.

A. Who Is at Risk?

1. Infants who are asphyxiated. The most common cause of metabolic acidosis in the newborn period is asphyxia. Other causes of tissue hypoxia, e.g., cardiac disease, hypovolemia, sepsis, hypotension, are also frequent causes of metabolic acidosis in the newborn.
2. Infants who are cold. Acidosis is due to an increase in lactate and pyruvate. Warmed infants recover from metabolic acidosis in 2 hours.
3. Infants whose mothers developed metabolic acidosis during delivery

TABLE 15–1.—CONDITIONS ASSOCIATED WITH METABOLIC ACIDOSIS IN THE NEWBORN*

CONDITION	CLINICAL FINDINGS	LABORATORY FINDINGS	MANAGEMENT
Asphyxia/shock	Perinatal asphyxia, low Apgar score, poor perfusion, tachypnea	Lactic acidosis	Resuscitate promptly (see chapter 3). Support intravascular volume (chapter 14–IIID).
Hypothermia	Exposure to cold stress, cold to touch	Increased lactate and pyruvate	Warm slowly; acidosis is corrected in approximately 2–3 hr (see chapter 6–IIIB).
Maternal acidosis	Maternal hypotension, hemorrhage, hypoxia	Maternal pH less than 7.25 with base excess less than 15 mEq/L	Expedite delivery and correct maternal acidosis/hemorrhage/ hypoxia.
Congenital adrenal hyperplasia (see Table 17–5)	21-hydroxylase deficiency is most common form (95%); virilization in genetic females; no external genitalia ambiguity in males; dehydration and vomiting are common	Serum: Increased K^+, decreased Na^+, decreased HCO_3^-; decreased serum 17-OH progesterone Urine: Decreased 17-OH corticosteroids and increased 17 ketosteroids and pregnanetriol	Correct dehydration, shock, and hyponatremia; administer cortisol and desoxycorticosterone acetate (DOCA) followed by fludrocortisone acetate (Florinef) or cortisone.
Distal renal tubular acidosis	Failure to thrive, vomiting, poor feeding, polyuria, dehydration; rickets and osteomalacia may occur	Metabolic acidosis; low level of urinary titrable acid excreted; alkalotic urine; Later: decreased concentration ability; nephrocalcinosis and nephrolithiasis	Correct metabolic acidosis with $NaHCO_3$.
Proximal renal tubular acidosis (infantile transient)	Healthy poorly growing premature: decreased ability to handle acid load due to acidifying defect and low tubular bicarbonate threshold	Metabolic acidosis; base excess −7 to −15 mmol/L, usually late onset	Reduce protein intake; condition spontaneously resolves or administer $NaHCO_3$, 5–10 mEq/kg/day, P.O., and follow pH.

Goat's milk acidosis	Administration of goat's milk	Metabolic acidosis	Withhold goat's milk.
Imperforate anus with colonic fistula (colonic reabsorption of chloride) (see chapter 17–VIII)	Acidosis occurs in about 50% of infants with high colonic fistula	Hyperchloremic acidosis; increased bicarbonate excretion into urine	Correct fistula surgically.
Renal failure (see chapter 18–IV)	Edema and/or abrupt weight gain, possibly flank masses, distended bladder or poor urinary output, ascites, seizures	Urine output less than 1 ml/kg/hr, increased BUN, increased creatinine, increased K^+; biochemical abnormality not present until second day of life; abdominal ultrasound may reveal cysts, hydronephrosis, etc.	Restrict fluids, correct metabolic acidosis with $NaHCO_3$, correct prerenal factors: shock, asphyxia, dehydration, etc. (see Chapter 18).
Congenital lactic acidosis	Tachypnea, poor feeding, lethargy, hyponatremia	Decreased pyruvate dehydroginase or decreased pyruvate carboxylase or increased serum lactate, increased pyruvate, and increased alanine	Specific enzyme deficiency must be determined before therapy. Low fat, high carbohydrate frequent feedings.
Transient methemoglobinemia	Cyanosis, lethargy	Chocolate brown blood	Correct acidosis with $NaHCO_3$ (see chapter 12–VI)

REFERENCE

*See Table 15–3 for other conditions with metabolic acidosis.

Barela T.D., Johnson J., Hayek A.: Metabolic acidosis in the newborn period. *Clin. Endocrinol. Metabol.* 12:429, 1983.

4. Infants who develop late metabolic acidosis of prematurity because of a decreased ability to handle an acid load and a low tubular HCO_3^- threshold
5. Infants who drink undiluted goat's milk
6. Infants with imperforate anus and rectourinary fistulas due to hyperchloremic acidosis secondary to urine passage into the colon. Colonic resorption of chloride and excretion of HCO_3^- result in hyperchloremic acidosis.
7. Infants with renal tubular acidosis due to a defect in renal acidification
8. Infants with renal failure (urine output less than 1 ml/kg/hour) due to shock, asphyxia, dehydration, congestive heart failure, or hemorrhage
9. Infants with inborn errors of metabolism (see Table 15–3).

Errors of carbohydrate metabolism	Glucose-6-phosphatase deficiency (Von Gierke's)
	Galactosemia
	Fructose intolerance
	Fructose-1,6-diphosphatase deficiency
Errors of organic and amino acid metabolism	Propionic acidemia
	Methylmalonic acidemia
	Maple syrup urine disease
	Isovaleric acidemia
	n-butyric/n-hexanoic acidemia
	Pyroglutamic acidemia
Errors of urea metabolism	Carbamylphosphate synthetase deficiency
	Arginosuccinase deficiency
Other	Methemoglobinemia
	Congenital lactic acidosis

B. Clinical Manifestations

Clinical features may include poor perfusion, vomiting, failure to thrive, feeding difficulties, apnea, cyanosis, tachypnea, hypotonia, seizures, and lethargy. Less common are dehydration, jaundice, hepatomegaly, and diarrhea. Cataracts may be seen in galactosemia. Infants with maple syrup urine disease may have an erythematous skin rash and maple sugar smell of urine. Profuse sweating is seen in hyperammonemia. Increased hair fragility may be seen in arginosuccinase deficiency.

C. Laboratory Findings

Laboratory findings are related to specific disease entities. Initial workup should include the following:

1. Blood gas to determine the degree of metabolic acidosis and degree of respiratory compensation.
2. Urine analysis. Look for characteristic odors, abnormal urine pH, presence of ketones, and/or amino acids.
3. Blood electrolytes. Determine anion gap, K^+ level, Cl^- level, glucose, BUN, and creatinine.

4. CBC
5. Blood amino acid level, organic acid level, lactate, and pyruvate. See Tables 15–1, 15–2, and 15–3 for laboratory findings in specific disease entities.

D. Supportive Management

Correct metabolic acidosis (see chapter 11–IIIB12).

E. Specific Therapy

Specific therapy depends upon the cause (see Tables 15–1 and 15–3).

REFERENCE

Schade D.S. (ed.): *Clinics in Endocrinology and Metabolism.* Philadelphia, W.B. Saunders Co., 1983.

VI. PERIVENTRICULAR-INTRAVENTRICULAR HEMORRHAGE

Periventricular-intraventricular hemorrhage (PVH-IVH) is the most common type of intracranial hemorrhage (ICH): 80% originate in the subependymal germinal matrix and 75% extend into the ventricular system. The hemorrhage then spreads to the basal cisterns of the posterior fossa where an obliterative arachnoiditis may develop, producing hydrocephalus. A few cases extend into the cerebral parenchyma (intraparenchymal hemorrhage) and subsequently form porencephalic cysts. CT scan has demonstrated a 40% to 50% incidence of ICH in less than 1,500-gm infants.

There is an inverse relationship between incidence and gestational age. The subependymal germinal matrix of the premature is poorly supported. The capillaries receive a disproportionately large blood flow. Any event that increases cerebral blood flow results in overperfusion of the area and PVH-IVH. This can happen with volume expanders, increased systemic blood pressure, impaired CNS autoregulation, elevation of Pa_{CO_2}, asphyxia, or local venous stasis.

A. Prevention

1. Prevent premature birth with the use of tocolytic agents to stop labor where indicated.
2. Use betamethasone antenatally to prevent respiratory distress syndrome and decrease the likelihood of PVH, IVH, and IPH.
3. Support premature infants: maintain neutral thermal temperature, maintain adequate blood gases, avoid pneumothorax, maintain systolic blood pressure, and correct apnea and bradycardia.
4. Do not rapidly infuse blood or hyperosmolar solutions.
5. Avoid physical manipulation of infant as much as possible so as not to raise CNS pressure.

6. The effect of prophylactic administration of phenobarbital, a muscle paralyzer (pancuronium), indomethacin, and ethamsylate is still under study.

B. Who Is at Risk?

1. Premature infants less than 32-weeks' gestation
2. Infants with birth asphyxia, shock, severe pulmonary disease, and persistent hypoxemia or hypercapnia
3. Infants who receive rapid infusion of blood products or hyperosmolar solutions
4. Infants who suffer pneumothorax with associated decreased cardiac output and increased central venous pressure
5. A "cerebral steal" syndrome secondary to a patent ductus arteriosus has been proposed.

C. Clinical Manifestations

Almost all PVH, IVH, IPH occurs in the first week of life, particularly in the first 3 days.

1. There are three basic clinical syndromes.
   a. Catastrophic syndrome
   Quickly occurring catastrophic neurologic deterioration consisting of coma, respiratory abnormalities, tonic seizures, unreactive pupils, and flaccid quadriparesis. There may be a falling hematocrit, bulging anterior fontanelle, lowered blood pressure, bradycardia, metabolic acidosis, and syndrome of inappropriate antidiuretic hormone.
   b. Saltatory syndrome
   A subtle deterioration characterized by hypotonia, lethargy, vertical drift of eyes with incomplete horizonal movements to an oculocephalic maneuver, and respiratory disturbances.
   c. "Silent" hemorrhage
   Clinically undetected PVH, IVH, IPH. The most common nonspecific symptoms are a fall in hematocrit, hypotonia, poor visual tracking, and activity.
2. Head circumference may increase if hydrocephalus develops.

D. Laboratory Findings

1. Xanthochromic CSF with increased crenated red blood cells, protein, and leukocytes
2. Decreased hematocrit/hemoglobin and platelet count
3. Hyperbilirubinemia
4. Metabolic acidosis
5. Scanning
   a. Ultrasound scanning
   Ultrasound real-time scanning through the anterior fontanelle has become the imaging technique of choice for the initial examination of the newborn.

This technique demonstrates hemorrhage, alterations in periventricular structure, and ventricular size. The instrument's portability is the major advantage. A scan in the first, third, and seventh day of life is preferable since almost all (90%) PVH, IVH, IPH occurs during the first week of life (40%–50% on day 1).

b. CT scanning
CT scan delineates the site and extent of the lesion, the size of the ventricles, and the presence of white matter involvement. The major disadvantage of CT is that the neonate must be transported to the scanner site.

c. Classification of intracranial hemorrhage by ultrasound or CT scanning (based on Papile et al.)
Grade I: PVH or subependymal hemorrhage (SEH); 25% of ICH; hemorrhage limited to ventricular wall with no evidence of intraventricular or parenchymal extension
Grade II: intraventricular hemorrhage without dilatation of the ventricles
Grade III: intraventricular hemorrhage plus dilatation of the ventricles with blood (rather than CSF)
Grade IV: IPH; 25% of ICH; extension of the hemorrhage into the periventricular white matter

6. Evidence of hydrocephalus usually occurs by scan at approximately 2 weeks after hemorrhage and prior to clinical manifestations of hydrocephalus but may occur as early as the time of hemorrhage.

E. Supportive Management

1. Avoid cerebral hyperperfusion by judicious use of bicarbonate to correct acidosis and the careful use of respiratory support measures to correct hypercapnia and hypoxia.
2. Maintain cerebral perfusion by maintaining systolic blood pressure. Transfusion of packed red blood cells followed by plasma should be given slowly. Rapid transfusion may increase cerebral blood pressure and extend the hemorrhage.
3. Reduce increased intracranial pressure in the acute stage by external ventricular drainage or lumbar puncture after determining the ventricular size by scanning (controversial).
4. See chapter 15–IIIB for "general supportive management for the infant with seizures."
5. See chapter 14–IIID for "general supportive management for the infant with anemia, hemorrhage, and/or shock."
6. See chapter 13–IIIC for "general supportive management for the infant with indirect hyperbilirubinemia."

F. Specific Therapy

1. Specific therapy for PVH, IVH, and IPH is not known.
2. Surgery for hydrocephalus may be required.

a. Monitor ventricular size by serial ultrasound or CT scanning. Measure head circumference daily.
b. If ventricular enlargement progresses:
   1) Serial lumbar puncture may be performed for prevention or treatment of posthemorrhagic hydrocephalus (controversial)
   2) Medical therapy with acetazolamide (100 mg/kg/day) and furosemide (1 mg/kg/day) has been reported to be beneficial, but not for infants with rapidly progressing hydrocephalus.
   3) Intervention with a ventriculoperitoneal shunt may be indicated.
   4) Drainage by external ventriculostomy has been used for infants with rapidly progressing hydrocephalus who are too small to receive a shunt.

G. Prognosis

The major anatomic sequelae of intracranial hemorrhage are subependymal cysts, porencephaly, and hydrocephalus (5% in grade I, 25% in grade II, 55% in grade III, and 80% in grade IV). The majority of subependymal cysts resolve completely without clinical residua; almost all parenchymal hemorrhages result in porencephaly. Posthemorrhagic hydrocephalus may return to normal ventricular size a few weeks after ventricular dilation. One quarter to one third of infants with hydrocephalus require a shunt. Newborns with PVH or IVH without hydrocephalus (grade I or II intracranial hemorrhage) usually have normal development. Grade IV intracranial hemorrhage has approximately a 50% mortality and a markedly increased risk of neurologic impairment at follow-up. In individual cases, however, there is no way to determine what the severity of neurologic deficit will be as related to the severity of periventricular hemorrhage.

REFERENCES

Allan W.C., Volpe J.J.: Pericentricular-intraventricular hemorrhage. *Pediatr. Clin. N. Am.* 33:47, 1986.

Dubowitz L.M.S., Dubowitz V., Palmer P.G., et al.: Correlation of neurologic assessment in the preterm newborn infant with outcome at 1 year. *J. Pediatr.* 105:452, 1984.

Papile L.A., Burstein J., Burstin K., et al.: Incidence and evolution of subependymal and intraventricular hemorrhage: A study of infants with birth weights less than 1,500 gm. *J. Pediatr.* 92:529, 1978.

Shankaran S., Slovis T.L., Bedard M.P., et al.: Sonographic classification of intracranial hemorrhage: A prognostic indicator of mortality, morbidity, and short-term neurologic outcome. *J. Pediatr.* 100:469, 1982.

Tarby T.J., Volpe J.J.: Intraventricular hemorrhage in the premature infant. *Pediatr. Clin. N. Am.* 29:1077, 1982.

Volpe J.J.: Neonatal intracranial hemorrhage. *Clin. Perinatol.* 4:77, 1977.

VII. SUBDURAL HEMORRHAGE

Subdural hemorrhage occurs primarily in fullterm infants who have suffered unusual stresses or trauma during labor and delivery. Bleeding sites include the straight sinus, vein of Galen, inferior sagittal sinus, superficial cerebral veins, lateral sinus, infratentorial veins, and occipital sinus.

A. Who Is at Risk?

1. Infants of mothers who are primiparous, who are of advanced age and multiparous, or who exhibit cephalopelvic disproportion
2. Infants born to women whose labor was precipitous or long
3. Infants who presented as breech, foot, or face presentation or who were born by difficult forceps extraction or rotation
4. Infants with large heads

B. Clinical Manifestations

1. Lacerations
   a. Tentorial lacerations: signs include stupor, coma, abnormal doll's head maneuver, unequal pupils
   b. Infratentorial lacerations: signs include nuchal rigidity, opisthotonus, respiratory arrest
2. Falx tears: bilateral cerebral signs
3. Subdural hemorrhage over the cerebral convexities: no clinical signs or focal seizures, hemiparesis, homolateral pupillary abnormality, or signs of a chronic subdural at a later date, i.e., enlarging head and failure to thrive

C. Laboratory Findings

1. CT scan or sonography will demonstrate the pathologic collection of blood.
2. A falling hematocrit and blood pressure may occur.

D. General Supportive Management

1. See chapter 15–IIIB for "general supportive management for the infant with seizures."
2. See chapter 14–IIID for "general supportive management for the infant with anemia, hemorrhage, and/or shock."

E. Specific Therapy

1. Lacerations of the tentorium and falx: rapid surgical correction
2. Acute convexity subdural: repeated subdural taps when the head is growing rapidly or surgical therapy

F. Prognosis

1. Lacerations of the tentorium and falx: nearly all die; the survivors develop hydrocephalus.
2. Convexity subdural hemorrhage: 50% to 80% are well on follow-up; the rest have hydrocephalus or focal neurologic signs.

REFERENCES

Abrams I.F., McLennan J.E., Mandell F.: Acute neonatal subdural hematoma following breech delivery. *Am. J. Dis. Child.* 131:192, 1977.

Rabe E.F., Flynn R.E., Dodge P.R.: Subdural collections of fluid in infants and children: Study of 62 patients with special reference to factors influencing prognosis and efficacy of various forms of therapy. *Neurology* 18:559, 1968.

Volpe J.J.: Neonatal intracranial hemorrhage: Pathophysiology, neuropathology and clinical features. *Clin. Perinatol.* 4:77, 1977.

VIII. SUBARACHNOID HEMORRHAGE

Hemorrhage within the subarachnoid space is a common type of neonatal intracranial hemorrhage and is usually venous in origin. It may be secondary to IVH, subdural hemorrhage, and/or intracerebellar hemorrhage.

A. Who Is at Risk?

1. Premature infants with hypoxic insults. This group comprises 75% of all infants with subarachnoid hemorrhage (secondary type).
2. Fullterm infants born with a traumatic delivery (primary type)

B. Clinical Manifestations

1. Hemorrhage, which may be silent
2. Seizures, especially in fullterm infants
3. Massive hemorrhage with a rapidly fatal course in infants with severe hypoxia and a traumatic delivery

C. Laboratory Findings

1. CT scan demonstrates blood in the subarachnoid space
2. Falling hematocrit and blood pressure
3. Blood in the subarachnoid space that can be documented by lumbar puncture

D. Supportive Management

1. See chapter 15–IIIB for "general supportive management for the infant with seizures."
2. See chapter 14–IIID for "general supportive management for the infant with anemia, hemorrhage, and/or shock."

E. Specific Therapy

No specific therapy exists.

F. Prognosis

In general, the prognosis is good for primary subarachnoid hemorrhage. Those with seizures have a 90% normal outcome on follow-up. A few develop posthemorrhagic hydocephalus.

REFERENCE

Volpe J.J.: Neonatal intracranial hemorrhage: Pathophysiology, neuropathology and clinical features. *Clin. Perinatol.* 4:77, 1977.

IX. HYPOCALCEMIA

Calcium is associated with a multiplicity of functions including muscle contraction, nerve impulse transmission, blood coagulation, enzymatic reactions, protein synthesis, bone structure, capillary permeability, and antibody-antigen reactions. Ionized calcium is the physiologically active fraction and should theoretically be determined, but current calcium-specific electrode systems are not generally in use. Deficiency of calcium can result in multiple abnormalities, especially those of neuromuscular transmission. Total serum calcium levels below 6.5 mg/dl in premature infants and 7.0 mg/dl in fullterm infants are considered hypocalcemia.

A. Prevention

1. Ensure adequate calcium and vitamin D intake in pregnant women.
2. Do not administer high-phosphate milk formulas to infants.
3. Systematically screen (preferable at 12 and 24 hours of age) infants at risk.
4. Ensure adequate calcium intake in the newborn.

B. Who Is at Risk?

1. Preterm infants: 30% to 35% develop hypocalcemia. The lower the birth weight of premature infants, the lower the plasma calcium tends to be and the more widely it fluctuates. Preterm infants exhibit impaired hydroxylation of vitamin D to 25 hydroxycholecalciferol (HCC) in the liver, poor calcium stores, and low postnatal calcium intake.
2. Asphyxiated infants: 30% of asphyxiated infants have hypocalcemia. Surprisingly, this may be associated with high parathyroid hormone. Calcitonin levels are elevated.
3. Infants who experienced a sudden rise in pH as a result of bicarbonate therapy.
4. Small-for-gestational-age infants with placental insufficiency whose mothers have hypertensive disease of pregnancy, postmature infants, etc.
5. Infants of diabetic mothers: 50% of infants of diabetics have hypocalcemia.
6. Infants whose mothers have osteomalacia.

7. Infants with transient hypofunction of the parathyroid gland. (Their mothers may have a parathyroid adenoma.) Hypocalcemia in this group usually occurs on the first day of life. Inherited hypoparathyroidism, an autosomal dominant disease (sometimes reported as sex linked), has also been described to cause hypocalcemia.
8. Infants with insufficient elemental calcium intake (less than 20 to 40 mg/kg/24 hours), e.g., those infants on long-term IV fluid therapy or prematures receiving breast milk.
9. Infants receiving lipid infusions. Free fatty acid elevations of 5 mM/L decrease ionized calcium by 0.6 mg/dl.
10. Infants fed high-phosphate milk formulas. Infants who develop hypocalcemia fed high-phosphate milk formulas have been shown to have maternal vitamin D deficiency, transient parathyroid insufficiency, and renal immaturity.
11. Infants who receive exchange transfusions with acid dextrose citrate blood and whose calcium is bound to citrate
12. Infants with DiGeorge's syndrome (absence of the parathyroid gland and thymus, intractable diarrhea, failure to thrive, lymphopenia, and immunologic deficiency)

C. Clinical Manifestations

Clinical manifestations include irritability, high-pitched cry, tremors, twitching, seizures, apnea, cyanosis, hypotonia, hypertonia, and vomiting. Early hypocalcemia in the first 3 days of life usually occurs in prematures, infants of diabetics, and asphyxiated infants. Late hypocalcemia in the fifth to the eight day of life usually occurs in large fullterm infants who are fed high-phosphate formulas and/or whose mothers are calcium or vitamin D malnourished and often is associated with hypomagnesemia and hyperphosphatemia.

D. Radiologic Features

Delayed skeletal mineralization occurs with relative frequency in very low-birth-weight infants since calcium intake and retention are much lower in extrauterine than intrauterine life. Overt rickets can also occur, but occurrence is less frequent.

E. Laboratory Findings

1. Specific findings
   A total serum calcium <6.5 to 7.0 mg/dl or ionized calcium less than 3.0 to 4.0 mg/dl. (The abnormal range varies slightly depending on studies.)
2. Prolonged QT_c interval greater than 0.425 seconds or QoT_c interval greater than 0.18 seconds for term infants and greater than 0.20 seconds for prematures. $Qtc = QT/\sqrt{RR}$ and $QoTc = QoT/\sqrt{RR}$ (QT = beginning of Q to end of T and QoT = beginning of Q to beginning of T). See chapter 19–VII.

3. Associated findings
   a. Hyperphosphatemia, especially with infants fed high phosphate loads
   b. Hypomagnesemia
   c. Parathyroid hormone insufficiency
   d. Elevated calcitonin
   e. Maternal vitamin D deficiency

F. Supportive Management

See chapter 15–IIIB for "general supportive management for the infant with seizures."

G. Specific Therapy

1. Immediate therapy
   Slowly administer 10% calcium gluconate, 100 to 500 mg/kg IV, over a 5-minute time period. Monitor the infant's cardiac rate carefully during the infusion as severe bradycardia can occur requiring curtailment of the infusion. Care must be taken not to inject subcutaneously as a subcutaneous injection can cause local necrosis. Admixtures with bicarbonate or phosphate should not be used because precipitation will occur.
2. Maintenance therapy
   a. Administer 10% calcium gluconate or lactate, 100 to 200 mg/kg, 4 times a day, at first IV and later orally. Calcium chloride is not recommended, despite a high percentage of elemental calcium, because of the complications of acidosis and necrosis and calcification of the gastric mucosa. Therapy should be maintained for at least 5 to 7 days. Recheck the serum calcium level before and after discontinuing therapy.
   b. Oral calcium supplements can be administered as 75 to 80 mg/kg/day of elemental calcium divided throughout the 24-hour period. Calcium lactate causes less GI irritability than calcium gluconate or Neo-Calglucon. The high sugar content and osmolality of Neo-Calglucon is not desirable. Some neonatologists do not use oral calcium because of complications.
   c. Feed fullterm breast milk or a formula with a low phosphorus load, e.g., PM 60/40, Enfamil Premature Formula, or Similac Special Care Formula.
3. When concurrent hypomagnesemia occurs, administer 50% magnesium sulfate (4.06 mEq/ml), IM, 0.1–0.2 ml/kg/dose.
4. For those infants who develop poor bone mineralization and/or rickets, administer vitamin D, 2,000 to 4,000 IU/day, feed formulas with a low phosphorus load, and ensure adequate calcium and phosphorus intake.

H. Prognosis

There are no carefully controlled studies demonstrating neurologic or other longterm sequelae of asymptomatic hypocalcemia.

Fifty percent of those infants with early onset hypocalcemic seizures have normal development. Of those infants with late onset hypocalcemic seizures, 80% to 100% have normal development.

REFERENCES

Forfar J.O.: Normal and abnormal calcium, phosphorus and magnesium metabolism in the perinatal period. *Clin. Endocrinol. Metabol.* 5:123, 1976.

Tsang R.C., Steichen J.J., Brown D.R.: Perinatal calcium homeostasis: Neonatal hypocalcemia and bone demineralization. *Clin. Perinatol.* 4:385, 1977.

X. HYPOGLYCEMIA

Glucose, the major substrate for brain oxidative metabolism, is extracted constantly at a given rate per unit of time. Failure of the metabolic processes to meet the infant's glucose requirement results in hypoglycemia and may result in neurologic sequelae when the infant is symptomatic. The incidence of hypoglycemia is 4 in 1,000 live births but higher in low-birth-weight infants and infants of diabetic mothers. Hypoglycemia is defined as follows:

In premature infants,

If the blood glucose value is

less than 20 mg/dl (< 25 mg/dl for serum glucose) during the first 72 hours of life, or

less than 40 mg/dl (< 45 mg/dl for serum glucose) after the first 72 hours of life

In fullterm infants,

If the blood glucose value is

less than 30 mg/dl (< 35 mg/dl for serum glucose) during the first 72 hours of life, or

less than 40 mg/dl (< 45 mg/dl for serum glucose) after the first 72 hours of life

Although the levels of blood glucose used to define hypoglycemia in preterm low-birth-weight and fullterm infants are substantially lower, there is general consensus that blood glucose levels should not be allowed to fall below 40 mg/dl of whole blood.

A. Prevention

1. Carefully monitor pregnant diabetics and keep their blood sugar levels within normal range. This will lessen the incidence of hyperinsulinemia and hypoglycemia in infants of diabetics.
2. Monitor the blood sugar levels of high-risk infants, e.g., low-birth-weight (small-for-gestational-age and premature) infants, infants of diabetics, and

other high-risk infants, until the glucose is stable (see specific therapy and management sections for time of monitoring).

3. Avoid hypothermia, hypoxia, perinatal stress, or other adverse conditions.
4. Supply adequate glucose to all infants (6 to 8 mg/kg/minute of glucose). Many infants require higher intake of glucose. Monitor at-risk infants frequently to be certain glucose demands are being met.

B. Who Is at Risk?

Infants with the following backgrounds are at risk to develop hypoglycemia:

1. Infants of diabetic mothers, especially during the first 6 hours of life, at about 18 hours of age, and again at 24 hours of age
2. The small-for-gestational age, dysmature infant, e.g., infants born to mothers with placental dysfunction, as early as 2 hours, and as late as 7 days of life
3. Infants with various perinatal illnesses such as asphyxia, perinatal distress, respiratory distress, hypothermia, erythroblastosis fetalis, infection, CNS hemorrhage or infection, adrenal hemorrhage, liver disease, leucine sensitivity, glycogen storage disease, galactose or fructose intolerance, islet cell adenoma, infant giantism, or congenital anterior midline defect
4. Infants of low birth weight: discordant twins, premature infants
5. Infants with a family history of neonatal hypoglycemia or unexplained infant death, or maternal history of prolonged β-adrenergic drugs.
6. Appropriate- or large-for-gestational-age infants with omphalocele, macroglossia, and giantism (Beckwith-Wiedemann syndrome) (see Table 9–4)

C. Clinical Manifestations

The infant may be asymptomatic. Symptomatic infants may have jitteriness, irritability, change in muscle tone, eye-rolling, convulsions, apnea, cyanosis, irregular respirations, tachypnea, high-pitched weak cry, poor feeding, hypotonia, lethargy, sweating, or hypothermia. Symptomatic episodes may be transient.

D. Laboratory Findings

1. Specific findings
   Low blood glucose levels with or without elevated insulin levels (greater than 12 units/ml)
2. Nonspecific associated findings
   a. Positive blood cultures or other laboratory findings of sepsis
   b. Laboratory findings of Rh incompatibility
   c. Laboratory findings of congestive heart failure
   d. High cord levels of C-peptide, maternal elevated hemoglobin A_{Ic}
   e. Hypocalcemia, hypomagnesemia, polycythemia, hyperbilirubinemia, and hyperviscosity may be associated.

E. Supportive Management

1. See chapter 15–IIIB for "general supportive management for the infant with seizures."
2. See chapter 11–IIIB for "general supportive management of the infant with respiratory distress."

F. Specific Therapy and Management

1. Screen infants at risk utilizing a glucose screening test (e.g., Glucoscan, Dextrostix or Chemstrip BG) every hour until 7 hours of age, then every 4 hours until 24 hours of age. An IV infusion of glucose, 6 to 8 mg/kg/minute, should be started if necessary to restore the glucose values to normal.
2. A blood sample should be obtained for glucose analysis while starting the IV.
3. If the blood glucose is low or if seizures ensue, administer 0.5 to 1.0 gm/kg of glucose in a 10% to 20% glucose solution over a 10-minute time interval. In the treatment of asymptomatic hypoglycemia, this is controversial. Some physicians feel this "push" will precipitate reactive hypoglycemia.
4. After the initial slow push of glucose, or as the initial therapy, infuse 6 to 8 mg/kg/minute of glucose. Monitor blood glucose levels every 15 to 30 minutes to ascertain that the blood glucose level is being maintained. Increase the rate of glucose infusion if necessary to keep the infant's blood glucose level normal.

   For example, to calculate glucose requirements for a 1-kg infant:

   1 kg $\times$ 6 mg/min = 6 mg/minute (360 mg/hour or 8,640 mg/24 hours)

   Note: A 10% glucose solution has 10 gm/100 ml, 10,000 mg/100 ml, or 100 mg/1 ml. Therefore, give 3.6 ml/hour of a 10% glucose solution to meet the maintenance requirements of 360 mg of glucose/hour.
5. Infants of diabetics often require 10 to 12 mg/kg/minute of glucose or greater quantities. Raise the percent of glucose from 10% to 15% as required. (Do not infuse glucose greater than 15% into the liver or into a peripheral vein; use a central vein or the umbilical artery.) Blood glucose should be monitored every 4 to 6 hours until normal glycemia persists.
6. Glucagon, 300 μg/kg, may be helpful in infants with good glycogen stores to raise the blood glucose while the glucose infusion is being started.
7. If symptoms persist after correction of hypoglycemia, search for an underlying pathological process (e.g., CNS disease, sepsis, congenital heart disease, asphyxia, adrenal hemorrhage, or administration of β-adrenergic drugs to the mother).
8. As a diagnostic test, administer glucagon, 30 μg/kg IV, IM, or SQ. Draw a baseline blood glucose level and a blood glucose level at 0.5, 1, and 2 hours postinjection. A rise of greater than 40 mg glucose/dl is normal.

a. At the same time, draw a baseline insulin level. If the hyperglycemic response exceeds 40 mg glucose/dl, the infant is large, and the plasma insulin is elevated (greater than 12 units/ml), hyperinsulinemia is the most likely diagnosis.
b. If the rise of glucose as a response to glucagon is less than 40 mg/dl, consider metabolic disorders or low glycogen stores in small-for-gestational-age infants.
c. If the response to glucagon is less than 40 mg glucose/dl in an appropriate- or large-for-gestational-age male infant with microcephaly, a midline deficit, jaundice, low thyroxine, low growth hormone, and resistant hypoglycemia, consider congenital hypopituitarism.
e. Obtain blood gases, bilirubin, uric acid levels, and urine analysis for reducing substance and ketones to consider the diagnoses of carbohydrate and amino acid abnormalities such as glycogen storage disease (see Table 16–5) and tyrosinemia, maple syrup urine disease, etc. (see Table 15–3).

9. If hypoglycemia persists, facilitate gluconeogenesis; glucocorticoids can be started. Give prednisone, 2 mg/kg/day orally, or hydrocortisone, 5 mg/kg/day, IM.
10. The infant should be weaned slowly from a hypertonic glucose infusion by lowering the concentration of glucose in the infusion slowly and starting oral fluids.
11. Withdraw steroids slowly if the infant has been on steroids more than 1 to 2 days.
12. Epinephrine, diazoxide, and growth hormone are only necessary in exceedingly rare instances.

G. Prognosis

The sequelae of asymptomatic hypoglycemia is controversial. A longterm prospective follow-up of symptomatic hypoglycemia in neonates showed that devastating neurologic consequences (CNS damage and/or abnormal ophthalmic examination) do not result from brief periods, up to 12 hours, of untreated hypoglycemia, but result from prolonged hypoglycemia with seizures in over 50% of infants.

REFERENCES

Cornblath M.: Hypoglycemia in infancy and childhood. *Pediatr. Ann.* 10:356, 1981.

Cowett R.M., Oh W., Pollak A., et al.: Glucose disposal of low birth weight infants: Steady state hyperglycemia produced by constant IV glucose infusion. *Pediatrics* 63:389, 1979.

Miranda L.E., Dweck H.S.: Perinatal glucose homeostasis: The unique character of hyperglycemia and hypoglycemia in infants of very low birthweight. *Clin. Perinatol.* 4:351, 1977.

XI. THE INFANT OF A DIABETIC MOTHER

Infants of diabetic mothers (IDMs) have greater mortality and morbidity than infants of age-matched, non-diabetic women. Perinatal mortality is directly related to the severity of maternal diabetes.

CLASS (MODIFIED WHITE'S CLASSIFICATION)	PERINATAL MORBIDITY AND MORTALITY
Gestational diabetes: glucose intolerance diagnosed during pregnancy that is controlled by diet alone, occasionally by insulin	Macrosomia and associated complications. Perinatal mortality: 4.8% uncontrolled
A. Chemical diabetes managed by diet and/or insulin	Macrosomia and associated complications
B. Insulin therapy Onset: age greater than or equal to 20 years or duration: less than 10 years	Macrosomia and associated complications Perinatal mortality: 10.4% uncontrolled
C. Onset: age 10 to 20 years or duration: 10 to 20 years	Same as A Perinatal mortality: 25% uncontrolled
D. Onset: Age less than 10 years or duration: greater than 20 years or chronic hypertension or benign retinopathy	Fetal macrosomia or intraurterine growth retardation. Perinatal mortality: 18.0% uncontrolled
F. Diabetic nephropathy with proteinuria greater than 500 mg/dl	Intrauterine growth retardation Perinatal mortality: 15% under optimal conditions, 47.8% uncontrolled
R. Malignant proliferative retinopathy	Severe intrauterine growth retardation. Perinatal mortality is high (50%)
H. Coronary artery disease	Grave fetal and maternal risk
T. Prior renal transplantation	

A. Prevention

1. Best neonatal results are obtained when meticulous obstetric medical care is rendered to the mother during pregnancy and maternal diabetes is well controlled with fasting blood glucose less than or equal to 100 mg/dl or 2-hour postprandial value less than 140 mg/dl or sequential hemoglobin A_{1C} 5% to 10%. HbA_{1C} correlates with mean daily glucose over a few weeks' duration. The better the maternal control, the less the incidence of neonatal complications (e.g., hypoglycemia, large for gestational age, or mortality; 24% perinatal mortality with average fasting glucose greater than 150 mg/dl, 12% with average glucose 100 to 150 mg/dl, and 3.8% with an average less than 100 mg/dl). Maternal hypoglycemia is common in early pregnancy and hyperglycemia and ketoacidosis may develop during the second and third trimester.
2. Obtain a baseline blood sugar level or a screening test on admission to the nursery and every hour until the infant is 7 hours of age, then every 4 hours during the first 24 hours of life. The higher the maternal glucose, the faster the glucose disappearance and the lower the plasma glucose level will be. Institute early oral feedings with formula. If oral feedings are not tolerated, administer IV glucose.

B. Who Is at Risk?

Infants born to diabetic mothers who are poorly controlled with elevated hemoglobin A_{1C} are at risk. Elevated hemoglobin A_{1C} reflects hyperglycemia over the previous 4 to 6 weeks.

C. Clinical Manifestations

Common problems seen in IDMs are as follows:

1. Inappropriateness of size
   Infants born to poorly controlled diabetics appear large for gestational age, obese, macrosomic, puffy, and plethoric. They have increased hemoglobin levels and a "tomato red" color. Infants whose mothers are in good control are appropriate for gestational age, while those whose mothers are class D, R, F, etc., are small for gestational age.
2. Macrosomia, asphyxia, and birth injury
   Macrosomia is associated with difficult vaginal delivery, shoulder dystocia, and brachial plexus injury. Diaphragmatic (phrenic nerve palsy) paralysis may occur. Difficulties in the intrapartum period and/or delivery may result in asphyxia with multiple organ system involvement. (see Table 5–3 and chapter 15–IV)
3. Congenital malformations in IDMs
   The incidence of congenital anomalies increases with increasing duration and severity of maternal diabetes. Approximately 10% of IDMs have major congenital anomalies; malformations account for 50% of perinatal mortality in IDMs. Strict normoglycemic control of the pregnant diabetic does not lessen the congenital malformation rate, possibly due to postconceptional or preconceptional hyperglycemia, fetal hyperinsulinemia, uteroplacental vascular disease, or genetic predisposition. Infants of diabetic fathers do not have an increased incidence of anomalies.
   The anomalies of IDMs include the following:
   a. Congenital heart disease
      1) Hypertrophic cardiomyopathy, hypertrophy of the intraventricular septum and walls of the right and left ventricles with or without subaortic stenosis
      2) Transposition of great vessels
      3) Ventricular septal defect
   b. Musculoskeletal deformities including caudal regression syndrome, agenesis of lumosacral spine, spina bifida, vertebral dysplasia
   c. Anencephaly, hydrocephalus
   d. Renal anomalies
   e. Small left colon syndrome
4. Respiratory distress due to respiratory distress syndrome and/or transient tachypnea of the newborn
   IDMs have a five to six times increased susceptibility to respiratory distress

syndrome. The presence of phosphatidylglycerol correlates with the absence of respiratory distress syndrome while the lecithin-sphingomyelin ratio is a poor predictor for respiratory distress syndrome. IDMs have an increased cesarean section rate at 36 to 37 weeks and are prone to develop transient tachypnea of the newborn with retained pulmonary fluid (see chapter II–IX).

5. Tremors, irritability, hypertonia, and convulsions as well as lethargy, poor feeding, and hypotonia
   a. Hypoglycemia (see chapter 15–X)
      The plasma glucose level falls as early as 30 minutes after birth and persists for 48 hours or longer. Rigorous control of maternal glucose levels during pregnancy and normoglycemia during labor and delivery tend to diminish hypoglycemic episodes. Hypoglycemia is due to hyperinsulinemia due to increased number and activity of pancreatic β-cells. A steady supply of glucose results in less hyperinsulinism.
   b. Hypocalcemia and hypomagnesemia (see chapter 15–IX and 15–XIII)
      Approximately 50% of the IDMs developed hypocalcemia (less than 7 mg/dl) during the first 72 hours of life. A high frequency and severity of clinical symptoms is usually not seen in class A diabetics. Symptomatology correlates with the maternal diabetic status. The pregnant diabetic is in a hyperparathyroid state; the rise in calcitonin, parathyroid hormone, and 1,25 hydroxycholecalciferol at birth in IDMs is sometimes sluggish, resulting in hypocalcemia. Hypomagnesemia occurs in one third of IDMs.
6. Jaundice
   The pathogenesis of hyperbilirubinemia in IDMs remains unknown. Decreased red blood cell survival time and polycythemia in IDMs have been suggested.
7. Plethora
   Venous hematocrits of ≥65% have been observed in 20% to 40% of IDMs. Umbilical cord erythropoietin levels are elevated. Hyperviscosity is often associated with neurologic problems (see chapter 12–V).
8. Abdominal distention and/or failure to pass meconium in the first few days of life. The incidence of meconium plug syndrome is increased in IDMs as is small left colon syndrome (see chapter 17–V, 17–IX).
9. Infection: IDMs have slightly increased incidence of infection.

D. Laboratory Findings

Laboratory findings depend on the effect of maternal diabetes.

1. Hypoglycemia less than 20 mg/dl in premature infants and less than 30 mg/dl in term infants during the first 72 hours of life and less than 40 mg/dl after 72 hours of life
2. Hyperinsulinemia greater than 12 units/ml
3. Hypocalcemia less than 7.0 mg/dl
4. Hypomagnesemia less than 1.5 mg/dl
5. Hyperbilirubinemia (see chapter 13)

6. Polycythemia (hyperviscosity) greater than 65% hematocrit
7. Blood gas derangement secondary to asphyxia, respiratory distress syndrome, transient tachypnea of the newborn, congenital heart disease, etc.
8. Ventricular enlargement on the ECG or echocardiogram

E. Radiologic/Echocardiographic Features

1. Chest x-ray film often reveals cardiomegaly, increased pulmonary markings, and the reticulogranular patterns of respiratory distress syndrome.
2. Radiologic features of spina bifida, agenesis of the sacrum, and shortened femur, tibia, and fibula may be present.
3. Septal hypertrophy on echocardiogram may be present.

F. General Supportive Management and Specific Therapy

For management see specific disease entities associated with IDMs, e.g., chapter 7 and 6III for large or small for gestational age, Table 5–3 for birth injury, chapter 11–XXVIII for congenital heart disease, or chapter 17–V for meconium plug syndrome. Long-term orthopedic support will be necessary for skeletal anomalies. See chapter 15–XF for specific therapy for hypoglycemia and Table 8–1 for admission studies and preventive management for high risk infants.

G. Long-term Prognosis and Follow-up

There is some evidence that macrosomia in IDMs may be a predisposing factor for later obesity.

There is an increased incidence of cerebral palsy and epilepsy in IDMs somewhat related to maternal severity of diabetes, maternal age, low birth weight for age, and complications of pregnancy. IDMs whose mothers had acetonuria have a higher incidence of intellectual impairment.

The empiric risk for IDMs to develop insulin-dependent diabetes is 1% to 5%. If both mother and father are insulin dependent, the risk is approximately 50%.

REFERENCES

Hare J.W., White P.: Gestational diabetes and the White classification. *Diab. Care* 3:394, 1980.

Cowett R.M., Schwartz R.: Infant of a diabetic mother. *Pediatr. Clin. N. Am.* 29:1213, 1982.

XII. HYPERGLYCEMIA

Hyperglycemia, a blood glucose level greater than 125 mg/dl, is seen in 20% to 80% of critically ill, low birth weight, less than 1,000-gm, premature infants. The reason for the greater degree of glucose intolerance in infants of very low birth weight is unknown. Smaller quantities of fat and skeletal muscle, stress, and immature pancreatic β-cells are factors that have been postulated.

A. Prevention

1. Avoid stress in low birth weight infants.
2. Carefully monitor glucose infusions. Try not to exceed 6 mg/kg/minute. Increase the quantity of administered glucose slowly: as little increment as 1% per day may be required for premature, less than 32 weeks' gestation infants.

B. Who Is at Risk?

1. Small-for-gestational-age, preterm, stressed, or intrauterine growth-retarded infants usually less than 3 days of age
2. Low birth weight infants receiving glucose infusions at rates greater than 6 mg/kg/minute. Occasionally, even lower rates will precipitate hyperglycemia.
3. Infants receiving parenteral nutrition with high glucose or lipid intake
4. Critically ill infants (e.g., intracranial bleeding and/or sepsis)
5. Infants with transient neonatal diabetes mellitus
6. Infants with a specific chromosomal aberration (e.g., Dq^- on no. 13)

C. Clinical Manifestations

Clinical manifestations include dehydration, frequent urination, and weight loss despite adequate fluid and calories. In addition, the infant may have intraventricular hemorrhage with seizures, apnea, and brain damage.

D. Laboratory Findings

1. Specific findings
   a. Blood glucose value greater than 125 mg/dl. The glucose screening test may not be accurate to detect severe degrees of hyperglycemia. Confirmatory blood or plasma glucose should be obtained.
   b. Hyperosmolality. Each rise of 18 mg/dl of glucose produces an increase in serum osmolality of 1 mOsm/L.
   c. Glucosuria with increased glomerular filtration rate and fluid and electrolyte loss in the urine due to osmotic diuresis
   d. Changes in CNS volume by CT scan
2. Associated findings
   Presence of red blood cells in CSF if serum osmolality increases more than 25 to 40 mOsm/L and serum glucose is over 500 to 800 mg/dl. At that level, CNS bleeding often occurs.

E. Supportive Management

1. Monitor glucose and electrolyte levels in all small-for-gestational-age, premature, stressed, and intrauterine growth-retarded infants carefully.

2. Monitor intake and output, osmolality, and weight loss/gain carefully.
3. Obtain a cranial sonogram at serial intervals.
4. See chapter 15–IIIB for "general supportive management for the infant with seizures."
5. If apnea ensues, see chapter 11–IIIB for "general supportive management for the infant with respiratory distress."

F. Specific Therapy

1. Reduce the concentration or rate of the glucose infusion while monitoring blood glucose levels.
2. Treat underlying causes for hyperglycemia, such as sepsis or asphyxia.
3. If necessary, institute insulin therapy cautiously to maintain adequate glucose level. Insulin, 0.25 to 0.50 units/kg, may be needed IV or SQ. Exogenous insulin should be used with caution because of its erratic effect. A dose that has no effect in one infant may produce profound hypoglycemia in another.

G. Prognosis

A serious risk of CNS hemorrhage with or without dehydration is associated with hyperglycemia and hyperosmolality.

REFERENCES

Brans Y.W.: Parenteral nutrition of the very low birth weight neonate: A critical view. *Clin. Perinatol.* 4:367, 1977.

Miranda L.E., Dweck H.S.: Perinatal glucose homeostasis: Unique character of hyperglycemia and hypoglycemia in infants of very low birth weight. *Clin. Perinatol.* 4:351, 1977.

XIII. HYPOMAGNESEMIA

Hypomagnesemia occurs when serum magnesium falls below 1.5 mg/dl. Hypomagnesemia is often associated with hypocalcemia and may be caused by insufficient replacement during total parenteral nutrition.

A. Prevention

1. Monitor high-risk infants.
2. Administer IV fluids and/or formulas with an adequate (2:1) calcium:phosphorus ratio. Add adequate magnesium to maintenance fluids.

B. Who Is at Risk?

Infants with the following problems are at risk of developing hypomagnesemia:

1. Transient hypoparathyroidism (usually occurs in the first day of life)

2. Chronic diarrhea or vomiting
3. Prolonged parenteral nutrition without the addition of magnesium
4. Hyperaldosteronism
5. Inborn error of magnesium metabolism
6. Renal tubular disease
7. Infants of diabetic mothers (hypomagnesemia in these infants is associated with neonatal hypocalcemia and decreased parathyroid function)
8. Premature or small-for-gestational age infants
9. Infants who have had intestinal resections or liver disease
10. Infants with increased phosphate intake or malabsorption defects
11. Infants who have had exchange transfusions with citrated donor's blood

C. Clinical Manifestations

1. Clinical manifestations are similar to those of hypocalcemia, such as tremors, seizures, tetany, etc.
2. Hypocalcemia is usually present concurrently and fails to respond to calcium therapy alone.

D. Laboratory Findings

1. Specific findings
   Magnesium levels less than 1.5 mg/dl
2. Nonspecific findings
   Associated hypocalcemia, hypoparathyroidism
3. Low amplitude EKG complexes, unstable cardiac rhythm, and inverted T waves over V_4 to V_6

E. Supportive Management

See chapter 15–IIIB for "general supportive management for the infant with seizures."

F. Specific Therapy

1. Administer 0.1 to 0.2 ml/kg of a 50% solution of $MgSO_4$ IM. Measure blood pressure. Observe for systemic hypotension and prolonged atrioventricular conduction time on the ECG. Repeat the dose every 8 to 12 hours as required. Be certain renal function is adequate.
2. If oral fluids are tolerated, give 50% $MgSO_4$, 0.1 ml/kg/day, diluted five-fold.
3. Check magnesium levels.

REFERENCES

Tsang, R.C., Chen I., Friedman M.A., et al.: Parathyroid function in infants of diabetic mothers. *J. Pediatr.* 86:399, 1975.

Tsang R.C., Steichen J.J., Brown D.R.: Perinatal calcium homeostasis: Neonatal hypocalcemia and bone demineralization. *Clin. Perinatol.* 4:385, 1977.

XIV. HYPONATREMIA

Sodium is the main extracellular ion. A serum sodium concentration of less than 130 mEq/L, but not always associated with a chloride level below 95 mEq/L, is considered hyponatremia in the newborn. Disturbances of sodium are usually associated with volume changes.

A. Prevention

1. Do not administer IV glucose/water solution to women in labor without adding adequate electrolytes.
2. Carefully calculate fluids and electrolytes administered to all infants.
3. Avoid perinatal asphyxia and stress and treat meningitis promptly to prevent syndrome of inappropriate antidiuretic hormone.
4. Treat diarrhea promptly and adequately.
5. Follow electrolytes carefully in all patients receiving diuretic therapy, having renal or adrenal disease, postsurgery, etc.

B. Who Is at Risk?

1. Infants with decreased sodium and decreased water
   a. Adrenogenital syndrome (adrenal cortical insufficiency)
   b. Hypotonic dehydration: post-GI surgery or diarrhea especially associated with malnutrition where more sodium than water has been lost
   c. Diuretic therapy
   d. Cystic fibrosis
   e. Renal disease
   f. Very low-birth-weight premature infants in the first few days of life
2. Infants with increased water
   a. Renal failure
   b. Excess vasopressin (syndrome of inappropriate antidiuretic hormone) (e.g., infants who are stressed or have chronic illnesses, malnutrition, meningitis, postsurgical procedures, etc; see chapter 18–XV).
   c. Infants with water intoxication. Commonly, an infant is fed a large quantity of diluted formula or an excess quantity of fluids are administered IV.
   d. Infants whose mothers received large quantities of dextrose in water without appropriate electrolytes

3. Infants with an increase in total body water and an increase in total body sodium as in nephrosis, cirrhosis, kwashiorkor, right-sided heart failure

C. Clinical Manifestations

Clinical manifestations include lethargy, coma, seizures, respiratory distress, poor skin turgor, jaundice and shock (due to decreased sodium and water). The infant may look well hydrated (due to increased water) or be edematous.

D. Laboratory Findings

1. Specific findings
   Serum sodium level of 130 mEq/L or less and hypo-osmolality less than 285 mOsm/L
2. Nonspecific findings
   Associated laboratory findings relate to the underlying disease process.
   a. Hyponatremia due to decreased sodium and decreased water.
      1) Adrenal insufficiency: increased serum K^+, decreased urinary steroids
      2) Diarrhea: positive stool culture
      3) Diuretic therapy: associated hypokalemia
      4) Cystic fibrosis: positive sweat test
      5) Renal disease: elevated BUN, K^+, creatinine
      6) Very low-birth-weight infant in the first few days of life due to increased urinary sodium and water excretion
   b. Hyponatremia due to increased water
      Diagnosis rests upon hyponatremia, hypo-osmolality of the plasma, elevated urine osmolality (greater than plasma), normal BUN, and K^+ levels.
      1) Renal failure: urine output less than 0.5 ml/kg/hour
      2) Excessive vasopressin (syndrome of inappropriate antidiuretic hormone): decreased blood pressure, positive chest x-ray film for pneumonia, positive CSF cultures, decreased right-sided heart pressure, increased head circumference, indomethacin therapy, hypo-osmolality of plasma
   c. Hyponatremia due to increased water despite increased total body sodium
      1) Nephrosis: low serum albumin with elevated urine albumin, elevated antidiuretic hormone
      2) Cirrhosis: elevated serum glutamic oxaloacetic transaminase (SGOT), serum glutamic pyruvic transaminase (SGPT), bilirubin, etc., elevated antidiuretic hormone
      3) Kwashiorkor: low serum albumin, elevated antidiuretic hormone
      4) Right-sided heart failure: elevated antidiuretic hormone
3. Hyperbilirubinemia possibly due to osmotic lysis of red cells.

E. Supportive Management

1. Monitor body weight every 8 hours.
2. Measure plasma and urine electrolytes and osmolality frequently (every 4 hours until normal, then every 12 to 24 hours until stable).
3. Monitor intake and urine volume carefully.
4. Obtain blood glucose, BUN, creatinine, etc.
5. Discontinue or reduce medications the infant is receiving especially diuretics (Lasix), phenobarbital, and indomethacin.
6. Obtain a sweat test if cystic fibrosis is suspected.
7. Obtain a chest x-ray film to consider cardiac disease with enlargement of the right atrium, congestive heart failure, or pneumonia.
8. Obtain a spinal tap to look for CNS infection if warranted.
9. If the infant develops seizures, see chapter 15–IIIB for "general supportive management for the infant with seizures."

F. Specific Therapy

1. Hyponatremia due to decreased sodium and decreased water
   a. Provide sodium (and chloride) in excess of that needed for maintenance. It is necessary to add 0.6 mEq of sodium per kg body weight for each 1 mEq/L increase in serum sodium concentration desired. Two thirds should be given as sodium chloride.
   b. Calculate the total body fluid deficit and provide therapy. To calculate the quantity of sodium required, subtract the actual serum sodium from the ideal serum sodium (135 mEq/L) and multiply the remainder by the infant's weight (kg) and by the extracellular volume (0.6). Supply half of the requirement slowly over a 12- to 18-hour period. For example, for a 3-kg infant with a serum sodium of 120 mEq/L:

   $$\left(\begin{array}{c}\text{Ideal serum sodium}\\ \text{(135 mEq/L)}\end{array} - \begin{array}{c}\text{Infant's}\\ \text{actual}\\ \text{serum sodium}\\ \text{(120 mEq/L)}\end{array}\right) \times \begin{array}{c}\text{Baby weight}\\ \text{(3 kg)}\end{array} \times \begin{array}{c}\text{Extracellular}\\ \text{volume}\\ \text{(0.6)}\end{array} = 27\ \text{mEq}$$

   Therefore, administer 13.5 mEq (27 ml) of 3% sodium chloride solution (0.5 mEq of sodium/ml) over a 12- to 18-hour period.
   c. Follow serum sodium levels carefully to ascertain that the sodium level is not rising too rapidly. Rapid correction may lead to severe brain damage.
2. Hyponatremia with increased water as in syndrome of inappropriate antidiuretic hormone (see chapter 18–XV)
3. Hyponatremia with an increase in total body water (see chapter 18–X)
   a. Treat as in *1* (hyponatremia due to decreased sodium and decreased water) only if CNS signs occur.
   b. Add diuretics (e.g., furosemide) to increase voiding of excessive water.

G. Prognosis

The prognosis depends upon the presence of CNS edema, hemorrhage, or seizure activity during the acute phase.

REFERENCE

Segar W.E., Chesney R.W.: Disorders of electrolyte metabolism. *Pediatr. Ann.* 10:288, 1981.

XV. HYPERNATREMIA

A serum sodium concentration greater than 160 mEq/L associated with an increased chloride level is considered hypernatremia in the newborn. Hypernatremia is seen commonly in dehydration due to diarrhea or inadequate fluid intake or when excessive salt has been provided.

A. Prevention

1. Prepare formulas and IV solutions carefully.
2. Monitor the infant's temperature and weight carefully.
   Do not overheat infant. Administer adequate fluid intake.
3. Treat diarrhea promptly.

B. Who Is at Risk?

1. Infants fed improperly prepared formula, e.g., one with excessive salt
2. Infants with high insensible water loss due to open infant warmer, high ambient temperature, or phototherapy
3. Infants given improperly prepared IV fluids
   a. Inadvertently, an overtired house officer adds electrolytes to glucose in saline rather than to glucose in water.
   b. The electrolytes are improperly calculated.
4. Infants with diarrhea who have been fed boiled skim milk or a powdered oral electrolyte solution
5. Infants receiving mannitol or urea in the treatment of cerebral edema
6. Infants with uncontrolled diarrhea caused by infection or enzyme deficiency
7. Infants with nephrogenic diabetes insipidus, especially males
8. Infants with renal medullary disease

C. Clinical Manifestations

Clinical manifestations include vomiting, diarrhea, GI disturbances, tremors, seizures, high fever, dehydration, apnea, lethargy, stupor, paralysis, and a "doughy" feel to the skin.

D. Laboratory Findings

1. Specific findings
   Serum sodium level greater than 160 mEq/L (newborns in the first few days of life can have elevated serum sodium normally; see normal values in appendix A–23, A–24)
2. Associated laboratory findings
   a. Decreased calcium, elevated chloride, reduced HCO_3^-
   b. Positive stool cultures, especially *E. coli* if diarrhea is present
   c. Increased red blood cells in the CSF
   d. Decrease or lack of antidiuretic hormone
   e. Hyperosmolality
   f. Intracellular dehydration
   g. Abnormal EEG, sometimes with seizure pattern
   h. Elevated specific gravity of urine

E. Supportive Management

See chapter 15–IIIB for "general supportive management for the infant with seizures."

F. Specific Therapy and Management

The goal is to provide an excess of fluid over solute so that sodium will be reduced to the normal range in 48 to 72 hours while treating the primary cause of hypernatremia.

1. Measure fluid intake and output. Obtain serum electrolyte levels, urine specific gravity, and serum and urine osmolality frequently.
2. Obtain culture of stool if diarrhea is present.
3. The "free water" deficit may be estimated from the elevation of the serum sodium. An increase of 1 mEq/L above 145 mEq/L would indicate a free water deficit of about 4.0 ml/kg. Therefore, multiply the elevation of the serum sodium above 145 mEq/L times 4.0 ml/kg to determine the amount of water needed per kilo to dilute the serum sodium to 145 mEq/L.
4. Although 5% D/W without added electrolytes can be given with extreme care, the possibility of cerebral edema ensuing with electrolyte-free solutes is great.
5. If the serum sodium is greater than 175 mEq/L, try to reduce not more than 15 mEq/L over a 24-hour period.
6. If seizures ensue, treat for seizures. Follow EEG, cranial sonogram, or cranial CT scan as required and treat for seizures (see chapter 15–III).
7. If the infant is severely dehydrated, administer Ringer's lactate, 20 ml/kg, or whole blood, 10 ml/kg, for the first 1 to 2 hours. Then, infuse 5% or 10% glucose/water in ¼ sodium chloride, 60 ml/kg, for the next 10 to 12 hours in

relation to the infant's state of hydration above maintenance. Do not correct hypernatremia rapidly or cerebral edema will ensue.

8. Administer calcium as required.
9. Digitalization is indicated if heart failure ensues (see chapter 11–XXIX).
10. Administer phenobarbital or Dilantin to control seizures (see chapter 15–III).
11. Administer potassium, 1 to 2 mg/kg/24 hours. Follow the infant's potassium level.
12. Peritoneal dialysis with glucose solution can be used to remove large quantities of sodium.
13. Exchange transfusion is not a desirable substitute for peritoneal dialysis since the sodium is high in citrate phosphate dextrose (CPD) or acid citrate dextrose (ACD) blood.

G. Prognosis

There is an appreciable mortality and a high incidence of longterm CNS dysfunction associated with hypernatremia.

REFERENCES

Paneth N.: Hypernatremic dehydration of infancy: An epidemiologic review. *Am. J. Dis. Child.* 134:785, 1980.

Segar W.E., Chesney R.W.: Disorders of electrolyte metabolism. *Pediatr. Ann.* 10:288, 1981.

XVI. HYPERAMMONEMIA

Hyperammonemia, the inability of the liver to clear the blood of preformed ammonia, occurs in association with inborn errors of the urea cycle enzymes and asphyxia, sepsis, hepatic failure, or parenteral nutrition. Although the acute form of genetically determined urea cycle disorders is almost always lethal, idiopathic self-limited hyperammonemia may have a normal outcome. Transient hyperammonemia is seen almost always in premature infants.

A. Prevention

1. Prevent perinatal asphyxia and monitor those infants with asphyxia for hyperammonemia.
2. Avoid use of excessive amino acids for parenteral nutrition in premature septic or hepatic impaired infants. Some protein hydrolysates contain a significant amount of preformed ammonia, which may account for hyperammonemia. Other intravenous nutrition solutions have a high concentration of glycine or alanine and may promote ammonia production as a result of deammonation of rapidly infused excess nonessential amino acids.
3. Do not feed high protein loads to premature, septic, or hepatic impaired infants.

B. Who Is at Risk?

1. Infants with severe perinatal asphyxia with or without shock (transient)
2. Infants with congenital disorders of the urea cycle or amino acid abnormalities
   a. Branch chain amino acid abnormalities
      1) Propionicacidemia (ketotic hyperglycemia)
      2) Methylmalonic aciduria (B_{12}-unresponsive)
      3) Beta-ketothiolase deficiency (congenital lysine intolerance)
   b. Urea cycle abnormalities
      1) Citrullinemia
      2) Argininosuccinicaciduria
      3) Argininemia
      4) Carbamylphosphate synthetase deficiency (congenital hyperammonemia type I)
      5) Ornithine transcarbamylase deficiency (congenital hyperammonemia type II)
   c. Dibasic amino acid abnormalities
      1) Ornithinemia
      2) Periodic hyperlysinemia with hyperammonemia
      3) Persistent hyperlysinuria (only in some patients)
      4) Familial protein intolerance (only in some patients)
3. Infants with hepatic failure, congestive heart failure, sepsis, etc.
4. Prematures with unexplained coma, respiratory distress, and normal enzymes
5. Low-birth-weight infants (appropriate and small for gestational age) (transient)
6. Infants receiving total parenteral nutrition (transient)

C. Clinical Manifestations

Infants affected with neonatal lethal variants of urea cycle defects are usually normal at birth and become acutely ill after 30 hours of life and after milk feeding is started. Infants with transient hyperammonemia usually have higher ammonia levels, lower birth weight, lower gestational age, and earlier respiratory distress, than infants with enzyme deficiency. Symptoms include poor feeding, apnea, irritability, stupor, hypertension, hyperthermia, wide neonatal heart rate oscillations, oliguria, neurologic and developmental abnormalities, seizures, coma, and death. Unusual posturing of the arms, similar to flapping asterixis of older patients, may be seen.

D. Laboratory Findings

1. Specific findings
   Blood ammonia levels greater than 150 μg/dl (normal values, 90 to 150 μg/dl). Hyperammonemia usually is associated with recent protein intake.
2. Deficiency of the enzymes previously listed (see chapter 15–XVIB) diagnosed by liver biopsy and/or fibroblast culture (see Table 15–3).

3. Urine amino acid and organic acid screen will delineate abnormality.
4. Urine orotic acid should be obtained to delineate hyperammonemia type 1 from type II (increased in type II).
5. Nonspecific findings
   a. Elevated SGOT, SGPT and bilirubin levels
   b. Hyponatremia, hypocalcemia, and hypoglycemia (may be concurrent)
   c. Increased rectal temperature
   d. Elevated arterial blood pressure
   e. Sinus arrhythmia, fetal heart rate oscillations, or nonreactivity
   f. Positive blood culture
   g. Metabolic acidosis (in association with branched chain amino acid catabolism)

E. Supportive Management

1. Support ventilation (see chapters 11–IV, and 11–VI).
2. Treat seizures as required (see chapter 15–III).
3. Treat infection vigorously and reduce protein intake during acute illness.
4. Provide genetic counseling.

F. Specific Therapy

1. When hyperammonemia is severe, no treatment is effective.
2. Reduce dietary intake of nitrogenous food; keep protein intake to 1.5 gm/kg/day. The degree of protein restriction is dependent on the severity of hyperammonemia.
3. Prevent catabolism by providing adequate caloric intake in the form of glucose and fat.
4. Reduce caloric reabsorption of ammonia by avoiding constipation, acidifying colonic contents with lactulose, or suppressing the breakdown of urea in the colon with antibiotics (Neomycin).
5. Direct supplementation of a deficient enzyme with a highly purified substitute enzyme has been tried.
6. Administer arginine, 0.5 to 1.0 mmol/kg/day, to provide arginine and enhance the removal of ammonia via the pyrimidine pathway.
7. Peritoneal dialysis and exchange transfusion may be effective temporarily for severe cases.
8. Liver transplant is under study.

G. Prognosis

Neonatal lethal variants of several urea cycle defects carry a grave prognosis. Infants with partial enzyme deficiency have a good prognosis for normal development with early treatment. Protein malnutrition and growth and developmental failure are common. The prognosis of infants with hyperammonemia secondary to asphyxia is related to the degree of asphyxia.

REFERENCES

Batshaw M.L., Brusilow S.W.: Asymptomatic hyperammonemia in low birthweight infants. *Pediatr. Res.* 12:221–224, 1978.

Goldberg R.N., Cabal L.A., Sinatra F.R., et al.: Hyperammonemia associated with perinatal asphyxia. *Pediatrics* 64:336–341, 1979.

Hudak M.L., Jones M.D., Brusilow S.W.: Differentiation of transient hyperammonemia of the newborn and urea cycle defects by clinical presentation. *J. Pediatr.* 107:712, 1985.

Shih V.E.: Congenital hyperammonemia syndromes. *Clin. Perinatol.* 3:3, 1976.

XVII. PYRIDOXINE (VITAMIN B_6) DEFICIENCY OR DEPENDENCY

Pyridoxine (B_6) is required for transamination, decarboxylation, deamination, and protein synthesis. Adequate CNS function is dependent on pyridoxine; its deficiency results in neonatal seizures.

A. Prevention

Administer vitamin B_6 concurrently with isoniazid (INH) to mothers with tuberculosis.

B. Who Is at Risk?

1. Deficiency
   a. Infants who are breast fed for prolonged periods of time by poorly nourished mothers
   b. Infants with inadequate general nutrition
   c. Infants whose mothers received pyridoxine antagonists, e.g., INH, with inadequate pyridoxine supplement
   d. Infants who are fed formula after accidental pyridoxine destruction during processing
2. Dependency
   a. Inborn errors of pyridoxine metabolism
   b. Infants whose mothers received large doses of pyridoxine during pregnancy have an increased requirement and are prone to develop pyridoxine dependency.

C. Clinical Manifestations

Clinical manifestations include irritability, convulsions, and weakness.

D. Laboratory Findings

Severely disorganized EEG pattern

E. Supportive Management

See chapter 15–IIIB for "general supportive management for the infant with seizures."

F. Specific Therapy

1. After elimination of common causes of seizures in the newborn, administer 50 mg of pyridoxine hydrochloride IM or IV.
2. If the seizures stop, vitamin B_6 deficiency or dependency should be suspected. For dependency, give pyridoxine 2–5 mg/day.
3. If EEG facilities are available, obtain an EEG tracing while injecting vitamin B_6. The abnormalities noted will immediately disappear, verifying the diagnosis.

REFERENCES

Bejsovec M., Kulenda Z., Ponca E.: Familial intrauterine convulsions in pyridoxin dependency. *Arch. Dis. Child.* 42:201, 1967.

Scriver C.R.: Vitamin B_6 dependency and infantile convulsions. *Pediatrics* 26:62, 1960.

XVIII. HYPERTHYROIDISM

Neonatal hyperthyroidism is acquired from the transplacental transfer of thyroid-stimulating immunoglobulins. Thyroid-stimulating immunoglobulins may readily cross the placenta and be demonstrated in the blood of infants born to mothers with Graves' disease. Fetal goiter or hyperthyroidism may occur in such infants and will usually subside as the immunoglobulins disappear. One half the infants born to mothers with Graves' disease are affected. Almost always the mothers have a past or present history of thyrotoxicosis. Thyroid-stimulating immunoglobulins remain high in the mother even after thyroidectomy.

A. Who Is at Risk?

1. Premature infants
2. Infants with tachycardia, tachypnea, and/or tremors
3. Infants born to mothers with Graves' disease or whose mothers have had a thyroidectomy

B. Clinical Manifestations

1. Irritability, restlessness, hyperactivity, fine tremors of hands, tachycardia, tachypnea with or without congestive heart failure, weight loss despite excessive feeding, plethora, elevated temperature, goiter, arrhythmias, advanced bone maturation, exophthalmos, hepatomegaly, jaundice, and thrombocytopenia
   a. All symptoms may be suppressed until 1 week after birth due to the effect of maternal antithyroid drugs.
   b. The disease is usually short-lived and coincides with the half life of the maternal thyroid-stimulating immunoglobulins.
   c. A second group of patients have the disease over a 5-year period.
2. Asphyxiation by tracheal compression can occur.
3. Congestive heart failure may occur.

C. Laboratory Findings

1. Specific findings
   a. Elevated thyroxine (T_4), triiodothyronine (T_3), and thyroid-stimulating immunoglobulins and suppression of thyroid-stimulating hormone
   b. Scan of thyroid showing enlarged thyroid
2. Associated findings
   a. Accelerated bone maturation
   b. Premature craniosynostosis
   c. Elevated basal metabolic rate/heart rate
   d. Increased Pa_{CO_2}, decreased Pa_{O_2}, and decreased pH due to goitrous encroachment on the trachea

D. Supportive Management

1. See chapter 11–IIIB for "general supportive management for the infant with respiratory distress."
2. Administer moist oxygen if required and follow blood gases.
3. See chapter 11–XXIX for the treatment of congestive heart failure.
4. Parenteral fluid administration may be required.
5. In more severe cases, sedation or β-adrenergic blocking agents, e.g., propranolol hydrochloride (Inderal), 0.5 to 2 mg/kg/24 hours in three divided doses, may be needed.

E. Specific Therapy

1. Lugol's solution (in mild cases), 1 drop three to six times per day
2. Propylthiouracil (in moderate and severe cases), 5 to 10 mg/kg/24 hours in three divided doses
3. Exchange transfusion in very severe cases

F. Prognosis

Permanent neurologic impairment may ensue. Hyperactivity has been described. In 20% to 30% of cases, the clinical manifestation may persist or recur for several years.

REFERENCES

Fisher D.A., Klein A.H.: The ontogenesis of thyroid function and its relationship to neonatal thermogenesis, in Tulchinsky D., Ryan K.J. (eds.): *Maternal-Fetal Endocrinology.* Philadelphia, W.B. Saunders Co., 1980, p. 281.

Lee W.N.P.: Thyroiditis, hyperthyroidism and tumors. *Pediatr. Clin. N. Am.* 26:53, 1979.

XIX. DRUG WITHDRAWAL SYNDROME IN THE INFANTS OF DRUG-ADDICTED MOTHERS (IDAM)

The increased incidence of drug addiction in women of childbearing age has increased the frequency of neonatal drug withdrawal syndrome. Because of its low molecular weight, heroin and other drugs cross the placenta and are distributed throughout fetal tissues. Both narcotics and nonnarcotic drugs can result in the neonatal withdrawal syndrome. Drugs that cause neonatal withdrawal include alcohol, amitriptyline (Elavil, Edep, Enovil), barbiturates, chlordiazepoxide (Librium), chlorpromazine (Thorazine), clomipramine, clonidine (Catapres), diazepam (Valium), diphenhydramine (Benadryl), ethchlorvynol (Placidyl), glutethimide, hydroxyzine (Atarax, Orgotrax, Vistaril), imipramine (Imavats, Tofranil, Sk-Pramine), lithium (Eskalith, Lithane, Lithobid, Lithonate, Lithotabs), meprobamate (Equanil, Meprospan, Miltown), methadone (Dolphine), pentazocine (Talwin), phenobarbital (Luminal, Sk-Phenobarbital, Sedadrops, Solfoton), propoxyphene (Darvon, Dolene, Sk-65), theophylline (Bronkodyl, Elixophylline, Slo-Phyllin, Theostat, Theolair, Theophyl), trifluoperazine (Stelazine), cocaine, amphetamines, LSD, etc. The accuracy of information provided by the drug dependent mother may be questionable. Multiple drug abuse, smoking and alcohol use is commonly involved.

A. Who Is at Risk?

1. Infants whose mothers are addicted to heroin, methadone, valium, cocaine, barbiturates, or other illegal drugs. (See drug listing above.)
2. If a history for drug addiction cannot be elicited from the mother, be suspicious of these situations:
   a. A mother unusually anxious to "sign out," or has
   b. Needle marks and/or ulcers, or has
   c. Poor prenatal care and/or unusual resistance to normal amounts of analgesics, or has
   d. Acquired immunodeficiency syndrome (AIDS) or HTLV-III antibody or other sexually transmitted disease.

B. Clinical Manifestations

1. There may be a history of poor to no prenatal obstetric care and perinatal infections, e.g., hepatitis, AIDS, syphilis, or gonorrhea. Prenatal care in the mothers on methadone is generally better than that received by heroin-addicted mothers.
2. There is an increased incidence of prematurity and small-for-gestational-age infants (more seriously affected by maternal heroin than other drugs). Normal birth weight is seen in infants of mothers receiving methadone.
3. With heroin, withdrawal usually occurs within the first 72 hours of life but may occur within the first week. A syndrome of late onset withdrawal has been described for methadone and phenobarbital occurring when the infant is 2 to 4 weeks of age, which is perhaps related to tissue binding and/or slow excretion of the drug.
4. Signs and symptoms are seen in 70% to 90% of infants and include the following:

   W—Wakefulness
   I—Irritability
   T—Tremulousness, temperature variation, tachypnea
   H—Hyperactivity, high pitched persistent cry, hyperacousia, hyperreflexia, hypertonia, hypertension
   D—Diaphoresis, disorganized suck and vomiting, diarrhea
   R—Rub marks, respiratory distress, rhinorrhea
   A—Apnea, autonomic dysfunction, skin abrasions
   W—Weight loss, failure to gain weight
   A—Alkalosis (respiratory)
   L—Lacrimation
   S—Sweating, sneezing, yawning, seizures

   The onset, duration and severity of withdrawal depends on the drug(s) the infant was exposed to in utero and the pharmacokinetics of the drug(s). Irritability and/or tremors may persist for 6 months or 1 year.
5. There is a decreased incidence of hyperbilirubinemia and respiratory distress syndrome in infants of drug- (heroin, barbiturates, etc) addicted mothers.
6. There is no increase in congenital malformations when mothers were on heroin or methadone.

C. Laboratory Findings

1. Heroin and/or methadone breakdown products and other drugs are excreted in the urine and may be detected by chromatography (positive urine toxicology studies). Quinine may be found in urine because heroin is cut with quinine.
2. Respiratory alkalosis is seen in some withdrawing newborns.
3. The infant's blood calcium, magnesium, sodium, and sugar levels are usually normal.

4. Elevated T_3 and T_4 have been described in infants of methadone-maintained mothers.
5. Thrombocytosis and increased platelet-aggregation activity have been reported in infants born to methadone-maintained mothers and those mothers who are multiple drug users.

D. Supportive Management

Prior to starting therapy obtain a detailed history from the mother regarding age, length of addiction, type of drugs taken, dosage, time of last dose during the present pregnancy, other habits (alcohol, smoking, marijuana, etc.), medications before and during labor and delivery, complications during this pregnancy and delivery, etc.

1. Attempt to keep the infant quiet.
   a. Keep the infant in a quiet, darkened environment.
   b. Swaddle the infant loosely.
   c. To prevent excessive crying, offer the infant a pacifier.
2. If the infant is not vomiting and does not have excessive tremors, oral administration of fluids is indicated. Feed the infant small amounts frequently. High caloric intake may be required.
3. Rule out other causes of tremors, convulsions, hyperthermia, diarrhea, electrolyte imbalance, hypocalcemia, hypoglycemia, hypomagnesemia, hyperthyroidism, CNS hemorrhage, infection, etc., that may exist.
4. If vomiting, diarrhea, marked tremors, or excessive weight loss occurs, IV administration of fluids is indicated.
5. Monitor vital signs, platelet count, and blood gases when withdrawal symptoms are severe.
5. See chapter 15–IIIB for "general supportive management for the infant with seizures."

E. Specific Therapy

Medical treatment is required when withdrawal symptoms are severe since tachypnea, hypertension, and alkalosis increase oxygen consumption and may cause failure to thrive. The criteria for pharmacologic intervention and the drug of choice varies among neonatologists.

1. A variety of drugs have been used to relieve the withdrawal symptoms and/or sedate the infant. The therapy must be individualized to balance the withdrawal symptoms against the quantity of drug required. Convulsions secondary to the withdrawal syndrome are frequently extremely difficult to control.
   a. Phenobarbital (sedatives):
   Phenobarbital is effective but is a CNS depressant, impairs sucking and

bonding and requires varying doses. Follow serum levels (20–40 μg/ml) to control withdrawal.
Dosage: 5 to 12 mg/kg/24 hours IM or orally divided into three or four doses. Dosage as high as 40 mg/kg/day may be utilized for severe withdrawal.

b. Tincture of paregoric (narcotics), 0.4 mg/ml morphine equivalent:
Paregoric is superior for treatment of diarrhea and seizures, rapidly normalizes sucking behavior, but requires longer duration of therapy. The drug has associated complications from composition (e.g., CNS depression from alcohol; CNS stimulation from camphor; acidosis, CNS depression, respiratory distress, renal failure, and death from benzoic acid, etc.).
Dosage: 0.2–0.5 ml (0.08–0.2 mg morphine equivalent) every 3–4 hours, increase by 0.05 ml increments to 1.0 ml until symptoms are controlled.

c. Tincture of opium (narcotics), 10 mg/ml morphine equivalent:
Dilute into the concentration as paregoric and use the same dose. Complications include constipation and CNS depression (no additives).

d. Diazepam (Valium) (neuroleptics):
Diazepam has no advantage over other drugs. It decreases or eliminates nutritive sucking behavior, and may be associated with the development of late onset of seizures. When hyperbilirubinemia is present, parenteral diazepam is contraindicated since the preservative, benzoate, competes with bilirubin for albumin binding sites and predisposes the infant to kernicterus. The composition of propylene glycol and ethyl alcohol gives complications of cerebral hepatic dysfunction and hyperosmolality.
Dosage: 0.1 to 1.0 mg/kg/day IM or IV slow infusion every 6–8 hours prn.

2. Observe for recurrence of withdrawal for approximately 7 days after gradual withdrawal and discontinuation of medications since recurrence is common.
3. The duration of therapy depends upon the degree of addiction of the infant and the type of drug used to withdraw or sedate the infant. The duration of therapy in neonatal heroin withdrawal varies from 4 days to 6 weeks; in methadone, the duration of therapy can be as long as 4 months.

F. Prognosis

1. Heroin: Mortality is less than 1%. There are some data supporting deficiencies in height, weight, and head circumference with generally normal intelligence, but somewhat lower scores in perception and cognition.
2. Methadone: A high incidence of hyperactivity, and learning and behavior disorders has been reported. An increased incidence of SIDS has been reported in infants born to methadone-maintained mothers.
3. Intravenous drug abuse: Increased incidence of AIDS.
4. Increased incidence of maternal (paternal) child abuse.
5. Behavioral disturbances (irritability, hyperactivity, feeding difficulties, abnormal Brazelton test), growth impairment, and slightly lower developmental scores have been reported.

REFERENCES

Goodfriend J.J., Shey I.A., Klein M.D.: The effects of maternal narcotic addiction on the newborn. *Am. J. Obstet. Gynecol.* 71:29, 1956.

Harper R.G., Solish G.I., Sang E., et al.: The effect of a methadone treatment program upon pregnant heroin addicts and their newborn infants. Fifth National Conference on Methadone Treatment, Washington, D.C., 1973.

Wilson G.S., McCreary R., Kean J.: The development of preschool children of heroin addicted mothers: A controlled study. *Pediatrics* 63:135, 1979.

Roberts R.J. (ed.): *Drug Therapy in Infants: Pharmacologic Principles and Clinical Experiences.* Philadelphia, W.B. Saunders Co., 1984, p. 337.

American Academy of Pediatrics Committee on Drugs: Neonatal drug withdrawal. *Pediatrics* 72:895, 1983.

XX. FETAL ALCOHOL SYNDROME, ALCOHOL-RELATED BIRTH DEFECTS, AND NEONATAL ALCOHOL WITHDRAWAL

Infants born to chronic alcoholic mothers who drink 1⅓ oz. (two standard drinks) of absolute alcohol per day during pregnancy are at risk for a variety of mental and physical impairments known as the fetal alcohol syndrome (FAS) and subtle birth defects and abnormal growth and development known as alcohol-related birth defects (ARBDs). The effect of maternal alcohol consumption on the developing fetus ranges from no apparent clinical signs to the fully developed FAS. The incidence has been reported to be 0.4 to 2.0 in 1,000 live births and 20% to 40% of alcoholic mothers for FAS and 3 to 5 in 1,000 live births for ARBDs.

A. Prevention

1. Dissemination of information about the harmful effects of alcohol on the fetus to prospective parents, supportive counseling, enrollment of the mother in a rehabilitation group, monitoring her compliance, general physical health, diet, etc., may prevent or ameliorate FAS.
2. A history of maternal individual drinking patterns to determine the frequency, type, variability, and absolute volume of consumption of alcohol should be taken with the aim of decreasing or eliminating alcohol consumption entirely during pregnancy.

B. Who Is at Risk?

1. Infants whose mothers consumed quantities in excess of 1⅓ oz. (two standard drinks) of absolute alcohol per day during the gestational period particularly during the first trimester. The incidence of FAS is dose dependent. Heavy smoking and caffeine consumption in association with excessive alcohol consumption are factors that increase risk for neonatal impairment.
2. Infants of mothers from low socioeconomic environments or minority groups,

infants of older single mothers (controversial), and infants of alcohol-dependent mothers who received little or no prenatal care are considered at risk.

3. Infants of alcohol-dependent and/or drug-dependent mothers whose general health and nutritional status are poor. Other conditions associated with chronic alcoholism include vitamin deficiencies, drug abuse, emotional disturbances, and socioeconomic deprivation.

C. Clinical Manifestations

1. Growth deficiency
   Intrauterine growth retardation (length more severely affected than weight), postnatal growth failure (weight more seriously affected)
2. Craniofacial abnormalities
   Microcephaly, short palpebral fissures, epicanthal folds, maxillary hypoplasia, cleft palate, micrognathia, hypoplastic philtrum, thinned upper vermilion, retrognathia, prognathia, ear anomalies (the helices of the ears are often undeveloped and the ear lobes small), strabismus, ptosis, microphthalmia
3. Limb malformations
   Joint anomalies, altered palmar crease pattern, camptodactyly, small nails
4. Cardiac anomalies
   Atrial septal defect (ASD), patent ductus arteriosus, ventricular septal defect, transposition of great arteries (TGA), tetralogy of Fallot, aplasia of the pulmonary artery, ventricular outflow tract obstruction
5. CNS deficiencies
   Developmental delays, psychomotor and intellectual retardation, gross motor and fine motor dysfunction (suck and grasp reflexes are weak), poor eye-hand coordination, seizures
6. Neuromuscular abnormalities
   Hypertonia, jitteriness, tremulousness, irritability
7. Other manifestations
   Anomalous external genitalia (hypoplastic labia and enlargement of the clitoris, septate vagina), capillary hemangiomas

A definite clinical diagnosis of FAS requires the presence of an abnormality in at least four areas: growth deficiency, CNS dysfunction, abnormal facies, and major and minor physical abnormalities in conjunction with a history of maternal alcohol abuse during pregnancy. Infants of alcoholic mothers may present signs of withdrawal in the first week of life that are similar to withdrawal symptoms from other drugs (see chapter 15-XIX).

D. Radiologic Features

Radiologic features include maxillary hypoplasia, micrognathia, camptodactyly, microphthalmia, microcephaly, and joint anomalies.

E. Laboratory Findings

1. Specific findings
   No biochemical markers are known.
2. Nonspecific findings
   Hypoglycemia within first hours of life

F. Supportive Management

Supportive management is directed toward correcting the correctable defects, e.g., patent ductus arteriosus, seizures, ventricular septal defect. Psychosocial support and counseling for further pregnancies are indicated.

G. Specific Therapy

No specific therapy for FAS is known. See chapter 15-XIX for treatment for withdrawal symptoms.

H. Prognosis

The majority (85%) of children with complete FAS have serious mental deficiency and growth retardation. The degree of growth deficiency and intellectual handicap is related to the extent of craniofacial abnormalities.

REFERENCES

Nichols M.M.: Acute alcohol withdrawal syndrome in a newborn. *Am. J. Dis. Child.* 113:714, 1967.

Peden V.H., Sommorn T.J., Downey D.A.: Intravenously induced infantile intoxication with ethanol. *J. Pediatr.* 83:490, 1973.

A Report to the Governor of the State of New York on Fetal Alcohol Syndrome by Task Force on FAS/ARBD. Shela B. Blume, Chairman, New York State Division of Alcoholism and Alcohol Abuse, November 1979.

Streissguth A.P., Clarren S.K., Jones K.L.: Natural history of the fetal alcohol syndrome: A 10-year follow-up of eleven patients. *Lancet* 2:85, 1985.

TABLE 15–2.—DISORDERS OF NEURONAL PROLIFERATION, MIGRATION, ORGANIZATION, AND MYELINATION

DISORDER	ANATOMIC CNS ABNORMALITY	CLINICAL MANIFESTATION	LABORATORY FEATURES
Disorders of neuronal proliferation			
Macrocephaly			
Autosomal dominant	Excessive proliferation	Macrocephaly, increased postnatal head growth	Increased familial head size
Autosomal recessive	Excessive proliferation	Macrocephaly, increased postnatal head growth, increased incidence of retardation	Increased familial head size
Beckwith-Wiedemann syndrome	Cerebral gigantism, pathologic lesion unknown	Macrocephaly, visceromegaly, macroglossia, omphalocele (see Table 9–4)	Hypoglycemia, polycythemia, hypocalcemia
Achondroplasia	Small foramen magnum, mild hydrocephalus	Macrocephaly, hypotonia, developmental delay, usually normal intelligence (see Table 9–4)	Short tubular bones (especially humeri), short trident hands, short femur
Neurocutaneous syndromes			
Tuberous sclerosis	Neuronal and glial excessive proliferation	White nevi, depigmented "ash leaf" skin lesions, seizures	CT scan: intercranial calcification in periventricular region, cysts of phalanges
Neurofibromatosis	Glia proliferation	40% cafe-au-lait spots at birth	Scoliosis, dysplastic nerve tumors
Sturge-Weber syndrome	Defect in vascular morphogenesis	Seizures, facial hemangiomas, macrocephaly	Intracranial calcifications, abnormal EEG
Klippel-Trenaunay-Weber syndrome	CNS hemangioma	Macrocephaly, asymmetric hypertrophy of limb and limb hemangioma	Brain or abdominal CT scan may show hemangioma of brain, eye, or viscera (see Table 9–4)
Unilateral macrocephaly	Localized neuron astrocyte proliferation	Unilateral cranial asymmetry, seizures, neurologic defects	CT scan: enlargement of hemisphere or portion, dilated lateral ventricles on the affected side
Disorders of neuronal migration			
Schizencephaly	Complete agenesis of a portion of the cerebral wall	Seizures, hypotonia, marked spasticity	CT scan: clefts in axis of cerebral fissure

(continued)

TABLE 15–2.—*(continued)*

DISORDER	ANATOMIC CNS ABNORMALITY	CLINICAL MANIFESTATION	LABORATORY FEATURES
Disorders of neuronal migration *(continued)*			
Lissencephaly	Few or no gyri	Hypotonia, spasticity, seizures, death in 3 years, myoclonic spasms, familial congenital heart disease, cloudy cornea, polydactyly	EEG: hypsarrhythmia. CT scan: Lack of gyri, thick cortical plate, dilated ventricles
Pachygyria	Few broad gyri, thick cortical plate	Seizures, spasticity, hypotonia, abnormal neurologic development; methyl mercury poisoning (?)	Associated with maternal history of methyl mercury ingestion
Polymicrogyria	Small plications in cortical surface	Zellweger's syndrome, (see Table 9–4), hypotonia, deafness, seizures, blindness	Renal cortical cysts, no response to visual or auditory stimuli
Neuronal heterotopias	Neuronal arrest during migration	Neurofibromatosis (?), Duchenne's muscular dystropies (?)	At autopsy
Agenesis of the corpus callosum	Failure of the formation of the corpus callosum	Mental retardation, hydrocephalus, seizures, antimongoloid slant to eyes	CT scan: displaced lateral ventricles, dilated occipital horns, large third ventricle
Disorders of organization			
Mental retardation with or without seizures	Maldevelopment of dendritic branching and spines	Infantile myoclonic seizures, hypsarrhythmia	EEG abnormalities
Trisomy 21 (Down's syndrome)	Abnormalities of dendritic and axonal development	Hypotonia, hyperflexibility of joints, mongoloid slants to eyes, brachycephaly	Chromosome study shows trisomy 21, mosaic or translocation (see Table 9–4)
Congenital rubella	Heterotopic neurons, decreased myelin	Small for gestational age, microcephaly, mental retardation	Increased antibodies to rubella (see chapter 16–IV)
Phenylketonuria	Decreased myelin, organization defects	No reliable signs in neonatal period	Plasma phenylalanine greater than 20 mg/dl
Trisomy 13–15	Prosencephalic cleavage, organization defects	Seizures, apnea, deafness, microphthalmia, cleft lip and palate, polydactyly	Chromosome study reveals trisomy 13–15
Perinatal insults	Decreased dendritic arborization, decreased synaptic development	Multiple (see chapter 15–IV)	Decreased Pa_{O_2}, decreased blood pressure, hypovolemia, or decreased heart rate

Disorders of myelination			
Central white matter hypoplasia	Deficient CNS white matter and myelin	Mental retardation, spastic quadriparesis, seizures	Deficient myelin formation
Alexander's disease	Deficient myelin, eosin in disordered astrocytes	Macrocephaly, abnormal development after 6 months of age, spastic quadriparesis	Disordered glial filaments in astrocytes
Canavan's disease	Deficient myelin, vacuolization of white matter in subcortical region	Hypotonia, macrocephaly, spasms, spasticity, seizures, optic atrophy	Deficient myelin
Krabbe's disease	Deficient myelin, deficient β-galactosidase	Spasticity, decerebrate posture, elevated CSF protein	Elevated CSF protein, large multinucleoid globoid cells
Pelizaeus-Merzbacher disease	Decreased myelin interspersed with islands of myelin	Pendular nystagmus, hypotonia, spasticity, blindness, optic atrophy, hearing deficits, intellectual failure	
Metachromatic leukodystrophy	Myelin deficiency and metachromatic material in CNS	Hypotonia, ataxia, spasticity, death at 3–6 years	Cerebroside sulfatase deficiency, severe myelin deficiency in central and peripheral nervous system
Amino and organic acidopathies, e.g., maple syrup urine disease, phenylketonuria, homocystinuria, nonketotic hyperglycemia	Vacuolization of myelin	See Table 15–3.	See Table 15–3
Perinatal undernutrition	20%–30% reduction in cerebrosides, 15%–20% reduction in plasmalogens (decreased normal myelin)	Small for gestational age, mental retardation	Decreased skin fold thickness (Ponderal index)
Potential disturbances			
Perinatal insults	Reduction and/or abnormalities in myelin (?), etc.	Seizures	See Chapter 15–IV

REFERENCE

Volpe J.J.: *Neurology of the Newborn.* Philadelphia, W.B. Saunders Co., 1981.

TABLE 15–3.—Inborn Errors of Metabolism Associated With Seizures in the Newborn*

DISEASE	ENZYMATIC DEFECT	CLINICAL BIOCHEMICAL FEATURES	THERAPY
Amino acidopathy			
Maple syrup urine disease	Branched-chain ketoacid decarboxylase	Stupor, seizures, hypoglycemia, retardation, vomiting, odor of maple syrup; metabolic acidosis, branched-chain amino/ketoacidemia (urea)	Control of acidosis and seizures, IV fluids, diet with no branched-chain amino acids
Nonketotic hyperglycinemia	Glycine decarboxylase	Stupor, seizures, myoclonus, hiccups, increased glycine, death	Exchange transfusion may be life-saving. Strychnine may be of benefit.
Methionine malabsorption	Unknown	Seizure, hypermethioninemia, odor of hops in the urine	Unknown
Hyper-β-alaninemia	β-alanine-α-ketoglutarate transaminase	Stupor, neonatal seizures	Large doses of vitamin B_6
Carnosinemia	Carnosinemia defect (?)	Seizures, delayed development	Unknown; zinc co-factors (?)
Hypervalinemia	Valine transaminase	Stupor, delayed development	Low valine diet
Urea cycle disorders			
Congenital hyperammonemia type I	Carbamylphosphate synthetase	Hyperammonemia, vomiting, seizures, stupor, coma; aminoacidemia (urea), elevated glutamine, lack of orotic aciduria, acidosis, hypoglycemia, elevated lactate, decreased biotin	Early detection: sterilization of the gut with Neomycin, cessation of protein feeds, high carbohydrate diet. When infant is stable, give 0.25–0.5 gm/kg/24 hours of protein, biotin 30 mg/day, α Ketoanalogues, correct hypoglycemia
Congenital hyperammonemia type II	Ornithine transcarbamylase	Severe in males in newborn period; vomiting, stupor, seizures, hypotonia, tachypnea, increased ammonia, increased orotic aciduria	Same as congenital hyperammonemia type I

Argininosuccinic acid synthetase deficiency (citrullinuria)	Argininosuccinic acid synthetase	Severe neonatal type: poor feeding, vomiting, tachypnea, hypotonia, seizures, increased ammonia, hypoglycemia, acidosis, increased citrulline	Same as congenital hyperammonemia type I plus arginine, 2–4 mmol/kg/24 hours
Argininosuccinase deficiency	Argininosuccinase	Severe neonatal type: poor feeding, tachypnea, vomiting, seizures, coma, increased ammonia, increased arginosuccinic acid, increased lactate, acidosis, decreased biotin, increased methemoglobin level	Same as congenital hyperammonemia type I plus arginine, 2–4 mmol/kg/24 hours
Disorders of pyruvate metabolism			
Pyruvate dehydrogenase deficiency	Pyruvate dehydrogenase	Stupor, tachypnea, hypotonia, seizures, increased lactic and pyruvic acid, hypoglycemia, hyperalaninemia	Early detection: treat acidosis promptly, peritoneal dialysis (?), or exchange transfusion, diet high in fat. Trial of thiamine.
Pyruvate carboxylase	Pyruvate carboxylase		
Disorders of carbohydrate metabolism			
Hereditary fructose intolerance	Fructose-1-phosphate aldolase	Vomiting, hypoglycemia, hypophosphatemia, hepatosplenomegaly, jaundice, liver failure, renal damage.	Exclusion of fructose from the diet, administer glucose.
Von Gierke's disease.	Glucose-6-phosphatase	Hypoglycemia, hepatomegaly, hyperlactacidemia, hyperurinemia, metabolic acidosis, negative glycogen stimulation test	Avoid fructose and galactose, administer a low-fat diet, treat hyperurinemia with allopurinol; use glucose with caution, since hypoglycemia can worsen.

(continued)

TABLE 15–3.—*(continued)*

DISEASE	ENZYMATIC DEFECT	CLINICAL BIOCHEMICAL FEATURES	THERAPY
Disorders of carbohydrate metabolism *(continued)*			
Galactose-1-phosphate uridyl transferase deficiency	Galactose-1-phosphatase uridyl transferase	Increased galactose, irritability, vomiting, diarrhea, hepatomegaly, amino aciduria, hypoglycemia, reducing substance in urine.	Avoid galactose.
Organic acid disorders			
Congenital lysine intolerance	β-ketothiolase	Vomiting, seizures, spasticity, hyperammonemia, ketonuria, hypoglycemia, metabolic acidosis	Early detection: restrict protein, correct hypoglycemia, administer $NaHCO_3$ to correct acidosis, exchange transfusion, low protein diet; biotin, 10 mg/day orally
Propionic acidemia	Propionyl-CoA carboxylase	Vomiting, stupor, tachypnea, seizures, coma, hypoglycemia, hyperammonemia, ketonuria, metabolic acidosis, neutropenia, thrombocytopenia.	Same as congenital lysine intolerance
Methylmalonic acidemia	Methylmalonyl-CoA racemase, methylmalonyl-CoA mutase apoenzyme.	Vomiting, stupor, tachypnea, seizures, ketonuria, metabolic acidosis	Early detection: vitamin B_{12}, and same therapy as congenital lysine intolerance
Isovaleric acidemia	Isovaleryl-CoA dehydrogenase	Vomiting, tachypnea, stupor, coma, odor of sweaty feet, isovaleric acidosis (-uria) isovaleric glycinuria, neutropenia, thrombocytopenia	Glycine 250 mg/kg. Then maintain 800 mg/day. Restrict protein from diet to 1.5 gm/kg/day.

REFERENCE

*Volpe J.J., *Neurology of the Newborn.* Philadelphia, W.B. Saunders Co., 1981.

Chapter 16

Poor Feeding, Poor Cry, and Poor Muscle Tone

Infection, neuromuscular diseases, metabolic disturbances, CNS abnormalities, drug effect, and chromosomal aberrations frequently present as poor feeding, poor cry, and poor muscle tone. The physician must keep in mind that even the smallest infants are normally vigorous; development of poor feeding, poor cry, and poor muscle tone indicates an ongoing disease process. Many features of infections are similar to those of many noninfectious conditions, and it is very difficult to diagnose infection on the basis of clinical manifestations alone.

I. CLINICAL EVALUATION: NORMAL DATA

Normally, the infant will move spontaneously even during sleep. Crying will continue poststimulation for a short period of time. The house officer must be aware of the normal neurologic examination of the newborn, the muscle tone as it develops with gestational age, and the environmental factors that may impinge on the infant's neuromuscular status (see Figs 6–1 and 6–2).

II. COMMON CAUSES OF POOR FEEDING, POOR CRY, AND POOR MUSCLE TONE

A. Infection

1. Common organisms acquired by the fetus in utero
   a. Rubella
   b. Cytomegalovirus (CMV)
   c. Toxoplasmosis
   d. Varicella
   e. Coxsackievirus

f. Syphilis
g. Tuberculosis
h. Hepatitis B
i. Malaria
j. Mumps
k. Rubeola
l. *Listeria monocytogenes*
m. HTLV-III

2. Common organisms and infections acquired during parturition or in the nursery
   a. Organisms
      1) Bacterial infection (gram-negative or gram-positive bacteria)
         Group B streptococcus, *Escherichia coli, L. Monocytogenes, Proteus, Staphylococcus aureus, staphylococcus epidermidis, Klebsiella, Pseudomonas aeruginosa, Hemophilus influenzae, Streptococcus pneumoniae, Neisseria meningitidis, Salmonella* sp., *Serratia marcescens,* tuberculosis
      2) Viral infections
         Herpes simplex, CMV (from human milk or transfusions), hepatitis B (from human milk or blood), rotavirus, enterovirus, adenovirus or respiratory syncytial virus, chlamydial trachomatis, HTLV-III
      3) Fungal infection
         Candida albicans
   b. Infections
      Sepsis, meningitis, urinary tract infection, pneumonia (see chapter 11–XI), conjunctivitis, diarrhea, omphalitis, dermatitis, acquired immunodeficiency syndrome (AIDS)

B. Neuromuscular Abnormalities (see chapter 16–XXIV)

1. Anterior horn cell disease (Werdnig-Hoffman disease)
2. Neuromuscular junction disease
   Neonatal myasthenia gravis
3. Muscle disease
   a. Congenital myopathy
   b. Myotonia dystrophy
   c. Glycogen storage disease

C. Metabolic Aberrations

1. Hyperglycemia or hypoglycemia
2. Hypercalcemia
3. Hypermagnesemia
4. Hypernatremia or hyponatremia
5. Hypokalemia

6. Hypoxia and/or hypercapnia
7. Hyperthermia or hypothermia
8. Acidosis

D. Cerebral Abnormalities

1. Intracranial hemorrhage
   a. Periventricular, intraventricular, or intracerebral
   b. Subdural
   c. Subarachnoidal
2. Hypoxic-ischemic encephalopathy
3. Congenital cerebellar ataxia
4. Kernicterus
5. Oculocerebrorenal syndrome (Lowe's syndrome)
6. Lipidoses
7. Prader-Willi syndrome
8. Drugs
   a. Narcotics, such as heroin or meperidine hydrochloride (Demerol)
   b. Barbiturates
   c. General anesthetic agents
   d. Local anesthesia

E. Chromosomal Aberrations

Trisomy 13–15, 18, and 21

F. Congenital Heart Disease With or Without Congestive Heart Failure

1. Hypoplastic left heart syndrome
2. Cyanotic heart disease

III. WHAT THE PHYSICIAN SHOULD DO WHEN CONFRONTED WITH AN INFANT SUSPECTED OF HAVING AN INFECTION

A. Diagnostic Workup for Intrauterine Infection

1. Review the maternal history to determine the possibility of the infant's exposure to known intrauterine infectious agents, such as syphilis, rubella, or hepatitis B. Check the maternal serologic status for toxoplasmosis, rubella, CMV, hepatitis, herpes, syphilis, etc. Determine if there was prolonged labor, prolonged rupture of membranes, fetal distress, etc.
2. Examine the infant carefully considering each of the common causes of in utero infection. Note carefully the presence of hepatosplenomegaly, jaun-

dice, petechiae, ecchymoses, chorioretinitis, microcephaly, or low birth weight. Eighty percent to 90% of infants with intrauterine infection are asymptomatic or mildly ill but unrecognized in the nursery.

3. Draw blood for IgM, complete blood count (CBC), platelets, and liver function test. TORCH (toxoplasmosis, rubella, CMV, herpes simplex) titers of both mother and infant may be obtained as a screening test. In addition, draw VDRL for syphilis.
4. Obtain fresh urine for cytomegalic inclusion bodies.
5. Obtain viral cultures from urine, cerebrospinal fluid (CSF), nasopharyngeal washings, and conjunctiva for CMV, rubella, and enterovirus.
6. Obtain CSF for viral cultures cell count and protein.
7. Draw blood for hepatitis B surface antigen and antibodies if hepatitis is suspected.
8. Note the infections acquired in utero and obtain the proper test if that infection is suspected (see chapter 16–IV to 16–VI, 16–VIII to 16–XIII).
9. Obtain skull x-ray films, cranial sonogram or CT scan to determine the presence of intracranial calcifications. Obtain long-bone x-ray films to determine the presence of periostitis, longitudinal radiolucency of "celery stalking," etc.

B. Diagnostic Workup for Infection Acquired During Parturition or in the Newborn Nursery

1. Review the perinatal history to determine if the infant was exposed to any of the known maternal or labor factors that may predispose the infant to infection, such as prolonged rupture of membranes, or prolonged labor.
   Note that early-onset infections occurring within a few days of life are often associated with obstetric complications.
2. Review the nurses' notes carefully to determine whether the infant developed poor feeding, irritability, lethargy, poor cry, hyperthermia or hypothermia, respiratory distress, abdominal distension, etc.
3. Examine the infant carefully noting especially signs of abdominal distension, diarrhea, jaundice, hepatomegaly, respiratory distress, tachypnea, apnea, retractions, cyanosis, pallor, hypotonia, neurologic depression, periumbilical erythema, petechiae, or sclerema.
4. If the infant has developed a fever, note whether his or her extremities are cold. The newborn with infection often has a warm trunk and cool extremities due to poor perfusion; the newborn who is overheated from the radiator or the sun will have a warm trunk and warm extremities.
5. Obtain a CBC including differential count, platelet count, and peripheral smear. Infants with infection will frequently have leukocytosis (greater than 25,000 white blood cells/cu mm) or leukopenia (less than 5,000 white blood cells/cu mm), an elevated immature neutrophil count, a depressed platelet count (less than 100,000 platelets/cu mm), a peripheral smear that suggests a hemolytic process, or an elevated absolute neutrophil count. A sudden

drop or increase in leukocytes and/or platelet count also suggests infection although values may be within normal limits.

6. Obtain cultures of blood, suprapubic urine, CSF, ear, endotracheal tube aspirate, gastric aspirate, and stool.
7. Determine the presence of meningitis before administering antibiotics. Perform a lumbar puncture to obtain a Gram's stain for bacteria and cell count, culture and sensitivity, and levels of glucose and protein in the CSF. See appendix A–39, A–40 for spinal fluid values in relation to the infant's age.
8. Serologic studies may help establish a diagnosis.
   These tests include countercurrent immunoelectrophoresis, coagglutination procedure, latex agglutination test, and limulus amebocyte lysate test. The house officer must be aware as to which tests are currently available in his institution.
9. Follow the bilirubin (total and indirect), hematocrit, CO_2, blood glucose, calcium, electrolytes, and urinalysis findings.
10. Obtain a blood gas study to consider metabolic acidosis.

C. General Supportive Management for the Infant With Infection Acquired In Utero, During Parturition, or in the Nursery

1. Handle the infant gently (as always).
2. Place the infant in the supine position with a roll under the shoulders to hyperextend the neck and open the airway.
3. Suction the infant as frequently as necessary.
4. Maintain the infant's abdominal skin temperature at approximately 36.5° C (97.7° F) and the rectal temperature at approximately 37.0° C (98.6° F). Work within a warmed environment to avoid precipitous drops in body temperature associated with procedures such as taking an ECG or inserting a catheter.
5. Measure intake and output.
6. Maintain serum and urine electrolytes and osmolality within normal limits.
7. Give the infant nothing by mouth and administer fluids and calories intravenously if the infant is unable to tolerate oral feedings.
8. Correct metabolic acidosis.
9. Transfuse with fresh whole blood, 10 ml/kg, if the infant is anemic (with a hematocrit less than 40%). This will improve tissue oxygenation and give nonspecific anti-infective factors. Granulocyte transfusions may be of value. Fresh frozen plasma may be administered for serious sepsis (controversial).
10. Be certain that all causes of poor feeding, poor cry, and poor muscle tone have been considered (see chapter 16–II).
11. If the infant develops convulsions, administer phenobarbital to control seizures and prevent additional hypoxia, decrease metabolic demands, and prevent cerebral edema (see chapter 15–IIIB).
12. If the infant develops respiratory distress, administer oxygen therapy and assisted ventilation as required (see chapter 11–IV, 11–VI).

13. If the infant develops shock, administer a volume expander to maintain adequate blood pressure (see chapter 14–IIID7).
    If shock persists and endotoxemia is suspected, administer hydrocortisone IV, 35 to 50 mg/kg over 10 to 15 minutes every 30 minutes not more than four times, and naloxone, 0.01 mg/kg IV.
    Hydrocortisone may interrupt the vasodilation effects of kallikrein released by granulocytes and vascular endothelial cells due to endotoxemia, and naloxone inhibits the hypotensive effect of the pituitary β-endorphin stimulated by endotoxin.
14. If the infant develops excessive hyperbilirubinemia, follow bilirubin levels and start phototherapy or perform exchange transfusion if needed (see chapter 13–V, 13–VI).
15. Specific Therapy
    Antibiotic therapy should be started even when only minimal signs of sepsis are present because of the nonspecific clinical signs of sepsis and high mortality. Initial antibiotic therapy may be started with penicillin or ampicillin in combination with an aminoglycoside while waiting for culture results.
    The choice of antibiotics for initial treatment depends on the type of infection (early vs. late onset) and the particular pattern of organism sensitivity in the hospital.
    Initial treatment may be started with the following antibiotics to cover gram-positive cocci and gram-negative bacilli.
    a. Penicillin G, 100,000 units/kg/day IV every 12 hours for first 7 days and 100,000 units/kg/day IV every 8 hours after 7 days; or ampicillin, 100 to 150 mg/kg/day IV every 12 hours for first 7 days and 100 to 150 mg/kg/day every 8 hours after 7 days of age; and
    b. Gentamicin, 5.0 mg/kg/day IM every 12 hours for first 7 days and 7.5 mg/kg/day IM every 8 hours after 7 days; or kanamycin, 15 to 20 mg/kg/day IM every 12 hours for first 7 days and 20 to 30 mg/kg/day every 8 hours after 7 days, or other aminoglycosides may be substituted for gentamicin if desired for the nursery. Therapeutic levels of gentamicin include peak (upper limit) of 4–8 μg/ml and a trough of 1–3 μg/ml. Although a single blood sample for a trough level at 8–12 hours after a dose given after 2–3 days of therapy may be helpful in adjusting dosage, micromethods are not generally available. Renal function and hearing screening should be followed.
16. Modify the antibiotic regimen according to the culture results of the organism and sensitivity if cultures are positive. See Table 16–1 for "dosage and complications of antibiotic therapy in the newborn."
17. When cultures are negative, continue antibiotic therapy if the infant remains symptomatic and discontinue antibiotics if the infant is asymptomatic.

REFERENCE

Remington J.S., Klein J.O. (eds.): *Infectious Disease of the Fetus and Newborn Infant.* Philadelphia, W.B. Saunders Co., 1983.

TABLE 16–1.—DOSAGE AND COMPLICATIONS OF ANTIBIOTIC THERAPY IN THE NEWBORN*

ANTIBIOTIC	INDICATIONS	ROUTE	DAILY DOSAGE/KG (NO. OF DOSES)			TOXICITY	COMMENTS
			PREMATURES < 1 WK	TERM INFANTS < 1 WK	INFANTS 1–4 WK		
Aminoglycosides							
Amikacin	Coliforms and pseudomonas resistant to other aminoglycosides	IM,IV	15 mg (2)	20 mg (2)	20–30 mg (2 or 3)	Nephrotoxicity and ototoxicity; transaminase elevations	Limited experience in newborns; indicated for gram-negatives; resistant to other aminoglycosides
Gentamicin	Broad-spectrum activity against gram-negative including pseudomonas and kanamycin-resistant organisms	IM,IV	5 mg (2)	5 mg (2)	7.5 mg (3)	Potential nephrotoxicity and ototoxicity with high serum levels or extended use	Good initial drug for unknown gram-negatives where kanamycin resistance is common; CNS levels unpredictable
Kanamycin	Broad-spectrum activity against gram-negatives	IM,IV	15 mg (2)	20 mg (2)	20–30 mg (3)	Potential nephrotoxicity and ototoxicity; avoid use for more than 12 days	Good broad-spectrum activity against gram-negatives; this is good initial drug in nurseries where resistance is uncommon; CNS levels unpredictable

(continued)

TABLE 16–1.—*(continued)*

ANTIBIOTIC	INDICATIONS	ROUTE	DAILY DOSAGE/KG (NO. OF DOSES) PREMATURES < 1 WK	TERM INFANTS < 1 WK	INFANTS 1–4 WK	TOXICITY	COMMENTS
Neomycin	Toxigenic *E. coli*	Orally	50 mg (4)	100 mg (4)	100 mg (4)	Ototoxicity and nephrotoxicity	Damage to small intestinal mucosa with secondary malabsorption syndrome and systemic absorption
Streptomycin	*Mycobacterium tuberculosis*	IM,IV	20 mg (1)	20 mg (1)	20 mg (1)	Nephrotoxicity and ototoxicity; cardiovascular collapse with excessive dose	Limited use in newborns due to toxicity and emergence of resistant organisms
Tobramycin	Coliforms and pseudomonas resistant to gentamicin	IM,IV	4 mg (2)	5 mg (2)	7.5 mg (3)	Nephrotoxicity and ototoxicity	Limited experience in newborns; many gentamicin-resistant organisms also tobramycin-resistant; CNS levels unpredictable
Amphotericin B	Systemic fungal infections	IV	0.25–1.00 mg (1)	0.25–1.00 mg (1)	0.25–1.00 mg (1)	Nephrotoxicity and hepatotoxicity	Limited experience in newborns

Cephalosporins							
Cephalothin	Gram-positive bacteria including penicillinase-producing staphylococci, many gram-negative bacteria	IM,IV	50 mg (3)	50 mg (3)	100 mg (4)	May aggravate existing renal failure; positive direct Coombs' test; transaminase elevations	Limited experience in newborns; does not penetrate CNS; positive Benedict's test in urine
Cefaclor	Pneumococci, *H. influenzae,* Enterobactericeae	IM,IV	45 mg (3)	45 mg (3)	45 mg (3)	Acute serum sickness	Poor penetration into CSF
Moxalactam	Gram-negative enterobacilli	IM,IV	50–100 mg (2)	100 mg (2)	150 (3)	Thrombocytopenia, platelet dysfunction, neutropenia	Good penetration into CSF
Chloramphenicol	Gram-negative and some gram-positive organisms, *Salmonella, H. influenzae*	IV, orally	25 mg (2)	50 mg (2)	50 mg (2)	Reversible bone marrow suppression, gray baby syndrome with high blood levels	Good CNS penetration makes this agent valuable in gram-negative meningitis
Colistimethate (Colistin)	Gram-negative organisms including *Pseudomonas*	IM	5 mg (2)	5 mg (2)	7.5 mg (3)	Ototoxicity and nephrotoxicity	Limited efficacy in systemic infection
Erythromycin	*Chlamydia trachomatis, Bordetella pertussis*	Orally	40 mg (3)	40 mg (3–4)	40 mg (3–4)	None	Not used parenterally due to tissue damage
Nystatin (Mycostatin)	*Candida* (thrush)	Orally	100,000–200,000 units (total) (4)	100,000–200,000 units (total) (4)	100,000–200,000 units (total) (4)	None	Not used in systemic infections

(continued)

TABLE 16–1.—*(continued)*

ANTIBIOTIC	INDICATIONS	ROUTE	DAILY DOSAGE/KG (NO. OF DOSES) PREMATURES < 1 WK	TERM INFANTS < 1 WK	INFANTS 1–4 WK	TOXICITY	COMMENTS
Penicillins							
Ampicillin	Gram-positive non-penicillinase-producing including *Listeria;* good gram-negative coverage including *E. coli, Proteus mirabilis,* enterococcus, *H. influenzae*	IM,IV	50–100 mg (2) 100 mg (2) (meningitis)	100–150 mg (2) 200 mg (2) (meningitis)	100–150 mg (3) 300 mg (3) (meningitis)	Uncommon in neonate elevation of transaminase; eosinophilia, irritability with excessive dosage	Use high dose with CNS infection, good broad-spectrum initial coverage; many gram-negative organisms resistant, so should be combined initially with an aminoglycoside
Carbenicillin	Same spectrum as ampicillin with addition of all *proteus* species and *pseudomonas;* sensitive to penicillinase	IM,IV	200 mg (2)	250 mg (3)	300–400 mg (4)	Transaminase elevations; coagulation abnormalities due to altered platelet function	Contains 4.7 mEq sodium per gm carbenicillin

Methicillin, oxacillin, nafcillin	Penicillin-resistant staphylococci only	IM,IV	50 mg (2) 100 mg (2) (meningitis)	100 mg (2) 150 mg (3) (meningitis)	75–150 mg (3) 200 mg (4) (meningitis)	Nephritis, watch for hematuria and rising BUN; transaminase elevations	Toxicity dose and duration dependent; used with gentamicin as drug of choice in nursery-acquired sepsis
Penicillin G	All susceptible gram-positive organisms, streptococci (group A, B, C), *S. pneumoniae, N. gonorrhoeae*	IM,IV	100,000 units (2) 150,000–200,000 units (meningitis) (2)	100,000 units (2) 150,000–250,000 units (meningitis) (2)	100,000 units (3) 150,000–250,000 units (3 or 4) (meningitis)	Uncommon	Use higher doses with CNS infection
Procaine penicillin	Congenital syphilis	IM	50,000 units (1)	50,000 units (1)	50,000 units (1)	Uncommon	Single dose for syphilis without neurosyphilis; 10 days therapy for neurosyphilis
Ticacillin	Same spectrum as carbenicillin and active against *P. aeruginosa*	IM,IV	150 mg (2)	150 mg (3)	225–300 mg (3 or 4)	Same as carbenicillin	Same as carbenicillin
Vancomycin	All aerobic and anaerobic gram-positive cocci and rods (e.g., *S. epidermidis*)	IV	30 mg (2)	30 mg (2)	45 mg (3)	Ototoxicity and nephrotoxocity; histamine-like response	Initial drug of choice for *S. epidermidis* infection

REFERENCE

Remington J.S., Klein J.O.: *Infectious Diseases of the Fetus and Newborn Infant.* Philadelphia, W.B. Saunders Co., 1983.

IV. CONGENITAL RUBELLA (GERMAN MEASLES)

Rubella, a common viral communicable disease of childhood, can cause a wide spectrum of abnormalities in the fetus and newborn if acquired before birth. These include spontaneous abortion, stillbirth, single or multiple congenital anomalies, and congenital infection. The fetus may be unharmed. Congenital rubella occurs in excess of 2% of deliveries after epidemic years and in 0.1% in endemic years.

A. Prevention

1. Expose girls to rubella before childbearing age or immunize young girls with rubella vaccine.
2. Avoid exposure of nonimmune pregnant females to rubella.
3. Immunize susceptible women of childbearing age.
   a. First demonstrate susceptibility to rubella (hemagglutination inhibition (HI) titers less than 1:10).
   b. Be certain that the recipient of the immunization is not pregnant (negative pregnancy test).
   c. Immunize
   d. Advise contraception for the next 3 months.
4. Termination of pregnancy, if desired, may be recommended if a woman is infected during the first trimester. Infection can be diagnosed by the rising titers of HI IgG antibodies from at least 2 weeks after contact.
5. Isolate infected newborns from nonimmune pregnant women, nonimmune nursery personnel, and other nonimmune newborns since rubella-infected infants are infectious to susceptible individuals.

B. Who Is at Risk?

Infants born to nonimmune pregnant women infected with rubella. Approximately 45% of those infants whose mothers are infected during the first month of the first trimester, 22% of those infants whose mothers are infected during the second month of the first trimester, and 7% of those infants whose mothers are infected during the third month of the first trimester are infected.

A maternal primary infection, not a past infection or reinfection, constitutes a hazard to the fetus and newborn.

C. Clinical Manifestations

The clinical manifestations of congenital rubella in the newbon vary widely from no evident disease to a chronic infectious state with multiple organ involvement persisting throughout the fetal period and the first few years of postnatal life. The time of exposure of the pregnant woman to rubella greatly influences the chance of defects. The disease is more severe and has a greater multiple organ involvement when acquired early, and subclinical infection is seen more frequently when acquired after the eighth week of gestation. Approximately 70% of subclinical infants develop evidence of disease at various times in the first 5 years.

Clinical manifestations include the following:

1. General
   Intrauterine growth retardation, delay in postnatal growth, poor weight gain, hypothermia or hyperthermia
2. Head
   Microcephaly
3. Eyes
   Cataracts, chorioretinitis, microphthalmos, rarely pigmentary retinopathy, cloudy cornea, glaucoma, hypoplasia of the iris and buphthalmus
4. Mouth
   Cleft palate, dental abnormalities
5. Ears
   Sensorineural deafness, central auditory impairment
6. Pulmonary
   Chronic diffuse interstitial pneumonitis
7. Cardiovascular
   Patent ductus arteriosus, branched pulmonary arterial stenosis, ventricular septal defect, myocarditis
8. CNS
   hypotonia
9. Skin
   Chronic rubelliform rash, thrombocytopenic purpura, "blueberry muffin" appearance (petechiae, purpura)
10. Abdomen
    Hepatosplenomegaly
11. Miscellaneous
    Autism, mental retardation, persistent adenopathy, recurrent infections, hypogammaglobinemia, abnormal dermatoglyphics, diabetes mellitus, chronic diarrhea, talipes equinovarus, syndactyly, hypospadias, speech defects

D. Radiologic Features

1. Poor mineralization of the skull with enlargement of the anterior fontanelle
2. Longitudinal radiolucent streaking of the long bones
3. Radiolucent areas at the knees
   (The skeletal abnormalities are self-correcting if the infant thrives.)

E. Laboratory Findings

1. In the mother during pregnancy
   a. Specific IgM antibodies measured by hemagglutination inhibition (HI), immunofluorescence, radioimmunoassay (RIA), or enzyme-linked immuno-

sorbent assay (ELISA) are detectable 5 to 10 days after the onset of the rash, peak rapidly at around 20 days, and decline and disappear by 50 to 70 days. A high titer of IgM antibodies indicates recent primary infection since reinfection does not usually give a booster IgM response.

   b. Specific IgG antibodies measured by hemagglutination inhibition, neutralization, RIA, ELISA, immunofluorescence, or precipitation assays become detectable 5 to 15 days after the onset of the rash, reach peak values at 15 to 30 days, and gradually decline over a period of years. Rising titers indicate recent disease.

2. In the newborn
   a. The virus can be isolated from nasopharyngeal washings, conjunctiva, urine, and spinal fluid at birth and up to 18 months of age.
   b. Specific IgM antibodies increase in the first 3 to 5 months after delivery while transplacental maternal IgG antibodies diminish. Thereafter, the IgM antibody decreases and IgG antibody becomes the dominant and persistent type for years. Therefore, the high specific IgM titer at birth or persistent, high, or rising HI IgG antibodies suggest intrauterine infection.
   c. Related laboratory findings include elevated cord serum total IgM (greater than 20 mg/dl), abnormal liver function tests, thrombocytopenia, increased CSF protein, impaired cell-mediated immunity, and occasional hypogammaglobulinemia.

F. Supportive Management

1. Isolate the infant from other infants and nonimmune pregnant women, as the infant sheds viruses for many months or years.
2. See chapter 16–IIIC for "general supportive management for the infant with infection."

G. Specific Therapy

No known chemotherapeutic or antibiotic agent will prevent or treat viremia in nonimmune persons exposed to rubella.

H. Prognosis

Extreme prematurity, gross cardiac lesion with early heart failure, rapidly progressive hepatitis, extensive meningoencephalitis, fulminant interstitial pneumonitis, and major life-threatening anatomic defects carry a poor prognosis for survival.

Sensorineural deafness, minimal-to-severe mental and psychomotor retardation, autism, failure to thrive, minimal-to-severe blindness, juvenile diabetes, and thyroid dysfunction are frequent sequelae.

REFERENCES

American Academy of Pediatrics, Committee on Infectious Diseases: Revised recommendations on rubella vaccine. *Pediatrics* 65:1182, 1980.

Dudgeon J.A.: Congenital rubella. *J. Pediatr.* 87:1078, 1975.

V. CYTOMEGALOVIRUS INFECTION

CMV is one of five known herpes viruses (herpesvirus hominis 1 and 2, herpesvirus varicellae, Epstein-Barr virus) that affect humans. In the United States, CMV can be isolated from approximately 3% to 28% of pregnant women at some time during pregnancy. Almost all infected women are asymptomatic. Congenital infection is present in 1% to 2% of newborns at the time of birth.

A. Prevention

1. If transfusion is necessary, give CMV antibody-negative blood.
2. Prevention depends on prevention of maternal infection presumably requiring the development of a safe, effective CMV vaccine that is under development, but not yet available.

B. Who Is at Risk?

The following infants should be closely observed for signs of CMV infection:

1. Infants whose mothers have had CMV infections with or without symptoms like a "cold" or "mononucleosis" during pregnancy
2. Infants exposed to perineal secretions from infected mothers during delivery
3. Infants who are premature or small for gestational age
4. Infants who are born to women of low socioeconomic status or women with multiple sexual partners
5. Small, sick, preterm infants in a neonatal intensive care unit setting who receive multiple blood transfusions
6. Infants receiving milk from women with CMV infection

C. Clinical Manifestations

1. Congenital CMV infection
   Maternal CMV immunity does not always protect against future intrauterine transmission, and approximately 50% to 82% of congenital infections are due to recurrent maternal infections. However, maternal immunity exerts a beneficial effect by reducing the virulence of fetal and neonatal infection. A congenital infection resulting from maternal primary infection is more serious than that resulting from recurrent maternal infection. CMV is not generally consid-

ered a teratogen; about 90% of infants with infection are asymptomatic, 5% of infants have atypical symptoms, and 5% of infants have typical symptoms of CMV infection.

a. Petechiae, hepatosplenomegaly, and jaundice are the most frequent signs.
b. Microcephaly with or without cerebral calcifications, intrauterine growth retardation, and prematurity are frequent signs.
c. Inguinal hernia and chorioretinitis are less common.
d. Pneumonitis is not common.
e. Hydrocephalus, strabismus, microphthalmia, optic atrophy, and cataracts may be seen.

2. Perinatal or postnatal CMV infection

A perinatal infection is acquired from exposure to infected maternal genital secretions during delivery (26% to 57%), from ingestion of infected breast milk (60%), or a transfusion that contains CMV. The incubation period ranges from 4 to 12 weeks. Infection from infected maternal cervical secretions or maternal milk is usually benign possibly due to transplacental transfer of maternal IgG. Perinatal CMV infection often manifests as the following:

a. Rapid deterioration, "septic" appearance, hepatosplenomegaly, interstitial pneumonitis, or exacerbation of pulmonary problems
b. Fatal or serious illnesses occur more frequently in perinatally infected infants of seronegative mothers than in infants of seropositive mothers (50% vs. 0%).

D. Radiologic Features

1. Periventricular calcifications in the subependymal region
2. Longitudinal radiolucent streaking of the long bones
3. Interstitial pneumonitis on chest x-ray film may be seen

E. Laboratory Findings

1. Specific diagnosis rests upon isolation of the virus from nasopharynx, conjunctiva, urine, or spinal fluid (best method of diagnosis). Viruria and pharyngeal shedding are present at brith in congenital infection and after 4 to 12 weeks of incubation in perinatal infection. Viruria is prolonged for years and may be intermittent, but is significant during the early months of life; lesser amounts of virus are excreted with time. Urine specimens for viral cultures should be stored at approximately 4°C for best result since storage and transportation at ambient temperature or freezing rapidly reduce infectivity.
2. Serologic test measuring CMV antibodies
   a. The complement fixation test detects primarily CMV-IgG antibody. Persistent rather than high titers during the first 4 to 6 months of age indicate congenital infection.
   b. The fluorescent antibody test detects CMV-IgM antibody. Specific CMV-IgM antibody can be interpreted as strong presumptive diagnosis of con-

genital CMV infection. Cross reactions to Epstein-Barr virus or varicella are seen. Antigen detected by immunofluorescence is diagnostic.

c. ELISA detects CMV-IgG and -IgM antibodies. This test is sensitive, rapid, and inexpensive.

3. Nonspecific laboratory findings
   a. Elevated cord serum IgM greater than 20 mg/dl (30% in asymptomatic infection and 3% in uninfected infants possibly due to maternofetal transfusion)
   b. Atypical lymphocytosis greater than 5%
   c. Abnormal liver function tests with elevated serum glutamic oxaloacetic transaminase (SGOT) greater than 80 mcU/ml and direct hyperbilirubinemia greater than 2 mg/dl
   d. Thrombocytopenia less than 100,000/cu mm
   e. Increased CSF protein greater than 180 mg/dl
   f. Typical enlarged cells containing intranuclear and cytoplasmic inclusions in the spinal fluid or freshly voided urine
   g. Hemolytic anemia
   h. Impaired cell-mediated immunity

F. Supportive Management

1. See chapter 16–IIIC for "general supportive management for the infant with infection."
2. Long-range plans to alleviate cerebral palsy and mental retardation are indicated. Monitor hearing and visual acuity. Support psychosocial needs of the family.

G. Specific Therapy

Presently, there is no effective treatment for CMV infections. Attempts have been made to treat severely infected newborns with adenine arabinoside (vidarabine, Ara-A) cytosine arabinoside (Ara-C) and Acyclovir. These drugs only temporarily suppress virus excretion and many infants already have irreversible damage before birth.

H. Prognosis

1. Congenital infection
   The mortality rate is 30% among seriously affected infants and the morbidity (handicap) rate is 90% of those with symptomatic congenital infection and 10% to 15% of those with asymptomatic infection.
   This morbidity includes delayed development (61%), neuromuscular disorders (35%), sensorineural hearing loss (30% to 50%), ocular abnormalities (22%), and dental anomalies with yellow discoloration and opaque and hypocalcified

enamel (40%). The progressive deterioration may increase the incidence and severity of developmental abnormality with time.
2. Perinatal infection
   The mortality rate is approximately 10%.

REFERENCES

Remington J.S., Klein J.O. (eds.): *Infectious Disease of the Fetus and Newborn Infant.* Philadelphia, W.B. Saunders Co., 1983, p. 104.

Stagno S., Pass R.F., Dworsky M.E., et al.: Congenital and perinatal cytomegalovirus infections. *Sem. Perinatol.* 7:31, 1983.

Stagno S., Pass R.F., Reynolds D.W., et al.: Comparative study of diagnostic procedures for congenital cytomegalovirus infection. *Pediatrics* 65:251, 1980.

VI. CONGENITAL TOXOPLASMOSIS

Toxoplasmosis is usually an asymptomatic protozoan disease of pregnant women but, through transplacental migration and invasion by the toxoplasma, may cause abortion, prematurity, congenital malformation, disseminated disease, or death of the fetus or newborn. The incidence of acquired toxoplasmosis is approximately 1 to 6 in 1,000 pregnant women and the incidence of congenital toxoplasmosis is about 0.5 to 3.0 in 1,000 live births. Ten percent of congenitally affected infants manifest disease in the newborn period; nearly all the remainder will eventually develop adverse sequelae.

A. Prevention

1. Serologically screen pregnant women as soon as possible for toxoplasmosis. Those at risk should be warned not to eat raw or uncooked meat or handle cat feces. Meat should be cooked to greater than 66°C. Touching the mucous membranes of the mouth and eyes should be avoided while handling raw meat. Transmission occurs during the acute infection in the pregnant woman, and toxoplasmosis could be almost entirely prevented if acquired infection during pregnancy was prevented.
2. Disinfect the cat litter box for 5 minutes with nearly boiling water every day.
3. Treatment of the mother during pregnancy results in approximately 50% reduction in infected infants.

B. Who Is at Risk?

1. Infants born to mothers who acquire toxoplasmosis during pregnancy through ingestion of raw meat (steak tartare) or from handling cat feces, especially during the third trimester. Most mothers are asymptomatic and diagnosis has to be made by rising antibody titers. The incidence of congenital toxoplasmosis is approximately 50% in these infants. Subsequent pregnancies are very rarely affected.

2. Transmission through human milk has not been demonstrated.
3. Prematures are at risk, particularly with low Apgar scores.

C. Clinical Manifestations

If toxoplasmosis is acquired during the last months of pregnancy, the protozoa is most frequently transmitted to the fetus, but the infection is subclinical in the newborn. If the mother is infected earlier, transmission to the fetus occurs less often, but frequently results in severe disease.

1. Neonatal disease
   CNS symptoms with or without generalized infection, hepatosplenomegaly, jaundice, anemia, chorioretinitis, lymphadenopathy, hypothermia, fever, vomiting, diarrhea, rash, petechiae, ecchymosis, nephrotic syndrome, pneumonitis, myocarditis, convulsions, hydrocephaly, microcephaly, etc.
2. Disease in the first months of life
   The disease is usually not recognized in the newborn period. Delayed onset during 2 to 3 months of life may be severe with severe CNS or eye lesions often in premature infants or mild with generalized symptoms, CNS involvement, or eye lesions in fullterm infants.
3. Sequelae or relapse of a previously undiagnosed infection during infancy, childhood, or adolescence
   a. Ocular lesions: chorioretinitis (central, bilateral, often recognized at 15 to 20 years of age), strabismus, cataracts, glaucoma, optic atrophy, microphthalmos, anisometropia
   b. Neurologic findings: convulsions, hydrocephaly, microcephaly, psychomotor and mental retardation, epilepsy, deafness
4. Subclinical infections

D. Radiologic Features

1. Diffuse, scattered nodular or lineal cerebral calcification (as opposed to bilateral periventricular calcifications in CMV, but overlap occurs) seen under 2 years of age in 80% of cases
2. Hydrocephalus
3. Bands of metaphyseal longitudinal lucency in long bones
4. Irregularity of the lines of provisional calcification in long bones
5. Computerized tomography (CT) scan that allows for neuroanatomic localization of intracranial calcifications, delineation of ventricular size, and recognition of cortical atrophy may be of value in evaluation of congenital toxoplasmosis.

E. Laboratory Findings

1. Isolation of the parasite from body fluid and tissues proves the diagnosis, but it takes approximately 4 to 6 weeks. Parasites persist in tissue for years.

2. Specific serologic test
   Demonstration of IgM antibodies to *Toxoplasma* in cord serum or infant's serum is diagnostic of congenital toxoplasmosis. However, in 25% to 75% of patients, specific IgM may not be detected until maternally transmitted antibody decreases to a low titer. Therefore, follow-up of specific IgG at birth and at 6 to 9 months of age may be the only means of diagnosis in some cases.
   a. IgM fluorescent test
      A high false negative test result in 50% to 75% of congenital toxoplasmosis, in immunodeficient patients, and in isolated ocular toxoplasmosis and a false positive test result in the presence of rheumatoid factor are noted.
   b. IgM ELISA
      The double sandwich IgM ELISA is positive in 73% of congenital toxoplasmosis and avoids a false positive test result due to rheumatoid factor.
   c. Sabin-Feldman dye test
      When parasites are incubated with methylene blue in the absence of antibodies, the parasites become swollen, whereas parasites with antibody plus methylene blue do not swell (single, most reliable test to detect antibodies).
   d. IgG ELISA test detects antigenemia in 65% of patients.
3. Nonspecific tests
   a. Elevated CSF protein (usually greater than 500 mg%)
   b. Increased IgM antibodies greater than 20 mg/dl in the first week of life
   c. Thrombocytopenia, anemia, leukopenia, leukocytosis, eosinophilia
   d. Delay in IgA development

F. Supportive Management

See chapter 16–IIIC for "general supportive management for the infant with infection."

G. Specific Therapy

An exact regimen for best results has not been established.

1. Pyrimethamine, 1 mg/kg/day in two divided doses orally for 3 to 4 days, then 0.5 mg/kg/day for 21 to 30 days; in addition, sulfadiazine, 50 to 100 mg/kg/day in two divided doses for 21 to 30 days, and folinic acid, 2 to 6 mg orally two to three times/week
   Therapy may be repeated up to three times in the first year of life, depending on clinical evidence of disease activity.
   Caution: Do not use sulfadiazine in the presence of jaundice in the newborn. Follow CBC and platelet count weekly as leukopenia and anemia may occur.
2. Isolation is not necessary.
3. Serologic follow-up of asymptomatic antibody-positive infants is recommended at 4- to 6-week intervals to allow treatment or retreatment. When the serologic titer is rising or unchanged, treatment is desirable.

H. Prognosis

The overall mortality rate is 12%.

The extraneural organs have slight or insignificant residual lesions because of regeneration while CNS and eyes have more severe permanent damage because of inability of nerve cells to regenerate.

Adverse sequelae including psychomotor retardation, intellectual deficits, cerebellar dysfunction, seizures, severe visual impairment, and deafness occur in more than 90% of the infected infants. There is no correlation between neurologic outcome and birth weight, race, or age.

REFERENCES

Balsari A., Poli G., Molina V., et al.: ELISA for toxoplasma antibody detection: A comparison with other serodiagnostic tests. *J. Clin. Pathol.* 33:640, 1980.

Stray-Pedersen B.: Infants potentially at risk for congenital toxoplasmosis: A prospective study. *Am. J. Dis. Child.* 134:638, 1980.

Wilson C.B., Remington J.S., Stagno S., et al.: Development of adverse sequelae in children born with subclinical congenital toxoplasma infection. *Pediatrics* 66:767, 1980.

VII. HERPES SIMPLEX

Herpes simplex virus (HSV) infection may be acquired at the time of delivery from maternal genital herpes by contact or ascending infection, rarely during pregnancy from transplacental infection, and not uncommonly after delivery from close contact with family members or nursery personnel with genital or labial herpes type I or II. An increased rate of abortion, stillbirth, prematurity, and small-for-date infants has been reported in mothers with genital herpes. The incidence of infection in the newborn is approximately 1 per 3,500 to 7,000 live births. The majority of infections in older individuals are insignificant or undetected while the majority of infections in newborns are disseminating and fulminant.

A. Prevention

When genital herpes is suspected because of clinical manifestations or diagnosed with positive cultures and/or Pap smear at term or within 1 week of delivery:

1. Obtain cultures and Pap smear at 32, 34, and 36 weeks of gestation and weekly thereafter.
2. Treat the mother with systemic antiviral (oral Acyclovir) therapy for primary and recurrent genital disease since maternal therapy may prevent neonatal infection although its effects on the fetus are not known.
3. Counsel the pregnant woman to avoid sexual contact including oral-genital contact with the partner with genital herpes during the last months of pregnancy.
4. Avoid fetal scalp monitoring.

5. Deliver the infant by cesarean section as soon as labor starts if the mother has primary genital herpes infection with intact membranes or rupture of the membranes for less than 4 to 6 hours or if the mother has had a recurrent infection within 1 to 2 weeks prior to delivery. Cesarean section does not always prevent infection particularly if there is prolonged rupture of the membranes.
6. Isolate the infant in a crib or incubator and isolate the mother in a private room with gown and glove precautions.
7. Avoid breast feeding if the mother has a history of herpetic breast lesions.
8. Educate the mother and other family members with regard to the risk of infection in the newborn.
9. Educate the mother to wear gloves and gown and adhere to strict handwashing precautions.
10. Permit the mother to handle her infant wearing gloves and gown.

B. Who Is at Risk?

1. Infants born vaginally to mothers with positive cultures and/or Pap smears for herpes or clinical genital herpes within 2 weeks of delivery. The risk is highest in a primary genital infection at the time of delivery with prolonged rupture of the membranes. About 40% to 60% of infants born to mothers with a positive culture at delivery develop HSV infection. At least half of mothers with primary genital herpes are subclinical.
2. Infants born vaginally to mothers with a prior history of genital herpes. Only one fourth of genital HSV infections are clinically diagnosable and recurrent genital herpes is common.
3. Infants born vaginally to mothers with HSV infection below the waist in the past or during current pregnancy since concommitant genital herpes infection is common
4. Infants born to mothers who have had sexual contact at any time with males with genital herpes
5. Infants who have contact with HSV infected personnel.

C. Clinical Manifestations

Neonatal infection with HSV is almost always associated with clinical findings. The infant usually (but not always) appears well at birth. Signs and symptoms develop within the first 2 weeks.

1. Disseminated infection

   Disseminated infection primarily involves liver, adrenal glands, lungs, and CNS (50%), but other organs including skin, oral cavity, and eyes may be involved.

   Clinical findings are nonspecific. These include poor feeding, vomiting, lethargy, fever, irritability, convulsions, jaundice, hepatomegaly, purpura, erythematous rash, apneic spells, cyanosis, respiratory distress, shock, herpetic skin vesicles in about one half of cases, ulcers in the oral cavity, and keratitis. More than one half of cases are prematures. Mortality is 80%.

2. Localized infections without disseminated infection
   Average onset is slightly delayed to 11 days.
   a. CNS: lethargy, irritability, tremors, convulsions in one half of patients with CNS involvement, 40% mortality
   b. Eyes: keratoconjunctivitis, chorioretinitis, microphthalmia, retinal dysplasia
   c. Skin: vesicular eruption to bullous type lesions, rarely erythematous macular exanthem, purpuric spots, petechiae. The skin lesions may rapidly denude.
   d. Oral cavity: ulcers
3. Subclinical infections
   Neonatal HSV infections are almost always associated with clinical findings.
4. Congenital infections
   Congenital infections are rare, but reported with congenital malformations; intracranial calcifications, microcephaly, hypertonicity, seizures, severe mental retardation, microphthalmos, retinal dysplasia, chorioretinitis, patent ductus anteriosus, short digits, and recurrent skin lesions. Abortion and prematurity have also been reported to be associated with congenital herpes infection.

D. Radiologic Features

Pneumonitis or pleural effusion is seen in approximately 20% of cases.

E. Laboratory Findings

1. Definite diagnosis rests upon isolation of the virus from skin lesions or urine, blood, CSF, throat, or eye specimens. Direct isolation or typing of the isolate as HSV-1 or HSV-2 or immunofluorescence demonstrating HSV 1 or 2 antigens can be utilized.
2. Cytologic tests and Pap smears (60% to 75% accuracy) establish a presumptive diagnosis. Cell scrapings from the base of skin vesicles, cervicovagina, oral ulcers, or conjunctival or corneal lesions show typical multinucleated giant cells and intranuclear inclusions.
3. Complement-fixation tests do not differentiate HSV-1 from HSV-2. Serologic tests for HSV-specific antibody are not useful in diagnosis of acute disease.
4. Nonspecific laboratory findings include thrombocytopenia, prolonged PT and PTT, elevated SGOT, SGPT, and direct bilirubin, increased CSF cells (usually lymphocytes) and protein, and normal or decreased CSF glucose. See appendix A–13, A–29, A–39, A–40 for normal values.

F. Supportive Management

See chapter 16–IIIC for "general supportive management for the infant with infection."

1. Avoid circumcision in the first 2 weeks of life.
2. Obtain baseline herpes serology, CBC, spinal tap, liver function test, and cultures of eye and mouth every 3 to 4 days for the first 2 weeks.
3. Observe the infant for clinical signs of HSV infection for 2 weeks (incubation period, 2 to 12 days) in the hospital if born vaginally and at home after discharge. If born by cesarean section, the infant needs to be observed for only a few days in the hospital.
4. Transplacental antibody has not yet proven effective so that active immunization of women prior to pregnancy or booster immunization in late pregnancy may not be of value.
5. Bar infected personnel from the nursery.
6. Administer topical antiviral eye ointment (adenine arabinoside A) for high-risk infants for 5 days to prevent herpetic keratoconjunctivitis (controversial).

G. Specific Therapy

1. Approximately 80% of infants with local disease progress to disseminated disease. There is no way to predict which infant will progress to the disseminated category. Therapy should be started as early as possible with one of the following:
   a. Acyclovir, 30 mg/kg/day IV divided into 3 doses is presently the therapy of choice. A number of clinical trials have shown that Acyclovir is equal or superior to iododeoxyuridine or vidarabin in healing herpes keratitis.
   b. Vidarabine (adenine arabinoside), 30 mg/kg/24 hours IV (vidarabine has less toxicity than iododeoxyuridine and cytosine arabinoside). Vidarabin is particularly utilized for localized disease.
   c. Iododeoxyridine can be used topically in the eyes if diagnosis is strongly suspected and has been shown to be of some benefit.
   d. Cytosine arabinoside has been used systematically for the treatment of infant herpes simplex. Toxicity includes depressed hematopoiesis and immune responses and prohibits usage now.
   e. Hyperimmune HSV globulin (available for research purposes at the present time).

H. Prognosis

The overall mortality rate is approximately 50% and neurologic sequelae are often devastating.

1. Disseminated infections, with or without CNS involvement, frequently result in death (in 70% to 80% of cases) or serious sequelae of psychomotor retarda-

tion, microcephaly, hydrocephaly, apnea, seizure disorder, optic atrophy, cataracts, and chorioretinitis.

2. Localized infection of the skin, oral cavity, or eyes is associated with a lesser mortality (less than 40%) and morbidity, but longterm CNS, psychomotor, and ocular derangement and late death up to 1.5 years after acute disease are common.

REFERENCES

American Academy of Pediatrics, Committee on Fetus and Newborn and Committee on Infectious Diseases: Perinatal herpes simplex virus infections. *Pediatrics* 66:147, 1980.

Kibrick S.: Herpes simplex infection at term. *J.A.M.A.* 243:157, 1980.

Remington J.S., Klein J.O. (eds.): *Infectious Disease of the Fetus and Newborn Infant.* Philadelphia, W.B. Saunders Co., 1983, p. 636.

VIII. VARICELLA (Chickenpox)

Varicella (chicken pox), an acute contagious disease of childhood, complicates 1 to 5 in 10,000 pregnancies. The effect upon the fetus or infant depends upon the time in pregnancy the disease was contracted.

A. Prevention

1. If the mother does not have a history of varicella, isolate the mother during pregnancy from any individual with varicella.
2. A mother with varicella with the onset of less than 5 days prior to delivery to 48 hours postdelivery should not have contact with her infant until all her vesicles are dry. If the mother had varicella during pregnancy before 5 days prior to delivery, it is not necessary to separate the mother from her infant because the infant is already exposed.
3. Isolate the infant with congenital varicella from other nonimmune infants because varicella is transmitted to susceptible newborns.
4. Prevent newborn contact with siblings, children, or adults who have contracted varicella.
5. Between 9 and 20 days, exclude the nonimmune nursery and delivery personnel with flourescent antibody membrane antigen (FAMA) antibody less than 1:4 from care of the varicella-affected infant.
6. Vaccines for varicella are under investigation.

B. Who Is at Risk?

1. Infants born to mothers with varicella in the first trimester may develop congenital malformations.
2. Infants born to mothers with varicella presenting less than 5 days prior to

delivery to 48 hours postdelivery can develop severe disseminated neonatal infection in about 17%, and the mortality is 30% if infants develop congenital varicella. Maternal varicella 5 days to 3 weeks prior to delivery results in mild disease with typical lesions of varicella (no deaths reported).

3. Infants born to mothers who have not had varicella and who come in contact with newborns, children, or adults with active disease may develop neonatal varicella.

C. Clinical Manifestations

Clinical manifestations vary from very mild with only a few crops to fulminant disease.

1. Perinatal varicella includes congenital varicella with the onset within 10 days of life (incubation period, 9 to 15 days) and postnatally acquired varicella with the onset between 10 and 28 days of life. Approximately 24% of infants of mothers with varicella with onset in the 21 days prior to delivery or within 17 days after delivery develop varicella.
2. Erythematous papules that develop into nonumbilicated vesicles appear at birth or within 1 to 2 weeks of age in infants born to mothers with active infection in the last month of pregnancy. Rarely, meningoencephalitis, hepatitis, pneumonia, and other visceral lesions ensue. The severity of the mother's illness does not appear to affect the course of illness in the infant.
3. Congenital varicella early in pregnancy (7 to 20 weeks of gestation) results in anomalies including skin scarring, muscle atrophy, hypoplastic extremity, atrophic digits, club feet, encephalitis, cortical atrophy, ocular anomalies, etc.

D. Radiologic Features

No distinctive features are seen.

E. Laboratory Findings

1. The virus may be isolated in tissue culture.
2. Viral (varicella zoster) antigen may be obtained from vesicular fluid by the countercurrent immunoelectrophoresis technique. This is the most rapid method.
3. Serologic tests for antibodies
   A complement fixation titer rise occurs in 2 weeks, but the test is insensitive. FAMA is the most sensitive and specific test. Immune adherence hemagglutination antibody or ELISA may be used.

F. Supportive Management

See chapter 16–IIIC for "general supportive management for the infant with infection."

G. Specific Therapy

1. For the infant born to the mother who developed varicella in the last 4 days of pregnancy or within 2 days after delivery
   a. Administer zoster-immune globulin (ZIG), 0.1 ml/kg IM, or varicella zoster immune globulin (VZIG), 1.25 ml (125 units) IM, within 48 hours postdelivery. ZIG or VZIG does not prevent the infection and is ineffective for the treatment of varicella, but may modify the infection.
   b. Isolate the infant in the hospital and discharge before 10 days of age. If the infant needs to stay in the hospital, strict isolation is necessary until 21 days of age.
2. For infants exposed to varicella postnatally in the nursery
   Normal fullterm infants do not require ZIG or VZIG, but premature infants less than 28 weeks of gestational age should receive 1.25 ml VZIG or ZIG because of inadequate transplacental antibodies.
3. For infants with varicella
   Adenine arabinoside (vidarabine), 15 mg/kg/day for 7 to 10 days, may be used for severe varicella. The efficacy and toxicity are not clear. Acyclovir and interferon have therapeutic potential. A multicenter control trial is in progress.

H. Prognosis

1. Transplacentally transmitted varicella: depends on time of presentation of varicella rash in the mother (chapter 16–VIIIB)
2. Postnatally acquired varicella: presenting within 10 to 28 days postbirth is generally mild

REFERENCES

American Academy of Pediatrics, Committee on Infectious Diseases: Expanded guidelines for use of varicella-zoster immune globulin. *Pediatrics* 72:886, 1983.

Evans E.B., Pollock T.M., Cradock-Watson J.E. et al.: Human anti-chickenpox immune globulin in the prevention of chickenpox. *Lancet* 1:354, 1980.

Frey H.M., Steinberg S.P., Gershon A.A.: Rapid diagnosis of varicella-zoster virus infections by countercurrent immuno-electrophoresis. *J. Infect. Dis.* 143:274, 1981.

IX. COXSACKIE B VIRUS INFECTIONS

The group B coxsackieviruses most commonly produce mild infection but on occasion may cause severe myocarditis, pleurodynia, or meningoencephalitis. Transplacental passage has been proven and intrauterine infection and infection acquired at birth have been reported. Neonatal infections are relatively common and several epidemics in newborn nurseries have been reported. There is a high incidence in July through October.

A. Prevention

1. Isolate newborns from adults with pleurodynia and upper respiratory infections.
2. Isolate infants with possible coxsackievirus infection (symptoms of upper respiratory infection or diarrhea).
3. Maintain good handwashing technique since transmission is via feces to skin (adult to infant or infant to adult).

B. Who Is at Risk?

1. Infants born to mothers with minor respiratory (coxsackieviral) infections in the third trimester (transplacental passage of the virus)
2. Infants exposed to infants, children, or adults with coxsackieviral infection, e.g., pleurodynia and/or myalgia

C. Clinical Manifestations

Clinical manifestations are nonspecific and usually occur between 5 to 7 days of life. Some patients exhibit a progressive course and some a diphasic pattern. Aseptic meningitis and encephalitis are frequent. Lethargy, irritability, vomiting, hypothermia or hyperthermia, diarrhea, anorexia, apnea, and convulsions have been associated with meningoencephalitis.

Myocarditis is the most prominent feature in the newborn and is characterized by cardiomegaly, tachycardia, dyspnea, rales, cyanosis, and hypertension. Hepatosplenomegaly, jaundice, and disseminated intravascular coagulation may be present, as may be diarrhea and signs of adrenal failure. A maculopapular rash is occasionally present.

D. Radiologic Features

1. Cardiomegaly
2. Patchy infiltration in the lung parenchyma

E. Laboratory Findings

1. Specific tests
   a. Isolation of virus from CSF, throat, rectal swabs, blood, and urine is diagnostic. Coxsackie B_2, B_3, and B_4 infections are associated with extremely severe disease and myocarditis.
   b. Serologic evidence of increasing antibody titers occurs during convalescence. (Hemagglutination inhibition or complement fixation tests require 2 to 4 weeks before a titer rise is present.)
   c. ELISA may be used for rapid detection of the virus antigen.

2. Nonspecific tests
   a. ECG findings of myocarditis
   b. Elevated white blood cell count and protein levels and decreased glucose in the CSF
   c. Elevated serum IgM level greater than 20 mg/dl
   d. Elevated peripheral white blood cells

F. Supportive Management

See chapter 16–IIIC for "general supportive management for the infant with infection."

G. Specific Therapy

1. No specific therapy is known.
2. Treatment with corticosteroids is contraindicated.
3. Treat congestive heart failure with digitalis and diuretics (see chapter 11–XXIX). *Caution:* With myocarditis, the heart is extremely sensitive to digitalis; start with small doses.
4. Administer 1.0 ml/kg IM of immune globulin to the infant with fulminating infection.

H. Prognosis

Infection may proceed rapidly to fatal outcome or complete recovery. Sequelae may include ocular abnormalities, spasticity, mental retardation, seizure disorders, spastic quadriplegia, hypertonicity, microcephaly, and delayed speech and language development.

REFERENCES

Kaplan M.H., Klein S.W., McPhee J., et al.: Group B Coxsackievirus infections in infants younger than three months of age: A serious childhood illness. *Rev. Infect. Dis.* 5:1019, 1983.

Marier R., Rodriguez W., Chloupek R.J., et al.: Coxsackievirus B5 infection and aseptic meningitis in neonates and children. *Am. J. Dis. Child.* 129:321, 1975.

X. CONGENITAL SYPHILIS

Congenital syphilis, a disease recognized since the 17th century, has an incidence of 1 in 5,000 live births today. Syphilitic infection of the pregnant female may result in fetal death, premature delivery, and/or an infected newborn. It is rare to make a definitive diagnosis with identified organisms, but a presumptive diagnosis may be made on the basis of high or rising serologic test for syphilis (STS) and/or clinical manifestations with positive STS.

A. Prevention

All pregnant woman should be tested for syphilis during the first trimester and the test repeated prior to delivery to detect infection.

B. Who is at Risk?

1. Infants born to inadequately or untreated syphilitic mothers (50% chance via transplacental or through contact with an infectious lesion during delivery)
2. Infants born to unmarried teenage, drug-addicted, or "no prenatal care" mothers

C. Clinical Manifestations

1. Infants usually are asymptomatic at birth but may be severely hydropic or become symptomatic several months later.
   Jaundice in the first 24 hours of life, associated with hepatosplenomegaly, is frequently the presenting sign. Congenital syphilis may present as nephrotic syndrome.
2. Physical findings in early congenital syphilis (first 2 years) include failure to thrive, alopecia areata, chorioretinitis, iritis, glaucoma, rhinitis, snuffles (mucopurulent bloody discharge), pneumonitis (pneumonia alba), hepatosplenomegaly, maculopapular rash (on palms or soles) with or without desquamation or bullae, lymphadenopathy, edema, deformed nails, and pseudoparesis of Parrot.

D. Radiologic Features

1. Metaphyseal and diaphyseal involvement of long bones is the most common manifestation.
   a. Metaphyseal dystrophy
      1) Enhanced zone of calcification (radiopaque bands) with osteoporosis under the dense zone
      2) Metaphyseal longitudinal radiolucency ("celery stalk" appearance)
      3) Wimberger's sign (bilateral demineralization and destruction of proximal medial tibial metaphysis)
      4) Saw tooth appearance due to irregular demineralization
   b. Periosteal dystrophy
      Single or multiple periosteal elevations, layers of new bone formation extending along the cortex of the entire diaphysis
2. Pneumonic infiltrations

E. Laboratory Findings

1. Dark-field demonstration of treponema from mucopurulent bloody nasal discharge, bullae, chondylomas, etc., is diagnostic.

2. STS

When the infant's STS titers are fourfold or greater than the maternal titer, rising or persistently elevated in weeks to months after birth, a presumptive diagnosis may be made.

   a. The VDRL test detects antibodies to cardiolipin, a constituent of treponema. False positives may occur with concurrent viral, mycoplasmal or protozoal infection, lupus, Hansen's disease, drugs, etc.
   b. Fluorescent treponemal antibody absorption test (FTA-ABS): This test uses non-*pallidum Treponema* to detect antibodies.
      All patients with disseminated and late infection and 90% of those with primary syphilis have a positive FTA-ABS test. The FTA-ABS test remains positive for life and is limited to the initial infection.
   c. The micro-*T. pallidum* hemagglutination antibody (TPHA) test is now coming into general use and is an easy quantitative test requiring a small volume of serum. MHA-TP is an automated version of the TPHA using minute quantities of serum and other reagents.
   d. RIA and ELISA are not yet standardized for clinical use in diagnosing syphilis but may be employed shortly.

3. Nonspecific laboratory findings
   a. Hemolytic anemia, thrombocytopenia, direct and/or indirect hyperbilirubinemia, leukocytosis or leukemoid reaction, lymphocytosis, monocytosis
   b. Azotemia, hematuria, or proteinuria in nephrosis (see Chapter 18–X)
   c. Increased CSF cells and protein
   d. Elevated IgM greater than 20 mg/dl in the first week of life

F. Supportive Management

See chapter 16–IIIC for "general supportive management for the infant with infection."

G. Specific Therapy

1. Maternal infection
   a. Early syphilis less than 1 year's duration: primary, secondary, or early latent
      Benzathine penicillin G, 2.4 million units IM for 1 dose; or aqueous procaine penicillin G, 600,000 units/24 hours IM for 8 days
   b. Latent syphilis more than 1 year's duration without neurosyphilis
      Benzathine penicillin G, 2.4 million units/week IM for 3 weeks; or procaine penicillin G, 600,000 units/24 hours IM for 15 days
   c. Latent syphilis with neurosyphilis
      Procaine penicillin G, 600,000 units twice per 24 hours IM for 2 to 3 weeks
      If mother is allergic to penicillin, cephaloridine, 0.5 gm daily orally for 10 days, or erythromycin, 40 mg/kg/24 hours orally for 10 days.
      Erythromycin may fail to cure the fetus.

2. Newborns
   a. Treat newborns with a positive VDRL test immediately in the following situations:
      1) When the infant has clinical manifestations such as hydrops fetalis, hepatosplenomegaly, jaundice, mucocutaneous or hematologic manifestations, or nephrotic syndrome
      2) When the infant's VDRL titers are a fourfold or higher than the mother's titer at birth even without clinical manifestations
      3) When the infant's VDRL titers are positive but not significantly higher than the mother's and the infant is asymptomatic, but has abnormal laboratory findings consistent with congenital syphilis such as elevated IgM at birth or abnormal hematologic, radiographic, or CSF findings
      4) When the mother was not treated or inadequately treated for early or latent syphilis
      5) When the mother is unreliable and adequate treatment is not assured
   b. Treatment schedule
      1) Without neurosyphilis
         Benzathine penicillin G, 50,000 units/kg IM in a single dose
      2) With neurosyphilis
         Aqueous penicillin G, 50,000 units/kg/24 hours divided into 2 doses IM or IV for 10 days; or procaine penicillin G, 50,000 units/kg/24 hours IM for 10 days
   c. Repeat VDRL titers monthly until 6 months of age.
      Additional spinal tap is required. Titers begin to fall 2 months after therapy.
   d. Observe newborns and follow and repeat VDRL test in the following situations:
      1) Seropositive newborns born of adequately treated mothers require a serologic test for syphilis at frequent intervals until 1 year of age. If at any time during the period of observation the infant shows a significant rise in titer, the titer remains positive, or any clinical signs appear, treatment should be instituted.
      2) Seronegative newborns born of inadequately treated mothers should be followed in a manner similar to no. G2d1) if the mother is reliable. If the mother is unreliable, the infant should be treated. If the results of the serology test become positive, the infant should be treated.
      3) Newborns with a negative cord serology born of adequately treated mothers need no specific treatment or period of observation.

H. Prognosis

Severity of infection and damage done prior to intrauterine or postnatal treatment influence the prognosis. The prognosis for symptomatic syphilis present at birth is usually poor. Prognosis is excellent if adequate treatment is given to the asymptomatic infant at birth.

REFERENCES

Bryan E.M., Nicholson E.: Congenital syphilis: A study of physical and biochemical aspects. *Clin. Pediatr.* 20:81, 1981.

XI. TUBERCULOSIS

Transplacental or hematogenous tubercular infection of the newborn is rare. The newborn infant, however, when exposed to the tubercle bacillus is quite susceptible to tuberculosis. Such exposure can occur transplacentally, during labor or delivery if the mother has miliary tuberculosis, or the infant can be infected directly from the maternal sputum if the mother has infected sputum. Routes of transmission are hematogenous from an infected placenta, ingestion from infected amniotic fluid, aspiration of amniotic fluid, and inhalation of tubercles from mother.

A. Prevention

1. Treat pregnant women who have active tuberculosis with isoniazid (INH) and/or other appropriate antibiotics.
2. Administer bacille Calmette-Guérin (BCG) vaccine at birth to infants born to mothers who have been adequately treated.

B. Who is at Risk?

1. Infants born to mothers with unrecognized and/or untreated active tuberculosis
2. Infants of families whose members have tuberculosis
3. Infants born to mothers in a low socioeconomic class

C. Clinical Manifestations

1. The infant usually appears well at birth, may feed well, but not thrive. Within the first 6 weeks or later, the infant can suddenly die or develop respiratory distress, usually with cyanosis, nasal discharge, cough, or generalized signs of sepsis, including poor feeding, poor cry, poor activity, lethargy, poor weight gain, hypothermia, hyperthermia, anemia, irritability, etc. Frequently, hepatomegaly with or without splenomegaly is present. Skin lesions (papular, pustular) may be present.
2. In prenatal infection, the liver is extensively involved early. Meningitis with CNS manifestation, lymphadenopathy, splenomegaly, and biliary obstruction are also common.

D. Radiologic Features

Chest x-ray films are abnormal in about 80% of cases. Chest x-ray films may show a miliary pattern if transmission is hematogenous, patchy infiltration, widespread areas of consolidation, and hilar gland enlargement, with or without cavitation and miliary spread. Segmental or lobar collapse may occur due to compression of the bronchi by hilar lymphadenopathy.

E. Laboratory Findings

1. Specific findings
   a. Recovery of the organism on smear and culture of nose, trachea, gastric washings (75%), urine, and spinal fluid is diagnostic.
   b. The tuberculin test is helpful if positive, but it is usually negative in 90% of newborns. It will become positive by 3 to 6 weeks of age.
   c. A liver biopsy may be positive if the infection is transplacental. A skin biopsy may be helpful if lesions are present.
   d. The value of complement fixation, hemagglutination, and lymphocyte stimulation tests is currently being explored.
2. Nonspecific findings
   a. Altered findings in CSF are rare.
   b. Liver function tests may be altered.
   c. Relative lymphocytosis

F. Supportive Management

See chapter 16–IIIC for "general supportive management for the infant with infection."

G. Specific Therapy

1. The infant born to a mother who has been adequately treated for tuberculosis and has a negative culture
   a. Maternal separation after birth is not necessary if the mother's sputum is negative.
   b. Obtain a chest x-ray film and perform a tuberculin test at birth and again at 6 weeks of age.
   c. Administer BCG vaccination at 6 weeks of age if the infant's tuberculin test and chest x-ray film are negative or follow the infant frequently to rule out postnatal infection.
2. The infant born to an untreated or inadequately treated mother whose sputum culture is positive for tuberculosis

a. Separate the mother from the infant if the mother has a positive sputum culture.
b. Obtain a tuberculin test and chest x-ray film at birth and again at 6 weeks of age.
c. If the tuberculin test and x-ray film are negative and the infant is asymptomatic at 6 weeks of age:
   1) Administer BCG vaccination.
   2) Separate the mother from the infant for 6 weeks after administration of BCG or until the maternal sputum is negative.
d. If the infant's reaction to the tuberculin test is positive, treat the infant with INH, 10 mg/kg/24 hours, if the maternal organism is sensitive to INH or if a sensitivity test is unavailable.

3. The clinically well infant born to a mother with miliary tuberculosis
   a. Separate the mother from the infant.
   b. Perform a tuberculin test and obtain a chest x-ray film.
      Also collect gastric washings and the infant's urine for smear, culture, and sensitivity.
   c. Depending upon the results of the maternal sensitivity tests, administer the appropriate drugs or INH, 10 mg/kg/24 hours, for 3 months if the maternal organism is sensitive to INH or if a sensitivity test is unavailable.
   d. If after 3 months of INH therapy, the results of the tuberculin test and chest x-ray film are negative, administer BCG vaccine.
4. The clinically ill newborn born to a mother with miliary tuberculosis
   a. Separate the mother from the infant.
   b. Perform a tuberculin test and obtain a chest x-ray film.
      Also obtain gastric washings and the infant's urine for smear, culture and, sensitivity. (Note: A false negative tuberculin test may be obtained.)
   c. Depending upon the results of the maternal sensitivity tests, administer the appropriate drugs or the following:
      1) INH, 10 to 20 mg/kg/24 hours once a day for a year, if the maternal organism is sensitive to INH or if a sensitivity test is unavailable; supplemental pyridoxin is not recommended since neurotoxicity is not generally encountered in infants with INH therapy, and
      2) Streptomycin, 40 mg/kg/2 days or 20 mg/kg/day IM once a day for 3 to 6 months if the maternal organism is resistant to INH or if the infant fails to respond to INH

H. Prognosis

Without therapy, death ensues within a few weeks to a few months. The mortality rate is recently reported to be about 50%. Early diagnosis and chemotherapy are essential to prevent morbidity and mortality. Infants presenting symptoms 4 weeks later have somewhat higher survival rate. It has been reported that surviving infants did not have obvious neurologic sequelae in the first year of life in a recent study.

REFERENCES

Avery M.E., Wolfsdorf J.: Diagnosis and treatment: Approaches to newborn infants of tuberculous mothers. *Pediatrics* 42:519, 1969.

Hageman J., et al.: Congenital tuberculosis: Critical re-appraisal of clinical findings and diagnostic procedures. *Pediatrics* 66:980, 1980.

Polansky S.M., Frank A., Ablow R.C., et al.: Congenital tuberculosis. *Am. J. Roentgenol.* 130:994, 1978.

XII. HEPATITIS

Viral hepatitis is caused by hepatitis A virus (with short incubation), hepatitis B virus (with long incubation), or hepatitis non-A, non-B virus. Hepatitis A and non-A, non-B viruses are no or little problem to the infant while hepatitis B virus (HBV) may cause chronic hepatitis, a carrier state or fulminating disease.

Vertical transmission of HBV infection from mothers with acute hepatitis during pregnancy or with hepatitis B surface antigen (HB_sAg) carrier state to the infant is possible. The incidence of HB_sAg carriers in the United States ranges between 0.1% and 0.5% while it is as high as 20% in hyperendemic areas such as Asia, sub-Saharan Africa, and the Pacific Islands. Maternal viral hepatitis has not been reported to increase the incidence of congenital malformations, stillbirths, spontaneous abortions, or low birth weight, but increases the prematurity rate to 25%–32%.

A. Prevention

1. When the mother has acute hepatitis B in the last trimester or chronic HB_sAg carrier state
   a. Administer hepatitis B immunoglobulin (HBIG), 0.5 ml within 12–24 hours of age and hepatitis B vaccine 0.5 ml (10 mcg) IM at birth, 1, and 6 months of age to infants.
   This will prevent perinatal infection or modify perinatal infection, prevent chronic HB_sAg carrier state, and prevent postnatal infection. Test for HB_sAg and anti-HB_s and/or IgM anti-HBc at 12–15 months of age.
   b. Use elective cesarean section, if desired, to minimize maternal fetal transfusion during delivery and to eliminate the ingestion of contaminated vaginal content if maternal HB_sAg and HB_eAg are positive.
   c. Avoid pharyngeal mucosal trauma with gentle resuscitation.
   d. Aspirate gastric content to remove infected fluid.
   e. Avoid breast feeding if possible (controversial) and avoid premastication of infant food (a common practice in the Orient).
   f. Instruct women with HB_sAg to carefully wash their hands prior to handling the baby. Infants need not be separated from their mothers or placed in special isolation. The newborn is rarely infectious at birth even if infected.
2. Screen pregnant women who are drug dependent or have signs of hepatitis for HB_sAg.

3. When the infant has HB_sAg
   a. Place the infant on "blood and secretion" precaution.
   b. Nursery personnel should maintain careful handwashing technique, wear disposable gloves, and maintain careful needle technique.
   c. Innoculate the needle-stuck personnel with HBIG.
4. Administer HBIG and HB vaccine to the susceptible personnel who are working in high-risk areas.

B. Who Is at Risk?

1. Infants born to women who are HB_sAg carriers (5%–50%) or who have contracted acute hepatitis B (50%–100%) in the last trimester of pregnancy or shortly after delivery.
   Mother-to-infant infections (vertical transmission) occur from micromaternal fetal transfusions during labor and/or infant contact with infectious maternal secretions in the birth canal or postnatal transmissions by saliva or possibly breast milk.
   Infants born to mothers with acute infection in the first trimester do not become carriers while 75% of infants born to mothers whose onset of acute hepatitis was in the third trimester or near the time of delivery become carriers.
   The presence of maternal hepatitis B e antigen (HB_eAg) is a good indicator that the infants may become infected and develop a consequent carrier state. HB_eAg is not found in the absence of HB_sAg and is present during the first month or two of acute HBV infection and usually is present during the first few years of the chronic HB_sAg carrier state. Approximately 90% to 100% of HB_eAg-positive mothers transmit infection to their infants and most of them (80% to 90%) become carriers, while HB_eAg-negative mothers less frequently infect their infants.
2. Infants born to mothers such as Asians or drug addicts are at risk. Perinatal infections occur most frequently (40%) among the Chinese, less frequently (7%) among African blacks, and least frequently among Caucasians.
3. Infants who receive a blood transfusion that has been infected with hepatitis B may acquire the infection.

C. Clinical Manifestations

The majority of infants who become HB_sAg-positive are asymptomatic and remain chronically HB_sAg-positive for long periods of time. They may have hepatosplenomegaly with persistently elevated bilirubin and transaminases and signs of chronic hepatitis. A few infants exhibit a severe fulminant form of hepatitis that is occasionally fatal. Low-birth-weight or premature infants often have fulminating disease (35%).

D. Radiologic Features

No specific radiologic pattern has been described.

E. Laboratory Findings

1. Specific findings
   The HBV contains surface antigen (HB_sAg), a core antigen (HB_cAg), and HB_eAg.
   In susceptible persons who are exposed to hepatitis B, jaundice and elevated SGOT and SGPT will be noted 6 to 12 weeks after exposure. Then, HB_sAg will be detected 2 weeks before onset of clinical symptoms and will persist for 2 weeks to 2 months; anti-HB_s antibody will be detectable 2 weeks to 2 months after HB_sAg disappears; anti-HB_c will be detected shortly after the onset of clinical disease; and detectable levels of anti-HB_c and anti-HB_s will be present for many years afterwards (Fig 16–1).

INTERPRETATION OF SEROLOGICAL MARKERS OF HEPATITIS B VIRUS INFECTION

HB_SAG	ANTI-HB_S	ANTI-HB_C	INTERPRETATIONS
+	–	–	Early (presymptomatic) acute type B hepatitis
+	±	+	Acute (anti-HB_CIgM present) or chronic type B hepatitis
–	+	+	Recovery from type B hepatitis
–	–	+	Long after hepatitis B virus infection, or immediate recovery phase from type B hepatitis, or "low level" carrier state
–	+	–	Long after hepatitis B virus infection or immunization with HB_SAg

2. Nonspecific findings
   a. Mild to moderate elevations of SGOT and SGPT may be noted.
   b. Liver biopsy may show chronic persistent hepatitis.
   c. Severe hepatic failure in fulminant hepatitis with elevation of SGOT, SGPT, γ-glutamyl transpeptidase, bilirubin, ammonia, etc.

F. Supportive Management

See chapter 16–IIIC for "general supportive management for the infant with infection."

G. Specific Therapy

No specific treatment for the chronic HB_sAg carrier is known.

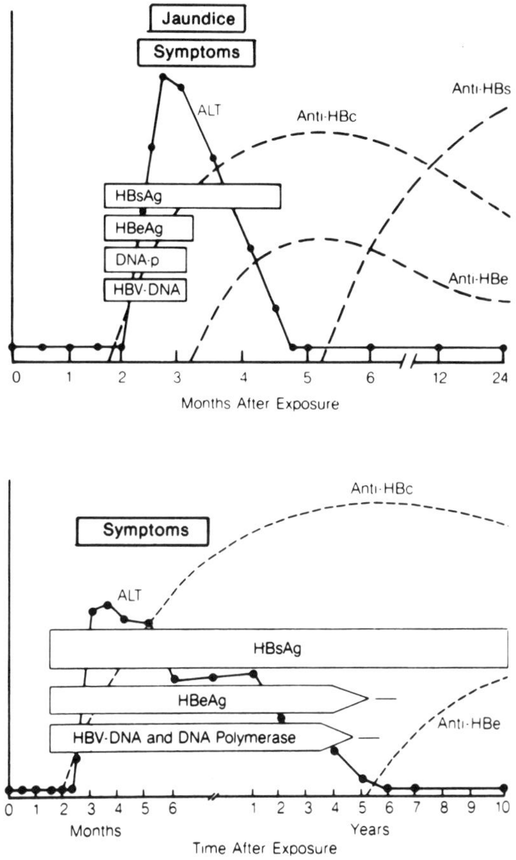

Fig 16–1.
The clinical, serologic, and biochemical course of typical acute *(top)* and chronic *(bottom)* type B hepatitis. *(ALT* = alanine aminotransferase; *HB_sAg* = hepatitis B surface antigen; *HB_eAg* = hepatitis B e antigen; *DNA-p* = serum hepatitis B virus DNA polymerase activity; *HBV-DNA* = serum hepatitis B virus DNA; *Anti-HB_s* = antibody to HB_sAg; *Anti-HB_e* = antibody to HB_eAg; *Anti-HB_c* = antibody to hepatitis B core antigen) (From Hoofnagle J.H.: Type A and B hepatitis. *Laboratory Med.* 14:705, 1983. Used by permission.)

H. Prognosis

1. HBV

   There are a few reports of neonatal severe fulminant hepatitis that was either from blood transfusions or from asymptomatic maternal carriers. Infected infants who develop antibody to HB_sAg (anti-HB_s) are presumably immune for life.

   The long-term effects of chronic neonatal HBV are unknown. Chronic HB_sAg carriers, particularly when acquired at birth or early in life, have an increased risk of subsequent liver disease such as chronic-active hepatitis, cirrhosis, and primary hepatocellular carcinoma as well as glomerulonephritis and systemic arteritis.

2. Hepatitis A

   Hepatitis A during pregnancy offers no risk for the fetus although it is recommended to administer a single dose of immune serum globulin, 0.5 ml IM, at birth if mother has acute hepatitis within 2 weeks prior to delivery.

3. Hepatitis non-A, non-B
   It is also recommended to administer a single dose of immune serum globulin at birth if mother has hepatitis non-A, non-B during the last trimester because indirect evidence, elevated liver enzymes, indicate maternal infant transmission.

REFERENCES

Centers for Disease Control: Recommendations for protection against viral hepatitis. *MMWR* 34:313, 1985.

Hoofnagle J.H.: Type A and type B hepatitis: *Lab. Med.* 14:705, 1983.

Stevens C.E., Toy P.T., Tong M.J., et al.: Perinatal hepatitis B virus transmission in the United States. Prevention by passive-active immunization. *JAMA* 253:1740, 1985.

XIII. LISTERIOSIS

Listeriosis, a non-acid-fast, gram-positive infection, is characterized by miliary granuloma and focal necrosis in many tissues and may cause habitual abortion, stillbirth, neonatal death, or death in early life. Although epidemics have occurred, most cases are sporadic in nature, particularly in late spring and summer.

A. Prevention

1. Administer prompt antibiotic therapy for the pregnant woman if the diagnosis is established or if flu-like symptoms occur in the second half of gestation when the pregnant woman works in the preparation of poultry.
2. Prophylactic treatment of women with repeated abortions particularly with serologic evidence of previous *Listeria* infection may give better outcome in subsequent pregnancies.
3. No effective methods of immunization are available for the newborn. Attempts to immunize animals with killed *Listeria* have failed.

B. Who Is at Risk?

1. Immune-deficient individuals of any age, newborns, and individuals over 45 years of age are at high risk for infection.
2. Infants born to women with vaginal colonization by *Listeria* have been reported to be at risk (not substantiated).
3. Low-birth-weight infants who suffered birth trauma are at high risk.
4. Infants born to women who handle sheep, cattle, swine, and poultry are at risk.

C. Clinical Manifestations

Clinical symptoms are variable and include premature birth, rash, respiratory distress (dyspnea, tachypnea, cyanosis), vomiting, poor feeding, and convulsions. The presence of roseoles (focal tiny granulomas) in the posterior pharyngeal wall is characteristic.

1. Early onset listeriosis is associated with a diffuse septic process involving the lungs, liver, CNS, skin, spleen, esophagus, posterior pharyngeal wall, and tonsils.
2. Late neonatal listeriosis is associated with infants who are asymptomatic at birth and develop meningitis several days to several weeks after birth.

D. Radiologic Features

No specific radiologic pattern has been described.

E. Laboratory Findings

1. Specific findings
   Isolation of *Listeria* from blood, CSF, urine, stool, gastric aspirate, cord, ears, etc., is the only reliable means of proving clinical disease.
2. Nonspecific findings
   a. The complement fixation reaction may be a useful adjunct in certain cases.
   b. The fluorescent antibody test can be used to demonstrate the presence of *Listeria* in smears and paraffin-embedded tissues.
   c. Elevated CNS protein and elevated CNS white blood count are nonspecific findings.

F. Supportive Management

See chapter 16–IIIC for "general supportive management for the infant with infection."

G. Specific Therapy

1. Ampicillin is the drug of choice: 100 mg/kg/day IV or IM in two divided doses for infants less than 1 week of age and 200 mg/kg/day IV or IM in three divided doses for infants 2 to 4 weeks of age.
2. Aminoglycosides in combination with ampicillin may be used for synergism.
3. Chloramphenicol and tetracycline are usually not suitable in the newborn period.

H. Prognosis

The prognosis depends upon early and effective antibiotic therapy. Without treatment, prognosis is poor and the mortality rate is as high as 70%. With antibiotic treatment, the mortality rate may be about 15%. Recovery can be complete or can be associated with permanent damage, e.g., hydrocephalus, cerebral palsy, and/or ptosis.

REFERENCES

Ahlfors C.E., Goetzman B.W., Halsted E.C., et al.: Neonatal listeriosis. *Am. J. Dis. Child.* 131:405, 1977.

Barresi J.A.: *Listeria monocytogenes:* A cause of premature labor and neonatal sepsis. *Am. J. Obstet. Gynecol.* 136:410, 1980.

Krause V.W., Embree J.E., MacDonald S.W., et al.: Congenital listeriosis causing early neonatal death. *Can. Med. Assoc. J.* 127:36, 1982.

Schlech W.F. III, Lavigne P.M., Bortolussi R.A., et al.: Epidemic listeriosis: Evidence for transmission by food. *N. Engl. J. Med.* 308:203, 1983.

XIV. CHLAMYDIAL INFECTION

Chlamydiae are obligate intracellular parasites that cause sexually transmitted infections: cervicitis, urethritis, and salpingitis in women and conjunctivitis and pneumonia in newborns. Many of the cervical infections are subclinical. The incidence of conjunctivitis in the newborn has been reported to be 7 to 40 per 1,000 live births and the incidence of pneumonia ranges from 3 to 10 per 1,000 live births.

A. Prevention

1. Test pregnant women for chlamydial infections and treat those found to carry the organism.
2. Reduce the reservoir by treating patients with gonorrhea with tetracycline since 20% of men and 30% of women with gonorrhea have concurrent chlamydial infection.
3. Substitute erythromycin for silver nitrate in ocular prophylaxis for neonates. However, topical erythromycin does not prevent chlamydial pneumonia and it may fail to prevent gonococcal ophthalmia.
4. There is no evidence to recommend isolation of the infant with chlamydial infection.

B. Who Is at Risk?

Infants born vaginally to mothers with chlamydial infection of the cervix or urethra (one third of exposed infants) are at risk. Young, unwed, sexually active mothers have high rates (25% to 30%) of cervical chlamydial infection.

C. Clinical Manifestations

1. The incubation period is 5 to 14 days. The conjunctivitis usually starts with a watery discharge from the eyes and rapidly and progressively becomes purulent. In addition, swollen eye lids and red conjunctiva with occasional pseudomembranes are seen.
2. Pneumonia may develop up to 3 to 4 months after birth. The course is usually benign. Symptoms include tachypnea, cough (often paroxysmal), irritability, and failure to thrive. Infants are not acutely or severely ill.

D. Radiologic Features

Hyperinflation and infiltration are common chest x-ray findings.

E. Laboratory Findings

1. The most useful diagnostic test is examination of Giemsa-stained conjunctival scrapings for inclusion bodies, which are seen within the epithelial cells.
2. A direct-slide fluorescence-tagged chlamydial monoclonal antibody test is as specific and sensitive as a culture.
3. Isolation of the chlamydia inoculated into tissue culture is diagnostic but expensive. Gonorrhea and CMV often co-exist.
4. Eosinophilia and increased IgG and IgM antichlamydial antibodies greater than 1:64 by microimmunofluorescence (not available commercially) are often seen in pneumonia.

F. Supportive Management

1. Clean the eyes with 0.9% NaCl as frequently as necessary.
2. See chapter 16–IIIC for "general supportive management for the infant with infection."

G. Specific Therapy

1. Topical ophthalmic tetracycline or erythromycin ointment, four times per day for 2 weeks, and oral erythromycin, 40 mg/kg/day divided into three doses for 2 weeks, should be administered because of the high failure rate (50%) of topical treatment.
2. Administer erythromycin, 40 mg/kg/day divided into three doses for 2 weeks, for pneumonia.
3. High levels of circulating antibody are not protective.

H. Prognosis

The conjunctivitis usually resolves spontaneously in a few months. Loss of vision is rare, but superficial corneal vascularization and conjunctival scar formation may occur. If treated early, the prognosis is excellent. Mortality from pneumonia is rare and recovery is usual and without residual effects.

REFERENCES

Fommell G.T., Rothenberg R., Wang S.P., et al.: Chlamydial infection of mothers and their infants. *J. Pediatr.* 95:28, 1979.

Hammerschlag M.R., Chandler J.W., Alexander E.R., et al.: Erythromycin ointment for ocular prophylaxis of neonatal chlamydial infection. *J.A.M.A.* 244:2291, 1980.

Schachter J., Holt J., Goodner E., et al.: Prospective study of chlamydial infection in neonates. *Lancet* 2:377, 1979.

Tam M.R., Stamm W.E., Handsfields H.H., et al.: Culture independent diagnosis of chlamydia trachomatis using monoclonal antibodies. *N. Engl. J. Med.* 310:1146, 1984.

XV. GROUP B STREPTOCOCCAL INFECTION

Shifts in the prevalence of etiologic agents producing neonatal bacterial infections have occurred in the past. In the 1970s, the incidence of group B streptococcus (GBS) infection in the newborn abruptly increased. In certain institutions, this organism has replaced *E. coli* as the single most common agent associated with bacteremia or meningitis during the first 2 months of life. The incidence is reported as 1.3 to 3.0 per 1,000 live births during the first week of life and 1.0 to 1.7 per 1,000 live births after the first week of life. Recently, the incidence seems to be lessening in some institutions.

A. Prevention

1. Routine chemoprophylaxis
   a. For the nonaffected sibling of a twin who is infected with GBS, start penicillin G, 200,000 units/kg/day IV, after cultures of blood and CSF are taken. Discontinue if cultures are negative in 72 hours.
   b. For the pregnant woman who previously delivered an infant with GBS infection
      1) Attempt to irradicate GBS from maternal vagina by penicillin and then deliver the infant electively, if possible, and/or
      2) Start ampicillin, 0.5 to 1.0 gm every 6 hours IV, or penicillin G, 1.0 to 1.5 million units every 4 hours IV, from the onset of labor or membrane rupture until delivery if vaginal or rectal cultures taken after the second trimester are positive or premature delivery occurs.
2. Immunoprophylaxis
   Active immunization to selected antibody-deficient women with type III GBS vaccine before or late in pregnancy and passive immunization of the newborn

with type-specific antibody (which is not available yet) may possibly prevent both early- and late-onset GBS infection.

B. Who Is at Risk?

1. Infants whose mothers have genital tract GBS microorganisms at delivery (1% to 2% develop symptomatic early-onset septicemia)
2. Premature infants (the incidence of disease is 15% if the mother is a GBS carrier)
3. Twins (35% incidence if the mother is a GBS carrier)
4. Infants with a maternal history of prolonged rupture of membranes (11% incidence if the mother is a GBS carrier) or having a previous infant with GBS infection
5. Infants born to mothers with postpartum fever and/or endometritis
6. Infants with a maternal history of prolonged labor or intrauterine devices
7. Infants who are deficient in type-specific antibody (opsonic antibody for native type III organisms) either from maternal low serum concentration or from failure to receive sufficient transplacental antibody prior to premature delivery since more than one half of maternal antibody is transported during the last 10 weeks of pregnancy
8. Infants who stay in a crowded nursery with poor handwashing techniques
9. Infants who are discharged to families with poor hygiene or many siblings

C. Clinical Manifestations

Two distinct clinical syndromes are recognized to be associated wtih GBS infections in newborn infants: early- and late-onset infection.

1. Early-onset infection within the first few days of age
   Respiratory distress in 90% (apnea, grunting, tachypnea, or cyanosis), hypotension with pallor and poor perfusion in 25%, lethargy, poor feeding, hypothermia or hyperthermia, abdominal distension, or jaundice. There has been equal frequency of septicemia (one third). Approximately one third of cases have meningitis, and the initial clinical manifestations are identical to those without meningitis. Approximately half of meningitis cases will develop convulsions in the first 24 hours. The onset of symptoms within 6 hours of birth and a 1-minute Apgar score of 5 or less may indicate in utero acquisition.
2. Late-onset infection after 1 week of age
   Fever (85%), irritability, lethargy, poor feeding, respiratory distress (20% to 30%), hypotension (15%), convulsions. Meningitis is the single most common clinical manifestation (85%).
3. Septic arthritis and osteomyelitis (early-onset acquisition but late-onset expression). The onset of symptoms varies between 1 and 8 weeks of age and it is somewhat delayed in osteomyelitis.
   Pain with passive motion, decreased spontaneous movement, mild swelling, occasional warmth and redness of the involved extremity. Usually systemic

involvement is absent. The most common site of involvement is the lower extremity (especially the hip joint) for septic arthritis and the proximal humerus for osteomyelitis. Single-bone involvement is usual in GBS osteomyelitis as opposed to neonatal osteomyelitis due to other organisms (*S. aureus* or gram-negative bacilli).

4. A miscellaneous syndrome is noted in infants who appear clinically well but who may have localized infections such as cellulitis, scalp abscesses, impetigo, breast abscesses, or conjunctivitis.

D. Radiologic Features

1. Chest x-ray film features are consistent with and indistinguishable from respiratory distress syndrome in more than one half of cases in premature infants.
2. Pulmonary infiltrates suggest congenital pneumonia in one third of cases.
3. Increased pulmonary vascular markings suggest transient tachypnea of the newborn or pulmonary edema in one sixth of cases.

E. Laboratory Findings

1. Isolation of the organisms from cultures of blood, CSF, urine, and/or suppurative focus is diagnostic.
2. Single, rapid presumptive diagnostic tests to detect GBS antigen include countercurrent immunoelectrophoresis (in hours), latex particle agglutination (in minutes), staphylococcal coagglutination (in minutes). Countercurrent immunoelectrophoresis provides a diagnosis in more than 90% of patients if blood, urine, and CSF specimens are tested.
3. Nonspecific tests are helpful in making the diagnosis. These are the same as those for sepsis.
   a. Leukocytosis (greater than 25,000/cu mm) or leukopenia (less than 5,000/cu mm)
   b. High or low neutrophils (see appendix Fig A–5 for normal values)
   c. Increased immature neutrophils and immature/total neutrophil ratio (greater than 0.16 in 24 hours; greater than 0.12 in 60 hours) (see appendix Fig A–6)
   d. Thrombocytopenia (less than 100,000/cu mm)

F. Supportive Management

See chapter 16–IIIC for "general supportive management for the infant with infection."

G. Specific Therapy

1. For septicemia without meningitis
   a. Initial therapy before culture results for the first 48 to 72 hours: penicillin G, 200,000/kg/day IV, or ampicillin, 150 to 200 mg/kg/day; and gentamicin, 7.5 mg/kg/day, or kanamycin, 15 mg/kg/day divided into two doses in infants less than 1 week of age and divided into three doses in infants over 1 week of age.
   b. Continue penicillin G, 200,000 units/kg/day, for a total of 10 days if cultures are positive for GBS.
2. For meningitis
   a. Initial therapy with gram-positive cocci for the first 24 to 48 hours: ampicillin, 400 mg/kg/day, plus gentamicin, 7.5 mg/kg/day, to cover GBS, *Listeria,* or pneumococcus (in vitro antagonism between ampicillin and chloramphenicol for GBS has been reported).
   b. Continue penicillin G, 400,000 units/kg/day, for a minimum total treatment course of 2 to 3 weeks with a positive culture.
   c. Repeat lumbar puncture in 24 to 48 hours after treatment is started to document sterility and at the completion of therapy in 2 to 3 weeks to document adequacy of treatment. Failure to achieve sterility suggests complications such as subdural empyema, brain abscess, obstructive ventriculitis, septic thrombophlebitis, etc.
   d. Perform careful periodic neurologic and developmental assessment test.
3. For septic arthritis or osteomyelitis
   To obtain a specific diagnosis, do a closed or open needle aspiration before or early in the course of treatment. This may be left open for drainage if required. Treat arthritis for 2 weeks, osteomyelitis for 4 weeks.

H. Prognosis

The mortality rate of the early-onset disease is reported to be 50% to 60% but less in greater than 1,500-gm infants.

The mortality rate among late-onset infections (approximately 20% to 30%) is lower than that of early onset infection. Approximately 30% to 50% of infants with meningitis develop permanent neurologic sequelae (e.g., cortical blindness, deafness, severe developmental retardation, seizure disorders, spasticity, hypothalamic dysfunction or subtle deficit). Convulsions, hypotension, leukopenia of 4,000/cu mm, and high CSF concentration of type III GBS antigen (greater than 3 μg/ml) are associated with fatal outcome or permanent neurologic sequelae.

REFERENCES

Edwards M.S., Rench M.A., Haffer A.A.M., et al.: Long-term sequelae of group B streptococcal meningitis in infants. *J. Pediatr.* 106:717, 1985.

Ingram D.L., Pendergrass E.L., Bromberger P.I., et al.: Group B streptococcal disease: Its diagnosis with the use of antigen detection, Gram's stain, and the presence of apnea, hypotension. *Am. J. Dis. Child.* 134:754, 1980.

Pass M.A., Gray B.M., Khare S., et al.: Prospective studies of group B streptococcal infections in infants. *J. Pediatr.* 95:437, 1979.

Pyati S.P., Pildes R.S., Ramamurthy R.S., et al.: Decreasing mortality in neonates with early-onset group B streptococcal infection: Reality or artifact. *J. Pediatr.* 98:625, 1981.

XVI. STAPHYLOCOCCAL INFECTIONS

Both *S. aureus* and *S. epidermidis* can cause infection in the newborn. Neonatal pyoderma occurs in about 3 to 6 infants per 1,000 live births. Disease since the 1970s has been characterized by mild illness and primarily impetigo. Conjunctivitis, pyoderma, or omphalitis are common during epidemic periods.

A. Prevention

1. Ensure handwashing technique of medical and nursing personnel.
2. Increasing the space allowance per infant in the nursery and utilization of the cohort system has not resulted in decreased infection.
3. Gowns, masks, and caps have little effect on the colonization rate.
4. Since infant-to-infant transmission is possible, those infants with pustules should be isolated.
5. Antimicrobial ointments (e.g., bacitracin) and antiseptic dyes (e.g., triple dye), and repeated use of hexachlorophene-containing washes have been utilized with varying degrees of success to decrease colonization.

B. Who Is at Risk?

1. Those infants colonized by staphylococci in the nursery by the hands of nursery personnel are at risk. Colonization with hospital strains does not always result in disease. Eighty-five percent of colonization results from an attendant's touch and 15% from air transfer. High colonization rates are not always associated with epidemics although colonized infants are more likely to develop infection than noncolonized infants.
2. Infants whose skin surface integrity has been broken or compromised due to bruises, cuts, or abrasions, which provide receptive sites for the bacteria to multiply. The circumcized penis, umbilical cord, and nares are particularly susceptible to infection.
3. Infants with indwelling catheters or endotracheal tubes are continually at risk.

C. Clinical Manifestations

1. Bullous impetigo
   Localized intraepidermal vesicles on a nonerythematous base around the um-

bilicus, diaper, and intertriginous areas, axilla, and neck occur usually within 2 weeks of life often by phage group II of staphylococci.

2. Staphylococcal scalded skin syndrome (toxic epidermal necrolysis)
   An initial scarlatina-form rash progresses into wrinkling and desquamation of large areas of skin with positive Nikolsky's sign followed by denudation, drying, and a secondary desquamation in 48 hours and lasts a few days. The skin manifestations are the results of toxin.
3. Toxic shock syndrome
   Sudden onset of fever, diarrhea, shock, hyperemia of the mucous membranes, a diffuse macular erythematous rash followed by desquamation of hands and feet
4. Otitis media, conjunctivitis, breast abscess
   Mastitis occurs usually at 10 to 14 days of life and is usually mild, but can progress into extensive involvement with systemic signs and symptoms of infection.
5. Septicemia and CNS infections
   Nonspecific poor feeding, respiratory distress, hypothermia, cyanosis, apnea, convulsions, jaundice, pallor, abdominal distension. *S. epidermidis* CNS infections may result from metastatic meningeal infection or ventriculoperitoneal shunts.
6. Pneumonia
   The incidence under 6 months of age is directly related to severe nursery outbreaks.
   Antecedent viral infection is followed by a rapid onset of tachypnea, dyspnea, tachycardia, hypothermia, and abdominal distension. The disease is often fulminating with a 12% to 15% mortality rate.
7. Osteomyelitis and arthritis
   Osteomyelitis is rare, but scapula and maxilla are often involved with absent clinical manifestations. Staphylococci are the common cause of arthritis under 1 month of age. Clinical manifestations are nonspecific. Irritability, edema, and discoloration surrounding the affected joint or bone may be present.

D. Radiologic Features

A chest x-ray film in the presence of pneumonia reveals pneumonic infiltrates, pneumothorax, pleural effusion, and pneumatoceles. In the presence of osteomyelitis, radiographic evidence of bone destruction and new bone formation is seen as early as 7 days after infection.

E. Laboratory Findings

1. Specific findings
   Diagnosis is established by a positive Gram's stain and culture of blood, CSF, urine, skin, conjunctiva smears, and needle aspirate of pleural or joint cavity.

2. Nonspecific findings
   a. Leukocytosis or leukopenia (see appendix A–12)
   b. Increased immature leukocytes (see appendix Figs A–5 and A–6)

F. Supportive Management

See chapter 16–IIIC for "general supportive management for the infant with infection."

G. Specific Therapy

1. Localized therapy with bacitracin ointment for mild superficial skin lesions is usually effective.
2. Drain established abscesses (i.e., incision and drainage for skin abscesses, closed underwater drainage for empyema).
3. Parenteral therapy
   In the case of more virulent infection, parenteral antibiotics are indicated once the pathogen is identified and/or there is a high index of suspicion.
   a. Parenteral methicillin, 50 to 150 mg/kg/24 hours divided into 2 doses for infants less than 7 days of age and 100 to 200 mg/kg/24 hours divided into three to four doses for infants more than 7 days of age (nafcillin may be used), should be started because approximately 50% of staphylococcal organisms are penicillin-resistant.
   b. If the organism is resistant to methicillin, administer vancomycin, 30 mg/kg/24 hours IV divided into two doses for infants less than 7 days of age and 45 mg/kg/24 hours divided into three doses for infants more than 7 days of age.

H. Prognosis

Prognosis depends upon location of the infection, resistance of the organism, virulence of the strain, and early initiation of therapy. Staphylococcal pneumonia frequently results in pulmonary abnormalities and pneumatoceles with a high mortality rate of 12% to 15%. Prognosis for osteomyelitis is good if the epiphyses are not destroyed.

REFERENCES

Elias P.M., Fritsch P., Epstein E.H. Jr.: Staphylococcal scalded skin syndrome: Clinical features, pathogenesis and microbiological and biochemical developments. *Arch. Dermatol.* 113:207, 1977.

Fox K.R., Golomb H.S.: Staphylococcal ophthalmia neonatorum and the staphylococcal scalded skin syndrome. *Am. J. Ophthal.* 88:1052, 1979.

Johnson J.D., Malachowski N.C., Vosti K.L., et al.: A sequential study of various modes of skin and umbilical care and the incidence of staphylococcal colonization and infection in the neonate. *Pediatrics* 58:354, 1976.

XVII. GONORRHEA

Neisseria gonorrhoeae, a gram-negative diplococcus, causes scalp abscesses, gonococcemia, septic arthritis, meningitis, vaginitis and/or gonorrheal ophthalmia neonatorum. The disease is contracted from the mother at delivery. Sixty percent to 80% of mothers are asymptomatic. Prevalency rates of gonococcal infection among pregnant women today have been reported to vary between 0.5% and 7.6%, depending on the populations studied. There is an increased incidence of chorioamnionitis, intrauterine growth retardation, and prematurity when mothers are infected with gonorrhea.

A. Prevention

Administer 1 drop of 1% silver nitrate ($AgNO_3$), 0.5% erythromycin, or 1% tetracycline ophthalmic ointment prophylactically in each conjunctival sac at birth to all newborns. Following instillation with $AgNO_3$, eyes should not be flushed. Failure of prevention may be due to occurrence of infection prior to delivery, irrigation with saline immediately, or subsequently acquired infection.

B. Who Is at Risk?

1. Infants born to mothers from low-income socioeconomic groups and unmarried teenagers who have been sexually promiscuous and who received little or no prenatal care
2. Low-birth-weight prematures, particularly male infants born to mothers with premature rupture of membranes or gonococcal chorioamnionitis
3. Infants born to mother who were not treated for acquired gonococcal infections in previous pregnancies or during the current pregnancy
   Gonococci are isolated from approximately 30% of infants of infected mothers.

C. Clinical Manifestations

1. In the newborn, 2 to 5 days postdelivery, gonococcal ophthalmia typically begins as a purulent conjunctivitis with a profuse discharge and fulminant course. Corneal ulcerations, perforation, fibrosis, and blindness frequently follow.
2. Neonatal gonococcal arthritis, possibly due to septicemia, may occur 1 to 5 weeks after delivery and must be differentiated from acute rheumatic fever.
3. Fetal sepsis in association with gonorrheal chorioamnionitis has also been reported. Occasionally, gonococcal scalp abscesses, attributable to intrauterine fetal monitoring are seen.

D. Radiologic Features

No typical radiologic features have been reported.

E. Laboratory Findings

1. A smear should be obtained and the conjunctival exudate or joint aspirate should be examined directly by Gram's stain technique. Detection of the characteristic gram-negative gonococcal diplococci intracellularly in polymorphonuclear leukocytes warrants the presumptive diagnosis of gonococcal conjunctivitis, although *Neisseria* species may be present.
2. Culture the organism by innoculating the conjunctival exudate or blood or joint aspirate directly onto blood, MacConkey, Thayer-Martin, or chocolate agar. (Thayer-Martin requires incubation in CO_2 environment.) Penicillin sensitivity or penicillinase production should be tested routinely because of increasing cases of penicillinase-producing *N. gonorrhoeae* infection.

F. Supportive Management

See chapter 16–IIIC for "general supportive management for the infant with infection."

G. Specific Therapy

1. Infants born to mothers with gonococcal infection
   Administer a single IV or IM injection of aqueous crystalline penicillin G: 50,000 units for fullterm infants and 20,000 units for prematures.
   a. Isolate infants for 24 hours after initiation of treatment. Observe strict handwashing technique.
2. Infants with gonococcal ophthalmia
   a. Isolate infants for 24 hours after initiation of treatment. Observe strict handwashing techniques.
   b. Irrigate the eyes with 0.9% NaCl immediately and then every hour until the discharge has abated.
   c. Treat gonorrheal ophthalmia with penicillin G, 50,000 units/kg/24 hours IM or IV divided into two doses for 7 days. Topical antibiotics alone are *not* sufficient.
   d. Consult an ophthalmologist.
3. Infants with arthritis and/or septicemia should be treated with aqueous crystalline penicillin G, 100,000 units/kg/24 hours IV divided into two doses for $<$ 7 days of age, three doses for $>$ 7 days of age. Adequate drainage of a septic joint by repeat aspiration or open drainage is important.
4. Treatment for meningitis requires aqueous crystalline penicillin G, 100,000

units/kg/24 hours divided into two doses for < 7 days of age and three to four doses for > 7 days of age for 10 days.

5. Both parents of newborns with gonococcal infections should be examined and treated.

H. Prognosis

Prior to the antibiotic era, *N. gonorrhoeae* was the leading cause of blindness in infants. With early and adequate therapy, prognosis for normal vision is excellent. No mortality and no permanent visual impairment with adequate treatment are reported.

REFERENCES

American Academy of Pediatrics, Committee on Drugs, Committee on Fetus and Newborn, and Committee on Infectious Diseases: Prophylaxis and treatment of neonatal gonococcal infections. *Pediatrics* 65:1047, 1980.

Edwards L.E., Barrada M.I., Hamann A.A., et al.: Gonorrhea in pregnancy. *Am. J. Obstet. Gynecol.* 132:637, 1978.

XVIII. CANDIDIASIS

C. albicans, a dimorphic gram-positive yeast, accounts for the majority of fungal infections in infants. Infection in the first few months of life is considered to result from colonization at the time of birth. Thrush is the most common clinical fungal disease. In debilitated or immunocompromised infants, *Candida* may cause widespread disease and death. The incidence of systemic candidiasis is approximately 4% in infants less than 1,500 gm at birth.

A. Prevention

1. Treatment of maternal vaginal candidiasis has not proven to be of preventive value.
2. Preventive measures include the avoidance of prolonged use of antibiotics and steroids. Oral nystatin has been recommended if prolonged antibiotics cannot be avoided.
3. Strict adherence to parenteral nutrition technique may reduce the incidence of candidiasis.

B. Who Is at Risk?

1. Infants who are severely debilitated are at risk since candidiasis is an opportunistic pathogen in humans.
2. Infants born to mothers who are vaginal carriers of candidiasis are at risk; the attack rate of thrush in newborns is 50%.

3. Systemic candidiasis
   a. Very low-birth-weight infants, small for gestational age infants, and those who are receiving long-term broad spectrum antibiotics or parenteral alimentation, and/or who have intravascular catheters or endotracheal tubes.
   b. Debilitated infants with local candidiasis (thrush or *Candida* dermatitis), e.g., infants with AIDS
4. Term infants receiving steroid therapy or infants with congenital malformations; malrotation, omphalocele, meningomyelocele, tetralogy of Fallot, sacrococcygeal teratoma, giant hemangioma, etc.

C. Clinical Manifestations

1. Thrush
   Whitish gray plaques on an inflammed base that are not easily scraped from the mucosa of the mouth and oral pharynx, soft palate, tongue, and gums. Oral thrush appears at 7 to 10 days of age. Suck is sometimes painful and the infant may refuse feedings.
2. Monilial dermatitis
   The skin lesions appear discrete, vesicular, or pustular, on an erythematous base and are usually found on the perineum, intertriginous areas, neck folds, and axilla. Rarely, lesions may be seen over the whole body including palms and soles.
3. Systemic candidiasis
   Clinical manifestations are nonspecific and not distinguishable from bacterial sepsis. These include apnea, bradycardia, respiratory deterioration, edema, abdominal distension, temperature instability, hypotension, abscesses, and erythematous rashes. Often multiple organs are involved: nephritis, meningitis, hepatitis, arthritis, osteomyelitis, pneumonia, endophthalmitis, endocarditis, etc. Systemic candidiasis occurs after 10 days of life, usually at about 5 weeks of age.

D. Radiologic Features

Patchy consolidation of the lungs can be seen.

E. Laboratory Findings

1. Specific findings
   a. Infection with *Candida* can be proven by direct microscopic examination by KOH or NaOH mounting or positive culture of scrapings from lesions of skin or mucous membranes.
   b. Demonstration of the fungus in blood, suprapubic urine, CSF, joint, pleural, or peritoneal fluid by direct microscopic examination or culture establishes the diagnosis of systemic candidiasis.

c. Isolation of *Candida* from sputum, feces, or clean-catch urine is difficult to interpret since *Candida* may be found in these specimens in the absence of clinical disease.
d. Serologic tests such as complement fixation and indirect fluorescent antibody techniques are not of value.

2. Nonspecific findings
Hyperglycemia, pyuria, hematuria, proteinuria, and multiple fluffy white lesions on both retina and viterous with a diffuse viterous haze may be seen.

F. Supportive Management

See chapter 16–IIIC for "general supportive management for the infant with infection."

G. Specific Therapy

1. Oral candidiasis (thrush)
Oral nystatin (Mycostatin) suspension, 1 to 2 ml of 100,000 units/ml four times daily for 10 days. Divide each dose in half and swab the mouth with one half and let the infant swallow the other half.
2. Systemic candidiasis
    a. Start amphotericin B, 0.1 mg/kg/day, and increase gradually to 1.0 mg/kg/day in 5 to 10 days. Administer the diluted dose 1 mg/10 ml by slow IV drip daily over 4 to 6 hours. If the infant develops nephrotoxicity (oliguria, increased creatinine and/or blood urea nitrogen (BUN), hyperkalemia or hypokalemia, renal epithelial cast, edema), which is a frequent complication of amphotericin B, interrupt the treatment for one or more days till the urine output is re-established.
    b. Fluorocytosine, 100 to 150 mg/kg/day in three to four divided doses IV or orally. Hepatotoxicity is common.

H. Prognosis

Oral thrush fades in about one week with therapy. Relapse may occur. Systemic candidiasis is associated with a high mortality rate (30% to 50%). Spontaneous recovery, without specific therapy, however, has been reported. In survivors, mental retardation and hydrocephalus have been noted.

REFERENCES

Baley J.E., Kliegman R.M., Fanaroff A.A.: Disseminated fungal infections in very low birth weight infants: Clinical manifestations and epidemiology. *Pediatrics* 73:144, 1984.

Kassner E.G., Kauffman S.L., Yoon J.J., et al.: Pulmonary candidiasis in infants: Clinical, radiologic and pathologic features. *Am. J. Radiol.* 137:707, 1981.

Keller M.A., Sellers B.B., Melish M.E., et al.: Systemic candidiasis in infants. *Am. J. Dis. Child.* 131:1260, 1977.

XIX. SEPSIS

Neonatal sepsis is characterized by systemic signs of infection associated with bacteremia in the first month of life. Not all infants with positive cultures are sick and not all infants with sepsis proven by postmortem examination have positive blood cultures. The incidence of sepsis is reported to be approximately 0.5 to 7.0 in 1,000 live births. As the newborn is often unable to localize infection, any minor lesion such as a pustule or omphalitis may disseminate into a generalized septic process. Frequently, the only clinical clue is that the infant is simply "not doing well." Early onset sepsis during the first few days of life is usually disseminating, fulminant, and associated with obstetric complications and a high infant mortality (10% to 25%), while late-onset infection occurring after 5 days of life is often focal and more slowly progressing.

A. Prevention

1. Mature infants whose mothers have had prolonged rupture of the membranes for more than 24 hours should be delivered promptly.
2. Premature infants whose mothers have had prolonged rupture of the membranes for more than 24 hours should be delivered when their lungs are mature or there is evidence of infection.
3. Every effort should be made to deliver the infant in sterile conditions.
4. Pregnant women should be treated immediately if they have acquired bacterial infections, such as diarrhea, cervicitis, vaginitis, amnionitis, or urinary tract infection.
5. Prolonged labor, traumatic delivery, and perinatal asphyxia should be avoided.
6. Personnel with infectious diseases should not be allowed to enter the nursery.
7. Infected infants, e.g., those with diarrhea, should be isolated from well infants.
8. Sterile technique must be maintained when inserting catheters or performing other procedures.
9. Use disposable individual equipment in the care of the newborn.
10. Avoid the unnecessary use of broad-spectrum antibiotics.

B. Who Is at Risk?

Bacteria responsible for early-onset infection are acquired from the birth canal during delivery and bacteria responsible for late-onset infection are acquired from the birth canal as well as from human contacts and contaminated equipment or materials after birth. The following infants are at high risk for infections:

1. Infants who are premature or of low birth weight
2. Infants whose mothers had prolonged rupture of the membranes or prolonged labor

3. Infants whose mothers had maternal peripartum infection: chorioamnionitis, urinary tract infection, pneumonia, endometritis, etc.
4. Infants of diabetic mothers
5. Infants born to mothers of low socioeconomic status
6. Infants who had fetal distress, were born by traumatic delivery, or were severely depressed at birth and required intubation and resuscitation
7. Infants who are the first born of twins
8. Male infants
9. Infants with a skin or mucosal defect (e.g., meningomyelocele)
10. Infants with indwelling catheters who are receiving parenteral alimentation
11. Infants with focal infections, omphalitis, superficial skin infection, etc., or necrotizing enterocolitis
12. Infants receiving iron therapy
13. Infants with galactosemia, immune defect, or asplenia

C. Clinical Manifestations

Clinical manifestations include hypothermia or hyperthermia, lethargy, hypotonia, tremors, irritability, occasional convulsions, poor feeding, poor cry, respiratory distress, (retractions, tachypnea, apnea, cyanosis), jaundice, hepatomegaly, abdominal distension, vomiting, diarrhea, failure to gain weight, petechiae, and sclerema.

Clinical signs of sepsis are usually subtle and nonspecific.

Many noninfectious conditions give similar clinical manifestations.

D. Laboratory Findings

1. Positive cultures of the offending organism from blood, urine, CSF, other body fluids, and tissues are the most valid method of diagnosing bacterial sepsis. Infectious organisms cultured from nose, throat, skin, umbilicus, endotracheal or gastric aspirate and stool indicate colonization and may become causative organisms, but do not indicate sepsis.
   a. Causative organisms (common)
      1) *E. coli*
      2) β-hemolytic streptococcus (groups B and D, rarely A)
      3) *L. monocytogenes*
      4) *Proteus* sp.
      5) *S. aureus* (especially during 1950 to 1963) or *S. epidermidis*
      6) *Klebsiella* and *Enterobacter* sp.
      7) *P. aeruginosa*
      8) *H. influenzae*
      9) *S. pneumoniae*
      10) *N. meningitidis*
      11) *Salmonella* sp.

2. Serologic studies may help establish a diagnosis rapidly. These tests should always be used in conjunction with smear and culture because cross reactions occur.
   a. Countercurrent immunoelectrophoresis (CIE) identifies bacterial antigens and may rapidly establish the etiologic diagnosis of septicemia or meningitis due to *H. influenzae, S. pneumoniae, N. meningitidis,* or group B streptococcus.
   b. The coagglutination (CA) procedure is commonly employed as a rapid slide agglutination test to identify group B streptococcus, *N. meningitidis, N. gonorrhoeae,* and *H. influenzae.*
   c. Latex agglutination (LA) is a rapid slide agglutination test of antibody-coated latex particles by bacterial antigens (β-hemolytic streptococci and other organisms) in the CSF.
   d. The limulus amebocyte lysate (LAL) test is a rapid detection test of bacterial endotoxins that are produced almost exclusively by gram-negative bacteria and are released into blood, CSF, and urine. However, this test cannot be used for the detection of gram-positive bacteria.
3. Nonspecific laboratory determinations are helpful.
   a. Leukocytosis (greater than 25,000/cu mm) or leukopenia (less than 5,000/cu mm) in less than half of infants with sepsis (see Appendix A–12)
   b. High or low neutrophil count (see Appendix Fig A–5 for normal values) in 75% to 90% of infected infants. Neutropenia (0 to 4,000/cu mm) may be helpful in differentiating sepsis (group B streptococcus, *H. influenzae,* pneumococcal or nonenterococcal group D streptococcal) from respiratory distress syndrome. Neutropenia is often seen in infants of toxemic mothers or in infants with CNS hemorrhage, isoimmune disease, asphyxia, congenital neutropenia, or drug ingestion.
   c. Increased immature neutrophils (bands, stabs) (greater than 1,100/cu mm in cord blood, greater than 1,500/cu mm in 12 hours, and greater than 600/cu mm by 60 hours of life) or an increased immature/total (I/T) neutrophil ratio (greater than 0.16 in 24 hours, greater than 0.12 in more than 60 hours) occurs in 85% of infants with sepsis. This increase of immature neutrophils is quite insensitive and delayed. While the increase is quite suggestive of infection, the elevation of I/T ratio has been seen in maternal fever, infants with asphyxia, convulsions, surgery or in infants of toxemic mothers. See appendix Fig A–6 for normal values.
   d. Thrombocytopenia (less than 100,000/cu mm). Thrombocytopenia is commonly seen in intrauterine and postnatal infections, birth asphyxia, meconium aspiration, and necrotizing enterocolitis.
   e. An abnormal peripheral smear of hemolytic process, Döhle inclusion bodies, or vacuolization of neutrophils and toxic granulations are associated with infection.
   f. Elevated serum IgM (greater than 20 mg/dl) is not as helpful for sepsis as for intrauterine infection because it is not sensitive, rapid, or specific enough to be used.

g. Metabolic acidosis with or without hyperkalemia secondary to hypoxia or hypoperfusion
h. Hyperbilirubinemia
i. Hypoglycemia or hyperglycemia
j. Micro ESR > 5 mm/hour in first week and > 10 mm/hour in second week of life

E. Radiologic Features

1. Radiologic examination is helpful to identify the focus of infection: pneumonia and infection in bones, joints, and genitourinary and GI tract.
2. CT scan with injection of contrast material is the most appropriate mode of diagnosis for brain abscess.
3. Real-time ultrasound has been of value in the diagnosis of ventriculitis.

F. Supportive Management

See chapter 16–IIIC for "general supportive management of the infant with infection."

G. Specific Therapy

Antibiotic therapy should be started at the discretion of the physician based on maternal history and clinial symptoms and signs of sepsis after cultures of blood, urine, and CSF are obtained. Even when minimal signs of sepsis are present, treatment should be started because of subtle nonspecific signs of sepsis, rapid progress of the disease, and high mortality.

1. Because any of the major pathogens may produce a similar clinical picture, it is not possible to identify the causative organism without laboratory aids. Therefore, while awaiting the results of cultures and sensitivity tests for the infant with suspected bacterial infection, start antibiotic therapy to treat gram-positive cocci, particularly group B streptococci and gram-negative bacilli. The choice of antibiotics for infection depends on the type of infection (early vs. late onset) and the particular pattern of susceptibility in the hospital or nursery during a recent period, particularly for gram-negative bacteria. See Table 16–1 for "dosage and complications of antibiotic therapy in the newborn."
   a. Ampicillin, 100 to 150 mg/kg/24 hours in two divided doses for less than 7 days of age and three divided doses for greater than 7 days of age; or sodium aqueous penicillin, 100,000 units/kg/24 hours in two divided doses for less than 7 days of age and 100,000 units/kg/24 hours in three divided doses for greater than 7 days of age, and
   b. Gentamicin, 5 mg/kg/24 hours IM in two divided doses for less than 7 days of age and 7.5 mg/kg/24 hours IM in three divided doses for greater

than 7 days of age; or kanamycin, 15 to 20 mg/kg/24 hours IM, may be substituted for gentamicin if desired.

2. If the results of the cultures are positive, modify the antibiotic regimen according to the etiologic agent and the sensitivity reports and continue antibiotic therapy for 7 to 14 days. Then discontinue antibiotic therapy and observe the infant 1 to 2 days before discharge.
3. If cultures are negative in 3 to 4 days, re-evaluate the infant's condition. Continue therapy if the infant remains symptomatic or if the infant was critically ill. Discontinue therapy if the infant is well. The house officer should be aware that some infants with significant bacterial infection may not have positive cultures.
4. Consider hyperimmune globulin, transfusion of whole blood or plasma, or exchange transfusion for fulminating cases and granulocyte transfusion for neutropenia.

H. Complications

Complications include shock, disseminated intravascular coagulation, respiratory arrest, acidosis, meningitis, otitis media, etc. Early onset sepsis is usually disseminating and fulminating with 10%–25% mortality and late onset sepsis is often slowly progressing, less fulminating, and has a lower mortality, but higher morbidity rate.

REFERENCES

Freedman R.M., Ingram D.L., Cross I., et al.: A half century of neonatal sepsis at Yale: 1928–1978. *Am. J. Dis. Child* 135:140, 1981.

Harris M.C., Polin R.A.: Neonatal septicemia. *Pediatr. Clin. N. Am.* 30:243, 1983.

Hodgman J.E.: Sepsis in the neonate. *Perinatol. Neonatol.* 5:45, 1981.

Spector S.A., Ticknor W., Grossman M.: Study on the usefulness of clinical and hematologic findings in the diagnosis of neonatal bacterial infections. *Clin. Pediatr.* 20:385, 1981.

Philip A.G.S., Hewitt J.R.: Early diagnosis of neonatal sepsis. *Pediatrics* 65:1036, 1980.

XX. NEONATAL MENINGITIS

Meningitis, an infection of the meninges, is more common and has a higher mortality and morbidity rate in the first month of life than any succeeding month. The incidence is reported as 0.4 to 1.0 in 1,000 live births.

A. Prevention

1. Aseptic technique must be maintained in the nursery.
2. Promptly treat neonatal sepsis.

B. Who Is at Risk?

1. Those infants at risk for developing septicemia are also at risk for developing meningitis (see chapter 16–XIX).
2. Infants born to mothers with prolonged rupture of membranes, amnionitis, pyelonephritis, or septicemia
3. Infants whose delivery was complicated by fetal distress, meconium-stained amniotic fluid, or traumatic or unsterile technique
4. Infants who developed pneumonia, otitis media, gastroenteritis, omphalitis, or skin, urinary tract, or other infections. Fifty percent to 75% of infants with meningitis have proven septicemia.
5. Infants with an open meningomyelocele
6. Low-birth-weight and male infants. Low-birth-weight infants have a higher incidence of meningitis and a higher mortality from meningitis probably due to the following:
   a. Lack of transplacental transfer of γ-globulin and opsonins
   b. Delay in appearance and transition of antibodies and relative inefficiency of early antibodies. (IgM is not produced by an infant who is less than 24 weeks' gestation.)
   c. Sparsity and delay in the appearance of plasma cells and lymphocytes
   d. Significantly diminished phagocytic ability of the polymorphonuclear leukocytes

C. Clinical Manifestations

The onset of meningitis is accompanied by general signs similar to those of nonspecific signs of sepsis: lethargy, temperature instability, poor feeding, vomiting, diarrhea, abdominal distension, respiratory distress, irritability, apnea, and cyanosis. Increasing irritability, an alteration in consciousness or poor tone, twitching, and convulsions are seen as the disease progresses. Opisthotonos and bulging fontanelle are rarely seen in prematures and only occasionally seen in fullterm infants because of open sutures.

D. Laboratory Findings

1. CSF fluid findings (see appendix A–39 and A–40 for normal values)
   Some infants will have one or more normal values but rarely will all values be normal in an infant with proven meningitis.
   a. Often turbid, cloudy
   b. Elevated white blood cell count with polymorphonuclear predominance. The median number of cells per cu mm is 2,000 with gram-negative meningitis and less than 100 with group B streptococcal meningitis. Occasionally, no pleocytosis is present in enteroviral and pneumococcal meningitis.
   c. Low spinal fluid sugar (less than 50% to 75% of simultaneous serum glucose)

d. Spinal fluid protein greater than 180 mg/dl.
e. Positive gram-stained smear of CSF in approximately 80% of cases. Group B β-hemolytic streptococci (usually subtype III) and *E. coli* (usually K_1) account for 65% of all cases. *L. monocytogenes* is the next most frequently occurring organism, followed by *H. influenzae, S. pneumoniae,* and groups D and A streptococci.

2. Blood
   Positive blood cultures occur in about 50% of cases.
3. White blood cell count
   Peripheral white blood cell counts are variable and similar to those in sepsis (leukocytosis, leukopenia, or normal).
4. Thrombocytopenia

E. Supportive Management

See chapter 16–IIIC for "general supportive management for the infant with infection."

F. Specific Therapy

Initial and subsequent therapy are the same as for sepsis since the causative organisms are the same but the duration of therapy is longer.

1. Institute antibiotic therapy as soon as cultures have been obtained with or without positive smear. Any delay aggravates prognosis. Initial choice of antibiotics can be guided by: a Gram's stain or CIE of the CSF fluid; the level of spinal fluid sugar, protein; CFS cell count; and positive maternal cultures or positive cultures from other infected sites of the infant.
   a. When organisms are seen on the CSF smear; start initial therapy with ampicillin, 100 to 300 mg/kg/day IV, plus gentamicin, 7.5 mg/kg/day IM, in two divided doses for less than 7 days of age and in three divided doses for greater than 7 days of age.
   b. When gram-positive organisms are seen on the CSF smear, initial therapy should include ampicillin and gentamicin because the combination therapy has a synergistic effect for group B streptococci and *L. monocytogenes* and it is difficult to differentiate streptococci from *L. monocytogenes* and pneumococci.
   c. When gram-negative organisms are seen on the CSF smear, moxalactam or chloramphenicol may be used for the initial therapy since the CSF levels of aminoglycosides (e.g., gentamicin) are low.
      1) Moxalactam, 100 mg/kg/day in two divided doses for less than 1 week of age, 150 mg/kg/day in three divided doses for 1 to 4 weeks of age, and 200 mg/kg/day in four divided doses for greater than 4 weeks of age after loading with 200 mg/kg.
      2) Chloramphenicol, 25 mg/kg/day in two divided doses in prematures less than 1 week of age, 50 mg/kg/day in two divided doses in fullterm in-

fants less than 1 week of age, and 50 mg/kg/day in two divided doses in infants greater than 1 week of age.

2. When cultures and sensitivity tests are obtained, appropriate antibiotics should be instituted. See Table 16–1 for "dosage and complications of antibiotic therapy in the newborn." The Neonatal Meningitis Cooperative Study (1979) reports no beneficial effect of intrathecal or intraventricular treatment of gram-negative meningitis.
3. Repeat examination and cultures of the CSF should be obtained every 24 to 36 hours until a sterile culture of the CSF is obtained. Therapy should be continued for a minimum of 2 weeks poststerilization of the CSF. This usually requires 3 weeks of therapy for gram-negative organisms and 2 weeks of therapy for gram-positive organisms.
4. Measure the head circumference weekly to determine abnormal head growth (hydrocephalus) (see Fig 6–2, 6–4, 6–5).
5. Transilluminate and/or obtain a sonographic examination of the infant's head weekly to determine the presence of subdural effusion, hydrocephalus, or other abnormality. Obtain a sonogram and/or CT scan prior to discharge.
6. Control convulsions if present (see chapter 15–III).
7. Watch for disturbances of fluids and electrolytes. Syndrome of inappropriate antidiuretic hormone frequently occurs. Follow daily weights, urine specific gravity, osmolality, and sodium along with serum electrolytes and osmolality (see chapter 18–XV).
8. Watch for hypoglycemia.
9. Before discharge, obtain audiologic, visual, developmental, and neurologic examination. Follow development of the infant carefully.

G. Complications

1. Subdural effusion
2. Hydrocephalus
3. Apnea
4. Neurologic sequelae

H. Prognosis

Overall mortality rate is 20% to 50%, but this varies with etiologic agent, population, and neonatal intensive care unit. Sequelae include mental and physical retardation, blindness, deafness, and/or seizures. Thirty percent to 50% of survivors will have some neurologic damage.

REFERENCES

Report of the Committee on Infectious Diseases, ed. 19. Evanston, Ill., American Academy of Pediatrics, 1982, p. 78.

Schaad U.B., McCracken G.H. Jr., Threlkeld N., et al.: Clinical evaluation of a new broad spectrum oxa-beta-lactam antibiotic, moxalactam in neonates and infants. *J. Pediatr.* 98:129, 1981.

XXI. URINARY TRACT INFECTION

Sepsis in the newborn is frequently associated with a hematogenous urinary tract infection. Conversely, an obstruction in the flow of urine may result in a urinary tract infection and generalized sepsis. The incidence of urinary tract infection is 1% in infants greater than 2,500 gm and 2% to 5% in infants under 2,500 gm.

A. Prevention

1. Treat sepsis promptly.
2. Treat maternal urinary tract infections adequately.

B. Who Is at Risk?

1. Those infants at risk for developing septicemia (see chapter 16–XIX) are also at risk for developing a urinary tract infection.
2. Male newborns have a higher incidence of urinary tract infections in contrast to other age groups.
3. Infants with partial or complete obstruction of the urinary flow are at risk although the incidence of associated structural genitourinary anomalies is low in newborns.
4. Infants with a neurogenic bladder usually caused by myelomeningocele are at risk for a urinary tract infection.

C. Clinical Manifestations

Generally, the symptoms are nonspecific. Poor feeding, failure to thrive, fever, diarrhea, abdominal distension, vomiting, jaundice, and abnormal weight loss may occur. Occasionally, a distended bladder is noted if urinary obstruction is responsible. Gray skin color and cerebral symptoms may be noted.

D. Laboratory Findings

1. Urinary findings (see Chapter 18–I, appendix A–34, A–35, and A–38 for normal values)
   a. Microscopic or gross pyuria and hematuria may be present, but these findings are not diagnostic.
   b. A Gram's stain of the unspun urine may identify bacteria. The finding of more than 10 organisms per high power field is significant.
   c. A positive culture of even one organism from the urine obtained by the suprapubic tap is diagnostic; *E. coli* (most common), *S. auerus, S. epidermidis, Klebsiella, Enterobacter,* and *P. mirabilis* are frequent. A culture of

greater than 100,000 organisms/ml of a single species indicates urinary tract infection in a clean-catch specimen.
   d. Albuminuria may be present.
2. Blood findings
   a. Peripheral white cell count is usually elevated.
   b. Positive blood culture and CSF cultures are frequently associated.
   c. Jaundice with direct hyperbilirubinemia is common.
   d. Elevated BUN and creatinine may be present.

E. Radiologic Features

Obstructive lesions of the urinary tract with or without parenchymal damage may be seen on x-ray film or by sonographic examination.

F. Supportive Management

See chapter 16–IIIC for "general supportive management for the infant with infection."

G. Specific Therapy

1. While awaiting the results of the urine culture, therapy should be started with the following:
   a. Ampicillin, 100 to 150 mg/kg/24 hours IV in two divided doses for less than 1 week of age and 100 to 150 mg/kg/24 hours IV in three divided doses for greater than 1 week of age, and
   b. Gentamicin, 5 mg/kg/24 hours IM in two divided doses for less than 1 week of age and 7.5 mg/kg/24 hours IM in three divided doses for greater than 1 week of age
      Other aminoglycosides may be used in place of gentamicin according to the sensitivity pattern of the nursery.
      Modify the antibiotic regimen according to the etiologic agent and sensitivity. Treatment should be continued for 2 weeks or longer.
2. Repeat and follow the urine cultures after 48 hours of antibiotic treatment to evaluate the efficacy and 1 week after cessation of therapy to be certain there is no recurrence.
3. Defer intravenous pyelogram to rule out obstructive uropathy until a few weeks of age. Administer urologic treatment appropriate to the obstruction if an obstruction is present.

H. Prognosis

Approximately 20% to 25% of infants with urinary tract infection have recurrence in a few months. Renal scars and atropic kidneys may occur.

REFERENCES

Edelman C.M., Ogivo J.C., Fine B.P., et al.: The prevalence of bacteremia in full-term and premature newborn infants. *J. Pediatr.* 82:125, 1973.

Ginsburg C.M., McCracken G.H. Jr.: Urinary tract infections in young infants. *Pediatrics* 69:409, 1982.

XXII. DIARRHEA OF THE NEWBORN

Often, isolated cases of diarrhea occur in nurseries; less often, epidemic diarrhea that involves a large number of infants in the nursery occurs. Because of the high mortality and morbidity associated with the disease, all nursery personnel must constantly be on the alert to diagnose, isolate, and treat any and all infants who develop diarrhea.

A. Prevention

1. Rigid adherence to the sanitary code and technique of the nursery is necessary. Wash your hands before and after handling each infant, since infection takes place by the fecal-oral route via hands.
2. Avoid overcrowding of infants.
3. Use individual equipment for each infant.
4. Carefully supervise the preparation and administration of formulas. Do not overfeed.
5. Bar all nursery personnel, including physicians, who have even mild gastrointestinal or upper respiratory infections from the nursery.
6. Do not allow nursery personnel, including physicians, who care for infants with diarrhea to concurrently care for infants who are well.
7. Isolate all infants born to mothers with diarrhea (*Salmonella, Shigella,* etc.) from the nursery.
8. Isolate *immediately* any infant with diarrhea from the remainder of the nursery population.
9. Breast feed infants if at all possible. Breast milk offers significant protection against neonatal diarrhea by supplying lactoferrin, lysozymes, phagocytes, specific secretory immunoglobulins, sensitized lymphocytes, and specific antibodies.

B. Who Is at Risk?

Newborns are highly susceptible to diarrhea since enteric flora is not acquired and local and systemic immune responses are poor. Diarrhea occurs before a few months of age while on formula particularly in a poor socioeconomic urban area and frequently only after 6 months of age while on breast feeding. Seasonal variations in the incidence of diarrhea seen frequently in the older infants is not commonly seen in newborns. The following infants are at risk:

1. Infants in an overcrowded nursery, particularly with improper hand washing
2. Premature low-birth-weight infants are not at higher risk but premature or debilitated male infants become sicker if infected.
3. Infants exposed to adults or children with diarrhea
4. Infants who have ingested maternal organisms through the birth canal (e.g., *Salmonella* or *Shigella*)
5. Infants who are overfed or fed improper formula
6. Infants with congenital or acquired lactase deficiency
7. Infants receiving phototherapy
8. Infants with narcotic withdrawal syndrome
9. Infants with congenital anomalies (e.g., Hirschsprung's disease or congenital adrenal hyperplasia)
10. Infants with cystic fibrosis

C. Clinical Manifestations

1. The infant passes explosive, frequent, yellow (later greenish), watery, mucoid stools. Occasionally, shock and death occur before a diarrheal stool is passed. Perianal excoriation caused by stool acidity is common. Flecks or streaks of blood are rarely seen with *E. coli* infection, but often with *Salmonella, Campylobacter,* or *Shigella.* Recurrence of diarrhea and vomiting after a period of initial improvement may occur as a result of sugar intolerance (secondary disaccharidase deficiency).
2. Signs of generalized illness such as listlessness, irritability, poor feeding, hyperthermia or hypothermia, vomiting, and abdominal distension ensue.
3. As the disease progresses, dehydration occurs. Dehydration can be categorized as mild, moderate, or severe.
   a. Mild dehydration with approximately 5% weight loss
      Dry mucous membranes and skin, slightly depressed anterior fontanelle, and decreased urinary output may be present.
   b. Moderate dehydration with approximately 10% weight loss
      Mottled skin, cold extremities, tachycardia, decreased urinary output, depressed fontanelle, sunken eye lids, and loss of abdominal skin turgor occur.
   c. Severe dehydration with approximately 15% weight loss
      The infant becomes cyanotic, shocky, lethargic, and comatose.
4. Complications are usually related to fluid and electrolyte imbalance and metabolic acidosis. Others include otitis media, bronchopneumonia, bacteremia, necrotizing enterocolitis, peritonitis (which may result from perforation of an intestinal ulcer), renal vein or cerebral sinus thrombosis, and secondary lactose intolerance.
5. Infants with diarrhea due to phototherapy almost always look well.
6. Infants with withdrawal syndrome have other signs of withdrawal, e.g., tremors or irritability (see chapter 15–XIX).

7. Infants with Hirschsprung's disease have diarrhea alternating with constipation (see chapter 17–XIV).
8. Infants with cystic fibrosis have steatorrhea (see chapter 17–VII).

D. Laboratory Findings

1. Specific Tests
   Positive cultures of organisms are diagnostic. Common etiologic agents include enteropathogenic *E. coli* (055:B5 and 0111:B4), *Salmonella, Shigella, Campylobacter, Staphylococci, Klebsiella, Pseudomonas, C. albicans,* and rotavirus. Occasionally, cultures of blood, urine, and CSF are positive for the same organism as that from the stool or for *Pseudomonas, E. coli,* or *Proteus* in the presence of *Salmonella* or *Shigella* gastroenteritis. Simultaneous excretion of virus and *Salmonella, Shigella,* or enteropathogenic *E. coli* may be present. *Salmonella* and *Shigella* that were not identified on admission may be cultured after oral antimicrobial therapy, which suppresses coliform overgrowth. *Campylobacter* needs at least 7 days of culture due to slow and inapparent growth.
2. Serologic tests
   a. The fluorescent antibody technique can rapidly identify enteropathogenic *E. coli.*
   b. ELISA can rapidly identify rotavirus and ELISA IgG and IgM antirotavirus antibody.
3. Nonspecific tests
   a. An elevated hematocrit is common.
   b. Urinalysis reveals protein, white cells, casts, and a high specific gravity.
   c. The infant may be severely acidotic.
   d. Smear of stool may show polymorphonuclear leukocytes or bacteria. Absence of stool polymorphonuclear leukocytes may be seen in enteropathogenic *E. coli* or rotavirus, while polymorphonuclear leukocytes are often seen with *Salmonella, Shigella, Campylobacter,* and invasive strains of *E. coli.*
   e. When dehydration ensues, an elevated BUN or creatinine may be present.

E. Diagnostic Workup

1. Review the infant's history carefully, including nurses' notes, to make sure the infant
   a. Was not overfed or fed a high osmolar, high-carbohydrate content formula. Ascertain if the formula was prepared carefully and if the infant was fed a protein formula or soy formula for which he or she could be intolerant.
   b. Actually had loose stools (the breast-fed infant has looser stools than the bottle-fed infant) or bloody, mucoid, or watery stools.

   c. Was on antibiotic therapy for a period of time. If so, mycotic enteritis, especially candidiasis, should be considered.
   d. Has a history of a concurrent infection.
   e. Has a family history of food allergy.
2. Examine the infant carefully to ascertain that no middle ear, urinary, or respiratory tract infection is present.
3. Note carefully the infant's hydration.
4. Obtain a stool culture for bacterial and viral pathogens and a smear of the stool for polymorphonuclear leukocytes and a stool specimen for reducing substances to rule out lactase deficiency.
5. Obtain cultures of urine, blood, and CSF.
6. Obtain blood for CBC, electrolytes, glucose, BUN, creatinine, blood gases, and osmolality.
7. Obtain urinary output, urinalysis, and urine specific gravity.
8. Consider other causes of diarrhea than infectious; phototherapy, Hirschsprung's disease, cystic fibrosis, adrenal hyperplasia, milk intolerance, narcotic withdrawal syndrome, etc.
   Review the infant's history to see whether the infant
   a. Has been on phototherapy.
   b. Has other signs of withdrawal syndrome.
   c. Has family history of cystic fibrosis.
   d. Has loose stools alternating with constipation.

F. Supportive Management

See chapter 16–IIIC for "general supportive management for the infant with infection."

1. Isolate immediately any infant with diarrhea with or without known cause from the remainder of the nursery population.
2. Monitor vital signs continuously and record hourly: heart rate, respiratory rate, temperature, and blood pressure.
3. Weigh the infant two to four times daily. The degree of hydration is ascertained by weight loss or gain in addition to the infant's skin turgor. Remember third space fluid loss into the bowel lumen does not reflect weight loss.
4. Maintain strict intake and output.
5. Discontinue oral feedings for severe diarrhea.
6. For mild to moderately severe uncomplicated diarrhea, start oral glucose electrolyte solution containing NaCl 3.5 gm, KCl 1.5 gm, $NaHCO_3$ 2.5 gm, and anhydrous glucose 20 gm per liter of boiled water. Two bottles of glucose electrolyte solution need to be alternated with one bottle of water and water is skipped when hyponatremia is present.
7. Support the fluid intake of the infant intravenously as required.
   a. Quanity
      Total fluid intake for 24 hours equals (1) maintenance fluid (see Table 6–1) and (2) replacement of the deficit calculated from the infant's weight loss.

5% weight loss (mild dehydration): Add 50 ml/kg/24 hours to maintenance fluid.
10% weight loss (moderate dehydration): Add 100 ml/kg/24 hours to maintenance fluid.
15% weight loss (severe dehydration): Add 150 ml/kg/24 hours to maintenance fluid.
Add to this (3) the predicted abnormal losses (caused by elevated temperature, vomiting, diarrhea, etc.) that will occur over the next 24 hours.
The sum of these three equals the quantity of fluid to be administered over the next 24 hours.

b. Quality
The quality of fluids administered depends upon the type of dehydration. Since the type of dehydration is not known at the commencement of therapy, administer a one-fourth to one-third isotonic NaCl solution to start. KCl, 2 mEq/100 ml of fluid intake, can be added after the infant voids. When the infant has isotonic, hypotonic, or mild hypertonic dehydration, a one-fourth to one-third isotonic solution can be administered. For hypertonic dehydration, some physicians prefer slow infusion of an isotonic solution (0.9% NaCl), which is hypotonic to the infant's blood.
The infant's electrolyte status must be followed frequently.

8. Maintain acid-base balance.
   a. The infant usually has mild or moderate metabolic acidosis that requires slow correction by IV administration of fluids, e.g., a one-fourth isotonic solution composed of one-half NaCl and one-half $NaHCO_3$ or all $NaHCO_3$.
   b. In cases of severe metabolic acidosis, correction with 4.2% $NaHCO_3$ may be used. To determine the quantity of mEq to be administered, multiply the infant's weight in kilograms $\times$ 0.3 (a constant factor) $\times$ the base deficit (see chapter 11–IIIB12).
   The hyperventilation associated with metabolic acidosis occasionally continues for approximately 12 to 24 hours after the correction of pH because of the time lag between equilibration of the serum pH and CNS pH.
   c. The pH should be followed serially.
9. Correct shock.
   a. Correct shock by administering 20 ml/kg of a volume expander (Plasmanate, dextran, salt-poor albumin, isotonic saline, or whole blood). If a volume expander does not correct shock and endotoxemia is suspected, administer hydrocortisone and naloxone. See chapter 14–IIID7 for "general management for the infant with anemia and/or hemorrhage."
   b. Monitor vital signs.
   c. Monitor the central venous pressure.
10. Administer diluted oral solution when dehydration, acid-base imbalance, and diarrhea are corrected.
   a. Administer small amounts of clear fluids, e.g., 5% dextrose in water or electrolyte solution.

b. If clear fluids do not precipitate an increased quantity of diarrhea, start diluted milk formula, e.g., a 13 calories/oz-formula.
c. Gradually decrease the quantity of fluid given IV while gradually increasing the quantity of fluid taken orally until the infant is taking fluids by mouth exclusively.
d. Since transient lactose deficiency may occur during diarrhea, the infant may require lactose-free formula (e.g., Pregestimil).

G. Specific Therapy

1. Administer parenteral antibiotics.
   a. Usually start with ampicillin, 50 to 100 mg/kg/day, divided into two doses for infants less than 7 days of age and three doses for infants greater than 7 days of age and aminoglycoside divided into two doses for infants less than 7 days and three doses for infants greater than 7 days of age. Selection of aminoglycoside depends on institutional sensitivity.
   b. When specific organisms are suspected, the following antibiotics may be administered before culture and sensitivity results are available. See Table 16–1 for "dosage and complications of antibiotic therapy in the newborn."

ORGANISM	ANTIBIOTIC
E. coli (enteropathogenic)	Neomycin, colistin, kanamycin, gentamicin, amikacin
Salmonella	Ampicillin, chloramphenicol
Shigella	Ampicillin, kanamycin, neomycin, colistin
Campylobacter	Gentamicin, amikacin, kanamycin
S. aureus	Cephalothin, cephaloridine, vancomycin, the penicillinase-resistant penicillin
Klebsiella	Kanamycin, gentamicin
Pseudomonas	Gentamicin, polymyxin B, colistin
C. albicans	Nystatin

   c. Modify the antibiotic regimen according to clinical response and culture and antibiotic sensitivity results.
   c. No specific antiviral agents are available yet.
   e. Sudden changes in clinical response may occur during the course of a single epidemic as drug-sensitive strains of enteropathogenic *E. coli* may be replaced by drug-resistant strains.

H. Management of Exposed Newborn Infants During a Diarrhea Epidemic

1. Close the nursery to new admissions.
2. Observe all exposed infants for signs of diarrhea and sepsis.

3. Obtain a stool culture and serology test for all exposed infants and the nursery personnel.
4. Treat carriers and all exposed infants with neomycin, 50 to 100 mg/kg/24 hours orally for 7 to 10 days or up to the day of discharge. The initial drug of choice depends upon local patterns of susceptibility and the subsequent continuation may be changed depending upon the result of sensitivity.
5. Repeat the stool culture every 3 days.
6. Isolate exposed infants in the nursery until discharge. Do not send exposed infants out of the nursery for feeding, mothering, etc.
7. Scrub the nursery after all infants have been discharged before reopening the unit.

I. Prognosis

Recovery from infectious diarrhea is usual. Occasionally, fluid and electrolyte imbalance or other complications cause severe sequelae, such as renal vein thrombosis or CNS hemorrhage.

REFERENCES

Finberg L.: The management of the critically ill child with dehydration secondary to diarrhea. *Pediatrics* 45:1029, 1970.

Pizarro D., Posada G., Mata L.: Treatment of 242 neonates with dehydrating diarrhea with an oral glucose-electrolyte solution. *J. Pediatr.* 102:153, 1983.

XXIII. ACQUIRED IMMUNODEFICIENCY SYNDROME (AIDS)

AIDS, a virus-induced immunodeficiency, is caused by the retrovirus, human T lymphotrophic virus Type III/lymphadenopathy-associated virus (HTLV-III/LAV). Most pediatric HTLV-III-infected infants acquire the virus transplacentally, during labor or delivery, or via breast feedings from their own infected mothers. Infants are more susceptible to the disease, have a more rapid onset of disease, and a higher mortality rate than adults (approximately 60% of antibody-positive infants die: 1985 data).

A. Prevention

1. Vaccines are not available.
2. Counseling of the general population, particularly women of the childbearing age, to decrease the risk of acquiring the HTLV-III virus by avoiding sex or transmission of bodily fluids with infected partners.
3. Counseling of IV drug users to avoid sharing of needles.
4. Premarital and prenatal screening for the HTLV-III antibody of women at risk and their sexual partners. If infected, counsel the infected person to modify her sexual practices, to avoid blood, organ, or sperm donations, to refrain

from sharing of needles and syringes, and to delay pregnancy until more about the disease is known.

5. If an HTLV-III antibody-positive mother delivers an infant:
   a. Avoid breastfeeding.
   b. Place the infant on "blood and secretion" precaution.
   c. Warn the nursery personnel to maintain thorough handwashing technique, wear disposable gloves, maintain careful needle technique, etc. Personnel should be advised to work carefully and slowly to prevent accidental injuries.
   d. Disposable syringes, needles, scalpel blades and other sharp items should be placed in puncture-resistant containers.
   e. Personnel should wear a gown, mask, and eye coverings (e.g., glasses) when personnel have extensive contact with blood or secretions.
   f. If personnel are stuck with a needle, cut, or splashed in the eye or mouth, perform an HTLV-III screening test at 1½, 3, 6, and 12 months after exposure.
6. If newborns (particularly prematures) require transfusions, transfuse blood or blood products that are negative for HTLV-III antibody, CMV antibody, and HB_S antigen.

B. Who Is at Risk?

The following infants are at risk to acquire perinatally transmitted AIDS:

1. Infants born to symptomatic or asymptomatic mothers who are HTLV-III antibody-positive.
2. Infants whose mothers have previous infants with AIDS.
3. Infants born to mothers at risk for AIDS. Approximately 75% pediatric AIDS cases are born to mothers at risk:
   a. IV drug users (48%)
      Infants who are born to IV drug-using mothers who reside in New York City (45%), Florida and New Jersey (32%) are at high risk to develop AIDS.
   b. Haitian immigrants (17%)
   c. infants born to a mother who had a sex partner at risk (either IV drug users or bisexual men) (10%)
   d. prostitutes
   e. hemophiliacs
4. Infants who received blood or blood products: red cells, platelets, plasma, whole blood, etc. (Approximately 10%–20% of transfusion-associated AIDS cases are infants.)

C. Clinical Manifestations

1. Asymptomatic
2. Transient nonspecific symptoms resembling infectious mononucleosis with fe-

ver 1–2 months after infection followed by asymptomatic period of a few months. Mild or severe symptoms develop after 1 month to 5 years (mean of 1 year for children and 2 years for adults) of incubation period. Symptoms due to perinatally acquired infection occur by 3 months of age. The mean incubation period is shorter for children than adults.

Mild symptoms—AIDS-related complex (ARC): fever, unexplained chronic lymphadenopathy, thrush, fatigue.

Severe symptoms—AIDS: chronic interstitial pneumonitis, failure to thrive, hepatosplenomegaly, lymphadenopathy, eczematoid rash, petechiae, recurrent diarrhea, melena, recurrent otitis media, low birth weight or small for gestational age at birth, associated one or recurrent opportunistic infections (candida, cytomegalovirus, hepatitis B, herpes, pneumocystis carinii pneumonia, syphilis, toxoplasmosis, tuberculosis, etc.).

3. Signs and symptoms are similar to cytomegalovirus, toxoplasmosis, herpes simplex, and congenital immunodeficiency disease (Di George syndrome or Wiskott-Aldrich syndrome, etc.).

D. Laboratory Findings

1. Specific
   Isolation of HTLV-III/LAV virus from blood, saliva, tears, maternal breast milk, urine, etc.
2. Presumptive
   The infant with HTLV-III antibody should be considered infected and/or infectious since HTLV-III virus has been isolated from 75%–95% of population with the antibody. However, it is not clear how long the infant can remain viremic or how many infants will eventually develop AIDS when asymptomatic, but antibody positive. Antibodies appear in 2–4 months after exposure. It is recommended to test for the antibody by the ELISA screening test (twice) in high-risk groups and by the ELISA (twice) and Western blot test in low-risk groups.
3. Nonspecific
   a. Reversal of the T4/T8 (helper/suppressor T-lymphocytes) ratio <1.0 (85%) as in Epstein-Barr virus and cytomegalovirus infection. The number of T helper cells is decreased in AIDS while suppressor cells are increased when Epstein-Barr virus and cytomegalovirus infection are seen. Toxoplasmosis, herpes in the first month, or cytomegalovirus in the first 6 months of age should be excluded.
   b. Absolute lymphopenia (<1500) (12%) (more common in adults).
   c. Marked hypergammaglobulinemia. Renal failure may develop due to immune complex deposition.
   d. B cell dysfunction with normal or increased levels (increased IgG), impaired antibody production to diphtheria, tetanus, or pneumococcal polysaccharides immunization
   e. Thrombocytopenia with normal platelet size.

E. Radiologic Features

1. Chronic interstitial pneumonitis.

F. General Supportive Management

1. Treat recurrent infections aggressively. Mucocutaneous candidiasis is difficult to treat and amphotericin B is the drug of choice.
   Pentamidine and TMP-SMZ are for pneumocystis carinii infection and some recommend chemoprophylaxis.
2. Monthly administration of parenteral gammaglobulin or interferons and interleukin 2 are under study.
3. Irradiate blood or blood products to prevent graft-versus-host reactions prior to transfusion into children with AIDS.
4. Test for HTLV-III antibody if children are born to mothers at risk for or with AIDS since live vaccine (e.g., MMR) are hazardous.
5. Support nutrition.
6. Psychoemotional support.

G. Specific Therapy

Antiviral agents are not available yet.

H. Prognosis

To date there is no evidence that AIDS is reversible. Clinical diagnosis prior to 6 months of age is usually fatal. The mortality is seen usually within 4 years in adults and within 1 month in newborns. Kaposi sarcoma is rare in children with AIDS.

REFERENCES

Shannon K.M., Ammann A.J.: Acquired immune deficiency syndrome in childhood. *J. Pediatr.* 106:332–342, 1985.

Scott G.B., Fischi M.A., Klimias N., et al.: Mothers of infants with acquired immunodeficiency syndrome. *JAMA* 253:363, 1985.

Scott G.B., Buck B.E., Leternon J.G., et al.: Acquired immunodeficiency syndrome in infants. *N. Engl. J. Med.* 310:76–81, 1984.

Centers for Disease Control: Recommendations for assisting in the prevention of perinatal transmission of HTLV-III/LAV and acquired immunodeficiency syndrome. *MMWR* 34:721, 1985.

TABLE 16–2.—OPHTHALMIA NEONATORUM

	ONSET OF SYMPTOMS (AGE)	CLINICAL SYMPTOMS	CAUSE	METHOD OF DIAGNOSIS	PREVENTION OR TREATMENT
Chemical conjunctivitis	6–24 hr	Purulent discharge lasting 24–48 hr	Failure of washing prophylactic 1% silver nitrate from the eye 15 seconds after administration	History plus negative eye culture	Wash eyes with normal saline 15 seconds after application of 1% silver nitrate
Acute purulent conjunctivitis	24–48 hr	Acute purulent discharge	*S. aureus*, Streptococcus group A and B, *S. pneumoniae*, pneumonococcus, *H. influenzae*, *E. coli*, *P. aeruginosa*	Smear and culture of the exudate	Appropriate antibiotic ointment, e.g., neosporin ophthalmic ointment
Gonorrheal conjunctivitis	2–5 days	Acute copious purulent discharge	N. gonorrhoeae	Smear and culture of the exudate on chocolate agar or transgrow medium	Systemic penicillin G, 50,000 units/kg/day divided into 2 doses for 7 days. Irrigate eyes with 0.9% NaCl every 1 hr until clear

Inclusion blennorrhea (chlamydial)	5 days–2 wk	Acute copious purulent discharge	*C.* trachomatis	Scraping (not smear) of the eyelid and Giemsa stain of the scrapings for characteristic inclusions or fluorescein—conjugated monoclonal antibody stain	Topical ophthalmic tetracycline or sulfonamides or erythromycin ointment four times daily for 2 weeks plus oral erythromycin, 40 mg/kg/day for 2 weeks
Herpes simplex virus conjunctivitis	2–3 days to 1 mo.	Slowly progressing conjunctivitis, keratitis, and corneal scarring	Herpes simplex virus	Fluorescein staining of corneal epithelia reveals dendritic or ameboid stain; viral culture	Topical use of acyclovir or vidarabine may be useful for prevention or treatment of ocular herpes

REFERENCES

Paentice M.J., Hutchinson G.R., Taylor-Robinson D.: Microbiological study of neonatal conjunctivitis. *Br. J. Ophthamol.* 61:9, 1977.

Tanner E.I.: Neonatal conjunctivitis, letter. *Br. Med. J.* 1:530, 1972.

Tam M.R., Stamm W.E., Handsfields H.H. et al.: Culture independent diagnosis of chlamydia trachomatis using monoclonal antibodies. *N. Engl. J. Med.* 310:1146, 1984.

TABLE 16–3.—Effects of Uncommon Maternal Infection on the Fetus and Neonate*

MATERNAL INFECTION	EFFECTS ON FETUS AND NEONATE	ASSOCIATED FACTORS
Influenza	Increased incidence of abortion and premature labor Occasional association of congenital malformations, especially anencephaly and meningomyelocele	Active immunization by an attenuated vaccine should not be given during pregnancy to prevent possible fetal damage.
Malaria	Direct transmission of *P. falciparum* occurs rarely Diminished growth with placental involvement	Placental involvement is 10 times more frequent than fetal involvement
Mumps	Abortion, premature birth, or stillbirth uncommon ? cause of endocardial fibroelastosis, transient diabetes mellitus	
Poliomyelitis	Abortion Rare congenital or acquired poliomyelitis Growth retardation in chronic, severe, maternal, paralytic poliomyelitis. Fetal and neonatal loss in 33%	Widespread use of immunization procedures has all but eliminated this disease as a pregnancy problem. Use of Sabin live virus vaccine during pregnancy is contraindicated. May safely administer Salk vaccine.
Rubeola	Interruption of pregnancy Congenital or neonatal measles with or without bronchopneumonia (typical dermal lesions are in same stage as those in mother) Maternal rubeola at any time during pregnancy is responsible for increased perinatal death rate. Great majority of infants are normal	Measles vaccine should be given to all nonimmune women prior to but not during gestation.
Smallpox and vaccinia	Increased fetal wastage in all stages of pregnancy Congenital malformations not more frequent, but congenital infections with skin lesions reported	Primary vaccination and revaccination against smallpox must be deferred until after delivery because vaccinia often causes fatal widespread fetal visceral and cutaneous lesions.

*Adapted by Rudolph from data of Desmond, in Klaus M.H., Fanaroff A.A. (eds.): Care of the high risk neonate, ed. 2. Philadelphia, W.B. Saunders Co., 1979, p. 272. Used by permission.

XXIV. POOR MUSCLE TONE: "THE FLOPPY INFANT"

Isolated poor muscle tone without poor feeding, poor cry, etc., may be present in the newborn infant. Since muscle tone increases with gestation, muscle tone should be evaluated according to the gestational age and can be assessed by using the gestational age assessment chart (See Figs 6–1, 6–2).

A. Who Is at Risk?

Infants with following conditions have hypotonia:

1. Proximal spinal muscular (neurogenic) atrophies
   Werdnig-Hoffman's disease
2. Congenital myopathies
   a. Central core disease
   b. Glycogen storage disease
3. Neuromuscular disorders
   a. Myasthenia gravis
   b. Congenital muscular dystrophy
   c. Congenital myotonic dystrophy
   d. Pseudohypertrophic muscular dystrophy (early onset Duchenne's dystrophy)
4. CNS disorders
   a. Hypotonic cerebral palsy
   b. Metabolic (e.g., amino-acid metabolism) disorders
   c. Trisomies (13–15, 18, 21, etc.)
   d. Birth trauma, perinatal asphyxia, CNS hemorrhage
5. Prader-Willi Syndrome
6. Connective tissue disorders, e.g., Marfan's syndrome, osteogenesis imperfecta
7. Metabolic or endocrine disorders
   Renal tubular acidosis, hypothyroidism
8. Acute illness
   Infection, hypoxia, acidosis, etc.
9. Benign congenital hypotonia

B. Clinical Manifestations, Laboratory Findings, and Supportive Management

See Table 16–4.

REFERENCES

Brans Y.W., Cassady G.: Neonatal spinal cord injuries. *Am. J. Obstet. Gynecol.* 123:918, 1975.

Fenichel G.M.: Clinical syndromes of myasthenia in infancy and childhood: A review. *Arch. Neurol.* 35:97, 1978.

Koch B.M., Eng G.M.: Neonatal spinal cord injury *Arch. Phys. Med. Rehab.* 60:378, 1979.

Zellweger H., Ionasescu V.: Early onset of myotonic dystrophy in infants. *Am. J. Dis. Child.* 125:601, 1973.

TABLE 16–4.—INFANTS WITH HYPOTONIA*†

DISEASE	ETIOLOGY	CLINICAL MANIFESTATIONS	EMG/CPK	MUSCLE BIOPSY	MANAGEMENT
Werdnig-Hoffman	Autosomal recessive trait	Weakness, tongue fasciculations, severe head lag Proximal limb girdle muscle paralysis, frog leg position Absent DTR	Degeneration of muscle/ normal	Atrophy of anterior horn cell and motor nerve root Single or multiple	Supportive management Chest PT NG tube feeding
Central core disease	Autosomal dominant	Diminished fetal movement Hypotonia and proximal weakness, no feeding and respiratory difficulties. Normal DTR, common CDH Associated with malignant hyperpyrexia	Normal/ ± normal	Central cores of myofibrils present Decreased central mitochondria, increased sarcoplasmic reticulum	Supportive management Chest PT Usually nonprogressive
Glycogen storage	See Table 16–5	Hypoglycemia, hepatomegaly, seizures, growth failure, mental retardation	Normal/normal	Abnormal glycogen	See Table 16–5
Myasthenia gravis	Passive transfer or autoimmune reaction	Hypotonia, ptosis, weak suck, swallow and/or breathing, inability to close the mouth Onset: 1–4 days 2–4 weeks in transient form, otherwise permanent	± Normal/ normal	Normal	Supportive management Prostigmin 0.1–0.2 mg IM 30 min before feeding (for 6 weeks in transient)‡ Common mental retardation if survive

Congenital muscular dystrophy	Autosomal recessive	Muscle atrophy, contractures, arthrogryposis, hypotonia, weakness Apnea, respiratory depression, ↓ DTR, abnormal CT scan	Myopathic pattern/ normal or ↑	Muscle atrophy nongrouped changes marked variation in fiber size, connective tissue and fat replacement	Usually nonprogressive or slow improvement Supportive management with PT
Congenital myotonic dystrophy	Autosomal dominant via mother	Hypotonia, poor suck, ptosis, weakness, and atrophy of facial, jaw and temporalis muscle, delayed motor develop, polyhydramnios, arthrogryposis	Abnormal/ normal or ↑	Muscle atrophy Small round fibers with large internal nuclei, sparse myofibrils, fetal myotonus	Procainamide or quinidine may be tried Death at 1 year of age Neonatal mortality (50%)
Pseudohypertrophic muscular dystrophy (Duchenne's)	X-linked dominant (50% carriers in females) (50% in males)	Slow motor development Weak hypertrophied muscle Rarely diagnosed before 3 years of age	Decreased amplitude and motor potentials/ ↑ (10X)	Muscle degeneration with fatty infiltration	Supportive management
Spinal cord injury (see Table 5–3)	Traumatic delivery (Breech)	Loss of function below the level of the lesion with priapism, ↑ or ↓ DTR	Normal/normal	Normal	Gentle neck traction Immediate cervical exploration

*Adapted from Klaus M., Fanaroff A.A. (eds.): Care of the high-risk neonate, ed. 3. Philadelphia, W.B. Saunders Co., 1986.

†Other entities listed in "who is at risk section" are in the text. CDH = Congenital dislocation of hip; CPK = creatine phosphokinase, PT = physiotherapy

‡Prostigmin 0.1–0.2 mg IM leads to a dramatic clinical improvement within 30 min.

TABLE 16–5.—COMMON GLYCOGEN STORAGE DISEASES (GSD)

TYPE/NAME	ENZYME DEFICIENCY	CLINICAL MANIFESTATIONS	COMMENTS
Type 0 (GSD 0)	Glycogen synthetase	Hypoglycemia, mental retardation, seizures	1% of normal glycogen present in liver. Treat with frequent protein rich meal
Type I (GSD I) Von Gierke's disease	Glucose-6-phosphatase	Hepatosplenomegaly, enlarged kidneys, normal mental development, tendency to hypoglycemia, lactic acidosis, hyperlipidemia, hyperuricacidemia, bleeding	Cardiac and skeletal muscle normal. Continuous NG tube feeding at night may be of value
Type IIa (GSD IIa) Pompe's disease, Cori type II	α-glucosidase	Cardiomegaly, progressive hypotonia and weakness, swallowing and respiratory difficulty, normal mental development, death in infancy, hepatomegaly	Abnormal ECG, increase in tissue glycogen, abnormal lysosomes in liver and skin, infantile fatal form
Type III (GSD III) Debrancher deficiency, Forbes' disease, limit dextrinosis, Cori type III	Amylo-1,6-glucosidase	Hepatomegaly, late onset of weakness, none to moderate cardiomegaly, no acidosis, no hypoglycemia	Cultured amniotic fluid cells abnormal, disease has benign course
Type IV (GSD IV) Brancher deficiency, Andersen's disease, Cori type IV	Amylo-1,4→1,6 transglucosidase	Hepatosplenomegaly, ascites, cirrhosis, liver failure, normal mental development, death in early childhood	Cultured amniotic fluid cells abnormal, death in early childhood
Type V (GSD V) McArdle's disease	Muscle phosphorylase	Myoglobinuria in later life, muscle cramps, normal mental development	No rise in blood lactate during ischemic exercise, begins in adolescence

Type VI (GSD VI) Hers' disease, Cori type VI	Hepatophosphorylase	Hepatomegaly, no splenomegaly, growth retardation, no hypoglycemia or acidosis, mild ketosis	Lack of glucagon-induced hyperglycemia
Type VII (GSD VII) Phosphofructokinase deficiency	Phosphofructokinase	Symptoms identical to Type V myophosphorylase deficiency, normal mental development, muscle cramps with exercise	Reduction of phosphofructokinase activity severe in skeletal muscle, mild in erythrocytes, no rise in blood lactate during ischemic exercise
Type VIII (GSD VIII) Phosphorylase kinase deficiency	Phosphorylase kinase or adenosine 3′,5′-AMP dependent kinase	Hepatomegaly, truncal ataxia, nystagmus, neurologic deterioration, hypertonia, spasticity, decerebration, death	Urinary epinephrine and norepinephrine increased during acute phase, cerebral glycogen increased
Type IX (GSD IX)	Inactive phosphophorylase kinase (content normal)	Hepatomegaly, no splenomegaly, hypoglycemia or acidosis	Urinary catecholamines normal, normal glucagon-induced hyperglycemia; x-linked recessive
Type X (GSD X)	Loss of activity of cyclic 3′-5′-AMP dependent kinase	Severe hepatomegaly, otherwise normal	Phosphorylase kinase activity 50% of normal

REFERENCE

Behrman R.E., Vaughan V.C.: *Nelson Textbook of Pediatrics,* Ed. 12. Philadelphia, W.B. Saunders Co., 1983. Used by permission.

Chapter 17

Vomiting and Abdominal Distention

Vomiting and abdominal distention are associated with various disturbances, both trivial and life threatening. It is imperative that the pediatric house officer differentiate minor gastrointestinal (GI) disturbances from major medical or surgical emergencies.

I. CLINICAL EVALUATION

A. Normal Data

1. Regurgitation
   When there is an effortless flow of gastric or esophageal contents from the infant's mouth during sleep or when the infant is prone or at the end of feeding, it is termed regurgitation. Regurgitation is associated with esophageal incoordination and poor esophageal sphincter tone. Regurgitation is not serious if weight gain is adequate and frequently stops gradually. Occasionally, the infant continues to regurgitate over many months.
2. Passage of meconium
   Ninety-four percent of infants pass meconium within 24 hours after birth; 99% pass meconium by 48 hours of age (see appendix A–36 and A–37).
3. Stool frequency
   Infants between 3 and 6 days of age fed milk feedings pass 4 ± 1.8 stools/24 hours (range, 1 to 12/24 hours).
4. Abdominal distention
   After feeding, small premature infants may appear to have mild abdominal distention that is benign. Fullterm and larger premature infants frequently appear to have abdominal distention after feeding but this "distention" should subside before the next feeding.

5. The presence of air in the GI tract
   Air is usually seen in the stomach immediately after birth. By 1 hour of age, the proximal portion of the small intestine is outlined. Air in the distal portion of the colon may be seen as early as the third hour of life. The passage of air through the GI tract may be retarded in compromised or premature infants. An abdominal film after 24 hours of age will normally show gas throughout the GI tract.

B. Abnormal Vomiting and Abdominal Distention

1. Vomiting
   Vomiting is the forceful flow of stomach contents with reversed gastric peristalsis.
   a. Projectile vomiting
      Forceful projectile vomiting is often associated with pyloric stenosis, antral spasm, and increased intracranial pressure.
   b. Bile-stained vomitus (green vomitus)
      Until proved otherwise, bile-stained vomitus must be assumed to be caused by intestinal obstruction beyond the ampulla of Vater. Bile-stained vomitus is a diagnostic emergency and requires immediate investigation to determine the cause of vomiting, no matter how well the infant appears.
   c. Blood-stained vomitus
      Blood-stained vomitus in the first 24 hours of life is most frequently caused by swallowed maternal blood, but the possibility that it is the infant's blood must always be considered. To differentiate maternal from infant's blood, perform an Apt test (see chapter 14–IIIB9). After the second day of life, fresh red blood in the infant's vomitus usually results from the infant bleeding but may be caused by ingested blood from the mother's nipple if the infant is breast fed.
   d. Vomiting associated with diarrhea
      Vomiting associated with diarrhea frequently indicates a localized or generalized infection. Diarrhea in the newborn is always a matter of concern, particularly if the infant is vomiting because dehydration may occur.
   e. Vomiting associated with abdominal distention
      Vomiting associated with abdominal distention frequently indicates a serious underlying abnormality such as a paralytic ileus, electrolyte imbalance, intestinal obstruction, and/or GI perforation.
2. Abdominal distention
   Abdominal distention may be associated with respiratory distress, sepsis or peritonitis caused by infection or chemical irritation, intestinal or urinary tract obstruction, Hirschsprung's disease, abdominal masses, ascites, hypokalemia, hypermagnesemia, and hemorrhage. Abdominal distention frequently follows an exchange transfusion or administration of positive-pressure breathing by bag and mask. Abdominal distention may be absent with a high intestinal obstruction.

II. COMMON CAUSES OF VOMITING AND ABDOMINAL DISTENTION IN THE NEWBORN

A. Normal Newborn

1. Irritative vomiting caused by excessive mucus
2. Feeding intolerance; disturbances related to the quality or quantity of the formula, e.g., excessive feeding or protein intolerance

B. Sick Infant

1. Infection
   a. Sepsis
   b. Necrotizing enterocolitis
2. Mechanical intestinal obstruction
   a. Congenital intrinsic
   Atresia, stenosis, duplication, imperforate anus, cysts, meconium ileus, webs, small left colon syndrome
   b. Congenital extrinsic
   Malrotation, fibrous bands, volvulus, duplications, cysts, tumors, annular pancreas, incarcerated hernia, adhesions, hiatus hernia
   c. Acquired
   Volvulus, intussusception, mesenteric thrombosis, necrotizing enterocolitis, tumors, polyps, meconium ileus (cystic fibrosis), meconium plug syndrome, bezoars or fecaliths
3. Disorders of neuromuscular control
   a. Pharyngeal incoordination
   b. Chalasia
   c. Achalasia
   d. Cardiospasm, antral spasm
   e. Pylorospasm/pyloric stenosis
   f. Hirschsprung's disease
   g. Familial dysautonomia
   h. Generalized hypotonia
4. Rupture of a hollow viscus; gastric, esophageal, or intestinal perforation
5. Intraperitoneal accumulation of fluid
   a. Ascites
   b. Exudate
   c. Blood
   d. Genitourinary transudate from genitourinary obstruction
6. Metabolic disorders
   a. Hypermagnesemia
   b. Hypokalemia
   c. Hyperammonemia
   d. Renal tubular acidosis

   e. Renal insufficiency
   f. Familial protein intolerance
   g. Hypothyroidism
7. Intracranial disorders
   a. Increased intracranial pressure
   b. Hydrocephalus
   c. Hypoxic encephalopathy
   d. Craniostenosis
   e. CNS bleeding or infection
8. Inborn errors of metabolism
   a. Congenital galactosemia
   b. Maple syrup urine disease
   c. Hyperammonemia
   d. Hypervalinemia
   e. Citrullinemia
9. Functional ileus
   Prematurity
10. Defects of GI development
   a. Omphalocele
   b. Gastroschisis
11. Miscellaneous
   a. Milk allergy
   b. Abdominal masses

III. WHAT THE PHYSICIAN SHOULD DO WHEN CONFRONTED WITH AN INFANT WITH VOMITING AND/OR ABDOMINAL DISTENTION

A. Diagnostic Workup

1. Determine if the infant is really vomiting. Review the onset, time, quantity, quality, and characteristics of the infant's vomitus.
   a. Is the vomitus small and effortless? Is it regurgitation?
   b. Was the infant overfed or fed improperly?
   c. Is the infant vomiting before feeding (as in upper GI obstruction)?
   d. Is the vomitus projectile and forceful (as in pyloric stenosis or upper GI obstruction)?
   e. What is the color of the vomitus? Green, blood-stained, composed of mucus, etc.? Perform an Apt test if bloody vomitus occurs when the infant is less than 24 hours old (see chapter 14–IIIB9).
   f. Does the infant vomit when placed in the semi-Fowler position or only when lying flat (as in hiatus hernia)? Does a change in the infant's position change the quantity of the vomitus?
2. Review the maternal history for the presence of polyhydramnios (commonly associated with a high intestinal obstruction). Note whether the mother re-

ceived magnesium sulfate for the treatment of pregnancy-induced hypertension or to stop labor.

3. Question the mother concerning a family history of pyloric stenosis, cystic fibrosis, Hirschsprung's disease, adrenogenital syndrome, or galactosemia.
4. Review the infant's prenatal and birth histories to determine if the infant had a history of fetal distress, birth trauma, or prolonged rupture of the membranes before delivery.
5. Request the nurse to save the infant's stools. Note carefully the quality and frequency of the passage of stools. Is the infant passing meconium and/or stools? Delay or absence of the passage of meconium may be seen in premature infants or infants with a low Apgar score or may indicate obstruction, infection, meconium plug syndrome, ileus (sepsis, metabolic abnormalities and maternal medications), small left colon syndrome, or cystic fibrosis. Even in complete atresia, however, some meconium may be passed. The onset of failure to pass stools after normal bowel movements for several days may indicate peritonitis, necrotizing enterocolitis, malrotation, or volvulus, etc. Blood in the stool may indicate necrotizing enterocolitis, volvulus with or without malrotation, hemorrhagic disease, milk allergy, or a purely local phenomenon such as an anal fissure.
6. Examine the infant completely, considering each of the common causes of abdominal distention and vomiting.
   a. Determine if the infant is lethargic or irritable or has a diminished cry, poor suck, poor muscle tone, respiratory distress, erythema around the cord, or other signs of sepsis.
   b. Note the infant's head size (see Figs 6–2, 6–4, and 6–5).
   c. Pay special attention to the presence of abdominal distention. (The vessels in the upper abdomen are frequently dilated and the skin is shiny when the infant has abdominal distention.) Are dilated loops of bowel present? Are bowel sounds present? Is peristalsis visible? Is a mass palpable? Is there gastric residual? Do the flanks bulge? Is a hernia present? During palpation, an infant who has peritonitis may flex his or her hips possibly due to tenderness, while an infant with generalized sepsis and abdominal distention will continue to lie still. Reddening of the abdominal wall indicates peritonitis.
   d. Is the anus patent? Perform a rectal examination with a catheter or the smallest finger possible. Rectal examination is sometimes followed by passage of a meconium plug.
7. Obtain a culture and sensitivity test of the infant's urine, blood, and cerebrospinal fluid.
8. Draw blood for electrolytes, magnesium, blood urea nitrogen (BUN), creatinine, blood gas, ammonia, and hematocrit determination.
9. Obtain a supine, left lateral decubitus, and/or upright x-ray film of the abdomen. (The upright may be difficult.)
   a. Air throughout the GI tract by 18 hours of age is normal.
   b. The presence of free air under the diaphragm or over the liver dome by upright or left lateral decubitus film, or a "football sign" in the supine film is seen in perforation.

c. The presence of distended loops of bowel with or without loss of haustration is seen in paralytic ileus or intestinal obstruction.
d. The presence of a homogenous flank opacity is seen when free fluid is in the peritoneal cavity. Loops of bowel are centrally located.
e. Intraabdominal calcifications are indicative of intrauterine perforation, adrenal hemorrhage, teratoma, or neuroblastoma.
f. Linear streaks or mottling of intramural air are seen in necrotizing enterocolitis.
g. A shifted gas pattern is caused by intrinsic or extrinsic compression.
h. Barium enema reveals whether small or large bowel is distended, whether there is microcolon or other anatomic abnormalities, and whether the position of cecum is normal or abnormal (malrotation). Upper GI series is helpful for the diagnosis of partial intestinal obstruction.

10. Consider mechanical intestinal obstruction (see chapter 17–IV) if
    a. A history of maternal polyhydramnios is elicited.
    b. The vomitus is bile-stained.
    c. Abdominal distention is present.
    d. The quantity of meconium passed is scanty or absent.
11. If no evidence of mechanical intestinal obstruction is present on radiologic evaluation, a functional intestinal obstruction should be suspected. Sepsis, respiratory distress, hypermagnesemia, hypokalemia, intracranial disorders, and inborn errors of metabolism can cause a functional obstruction.
12. Consider pyloric stenosis if the infant sucks vigorously and vomits undigested food shortly after feeding, especially during the first 2 to 6 weeks of life in a male (see chapter 17–XIII).
13. If peritoneal fluid is present, perform a paracentesis to determine whether the fluid is meconium, pus, bile, blood, urine, or ascitic fluid.
14. Consult the pediatric surgeon if signs of intestinal perforation or obstruction are present.
15. Obtain abdominal sonogram to study abdominal cystic or solid masses.

B. General Supportive Management of the Infant With Vomiting and Abdominal Distension

1. Handle the infant gently (as always).
2. Maintain the infant's abdominal skin temperature at approximately 36.5° C (97.7° F) and the rectal temperature at approximately 37.0° C (98.6° F). Work within a warmed environment to avoid precipitous drops in body temperature associated with procedures, such as taking an x-ray film or inserting an intravenous line.
3. Monitor vital signs.
4. Discontinue all oral feedings while vomiting and/or abdominal distention persists.
5. Pass a soft, polyethylene nasogastric tube (see chapter 19–VA) and aspirate the stomach to empty it. Aspirate the stomach contents frequently to avoid aspiration and subsequent pneumonia. Pass a Replogle or nasogastric feed-

ing tube and attach to low pressure suction for continuous decompression.
6. Weigh the infant daily or more frequently if necessary.
7. Monitor the infant's electrolyte, hematocrit, and blood gas levels.
8. Administer IV fluids to maintain fluid and electrolyte status.
9. Correct electrolyte imbalance and dehydration.
10. Record intake and output (urine, stool, and GI aspirate) every 2 hours. Replace excessive fluid and electrolyte loss.

C. Preoperative Management of the Infant

1. Explain to the parents the meaning and nature of the surgical procedure and obtain consent for the surgical procedure.
2. Withhold oral feedings.
3. Administer vitamin K_1, 1.0 to 2.0 mg, IM.
4. Draw blood for hematocrit, CBC, platelets, glucose, electrolytes, calcium, magnesium, BUN, protein, osmolarity, blood gas studies, and type and cross-match.
5. Correct fluid, electrolyte, glucose, blood gas and/or hematologic imbalances if present.
6. Start broad-spectrum antibiotics.
7. Place an IV angiocatheter or percutaneous central venous line.

D. Intraoperative Management of the Infant

A pediatric house officer, a member of the neonatal staff, or a pediatric anesthesiologist experienced in handling newborns should attend the operation to do the following:

1. Monitor the infant during the procedure.
   a. Maintain the infant's rectal temperature at 37.0° C (98.6° F) by use of a radiant heater with a thermistor probe since inadvertent hypothermia occurs frequently in modern, air-conditioned operating rooms.
   b. Monitor continuously heart rate, respiratory rate, and blood pressure.
   c. Monitor blood gases. Transcutaneous PO_2 may be useful but poor perfusion during anesthesia may preclude its use.
   d. Ascertain that the IV route is patent so that significant blood losses can be replaced.
2. Be prepared for cardiorespiratory emergency support.
3. Observe the procedure so that the infant can be handled correctly after the operation.

E. Postoperative Management of the Infant

1. Monitor the infant. Follow vital signs, weight, abdominal girth, hematocrit, electrolytes, calcium, blood pressure, and fluid balance and correct as required.

2. Give the infant nothing by mouth and maintain caloric and fluid requirement via the IV route. Watch carefully for third space losses and adjust fluid input accordingly with plasma, Plasmanate, or 5% albumin. Start TPN as required.
3. Resume antibiotic therapy.
4. Maintain oxygenation, ventilation, and acid-base status.
5. Empty the gastric contents with an orogastric tube attached to low pressure suction continuously.
6. Maintain adequate vitamin K levels. Give 1 mg every 5 to 7 days while infant is receiving nothing by mouth.
7. Obtain results of cultures taken preoperatively or intraoperatively.
8. Start feedings and advance feeding slowly after infant has good bowel sounds and is passing stool.
9. Support the psychosocial needs of the family through this difficult period.

REFERENCES

Holder T.M., Leape L.L.: The acute surgical abdomen in the neonate. *N. Engl. J. Med.* 278:605, 1968.

Lemoh J.N., Brooke O.G.: Frequency and weight of normal stools in infancy. *Arch. Dis. Child.* 54:719–720, 1979.

Talbert J.L., Felman A.H., DeBusk F.L.: Gastrointestinal surgical emergencies in the newborn infant. *J. Pediatr.* 76:783, 1970.

IV. MECHANICAL INTESTINAL OBSTRUCTION

Obstruction may occur at any site along the intestinal tract and may be partial or complete. Mechanical obstruction must be differentiated from functional obstruction. Salvage of viable bowel is frequently possible only if emergency investigation and surgical correction are immediately undertaken.

A. Prevention

1. Since most causes of mechanical obstruction are congenital, no known methods of prevention are available.
2. To prevent bezoars, do not feed excessively high caloric formulas or improperly diluted formulas to premature infants.
3. To prevent mesenteric emboli/thrombi, do not push clots or air into umbilical artery catheters.
4. Prevent perinatal asphyxia and treat sepsis promptly to prevent necrotizing enterocolitis (controversial).
5. Observe passage of meconium in those infants whose mothers received magnesium sulfate and are at risk for drug-induced meconium ileus.

B. Who Is at Risk?

1. Infants with a maternal history of polyhydramnios are at risk for congenital obstruction (one half of infants with obstruction have a history of polyhydramnios).

2. Infants with a family history of cystic fibrosis, intestinal atresia, Hirschsprung's disease, or pyloric stenosis
3. Infants with Down's syndrome with duodenal atresia, annular pancreas and/or imperforate anus
4. Infants with prolonged hyperbilirubinemia
5. Infants with omphalocele due to coexisting malrotation and volvulus
6. Infants with sepsis and/or necrotizing enterocolitis (due to acquired stenosis)
7. Infants with prune belly syndrome
8. Infants with exstrophy of bladder or cloaca
9. Premature infants are at risk of developing incarcerated inguinal hernias and obstruction secondary to the hernia
10. Premature infants who receive 24-calories/oz or improperly diluted formulas are at risk for bezoars.

C. Clinical Manifestations

1. Bilious vomiting may occur shortly after birth in upper intestinal obstruction and may be delayed in lower intestinal obstruction.
2. Abdominal distention. Epigastric distention and peristaltic waves are seen in upper GI obstruction, while bulging of the flanks and vomitus with a fecal odor occur in lower GI obstruction.
3. Bowel sounds may be normal, hypoactive, or hyperactive.
4. There may be failure to pass meconium (or white meconium). Infants may pass meconium two to three times in the first 1 to 2 days with partial or upper GI obstruction.
5. Dehydration with decreased urinary output, respiratory difficulty and excessive salivation may occur.

D. Laboratory Findings

1. Specific findings
   There are no specific laboratory findings.
2. Associated findings
   a. A large residual gastric aspirate
   b. Electrolyte and acid-base imbalance (often hypokalemia, hypochloremia, and alkalosis)
   c. Increased hematocrit and/or osmolality as a result of dehydration
   d. Hyperbilirubinemia
   e. Increased urine osmolality and specific gravity

E. Radiologic Features

Air present in the GI tract is frequently sufficient for proper evaluation. If not, 10 to 20 ml of air may be injected after aspiration of fluid.

1. Air extending only to the pylorus after a few hours of age signifies a pyloric web or obstruction.
2. A "double-bubble sign" (air in the proximal duodenum superimposed upon the dilated stomach) may be present in cases of duodenal obstruction.
3. A "stepladder pattern" (dilated loops of bowel with air fluid levels) is seen in lower intestinal obstruction.
4. A barium enema is essential for the diagnosis of colonic atresia and is recommended when small-bowel obstruction is suspected to determine meconium ileus or malrotation of the intestines with or without midgut volvulus (see chapter 17–VI and 17–X).
5. If an upper GI examination is required, the examination should not be performed with water-soluble iodinated contrast medium (Gastrografin) given orally because it can lead to progressively severe vomiting, hypovolemia, and shock. It is unlikely that barium will inspissate in an obstructed loop of small intestine because of the increased fluid of these loops.
6. In paralytic ileus, both the small and large bowels are dilated.
7. Duodenal and high intestinal obstruction may be identified in utero by ultrasound.

F. General Supportive Management

See chapter 17–IIIB-E for "general supportive management for the infant with vomiting and abdominal distention," including preoperative, intraoperative, and postoperative management of the infant.

G. Specific Therapy

1. Immediate surgical repair of mechanical obstruction is the definitive therapy.
2. Postoperative diarrhea is frequent, necessitating close attention to fluid-electrolyte status, especially hypokalemia, hyponatremia, hypernatremia, hypocalcemia, and hypomagnesemia.
3. See chapter 17–VI for meconium ileus, 17–V for meconium plug syndrome, 17–VIII for imperforate anus, 17–IX for small left colon syndrome, etc.

REFERENCES

Ghory M.J., Sheldon C.A.: Newborn surgical emergencies of the gastrointestinal tract. *Surg. Clin. North Am.* 65:1083, 1985.

Holder T.M., Leape L.L.: The acute surgical abdomen in the neonate. *N. Engl. J. Med.* 278:605, 1968.

Santulli T.V.: Intestinal obstruction in the newborn infant. *J. Pediatr.* 44:317, 1954.

V. MECONIUM PLUG SYNDROME

Meconium plug syndrome refers to a temporary obstruction of the distal colon by tenacious meconium. The simple plug (or plugs) is gelatinous, yellow-white, and composed of mucus and other intestinal secretions. The disease has been attributed to transient deficiency in colonic maturity due to immature ganglion cells.

A. Who Is at Risk?

1. Premature infants (25% of cases occur in premature infants)
2. Infants with cystic fibrosis
3. Hypotonic infants
4. Infants with Hirschsprung's disease (10% to 15% of patients with meconium plugs have Hirschsprung's disease)
5. Infants of diabetic mothers and those with small left colon syndrome

B. Clinical Manifestations

1. No meconium passage for more than 24 hours
2. Abdominal distention with clear and later bilious vomiting
3. Hyperactive bowel sounds
4. Rectal examination may result in the passage of the gelatinous meconium plug.

C. Radiologic Features

1. Distention of bowel loops without air fluid level (features compatible with low intestinal obstruction)
2. A small left colon may be present especially in infants of diabetic mothers.
3. Barium enema may reveal a normal-sized colon with multiple elongated filling defects due to meconium.

D. Supportive Management

See chapter 17–IIIB for "general supportive management for the infant with vomiting and abdominal distention."

E. Specific Therapy

1. If rectal examination does not dislodge the plug, warm saline, Gastrografin, or 4% N-acetyl cysteine (Mucomyst) enemas may be administered and usually result in passage of the plug.
2. Do not use hydrogen peroxide enemas.
3. All patients should have a rectal biopsy to exclude Hirschsprung's disease and a sweat test to rule out cystic fibrosis.

F. Prognosis

The prognosis is good if no underlying disease exists.

REFERENCES

Berdon W.E., Slovis T.L., Campbell J.B., et al.: Neonatal small left colon syndrome: Its relationship to aganglionosis and meconium plug syndrome. *Radiology* 125:457, 1977.

LeQuesne G.W., Reilly B.J.: Functional immaturity of the large bowel in the newborn infant. *Radiol. Clin. N. Am.* 13:331, 1975.

Wagget J., Johnson D.G., Borns P., et al.: The nonoperative treatment of meconium ileus by gastrograffin enema. *J. Pediatr.* 77:407, 1970.

TABLE 17–1.—CAUSES OF DIFFICULTIES WITH SUCK AND SWALLOW*

ABSENT OR DIMINISHED SUCK	MECHANICAL PROBLEMS WITH SUCK	DIFFICULTY IN SWALLOWING	
Anoxia	Ankyloglossia superior syndrome	High lesions: aspiration with swallowing or nasal regurgitation of formula	Low lesions: associated with aspiration after feeding or pain during feeding
Kernicterus	Fusion of gums	Cleft palate	Esophageal motor dysfunction
Trisomies 13–15, 21	Macroglossia	Choanal atresia	Familial dysautonomia
Amyotonia congenita syndrome	Aglossia	Pharyngeal tumors	Achalasia
Prader-Willi syndrome	Ankylosis of the temporomandibular joint	Pharyngeal cysts	Chalasia
Werdnig-Hoffmann disease	Cleft lip	Tracheoesophageal fistula	Postvagotomy
Myasthenia gravis	Tumors	Laryngotracheo-esophageal cleft	Congenital lesions of the esophagus
Congenital muscular dystrophy		Infectious diseases of the pharynx	Vascular compression
Bulbar palsy		Micrognathia	Duplication cyst
		Pharyngeal diverticulum	Esophageal stenosis or web
		Pharyngeal perforation	Acquired lesions of the esophagus-
		Myotonic dystrophy	Leukemic infiltrate
		Palatal paralysis	Caustic burns
		Bulbar paralysis	Peptic esophagitis
		Transient palatal or pharyngeal dysfunction	Esophageal stricture
		Laryngeal nerve paralysis	Infection
		Cricopharyngeal dysfunction or achalasia	
		Post tracheotomy	

*From Gryboski J., Walker W.A.: *Gastrointestinal Problems in the Infant,* ed. 2. Philadelphia, W.B. Saunders Co., 1983. Used by permission.

TABLE 17–2.—Disorders of Neuromuscular Control of the Pharynx, Esophagus, and Pylorus*

Neuromuscular Disorders	Onset	Clinical Manifestations	Radiologic Findings	Specific Therapy
Transient pharyngeal muscle incoordination	First day of life	Respiratory distress (choking, coughing, cyanosis, especially at feeding)	On fluoroscopy, a pooling of contrast material in the hypopharynx with resulting overflow into the larynx and trachea	Gavage feeding until pharyngeal incoordination has disappeared. Rule out other neurologic impairment. Give oro-motor physical therapy.
Cardiospasm	First day of life	Repeated choking spells; regurgitation, vomiting of small quantity of unaltered food	On esophogram, a constricted point above the cardia is seen with dilation and hypertrophy of the lower part of the esophagus	Atropine, 1:1000 solution, 1 drop before each feeding, increasing by 1 drop a day up to the point of flushing
Achalasia (failure of the lower esophagus to relax with swallowing)	First day of life	Recurrent vomiting, pneumonia, poor weight gain, may be associated with trisomy 21	On esophogram, narrowing of the esophagus at the hiatus with dilation (megaesophagus) above the stenotic point caused by stagnation of ingested food	Dilation of the cardia by a pneumatic bag or bougie. Myotomy may be of value. Rule out trisomy 21.
Chalasia (relaxation of the lower esophageal sphincter; normal in young infants)	First week of life	Regurgitation, vomiting, poor weight gain, choking, apnea, aspiration pneumonia, often in prematures	On esophogram, a dilated, thin, flaccid lower esophagus. Crying, struggling or light pressure upon the abdomen in the supine position will increase vomiting. Reflux demonstrated by pH probe or barium studies	Small, frequent thickened feedings. Position the infant on the abdomen at a 45-degree angle for at least 1 hour after feedings. Do not use "feeding chair." Look for "soft" signs of CNS dysfunction. See chapter 17–XII.
Pylorospasm or antral spasm	First weeks of life	Vomiting, intermittent or after each feeding, with visible gastric bubble pattern; no palpable mass	On right oblique film after barium swallow, a short delay in peristaltic activity and emptying of the stomach occurs; results are variable	Atropine, 1:1000 solution, 1 drop 10 or 15 minutes before each feeding. Increase by 1 drop a day up to the point of flushing.

*From Harper R.G., Yoon J.J.: *Handbook of Neonatology*. Chicago, Year Book Medical Publishers, 1974. Used by permission.

VI. MECONIUM ILEUS

Thick, viscid meconium can cause a mechanical obstruction of the small intestine with or without intestinal wall necrosis, perforation, or peritonitis. The distal bowel collapses while the proximal is dilated with gas. Meconium ileus is seen in 10% to 15% of infants with cystic fibrosis and is an early manifestation. All infants with meconium ileus do not have cystic fibrosis. See chapter 17–VII for cystic fibrosis.

A. Who Is at Risk?

1. White infants (very rare among non-whites)
2. Infants with a family history of cystic fibrosis or intestinal obstruction (10% to 20% have intestinal atresia)
3. Infants with a history of maternal polyhydramnios (20% of meconium ileus)

B. Clinical Manifestations

1. Abdominal distention in the first 12 to 24 hours associated with dilated intestinal loops and numerous movable hard masses, which may be seen or palpated through the abdominal wall
2. Bile-stained vomitus usually on the second day
3. Failure to pass meconium and absence of meconium in normal anus and rectum on rectal examination
4. Increased peristalsis
5. Occasional tachypnea, retractions, grunting

C. Laboratory Findings

Specific findings (most cases due to cystic fibrosis):

1. A sweat test is necessary to confirm the diagnosis of cystic fibrosis, but it is difficult to obtain the necessary minimum of 40 mg of sweat in the newborn. A sweat chloride level of 60 mEq/L or more is diagnostic of the disease. Falsely reduced NaCl may be present due to hypoproteinemia and edema in the newborn.
2. Increased albumin in the first meconium tested by BM-test or Albustix (high rate of false positive and false negative results).

D. Radiologic Features

1. A flat plate of the abdomen will often show the following:
   a. Inspissated meconium, with air bubbles trapped in the meconium, and a ground glass appearance
   b. Dilated loops of bowel of varying size with air fluid levels

c. Meconium peritonitis may be seen in the form of scattered, irregular, calcified densities in the abdomen.
d. Evidence of volvulus, atresia, or perforation in 25% of cases

2. Barium enema may show the presence of microcolon.

E. Supportive Management

See chapter 17–IIIBE for "general supportive management of the infant with vomiting and abdominal distention," including preoperative, intraoperative, and postoperative management.

F. Specific Therapy

1. Medical therapy
   a. If signs of obstruction are mild, 4% N-acetyl-cysteine (Mucomyst) enemas may be used. Oral doses of acetyl-cysteine may also be given. Care must be taken not to administer a 10% or more Mucomyst solution because this strength solution can cause hyperemia, hemorrhage, and necrosis of the bowel mucosa.
   b. Water-soluble iodinated contrast medium (Gastrografin) enemas have been used to relieve the obstruction under fluoroscopic control. Care must be taken to hydrate the infant well before administering Gastrografin.
   c. Do not use hydrogen peroxide for enemas.
   d. Oral feeding of pancreatic enzyme (pancreatin, Viokase, Pancrelipase) may be of value. Dosage must be individualized.
   e. Evaluate the infant for possible cystic fibrosis. Measure the electrolytes in the infant's sweat.
2. Surgical therapy
   Patients with volvulus, gangrene, perforation, and peritonitis require immediate surgical correction. Surgical therapy should not be delayed unless progress is being made with medical therapy. Acetyl-cysteine (Mucomyst) may be administered by nasogastric tube or enema to promote evacuation of any remaining meconium. Since respiratory complications are common after surgery, chest physiotherapy and humidification may need to be started to prevent thick secretions.
3. After medical or surgical correction of the ileus an easily digestible formula (e.g., Pregestimil) with hydrolyzed protein, medium-chain triglycerides, and glucose or regular formula with pancreatic enzymes (e.g., Viokase) may be started.

G. Mortality and Prognosis

Mortality is between 50% and 60%. A small percent of infants who survive develop short gut syndrome and/or severe intestinal malabsorption. Almost all infants with meconium peritonitis have cystic fibrosis.

REFERENCES

Allan J.L., Robbie M., Phelan P.D., et al.: Familial occurrence of meconium ileus. *Eur. J. Pediatr.* 135:291, 1981.

Donnison A.B., Schwachman H., Gross R.E.: A review of 164 children with meconium ileus seen at the Children's Hospital Medical Center, Boston. *Pediatrics* 37:833, 1966.

VII. CYSTIC FIBROSIS

Cystic fibrosis, an inherited disorder in which the viscosity of the mucus is increased, is the commonest genetic disease in whites. The incidence of the disease is 1 in 1,000 to 2,000 live white births and 1 in 17,000 live black births. The basic defect and the cure are unknown. See chapter 17–VI for meconium ileus.

A. Who Is at Risk?

1. Five percent of the white population are carriers of the disease.
2. Infants with meconium ileus, especially those who become obstructed or who have intestinal atresia
3. Infants with diarrhea, edema, hypoproteinemia, and failure to thrive—80% have pancreatic insufficiency.

B. Clinical Manifestations

1. Newborn
   Failure to pass meconium, persistent jaundice, abdominal distention, and vomiting that eventually becomes bilious in nature may occur. Rectal sphincter tone is normal. Bulky malodorous steatorrhea and failure to thrive are common.
2. Beyond the newborn period
   Diarrhea, edema, low serum protein, and failure to thrive may occur along with a more specific skin rash. Most diseases of malabsorption occur after the newborn period. Salty sweat may be present. Repeated respiratory infection is common, as is failure to gain weight.

C. Laboratory Findings

1. The prenatal diagnosis of cystic fibrosis is strongly (but not absolutely) supported by the absence of arginine esterase activity in midtrimester amniotic fluid.
2. A sweat test is necessary to confirm the diagnosis of cystic fibrosis (see chapter 17–VIC).
3. Increased albumin in the first meconium tested by BM-test or Albustix (high

rate of false positive and false negative results). Hypoproteinemia may result from protein malabsorption.

4. Increased fat in the stools and deficiency of fat soluble vitamins due to decreased lipase
   a. Vitamin K malabsorption results in hemorrhagic diathesis.
   b. Vitamin A deficiency (may present as xerophthalmia)
   c. Vitamin E deficiency is seen with "brown bowel syndrome" or may present as neonatal hemolytic anemia.
   d. Hypocalcemia occurs secondary to saponification of calcium with unabsorbed fats. (Vitamin D deficiency is rare because of direct absorption via lymphatics.)
5. Hyperbilirubinemia (persistent)
6. Increased intracranial pressure
7. Hyperelectrolytemia and metabolic alkalosis have been reported in warm weather.
8. Other laboratory findings include biliary cirrhosis, lactose intolerance, and pulmonary infection. Hepatic biliary cirrhosis has been seen as early as the third day of life.
9. γ-Glutamyl transpeptidase is considered the most sensitive indication of liver disease associated with cystic fibrosis. Other liver function tests are usually normal.

D. Radiologic Features

1. For x-ray film findings, see chapter 17–VI. In addition, abnormal metaphyseal bands have been seen in x-ray films of the iliac crest and femur.
2. Nonspecific changes are seen in the small bowel.
3. Barium enema may show a shaggy and nodular appearance (chrysanthemum effect) or filling defects in cecum and ascending colon or microcolon.

E. Therapy

1. See treatment of meconium ileus (see chapter 17–VI). Operative resection may be necessary.
2. Infants usually require Pregestimil.
3. Pancreatic enzyme replacement is usually necessary for optimal absorption (Cotazym or Viokase).
4. Cimetidine, to reduce gastric acidity, has been advocated.
5. Additional vitamin K and E, should be given.
6. Do not give iron supplement; absorption is elevated.

F. Prognosis

Prognosis depends upon the degree of pulmonary involvement. Those who present with meconium ileus have the worst prognosis. More than ⅓ of infants with meconium ileus die of pulmonary complications during the first 6 months of age. Those with no pulmonary disease and only pancreatic insufficiency have the best prognosis. Volvulus or perforation may occur at any time. The degree of lung involvement does not seem to be related to the degree of GI obstruction.

REFERENCES

Arvanitakis C., Cooke A.R.: Diagnostic tests of exocrine pancreatic function and disease. *Gastroenterology* 74 (1):932, 1978.

Hellsing K., Barrljung K., Ceder O., et al.: Meconium screening for cystic fibrosis: An eight year follow-up study. *Acta Paediatr: Scan.* 71:827–832, 1982.

Katznelson D.: Increased intracranial pressure in cystic fibrosis. *Acta. Paediatr. Scand.* 67:607, 1978.

Rosenstein B.J., Langbaum T.S.: Incidence of meconium abnormalities in newborn infants with cystic fibrosis. *Am. J. Dis. Child.* 134:72, 1980.

VIII. ATRESIA AND STENOSIS OF THE ANAL CANAL (IMPERFORATE ANUS)

Stenosis of the anorectal canal may occur at any point along the canal. The incidence of imperforate anus is 1 in 5,000 live births. (Infants with anorectal anomalies often have associated congenital heart disease, esophageal atresia, hydronephrosis, spinal anomalies, etc.) Atresia and stenosis of the anorectal canal are related to incomplete resolution of the anorectal membrane. A simple perineal incision will rarely suffice to correct the anomaly.

A. Who Is at Risk?

1. Males
2. Infants born to a family with affected siblings (25% chance)
3. Infants with a perineal fistula or urologic anomaly
4. Infants with triphalangeal thumbs, abnormalities of hands and feet, and sensorineural deafness
5. Infants with a tracheoesophageal fistula or VATER syndrome

B. Clinical Manifestations

1. An imperforate anus.
2. Perineal fistula between the rectum and genitourinary tract.
   Meconium may be seen coming from the vagina or urethra.
3. Anal stenosis
   The anus may be anterior. As stools become firmer after transitional stools, stools may be small and thin or absence of meconium with progressive abdominal distention may develop.

4. Anal stenosis may be associated with hand and foot abnormalities and sensorineural deafness.
5. Signs of intestinal obstruction may be present with vomiting and abdominal distention.

C. Classification of Anorectal Anomalies

1. Ladd's classification of the anatomic anomaly
   a. Type I: stenosis of the anus or lower rectum with both patent
   b. Type II: persistence of the anal membrane
   c. Type III: imperforate anus with the rectum ending blindly as a pouch. Type III is 10 times more common than types I, II, or IV; 75% are associated with rectourethral, rectovesical, or rectoperineal fistula in the male and rectovaginal or rectoperineal fistula in the female.
   d. Type IV: the anal canal and lower rectum form a pouch and are separate from the blind upper rectal pouch.
2. International classification
   a. Low (translevator)
      1) At normal anal site
         Anal stenosis or completely covered anus
      2) At perineal site
         Anocutaneous fistula or anterior perineal anus
   b. Intermediate
      1) Anal agenesis
         With or without rectobulbar fistula (in males), rectovestibular or rectovaginal fistula (in females)
      2) Anorectal stenosis
   c. High (supralevator): absent internal sphincter
      1) Anorectal agenesis
         With or without rectourethral fistula (in males), rectovesical (in males and females), rectovaginal, or rectocloacal fistula (in females)
      2) Rectal atresia
   d. Miscellaneous
      1) Imperforate anal membrane
      2) Cloacal exstrophy

D. Laboratory Findings

Meconium or epithelial debris may be found in the urine.
Hyperchloremic acidosis in infants with rectovesical or urethral fistula.

E. Radiologic/Ultrasonic Features

1. The classic upside down x-ray film may be helpful in low lesions after 24 hours. It is not diagnostic because air may not go into the rectum, the film

cannot be performed when the infant is less than 24 hours of age, and the marker may suggest a greater space between the segments than what exists.
2. Air in the bladder suggests rectovesical fistula and injection of contrast material into the vagina or urethra confirms the fistula.
3. Intravenous pyelogram and cystography are required to rule out genitourinary anomalies.
4. Ultrasonogram may be helpful in differentiating high and low anorectal anomalies

F. General Supportive Management

See chapter 17–IIIBE for "general supportive management for the infant with vomiting and abdominal distension," including preoperative, intraoperative, and postoperative management.

G. Specific Therapy

1. For anal stenosis, dilate repeatedly.
2. For persistent anal membrane, excise surgically.
3. For low (translevator) anomalies, a direct perineal repair is sufficient.
4. For high (supralevator) anomalies, an abdominal repair is indicated to preserve any sphincter potential of muscles.
5. In the type III anomaly, correction rarely requires immediate repair at time of delivery. If a fistula is present in the female, operation may be delayed as long as 6 months.
6. If complications exist, a colostomy is performed and the repair is postponed.

H. Complications

Complications include rectal prolapse or stenosis, separation of anastomosis, urethral injury and stricture, urinary retention and infection, small bowel obstruction, fecal impaction or incontinence, etc.

I. Prognosis

Prognosis generally depends upon extent of associated anomalies with a poorer outcome if >3 anomalies are present. Function depends on accurate placement of the rectal pouch through the levator sling.

REFERENCES

Kottmeier P.K., Dziadiw R.: The complete release of the levator ani sling in fecal incontinence. *J. Pediatr. Surg.* 2:111, 1967.

Ladd W.E., Gross R.E.: Congenital malformations of anus and rectum: Report of 162 cases. *Am. J. Surg.* 23:167, 1935.

Santulli T.V., Kiesewetter W.B., Bill A.H. Jr.: Anorectal anomalies: A suggested classification. *J. Pediatr. Surg.* 5:281, 1970.

Santulli T.V., Schullinger J.N., Kiesewetter W.B., et al.: Imperforate anus: A survey from the members of the surgical section of the American Academy of Pediatrics. *J. Pediatr. Surg.* 6:484, 1971.

IX. SMALL LEFT COLON SYNDROME

The small left colon syndrome is characterized by a decreased caliber of the descending left colon with low colonic obstruction. The cause is thought to be related to decreased jejunal and sigmoid motor activity in response to increased glucagon or increased magnesium. Rarely it may be difficult to differentiate Hirschsprung's disease. The incidence is 1 in 855 deliveries.

A. Who Is at Risk?

1. Infants of diabetics, usually insulin-dependent (40%)
2. Infants of women who have had hypertensive disease of pregnancy and/or polyhydramnios
3. Septic infants

B. Clinical Manifestations

1. Failure to pass meconium
2. Respiratory distress, cyanosis, and abdominal distention may be present.

C. Laboratory Findings

1. Hypoglycemia (see chapter 15–X)
2. Hypoxia (persistent pulmonary hypertension of the newborn may be present). See chapter 11–XIII.

D. Radiologic Features

1. Plain films may show low colonic obstruction.
2. Barium enema is diagnostic and shows a decreased colon caliber from splenic flexure with proximal colonic dilation and a normal size rectum.
3. Previously perforation occurs in one half the patients but is now rare. Pneumoperitoneum may be present.
4. Chest x-ray film may reveal cardiomegaly.

D. Supportive Therapy

See chapter 17–IIIB for "general supportive management for the infant with vomiting and abdominal distension."

E. Specific Therapy

A water-soluble contrast enema (Hypaque) is both diagnostic and therapeutic. Surgery is usually not indicated except if perforation occurs. Surgical closure is then required.

E. Prognosis

With early therapy, mortality is negligible. With perforation, mortality is 50%. In most infants the clinical obstruction clears in 24 hours.

REFERENCE

David W.S., Campbell J.B.: Neonatal small left colon syndrome. *Am. J. Dis. Child.* 129:1024, 1975.

David W.S., Allen R.P., Favara B.E., et al.: The neonatal small left colon syndrome. *Am. J. Roentgenol. Radium Ther. Nucl. Med.* 120:322, 1974.

X. MALROTATION WITH VOLVULUS

Malrotation, a congenital anomaly in which the cecum is incompletely rotated and located in the upper right quadrant, is often found in association with volvulus of the midgut. Volvulus occurs because the small intestine lacks a fixed position and results in obstruction of the duodenojejunal junction and the transverse colon. Two thirds of the patients with malrotation and volvulus show symptoms before 1 month of age. A partial or complete occlusion of the superior mesenteric artery follows, causing infarction of the entire midgut. Malrotation is encountered in 0.2% of barium studies of the GI tract at any age.

A. Who Is at Risk?

1. Male infants (twice the risk of females)
2. Infants with diaphragmatic hernia, omphalocele, gastrochisis, duodenal atresia, ileal atresia, pyloric stenosis, mesenteric cyst, polysplenia, and asplenia
3. Infants with a family history of midgut volvulus

B. Clinical Manifestations

Symptoms are related to duodenal obstruction or volvulus.

1. Bile-stained vomitus, which may be intermittent or persistent usually not at birth but within the first month of life
2. Abdominal distention, initially limited to the stomach and duodenum (may be severe and generalized in acute volvulus)
3. Dehydration and electrolyte imbalance are common.
4. Stools are decreased in quantity and frequently become bloody. Diarrhea may be the presenting sign.

5. Ecchymosis of the fascial planes of the abdomen and around the umbilicus is sometimes seen if a superior mesenteric artery thrombosis with hemorrhage has occurred (Cullen's sign).
6. Signs of peritonitis, sepsis, and shock may occur abruptly with vomiting and irritability if midgut volvulus occurs with malrotation.
7. A history of "colic" with intermittent vomiting and abdominal distention or chronic diarrhea due to blind loop syndrome may be present.
8. Asymptomatic (15% of malrotation)

C. Laboratory Findings

1. Specific findings
   There are no specific laboratory findings.
2. Associated findings
   a. Decreased hemoglobin secondary to intestinal hemorrhage with bloody stools
   b. A severe leukocytosis occurs with gangrene of the gut.
   c. Fluid and electrolyte imbalance; metabolic acidosis
   d. Hyperbilirubinemia
   e. Positive blood culture

D. Radiologic Features

1. A flat plate of the abdomen may reveal a gas-filled stomach and slightly dilated duodenum.
2. A barium enema will show abnormal positioning of the cecum and ascending colon or may fail to penetrate beyond the transverse colon.
3. An upper GI series will define the site of obstruction, the duodenojejunal junction, and jejunum.
4. Gaseous distention of the intestines may show multiple dilated air-filled loops of small bowel and air fluid levels if complete intestinal obstruction has occurred.

E. Supportive Management

See chapter 17–IIIB for "general supportive management for the infant with vomiting and abdominal distension," including preoperative, intraoperative, and postoperative management.

F. Specific Therapy

Immediate surgical correction is required if volvulus occurs (run, do not walk, to the nearest pediatric surgeon).

G. Prognosis

Complete volvulus in the neonate is associated with 80% mortality. Volvulus will recur in 5% of cases. Short bowel syndrome is a frequent complication.

REFERENCES

Rowe M.I. (ed.): Symposium on neonatal surgery. *Clin. Perinatol.* 5:1, 1978.

Stewart D.R., Colodny A.L., Daggett W.C.: Malrotation of the bowel in infants and children: A 15 year review. *Surgery* 79:716, 1976.

XI. ANNULAR PANCREAS

Annular pancreas, the most common cause of extrinsic duodenal obstruction in infancy, is secondary to persistance of the left bud of the ventral pancreas attached to or rotated around the duodenum.

A. Who Is at Risk?

1. Infants with Down's syndrome (approximately 25%)
2. Infants with congenital heart disease, especially tetralogy of Fallot (20%)
3. Infants with duodenal obstruction, 50% of which are small for gestational age and 40% of which develop hyperbilirubinemia

B. Clinical Manifestations

1. Asymptomatic if incomplete
2. History of "colic" may be present.
3. Bilious vomiting with peristaltic waves from left to right, abdominal distention, and small and infrequent stools if obstruction is complete

C. Laboratory Findings

Hyperinsulinism has been reported; elevated amylase or bilirubin may occur.

D. Radiologic Features

1. With complete obstruction, plain films show "double bubble" sign.
2. Without complete obstruction, compression is confirmed by contrast studies.

E. Supportive Management

See chapter 17–IIIBE for "general supportive management for the infant with vomiting and abdominal distention," including preoperative, intraoperative, and postoperative management.

F. Specific Therapy

Duodenojejunostomy is the treatment of choice.

G. Prognosis

The prognosis depends upon associated malformations.

REFERENCES

Ravitch M.M.: The pancreas in infants and children. Surg. Clin. North Am. 55:377, 1975.

Johnston D.W.B.: Annular pancreas: A new classification and clinical observations. *Can. J. Surg.* 21 (3):241–244, 1978.

XII. GASTROESOPHAGEAL REFLUX (CHALASIA)

Approximately 40% of normal healthy infants regurgitate in early infancy. Some infants develop respiratory distress, intractable asthma, chronic bronchitis, apnea, recurrent pneumonia, esophagitis, and failure to thrive in association with gastroesophageal reflux (GER). GER may occur with low, normal, or hypertonic lower esophageal sphincter tone.

A. Prevention

Maintain the infant in the prone position at a 30- to 45-degree angle. (Do not sit the infant in an infant seat during awake periods; this method is ineffective.) Keep the infant prone with the head elevated.

B. Who Is at Risk?

1. Premature infants (often have lower esophageal sphincter above the diaphragm and lower esophageal sphincter moves into the abdomen with growth)
2. Infants with delayed gastric emptying with or without antral or pylorospasm
3. Infants with increased intragastric pressure
4. Infants with severe mental retardation, e.g., Down's syndrome

C. Clinical Manifestations

1. A history of "spitting" since birth
2. As the feeding volume increases, the postprandial regurgitation increases.
3. Feeding is difficult because of arching, crying, and refusal to feed.

4. Failure to thrive and recurrent pneumonia is common. Severe asthmatic attacks and/or chronic bronchitis may ensue.
5. Pale, anemic appearance with positive occult blood in the stool may be present when esophagitis occurs.

D. Laboratory Features

1. Anemia with occult melena is frequent.
2. The acid reflux tests may be positive (most sensitive means of detecting GER). Reflux is considered to be present when the intraesophageal pH is less than 4.
   a. Tuttle test: After introduction of 0.1N HCl into the stomach, the esophagus is cleared of acid and a pH probe is placed in the esophagus. pH with spontaneous and induced reflux is then measured over 2 hours.
   b. Intraesophageal pH: A pH probe is placed in the esophagus and apple juice is given by mouth and the number of refluxes (pH less than 4)/hour and reflux time/hour is calculated. In mild reflux, reflux time is 16% of time observed; severe is approximately 40% to 50% of the time.
3. Endoscopy is utilized to establish the diagnosis of esophagitis and is reserved for infants who fail to respond to medical management.

E. Radiologic Features

1. Barium swallow is the least accurate means to obtain the diagnosis of GER. An upper GI series is recommended to rule out obstructive and motility disorders.
2. Mega-aeroesophagus is indicative of reflux.
3. After the stomach has filled with barium, fluoroscopy reveals reflux with swallowing.
4. Technetium-99m sulfur colloid added to the feeds can be utilized to scan for reflux and gastric emptying time.

F. Supportive Management

See chapter 17–IIIBE for "general supportive management for the infant with vomiting and abdominal distension," including preoperative, intraoperative, and postoperative management.

G. Specific Therapy

1. Maintain the infant in the prone position so noted in *A.*
2. Do not administer acid juices or fruits.
3. Administer small, frequent, thickened (with cereal) feedings.

4. If symptoms persist after 2 weeks of therapy, administer aluminum hyroxide antacids, 0.5 to 1.0 tsp 15 to 30 minutes after feedings.
5. Other drugs that have been utilized include the following:
   a. Bethanechol chloride, 8.7 $mg/mm^3/day$ in three divided doses to stimulate gastric emptying (side effects of diarrhea and irritability may be severe), and metoclopramide HCl may also be used.
   b. Cimetidine, 10 to 20 mg/kg/day in four divided doses over 10 to 20 minutes to decrease gastric acid production (no controlled studies are available in infants)
6. If regurgitation persists despite medications or if pneumonia, serious apnea, and/or stricture is present, surgical therapy, e.g., Nissen fundoplication, may be necessary.

H. Prognosis

Prognosis depends upon the concurrent presence of neurologic disease.

Sudden infant death syndrome, esophageal stricture, and hiatal hernia are rare complications.

REFERENCE

Herbst J.J., Minton S.D., Book L.S.: Gastroesophageal reflux causing respiratory distress and apnea in newborn infants. *J. Pediatr.* 95:763, 1979.

XIII. PYLORIC STENOSIS

Pyloric stenosis, the hypertrophy and hyperplasia of the pyloric musculature, impairs gastric emptying, may result in complete obstruction of the GI tract, and occurs in 4 to 5 per 1,000 live births. Although thought to be congenital, the disease usually does not manifest until the infant is 4 to 5 weeks of age.

A. Who Is at Risk?

1. Male infants (five times the risk of females)
2. Infants with a familial history of pyloric stenosis
3. The firstborn is not especially at risk.

B. Clinical Manifestations

1. The infant is hungry, irritable, and sucks vigorously.
2. Vomiting may begin within 1 week of life, but usually commences at 2 to 6

weeks of age. The vomiting increases in frequency and may become projectile, but is not bile-stained.
3. Constipation is frequent.
4. The pyloric tumor may be palpated in 40% to 100% of infants as an ovoid mass between the umbilicus and right lower costal margin along the lateral border of the rectus muscle. A gentle, unhurried examination should be performed during a feeding or immediately after vomiting when the abdominal musculature is relaxed.
5. Gastric peristalsis may be visible across the abdomen from left to right when the stomach is distended after feeding.
6. Weight loss and dehydration are common.
7. Prolonged jaundice may occur.

C. Laboratory Findings

1. Hypochloremic alkalosis with electrolyte derangement; increased pH, increased HCO_3^-, decreased Cl^-, decreased K^+
2. Increased hematocrit resulting from dehydration
3. Indirect hyperbilirubinemia

D. Radiologic Features

Radiologic studies provide the diagnosis.

1. A flat film of the abdomen will often show a large dilated stomach with relatively little gas in the intestines.
2. A GI x-ray film with contrast medium will show
   a. An enlarged stomach
   b. A delay in pyloric opening time
      1) With less than a 10-minute delay, the diagnosis of pyloric stenosis is questionable.
      2) With more than a 20-minute delay, the diagnosis of pyloric stenosis or upper intestinal obstruction is certain.
   c. A narrowed pyloric canal; the "string" sign is a tract of barium in the canal.
   d. The "beak" sign, which is the beginning of the elongated pyloric canal, is usually seen with the string sign.
   e. The "double tract" sign, which is the folded mucosa in the pyloric canal.
3. Abdominal sonogram with high frequency system (7 MHz or more) accurately demonstrates hypertrophic pyloric stenosis.

E. General Supportive Management

See chapter 17–IIIBE for "general supportive management for the infant with vomiting and abdominal distension" including preoperative, intraoperative, and postoperative management.

F. Specific Therapy

1. Medical therapy
   Administer small, concentrated, thickened feedings and tincture of belladonna, 0.1 ml (0.03 mg atropine)/kg/dose orally every 4 hours, 10 to 30 minutes before feedings. Therapy must usually be continued for several months.
2. Surgical therapy
   a. Perform a Fredet-Ramstedt pyloromyotomy after hydration and blood gas and electrolyte status have returned to normal.
   b. Parenteral fluids are indicated the first 24 hours postoperatively.
   c. Small amounts of oral feeding may be started 12 hours after surgical repair.

G. Prognosis

Complete recovery is common several days after surgical therapy. Patients treated medically may develop dyspepsia, vomiting, and/or gastric ulcers.

REFERENCES

Blumhagen J.D., Noble H.G.S.: Muscle thickness in hypertrophic pyloric stenosis: Sonographic determination. *A.J.R.* 140:221, 1983.

Shuman F.I., Darling D.B., Fisher J.H.: The radiographic diagnosis of congenital hypertrophic pyloric stenosis. *J. Pediatr.* 71:70, 1967.

XIV. HIRSCHSPRUNG'S DISEASE

Hirschsprung's disease, the most frequent cause of lower intestinal obstruction in the newborn, is due to an absence of ganglion cells in Meissner's and Auerbach's plexus and the presence of hypertrophic nonmyelinated nerve fibers in the submucosal and intramucosal areas. It has been reported that acquired Hirschsprung's disease (degeneration of preexisting nerve cell) may occur in an infant with systemic stress, e.g., hypoxia. The area of aganglionosis may vary from a limited segment of the rectosigmoid to the total colon and part of the ileum. Absence of peristalsis in the aganglionic segment causes functional intestinal obstruction and narrowing of the segment. The incidence is 1 in 5,000 newborns.

A. Who Is at Risk?

1. Male, most are fullterm infants; four times the risk of females.
2. Infants with a family history of Hirschsprung's disease; the risk is higher for siblings of affected females than siblings of affected males.

3. Infants with Down's syndrome, pyloric stenosis, achalasia, Klinefelter's syndrome, congenital rubella, imperforate anus, megaureters, or colonic atresia are at risk for Hirschsprung's disease.

B. Clinical Features

1. Failure or delay in the passage of meconium due to absence of peristalsis in the aganglionic segment
2. Abdominal distention with later bilious vomiting
3. Diarrhea may be seen with vomiting and abdominal distension in 25% of the patients alternating with constipation.
4. There may be days or weeks of normal bowel movements, persistent constipation, intermittent distention, or feeding problems.
5. Obstruction without vomiting may lead to perforation or peritonitis. Sudden marked abdominal distention, fever, dehydration, and shock with or without diarrhea are signs of enterocolitis, which is the major cause of death.
6. Rectal examination reveals an empty ampulla (60% of cases), but a high impaction is often palpable. Explosive passage of gas or stool after rectal examination follows.

C. Laboratory Findings

1. Specific findings
   a. The definitive method of diagnosis is suction or deep-wedge biopsy that shows the absence of intramural ganglion cells and the presence of an abnormal configuration of nerve fibers. Care must be taken to obtain the specimen from above the dentate line because a normal hypoganglionic area exists below the line. If ganglion cells are not seen with suction biopsy, a surgical biopsy is necessary.
   b. Acetylcholinesterase levels of aganglionic tissue are elevated; the serum acetylcholinesterase level is also elevated.
2. Associated findings
   a. Manometric studies may show nonrelaxing of the external sphincter with increased activity of the internal sphincter with dilation of the rectum. False positive and false negative results occur.
   b. Electrolyte imbalance due to excessive intraluminal loss of electrolytes may occur. Hypoproteinemia may be present.

D. Radiologic Features

1. Plain films may show characteristic distended gas-filled loops of sigmoid colon ending in an unexpanded rectum.
2. Barium is used to demonstrate the transitional zone. Barium enema will not show the characteristic narrowed aganglionic segment until several weeks or

months after birth. Retention of barium for more than 24 hours past the examination is a significant finding and suggests that rectal biopsy should be obtained.

3. Typically, a distended colon ending in an unexpanded rectum or intraperitoneal air may be present.

E. General Supportive Management

See chapter 17–IIIBE for "general supportive management for the infant with vomiting and abdominal distention," including preoperative, intraoperative, and postoperative management. Prior to surgery administer isotonic enemas to prevent enterocolitis.

F. Specific Therapy

1. Surgical removal of the aganglionic, nonfunctioning segment of bowel. A colostomy is placed and definitive repair is undertaken when the infant is larger.
2. A one-stage complete repair is performed at some centers.

G. Prognosis

Mortality varies from 5% to 43%, usually associated with enterocolitis, which may occur prior to or after surgery. Other complications include hydroureter, hydronephrosis, cecal perforation, and incontinence.

REFERENCES

Andrassy R.J., Isaacs H., Weitzman J.J.: Rectal suction biopsy for the diagnosis of Hirschsprung's disease. *Ann. Surg.* 193:419, 1981.

Boley S.J., Dinari G., Cohen M.I.: Hirschsprung's disease in the newborn. *Clin. Perinatol.* 5:45, 1978.

Chow C.W., Chan W.L., Yue K.C.: Histochemical criteria for the diagnosis of Hirschsprung's disease in rectal suction biopsy of acetylcholinesterase activity. *J. Pediatr. Surg.* 12:675, 1977.

XV. GASTRIC PERFORATION

Gastric perforation usually occurs suddenly in 3- to 8-day-old premature infants who have had a previous hypoxic episode. The cause is unclear; congenital muscular defects, ischemia, enterocolitis, and trauma have all been postulated.

A. Prevention

1. Avoid oxygen administration by nasal catheter at high flow rates. Do not administer oxygen via a tight face mask without a blow-off catheter in place.

2. Prevent perinatal asphyxia (63% have this history).
3. Do not use stiff feeding tubes.

B. Who Is at Risk?

1. Premature, male, black, or twin infants
2. Infants with a congenital defect of the gastric musculature, especially on the greater curvature near the cardia
3. Infants with low Apgar scores and resulting gastric necrosis
4. Infants with sepsis and ulceration of the gastric mucosa
5. Infants receiving intermittent positive-pressure breathing through a tight face mask
6. Occasionally, no known predisposing factors are present.

C. Clinical Manifestations

The infant is usually premature and appears well for several days after hypoxic stress. The infant then refuses to feed and is more fretful than usual. Impressive abdominal distention and bilious or blood-tinged vomiting follow shortly after. Subcutaneous emphysema frequently occurs. Dyspnea and cyanosis are common. Temperature instability, sepsis, and shock may occur.

D. Laboratory Findings

1. Specific findings
   There are no specific findings.
2. Associated findings
   a. Elevation in the white blood cell count occurs with peritonitis.
   b. Anemia may occur with bleeding while elevated hemoglobin may also occur with dehydration.
   c. Gastric aspirates are grossly bloody or have positive occult blood on testing.

E. Radiologic Features

Perforation is demonstrated in the upright film by free air under the diaphragm and above the dome of the liver ("saddle bag" sign) or in the supine film where the falciform ligament is outlined against radiolucent abdominal air, which is the shape of a large bubble ("football" sign). The gastric air bubble is absent.

F. Supportive Management

See chapter 17–IIIBE for "general supportive management for the infant with vomiting and abdominal distension," including intraoperative and postoperative management. Cautious feedings are usually started within a few days after surgery.

G. Specific Therapy

1. Immediate surgical correction
2. Preoperative paracentesis if pneumoperitoneum is life-threatening

H. Prognosis

Seventy percent of the patients will survive.

REFERENCES

James A.E. Jr., Heller R.M., White J.J., et al.: Spontaneous rupture of the stomach in the newborn: Clinical and experimental evaluation. *Pediatr. Res.* 10:79, 1976.

Marchildon M.B.: Meconium peritonitis and spontaneous gastric perforations. *Clin. Perinatol.* 5:79, 1978.

Shashikumar V.L., Bassuk A., Pilling G.P., et al.: Spontaneous gastric rupture in the newborn: A clinical review of nineteen cases. *Ann. Surg.* 182:22, 1975.

XVI. NECROTIZING ENTEROCOLITIS

Necrotizing enterocolitis is primarily a disease of low-birth-weight infants. The incidence (0% to 5% of newborn intensive care unit admissions; 1.0 to 2.5 in 1,000 live births) varies among institutions and cases are clustered in time and location. The overall mortality varies between 30% and 40%.

A. Prevention

Eliminate circulatory derangements that result in bowel ischemia and minimize bacterial proliferation in the presence of bowel ischemia.

Late initiation of feedings at 5 to 7 days of age with 2 to 4 ml of water and slow increments of 1 to 2 ml, preferably of human milk, for the first week of feeding in high-risk infants (controversial).

B. Who Is at Risk?

1. Premature infants (75% to 90% of cases)
2. Small for gestational age or dysmature infants in half of term infants
3. Infants who have sustained periods of stress or hypoxia (fetal distress, peri-

natal asphyxia, respiratory distress syndrome, hypothermia, hypoglycemia, hypovolemia, shock, or congenital heart disease)
4. Infants who had an umbilical vessel (arterial or venous catheterization), particularly infants who received an exchange transfusion via an umbilical vessel catheter
5. Infants who have sepsis
6. Infants who have polycythemia
7. Infants who received enteral feeding of hyperosmolar formula and/or sudden increment of feeding
8. Infants who have a patent ductus arteriosus

C. Clinical Manifestations

Onset is usually at less than 5 days of age and less than 3 days of feeding although necrotizing enterocolitis may occur after 4 days of feeding in very ill newborns or very low-birth-weight infants with or without problems. The onset may be explosive and dramatic with rapid deterioration or simply abdominal distension and retention of feedings.

1. Abdominal distension
2. Lethargy
3. Temperature instability
4. Apnea
5. Retained gastric content
6. Vomiting, regurgitation
7. Guaiac positive stool and/or presence of reducing substances
8. Progressive, massive abdominal distension, acidosis, generalized bleeding (disseminated intravascular coagulation), and shock

D. Laboratory Findings

1. Leukocytosis or leukopenia
2. Thrombocytopenia
3. Hyponatremia
4. Hypoalbuminemia
5. Prolonged prothrombin time and partial thromboplastin time
6. Decreased factor V

E. Radiographic Features

1. Dilated, fixed loops of bowel
2. Enteric edema and wide separation of gas in adjacent bowel segments
3. Pneumatosis intestinalis and gas within portal venous system in one third of those with pneumatosis intestinalis
4. Pneumoperitoneum (free air within the peritoneal cavity if perforation has occurred)

F. Supportive Management

1. Give the infant nothing by mouth for 7 to 14 days after acute hypoxic/hypotensive episode.
2. See chapter 17–IIIB for "general supportive management for the infant with vomiting and abdominal distension."
3. Obtain appropriate cultures and administer antibiotics.
   a. Parenteral antibiotics (penicillin or penicillin derivates in addition to aminoglycosides) after cultures are obtained
   b. Enteral antibiotics (kanamycin, 15 to 20 mg/day divided into four doses) by gavage and clamp Replogle tube for 30 minutes to 1 hour after administration of antibiotics (controversial)
4. Fresh frozen plasma daily until sepsis, shock, and disseminated intravascular coagulation are controlled
5. Abdominal x-ray film every 6 to 8 hours to determine if perforation has occurred
6. For therapy for shock, see chapter 14–IIID7.
7. Monitor coagulation factors.
8. Indications for surgery
   a. Absolute indication: perforation
   b. Strong indications: infants with rapid deterioration, no improvement after medical management of 4 to 12 hours, increasing abdominal tenderness, persistent loop of dilated bowel
   c. Possible indications: thrombocytopenia, persistent acidosis, decreasing urinary output

G. Complications

1. Early acute complications: perforation, shock, disseminated intravascular coagulation, sepsis
2. Late complications: intestinal strictures in 25% to 36% of cases, often in the large bowel in 75%, within 6 months of acute episodes
3. Intestinal malabsorption; peritoneal, often pericolic, or retroperitoneal abscess; enterocolic fistula; enterocyst formation between strictures
4. Short gut syndrome

H. Prognosis

High mortality (30% to 50%) has been reported. Short gut syndrome as a result of bowel resection may complicate feeding and require total parenteral nutrition for years.

REFERENCES

Brown E.G., Sweet A.Y.: Neonatal necrotizing enterocolitis. *Pediatr. Clin. N. Am.* 29:1149, 1982.

Egan E.A., Mantilla G., Nelson R.M., et al.: A prospective controlled trial of oral kanamycin in the prevention of neonatal necrotizing enterocolitis. *J. Pediatr.* 89:467, 1976.

Schwartz M.Z., Hayden C.K., Richardson J., et al.: A prospective evaluation of intestinal stenosis following necrotizing enterocolitis. *J. Pediatr. Surg.* 17:764, 1982.

XVII. HYPERMAGNESEMIA

Hypermagnesemia (> 2.8 mg/dl) in the fetus and newborn results primarily from the administration of magnesium sulfate ($MgSO_4$) to mothers for the treatment of hypertensive disease of pregnancy or to allay premature labor. Normally, the serum magnesium level in the newborn is 1.5 to 2.8 mg/dl.

A. Prevention

1. Administer $MgSO_4$ cautiously to women in labor.
2. Monitor maternal magnesium levels and renal excretion rate when administering $MgSO_4$ to treat hypertension or allay premature labor.

B. Who Is at Risk?

1. Infants born to mothers receiving $MgSO_4$
2. Infants with low Apgar scores. Since acidosis results in a shift of intracellular magnesium to the extracellular compartment, asphyxia and acidosis may be the cause of this correlation.
3. Premature infants have higher magnesium levels perhaps related to low glomerular filtration rates and poor urinary excretion of magnesium.
4. Infants with renal failure

C. Clinical Manifestations

A high serum magnesium level may cause decreased muscle tone, respiratory depression, generalized lethargy, abdominal distention, hypotonia, and weak cry because of peripheral neuromuscular blockage and CNS depression. Smooth muscle contraction is also altered with resultant vasodilation and hypotension. Elevated levels of magnesium, however, do not correlate well with symptomatology in the newborn, as serum magnesium concentrations may not reflect intracellular and/or total body magnesium.

D. Laboratory Findings

1. The level at which newborns become symptomatic is not known.
2. ECG changes include early tachycardia and later bradycardia. There is increased atrioventricular and ventricular conduction time.
3. A rise in serum magnesium will inhibit secretion of parathyroid hormone resulting in increased urinary excretion of calcium with resultant hypocalcemia.
4. Decreased blood pressure

E. Radiologic Features

There are no specific radiologic features.

F. Supportive Management

1. Obtain serum magnesium and calcium levels of cord blood and at 2, 12, and 24 hours of age in infants at risk.
2. Administer respiratory support as required (see chapter 11–IV and 11–VI).
3. Follow blood pressure carefully (See chapter 14–IIIC for shock).

G. Specific Therapy

1. Maintain adequate hydration to hasten the excretion of magnesium.
2. If the infant is symptomatic, administer 200 to 500 mg of calcium gluconate IV. Give slowly to prevent bradycardia. Calcium salts are antagonistic to both the central and peripheral depressant effect of magnesium.
3. Exchange transfusion may be of value.

REFERENCES

Donovan E.F., Tsang R.C., Steichen J.J., et al.: Neonatal hypermagnesemia: Effect on parathyroid hormone and calcium homeostasis. *J. Pediatr.* 96:305, 1980.

Tsang R.C.: Neonatal magnesium disturbances. *Am. J. Dis. Child.* 124:282, 1972.

XVIII. HYPOKALEMIA

Potassium (K^+) is the principal intracellular ion, the intracellular concentration varying from 140 to 160 mEq/L. Hypokalemia usually indicates reduction in total body (intracellular) K^+ stores and intracellular K^+ deficit. Intracellular hypokalemia in the presence of normal total potassium can occur due to an abrupt shift in extracellular pH or glucose concentration. Normal serum potassium can be seen despite considerable intracellular loss due to the relatively small extracellular potassium content.

A. Prevention

1. Supply adequate dietary intake of K^+. Newborns require 2 to 3 mEq of K^+/kg/24 hours. Avoid exclusive feeding of Cl-deficient soy formulas since they may produce a high NaCl and KCl renal loss (Bartter-like syndrome).
2. Replace excessive GI potassium losses due to diarrhea or vomiting.
3. Replace excessive renal potassium losses.
4. Carefully monitor the serum potassium of those infants at risk for transcellular shifts, i.e., those infants with metabolic or respiratory alkalosis and insulin or glucose therapy. Supply additional potassium as required.

B. Who Is at Risk?

1. Infants receiving parenteral fluids inadequate in potassium or foods containing inadequate potassium, or chloride deficient soy formulas.
2. Infants with excessive GI losses, e.g., diarrhea or vomiting
3. Infants with excessive renal losses due to the following:
   a. Direct renal tubular damage from pyelonephritis, chronic interstitial nephritis, or the direct toxic effect of amphotericin B, polymyxin, or outdated tetracycline or gentamicin
   b. Enhanced distal tubule sodium-potassium exchange, i.e., that seen with glucocorticoids, mineralocorticoids, or aldosterone
   c. Increased distal tubule sodium delivery with enhanced potassium excretion, e.g., thiazide diuretics, loop diuretics (furosemide or ethacrynic acid), or Fanconi's syndrome
   d. Agents that increase the negativity of the distal tubule lumen, e.g., carbenicillin or massive penicillin or nafcillin therapy
   e. A defect in the thick ascending limb of the loop of Henle, e.g., Bartter's syndrome
4. Infants with transcellular shifts, e.g., metabolic or respiratory alkalosis or insulin or glucose therapy

C. Clinical Manifestations

Clinical manifestations include skeletal muscle weakness, depressed deep tendon reflexes, smooth muscle weakness, and paralytic ileus (abdominal distention, absent peristalsis). Cardiac arrhythmias may occur.

D. Laboratory Findings

1. Specific findings
   a. Decreased serum potassium levels less than 3.5 mEq/L
   b. Severe defects of total body K^+ can best be estimated by ECG changes that include broad flat T waves, inverted T waves, depressed ST segment, prolonged PR interval, and prominent P waves (chapter 19–VII).
2. Nonspecific findings
   Associated laboratory findings are related to the underlying disease process.

E. Specific Therapy

1. Administer K^+, 2 to 3 mEq/kg/24 hours, as maintenance therapy for infants receiving IV fluids. The K^+ concentrate in parenteral fluid should not exceed 40 mEq/L. Adequate urine output must be confirmed prior to starting K^+.
2. Monitor K^+ levels daily in all infants on IV fluids.
3. If hypokalemia occurs, supplement K^+ intake at two or three times the maintenance requirement orally or intravenously.

4. If severe ECG changes are present, administer K^+, 0.2 to 0.5 mEq/kg/hour as a *slow* infusion. Do not give K^+ by IV push as sudden death may occur.
5. Correct or remove predisposing cause, if possible.

REFERENCE

Segar W.E., Chesney R.W.: Disorders of electrolyte metabolism. *Pediatr. Ann.* 10:288, 1981.

XIX. HYPOTHYROIDISM

Congenital hypothyroidism, or cretinism, is a deficiency of thyroid hormone, usually characterized by low serum thyroxine (T_4) and elevated serum thyroid-stimulating hormone (TSH). Hypothyroidism is difficult to diagnose in the first 28 days of life since only 10% to 15% of affected newborns present sufficient findings to alert the examining physician to the disease state. With the advent of mass neonatal screening programs, asymptomatic hypothyroid neonates are now identified. Early diagnosis permits replacement therapy to commence prior to the development of long-term growth and CNS abnormalities.

A. Levels of Triiodothyronine, Thyroxine, and Thyroid-Stimulating Hormone (see Appendix A–30 and Fig 17–1)

The fetal pituitary-thyroid axis functions autonomously throughout gestation, the placenta being relatively impervious to iodothyronines and TSH. Rapid changes in triiodothyronine (T_3), T_4, and TSH levels occur in fullterm and premature infants in the immediate postpartum period.

1. Fullterm infants
   In the fullterm infant, the cord blood T_3 is in the range of 15 to 88 ng/dl, while that of T_4 is 6.9 to 16.7 μg/dl and TSH is 3 to 22 μU/ml. By a few minutes after birth, TSH rises rapidly as a response to cooling postdelivery. TSH then slowly declines over the next 48 hours to 12.8 μU/ml. The TSH increment is followed by a rise in T_3 to 115 to 285 ng/dl and T_4 to 23 μg/dl. PBI levels (4.3–9.5 μg/dl) gradually increase to 9.6–16.8 by 48 hours of life and then declines to 4–11 in 2 weeks. The level of TBG ranges 1.4 to 4.1 mg/dl and FT_4 (free T_4) ranges 1.3 to 3.8 ng/dl.
2. Premature infants
   The postpartum changes in serum T_3, T_4, and TSH levels for premature infants are qualitatively similar to that of fullterm infants but of a lesser magnitude. In healthy premature infants, the cord blood T_3 is 39 ± 12 ng/dl while that of T_4 is 6.5 ± 1.2 μg/dl and TSH is 5.6 ± 0.80 μU/ml. By 24 hours after birth, T_3 is 76 ± 10 ng/dl, T_4 is 9.7 ± 1.12 μg/dl, and TSH is 10.5 ± 3.12 μU/ml. These levels then fall over the next 72 hours.
   In the sick prematures, T_3, T_4, and TSH levels gradually increase over the first few days of life, but the rate of increase is delayed.

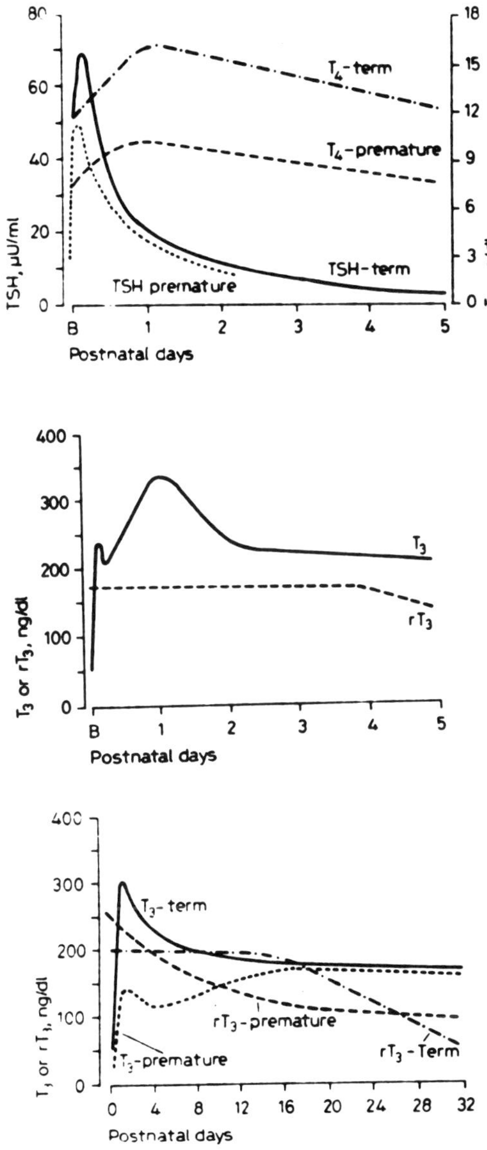

Fig 17–1.
Changes in serum TSH and T_4 *(top)* in full-term and premature infants; T_3 and rT_3 *(middle)* in infants during the first 5 days of life, and T_3 and rT_3 in term and premature infants during the first month of life *(bottom)*. (From Malvaux P.: Thyroid function during the neonatal period, infancy, and childhood. *Peditr. Adolesc. Endocrinol.* 14:33, 1985. Used by permission.)

B. Causes of Congenital Hypothyroidism

1. Transient hypothyroidism
   Premature infants who are ill or stressed have low levels of T_4 and free T_4 and normal levels of TSH and thyroid-binding globulin (TBG) when compared with fullterm infants. The level of T_4 can remain depressed for up to 3 to 4 weeks but eventually rises to the normal range.

2. Defective embryogenesis: agenesis, dysgenesis, or ectopia of the thyroid gland
   Failure in the anatomic development of the thyroid gland accounts for 80% of all cases of cretinism. Ectopic thyroid tissue is usually midline, often at the base of the tongue. The cause of defective embryogenesis is unknown.
3. Dyshormonogenesis
   Ten percent to 15% of all cases of hypothyroidism are due to dyshormonogenesis, an enzymatic defect in the production, release, or action of thyroid hormone. Eight inborn errors of thyroid synthesis or metabolism are known:
   a. Insensitivity of thyroid to TSH
   b. Iodide-trapping defect
   c. Iodide-organification defect
   d. Coupling defect of iodotyrosines
   e. Deiodination defect
   f. Thyroglobulin defect
   g. Failure of throid hormone secretion
   h. Peripheral tissue unresponsive to thyroid hormone
4. Pituitary-hypothalamic hypothyroidism
   Hypothalamic defects are often associated with other pituitary defects. This condition occurs in 1 in 66,000 infants and is associated with midline deficit such as cleft palate, micropenis, and undescended testes as well as hypoglycemia and nystagmus.
5. Maternal ingestion of antithyroid drugs
   Maternal ingestion of thiocarbamides, potassium perchlorate, and inorganic iodides can produce congenital goiter and neonatal hypothyroidism.
6. Deficiency of iodine
   Endemic goiter occurs in areas where iodine is deficient. The incidence of congenital hypothyroidism, however, is not high in the United States.
7. Maternal thyroiditis
   Destruction of the fetal thyroid by maternal antibodies has been postulated to cause hypothyroidism.
8. TBG deficiency
   A few patients have been reported in which the TBG has been deficient.

C. Who Is at Risk?

1. Infants whose mothers have thyroiditis or have been on antithyroid drugs, e.g., potassium perchlorate, thiocarbamides, and inorganic iodides
2. Infants who have a familial history of hypothyroidism or goiter or enzymatic defects of the thyroid
3. Sick premature infants are at risk for transient hypothyroidism.
4. Infants who have midline defects
5. Infants whose mothers have a deficiency or excess of iodine
6. Infants with Pendred's syndrome: congenital deafness, goiter, and an iodide organification defect

D. Clinical Manifestations

Clinical findings are often subtle or absent in the neonatal period. Length and weight are usually normal at birth. The anterior fontanelle size is usually increased. A patent posterior fontanelle with widely open cranial sutures may be present. Unconjugated hyperbilirubinemia is sometimes persistent. Slow feeding, constipation, little tendency to cry, and hypotonia can be seen. Signs include goiter, umbilical hernia, protruding tongue, poor circulation, hypothermia, and reduced growth rate. Later features (not usually seen in the newborn nursery) include hoarse cry, nasal congestion, choking episodes during feeding, dry skin with carotenemia, and large tongues with puffy faces.
Skeletal features such as delayed skeletal maturation and open posterior fontanelle are diagnostic as well as prognostic and indicate a significant intrauterine hypothyroidism with less favorable outcome.

E. Laboratory Findings

Laboratory results should be evaluated in relation to gestational age of the infant and the clinical situation.

1. Transient hypothyroidism
   Low T_4 (and normal TSH) in premature infants that reverts to normal in approximately 3 weeks
2. Defective embryogenesis
   Agenesis, dysgenesis, and ectopia of the thyroid gland
   a. Agenesis
      Diagnosis made by thyroid scan with ^{123}I or ^{99m}Tc, which fails to visualize the gland
   b. Dysgenesis
      Diagnosis made by visualizing a remnant of thyroid tissue by thyroid scan. TSH may be normal or moderately elevated.
   c. Ectopic gland
      Diagnosis made by visualization of thyroid gland in upper portion of the neck or elsewhere by scan. Oral inspection may be sufficient to visualize the gland at the base of the tongue. TSH is usually elevated.
3. Dyshormonogenesis
   a. Insensitivity of throid to TSH
      Hypersensitivity of TSH usually presents with compensatory hyperplasia of the thyroid.
   b. Iodide trapping defect
      Administrated ^{123}I does not concentrate in the neck, goiter present, and saliva fails to concentrate radioiodine; autosomal recessive trait
   c. Iodide organification defect
      Deficient iodide peroxidase or iodide transferase, the latter associated with Pendred's syndrome; autosomal recessive trait

d. Coupling defect
   Decreased T_3 and T_4
e. Deiodination or dehalogenase defect
   Wastage of iodotyrosine in the urine
f. Thyroglobulin defect
   Abnormal iodoproteins in the sera
g. Failure of thyroid hormone secretions
   Goiter with calcification
h. Peripheral tissue unresponsiveness
   Elevated TSH; no response to TSH stimulation test.

4. Pituitary-hypothalamic hypothyroidism
   TSH and T_4 are decreased. Growth hormone deficiency, adrenocorticotropin deficiency, and gonadotropin deficiency are present. TSH deficiency is usually partial. Thyrotropin releasing hormone test does not produce a sharp rise in T_4.
5. TBG deficiency
   In these infants, T_4 and T_3 are low but TSH is normal. Free T_4 is within the normal range.

F. Specific Therapy

1. Premature infants with transient hypothyroidism do not require therapy (controversial).
2. All hypothyroid infants with low T_4 and increased TSH with or without goiter should be started on substitution therapy.
   a. Thyroid replacement should begin immediately. Give L-thyroxine, 10 μg/kg/24 hours. This dose is increased by increments of 12.5–25 μg/24 hours every 2 weeks while serum T_4 is maintained in the range of 9 to 12 μg/dl and TSH is suppressed. Usually a dose of 75 μg/day is sufficient. Maximum effect occurs 10 days to 2 weeks after therapy is begun.
   b. Do not attempt to bring initial TSH to normal range quickly or thyrotoxicosis will result. In some cases, TSH will remain elevated despite normal T_4 levels.
   c. Overtreatment is as bad as inadequate therapy because overtreatment will result in premature synostosis.
   d. Monitor T_4 closely and keep T_4 within the normal range.
3. Compensated hypothyroid infant with normal T_4 and elevated TSH requires therapy also.
4. Hypothyroidism due to maternal antithyroid drugs requires therapy for approximately 4 weeks.
5. Infants with TBG deficiency do not require therapy.

G. Prognosis

Congenital hypothyroidism often results in irreversible mental retardation if thyroid replacement therapy is not begun during the first few months of life.

REFERENCES

Erenberg A.: Thyroid function in the preterm infant. *Pediatr. Clin. N. Am.* 29:1205, 1982.

Fisher D.A., Klein A.H.: Thyroid development and disorders of thyroid function in the newborn. *N. Engl. J. Med.* 304:702, 1981.

Fort P., Lifshitz F.: Screening for congenital hypothyroidism. *N. Sh. Univ. Hosp. Clin. J.* 4:24, 1981.

La Franchi S.H.: Hypothyroidism. *Pediatr. Clin. N. Am.* 26:33, 1979.

Malvaux P.: Thyroid function during the neonatal period, infancy and childhood. *Pediatr. Adolesc. Endocr.* 14:33, 1985.

XX. NEONATAL ASCITES

Ascites, an accumulation of fluid in the peritoneal cavity, can result from many causes. The most common cause in the newborn is urinary tract obstruction and the next common is meconium peritonitis. Rh incompatibility, formerly a more frequent cause of neonatal ascites, is considerably less common.

A. Who Is at Risk?

1. Infants with obstructive uropathy, usually males
2. Infants with meconium peritonitis (family history of cystic fibrosis, etc.)
3. Infants with lymphatic obstruction (chylous ascites) (males, twice the risk of females) and family history of abnormal lymphatic drainage
4. Infants with perforation of the biliary tree (bile ascites)
5. Infants with intraperitoneal or ovarian cysts
6. Infants with acute peritonitis (bacterial, viral, or toxoplasmosis): primary peritonitis (males, twice the risk of females) tuberculous peritonitis, secondary bacterial peritonitis, hypersensitivity peritonitis
7. Infants with generalized edema or anasarca
   a. Severe Rh incompatibility
   b. Homozygous α-thalassemia
   c. Cardiac failure secondary to severe anemia (twin-to-twin transfusions, Diamond Blackfan syndrome, cardiac arrhythmias, etc.)
   d. Pulmonary lymphangiectasia
   e. Cystic adenomatoid malformation of the lung
   f. Congenital nephrosis

B. Clinical Manifestations

Clinical manifestations vary depending upon the cause (see Table 17–3).

C. Laboratory Findings: Radiologic Features and Isotopic Studies

Laboratory findings depend upon the underlying disease entity (see Table 17–3).

TABLE 17–3.—Ascites: Causes, Manifestations, and Management

CAUSE	CLINICAL MANIFESTATIONS	RADIOLOGIC FEATURES	MANAGEMENT
Obstructive uropathy from rupture of fornix	Abdominal distension (at birth), dystocia, generalized edema Respiratory distress	Abdominal sonogram, intravenous pyelogram, or VCU may reveal obstructive lesion. Hippuric acid or iodine 131 scan may show extravasation of urine into the peritoneum.	Immediate drainage of the obstructed area (ureterostomy/pyelostomy/vesicostomy) and/or peritoneal fluid
Meconium peritonitis (fibroadhesive, cystic, or generalized types)	Marked abdominal distension with labored breathing Obstipation and bilious vomiting Ascites and/or flank edema Scrotal swelling in males Distended abdominal wall veins Paraumbilical ecchymosis Hypothermia, cyanosis, shock	Opaque ground-glass appearance with scattered flecks/masses of calcium or intraluminal concretion Pneumoperitoneum if perforation is recent	Laparotomy Supportive management
Chylous ascites	Abdominal distension Edema (pedal or periorbital, etc.) due to hypoproteinemia Respiratory distress (with pneumonia and/or chylothorax) Hypogammaglobulinemia Intercurrent infection	Separation of small bowel loops with edematous bowel wall Lymphangiogram: high rate of complications, not for newborn	Supportive management with low fat diet (Pregestimil) until spontaneous remission (common)
Bile ascites due to perforated common bile duct, choledochal cyst, and gallstones (hepatitis, syphilis)	Abdominal distension Pale-colored stool Prolonged jaundice Inguinal hernia Occasional anorexia, vomiting Decreased or normal bowel sounds	HIDA or PIPIDA Scan may reveal extravasation of the bile into the peritoneum.	Exploration of biliary tree and anastomosis
Intraperitoneal cyst	Abdominal distension Respiratory distress	X-ray film or sonogram may localize a soft tissue mass or cyst and reveal displacement of bowel (75%)	Excision of the cyst
Acute peritonitis (from transmural perforation of bowel, NEC, gastroschisis, omphalocele, or sepsis)	Abdominal distension Vomiting, tachycardia, tachypnea, fever, diarrhea, tender abdomen, increased, decreased, or normal bowel sounds	Dilated and separated loops of bowel, edema of the bowel wall, obliterated psoas shadow, with or without intraperitoneal air	Laparotomy for perforation, etc. Ampicillin and an aminoglycoside until sensitivity result of peritoneal aspirate. Then give appropriate antibiotics. Supportive management (continuous suction, etc.), correct hypovolemia

D. Diagnostic Workup

1. Obtain a flat plate and/or sonogram of the abdomen to demonstrate ascitic fluid and rule out cysts, tumors, stones, necrotizing enterocolitis, obstruction, perforation, etc.
2. Obtain ascitic fluid for bacterial and viral culture, bile, pH, smear, protein, fat globules, cell count, and serology.
3. Obtain complete blood count, blood culture, and urine culture.
4. Obtain ECG and chest x-ray film.
5. Obtain an intravenous pyleogram and voiding cystourethrogram (VCU) if obstructive nephropathy or nephrosis is suspected.
6. Obtain urinalysis.
7. Obtain a liver scan if choledochal cyst or biliary stone is suspected.
8. Obtain type and Rh of infant's and mother's blood if Rh incompatibility is suspected.

E. Supportive Management

1. See chapter 17–IIIB for "general supportive management for the infant with vomiting and abdominal distension."
2. Paracentesis is indicated to reduce respiratory distress, if present, but is only of temporary benefit. Treat root cause!

F. Specific Therapy

Perform surgical procedures as required in relation to the cause.

For infants with generalized edema, see chapter 13–VII for "Rh incompatibility," see chapter 11–XXIX for "congestive heart failure," see chapter 18–X for "congenital nephrotic syndrome," and see chapter 18–XII for "hydrops fetalis."

G. Prognosis

The prognosis depends on the underlying cause.

REFERENCES

Evans R.J., Brown H.E.: Ascites in newborn infants. *Urology* 1:386, 1973.

Griscom N.T., Colodny A.H., Rosenberg H.K., et al.: Diagnostic aspects of neonatal ascites: Report of 27 cases. *Am. J. Roentgenol.* 128:961, 1977.

XXI. OMPHALOCELE

Omphalocele, a central defect of the abdominal wall with protruding abdominal viscera covered with a translucent membrane, is seen in 1 in 3,000 to 9,000 live births. Life-threatening congenital malformations are often associated.

A. Who Is at Risk?

1. Males, especially premature males
2. Infants with Beckwith-Wiedemann syndrome (14%)
3. Infants with trisomy 13–15, 18, or 21 (20% of omphalocele)
4. Infants with congenital heart disease (20%)

B. Clinical Manifestations

1. Failure of lateral fold closure
   a. Central abdominal wall defect is recognizable at birth.
   b. The size of the defect varies from 2 to 12 cm.
   c. The membraneous covering is underdeveloped and may be ruptured.
   d. The umbilical cord arises from the apex of the sac.
2. Failure of cephalic and lateral fold closure
   Pentalogy syndrome, (thoracoabdominal omphalocele, ectopia cordis, intracardiac malformations, and defects of sternum, pericardium, and diaphragm)
3. Failure of caudal and lateral fold closure
   Vesicointestinal fissure (exstrophy of the cloaca, exstrophy of bladder, agenesis of hind gut and colovesical fistula)
4. Heat and fluid loss
   a. Hypothermia
   b. Dehydration
5. Inflammation around wound (postoperatively or preoperatively if ruptured)

C. Laboratory Findings

1. Dehydration and hemoconcentration
   a. Polycythemia
   b. Increased urine osmolality and specific gravity
   c. Increased serum osmolality
   d. Electrolytes imbalance (hypernatremia, etc.)
2. Hypoglycemia: associated with Beckwith-Wiedemann syndrome.

D. Radiologic Features

1. Radiologic films may reveal malrotation (25%) or atresia as a consequence of omphalocele (see chapter 17–X and 17–IV).
2. Cardiac, vascular, and genitourinary studies may reveal anomalies.

E. Supportive Therapy

1. See chapter 17–IIIB for "general supportive management for the infant with vomiting and abdominal distension," including the preoperative, intraoperative, and postoperative management of the infant.

2. Cover the omphalocele with slightly moistened sterile dressing.
3. Decompress the GI tract with a Replogle tube to low pressure suction.
4. Enclose the omphalocele in a plastic covering to prevent evaporation.
5. Monitor the infant's temperature carefully since hypothermia is a frequent cause of death.
6. Prevent and replace excessive insensible water loss.
7. Antibiotic therapy before and during surgery.
8. Supply early and adequate nutrition by parenteral route.
9. Recognize the associated life-threatening anomalies.

F. Specific Therapy

Therapy and prognosis are related to the size of the omphalocele.

1. For the less than 5-cm omphalocele (at the base), without liver, primary closure is possible.
2. For the more than 5-cm omphalocele (at the base), inject air into the peritoneal cavity to gradually stretch the abdominal wall prior to surgery or surgically enlarge the abdominal opening and deliver the omphalocele into the abdominal cavity. With a Teflon, Silastic, or polymer membrane (Silastic silo) cover the excessive omphalocele. The polymer is then gradually reduced in size and removed in 3 weeks.
3. Enterostomy rather than primary anastomosis if resection is necessary.
4. Medical therapy: daily painting with 0.5% $AgNO_3$ for 6 to 8 weeks

G. Prognosis

Overall survival is 70%. The major cause of mortality is related to the associated malformations.

REFERENCES

Seashore J.H.: Congenital abdominal wall defects. *Clin. Perinatol.* 5:61, 1978.

Wesselhoeft C.W., Randolph J.G.: Treatment of omphalocele based on individual characteristics of the defect. *Pediatrics* 44:101, 1969.

XXII. GASTROSCHISIS

Gastroschisis, an antenatal evisceration of the abdominal contents without a sac through a paraumbilical defect, has been estimated to occur in 1 in 6,000 to 50,000 live births. The associated congenital malformations are far less often than in omphalocele.

A. Who Is at Risk?

1. Males and females are equally affected.
2. Prematues (75%)

3. Slightly less than one fifth of cases are seen in siblings of infants who have had gastroschisis.
4. Infants born to young primiparous mothers

B. Clinical Manifestations

1. Evisceration of the abdominal viscera through a paraumbilical defect ranging 2 to 5 cm usually to the right of normally inserted umbilical cord
2. There is no sac.
3. Hypoplastic abdominal cavity
4. Thickened and edematous bowel due to chronic inflammation, which may lead to mesenteric vascular obstruction (antenatal infarction leads to intestinal atresia)

C. Laboratory Findings

Laboratory findings include fluid loss and hemoconcentration, polycythemia, hyperosmolality, hypernatremia, acidosis, and oliguria with high specific gravity

D. Radiologic Features

Radiologic features of malrotation (always present) and atresia may be seen.

E. Supportive and Specific Therapy

Supportive and specific therapy is similar to that for omphalocele (see chapter 17–XXI).

F. Prognosis

Mortality is about 20% to 30%. Prolonged feeding intolerance is common postoperatively and may require prolonged parenteral nutrition. Complications include sepsis, electrolyte imbalance, ileus, perforation, and malabsorption.

REFERENCE

Stringel G., Filler R.M.: Prognostic features in omphalocele and gastroschisis. *J. Pediatr. Surg.* 14:515, 1979.

TABLE 17–4.—TUMOR MASSES OF THE NEONATE

Hemangioma	Found throughout the body. Variable size, depth, growth, tendency to ulcerate, and degree of resolution. Most regress spontaneously and need no therapy. Large ones trap platelets. Those of the airway are life-threatening; those of the eyes are vision-threatening. Therapy when indicated: dexamethasone every other day for 1–2 weeks.

Subcapsular liver hemangioma	Frequently associated with cutaneous hemangiomas. Bruit may be heard. Congestive heart failure is common. Therapy with steroids, radiation, or surgery has been utilized.
Cystic hygroma	Benign, multilobulated tumor usually present in neck. Composed of lymphangiomatous and hemangiomatous elements. Spontaneous regression does not occur; tumors tend to increase in size; surgical excision required. May cause airway obstruction.
Hydronephrosis	Second most common abdominal mass in the neonate. Usually secondary to obstruction of the ureter. Drainage frequently results in salvage of hydronephrotic kidneys. See chapter 18–XI.
Cystic renal disease	Most common abdominal mass in the neonate. Usually unilateral. Surgical resection prevents future complications. See chapter 18–IX.
Renal vein thrombosis	A palpable smooth flank mass with hematuria and history of shock, dehydration, or maternal diabetes suggest the diagnosis. See chapter 18–VIII.
Neuroblastoma	Rare, incidence: 1 in 10,000. Arises from adrenal medulla and is malignant in the newborn. Widespread metastasis common (60%–70%). Skin metastasis seen in blueberry muffin spots. Hypertension and catecholamines positive in 95% of patients. Therapy includes surgical excision plus chemotherapy. Overall survival, 60% to 70%. The younger the patient, the better the prognosis.
Wilms' Tumor	Solid smooth, mobile tumor palpable in the anterior flank with distorted splayed out renal collecting system. Usually unilateral. Bilateral Wilms' tumor is often (70%–80%) associated with anomalies; GU anomalies, hemihypertrophy, Beckwith-Wiedemann syndrome, aniridia, or the ARG syndrome (aniridia, retardation, GU anomalies).
	After surgical excision those beyond stage 1 require chemotherapy. Survival rate, 90%.
Hydrometro-colpos	Large midline lower abdominal mass that persists after voiding. Often associated with imperforate hymen, distal vaginal atresia, or absence of the vagina. Surgical incision usual therapy. Ascertain normality of other genital organs.
Inguinal hernia/ hydrocele	Infants of low gestational age more prone to develop inguinal hernia. In general, repair in the newborn period. Surgery for hydrocele and undescended testes should be delayed until infant is at least 6 months of age.
Pigmented nevi	Deeply pigmented tumors, covered with fine black hair, rough and warty. Usually benign but occasionally malignant. Surgical therapy indicated.
Teratoma	Sacrococcygeal most common solid tumor of neonatal period. Usually seen as a mass just anterior to the sacrum and behind the rectum. 15% malignant. Early excision indicated in all cases. Teratoma of the thorax may present with respiratory symptoms. Those of the neck may interfere with deglutition and respiration.
Intestinal duplication	Duplications are often in small bowel around ileum, may be cystic, decompressed or tubular, and may lead to intussusception. Ultrasound may be helpful for diagnosis and surgery is the treatment of choice.
Cysts	Follicular ovarian, choledocal or liver cysts, or hydrops of gallbladder are benign conditions. Ultrasound is useful for the diagnosis.

REFERENCES

Allen R.G.: Tumor masses of the neonate. *Clin. Perinatol.* 5:115, 1978.

Stevenson R.J.: Abdominal masses. *Surg. Clin. North Am.* 65:1481, 1985.

TABLE 17–5.—CLINICAL AND BIOCHEMICAL FEATURES IN NEWBORN ADRENAL INSUFFICIENCY*†

		AMBIGUOUS GENITALIA		SERUM				URINE		
ADRENAL INSUFFICIENCY DISORDERS	ELECTROLYTE DISTURBANCE	VIRILIZED FEMALE	INCOMPLETE MALE	CORTISOL	ALDOSTERONE	17-OHP	DHEA	17-OHCS	17-KS	PREGNANETRIOL
Hypoplasia	Severe	No	No	Decrease	Decrease	Decrease	Decrease	Decrease	Decrease	Decrease
Hemorrhage	Moderate to severe	No	No	Decrease	Decrease	Decrease	Decrease	Decrease	Decrease	Decrease
Desmolase (20, 22)	Severe	No	Yes	Decrease	Decrease	Decrease	Decrease	Decrease	Decrease	Decrease
3 βHSD	Severe	Yes	Yes	Decrease	Decrease	Decrease	Increase	Decrease	Increase	Decrease
21-hydroxylase‡	Moderate to severe	Yes	No	Decrease	Decrease	Increase	Increase	Decrease	Increase	Increase
Aldosterone synthesis block	Severe	No	No	Normal	Decrease	Normal	Normal	Normal	Normal	Normal
Pseudohypoaldosteronism	Severe	No	No	Normal	Increase	Normal	Normal	Normal	Normal	Normal
11-Hydroxylase‡	None	Yes	No	Decrease	Decrease	Normal-slight increase	Normal	Increase	Increase	Normal-slight increase
17-Hydroxylase	None	No	Yes	Decrease	Normal or decrease	Decrease	Decrease	Decrease	Decrease	Decrease
Unresponsiveness to ACTH	None	No	No	Decrease	Normal or low	Normal	Normal	Decrease	Decrease	Decrease

*3β HSD = 3β-hydroxysteroid dehydrogenase; ACTH = adrenocorticotropin; 17-OHP = 17-hydroxyprogesterone; DEAH = Dehydroepi androgen; 17-OHCS = 17 hydroxycorticosteroids; 17-KS = 17-ketosteroids.

†From Sperling M.A.: Newborn adaption, adrenocortical hormones and ACTH, in Tulchinsky D., Ryan K.J. (eds.): *Maternal-Fetal Endocrinology*. Philadelphia, W.B. Saunders Co., 1980. Used by permission.

‡Lack of one or more of these enzymes results in the accumulation of intermediate steroid metabolites, including androgens, and adrenogenital syndrome.

TABLE 17–6.—COMPARATIVE SUMMARY OF DISORDERS OF SEXUAL DIFFERENTIATION‡

DISORDER	CHROMOSOMES	GENES	GONADA	DUCTS	EXTERNAL GENITALIA	HORMONES	CAUSE
Gonadal agenesis	Majority 46,XY	. . .	Absent	Rudimentary; ambiguous	Small; ambiguous	—	Polygenic defect or teratogen*
Gonadal dysgenesis with normal karyotype	46,XY	H-Y antigen positive in one patient	Streak, or degenerated testis	Immature female	Female, may have clitoral enlargement	Elevated gonadotropins	Mutant gene*
	46,XX	. . .	Streak	Immature female	Female	Elevated gonadotropins	Mutant gene*
46,XX males	46,XX	H-Y antigen positive	Small testes	Male	Male, but small	Testosterone low, gonadotropins normal or elevated	Gene translocation, mutation, mosaicism or chimerism*
Turner's syndrome	45,X	Deficiency of gene for further ovarian development*	Streak	Hypoplastic female	Female, but small	Estrogens low, androgens low, gonadotropins elevated	Nondisjunction in prenatal gametogenesis or in early embryo*
Klinefelter's syndrome	47,XXY	. . .	Testes, germinal epithelium degenerates	Male	Male	Testosterone low, gonadotropins elevated	Nondisjunction in gametogenesis or in early embryo*
True hermaphroditism	46,XX	H-Y antigen positive in some cases	Testicular and ovarian tissue	Female and male, variable	Ambiguous or predominantly male	FSH normal	Translocation of testicle differentiating gene, mutant gene, or mosaicism*
	46,XY	. . .	Testicular and ovarian tissue	Female and male	Male	FSH normal	Translocation of ovary-differentiating gene, mutant gene, or mosaicism*
	46,XX/46,XY	. . .	Testicular and ovarian tissue	Female and male	Ambiguous or male	FSH normal	Union of two zygotes*
Male pseudo-hermaphroditism							
Sex chromosomal mosaicism	45,X/46,XY or other with at least one Y	. . .	Streak or dysgenetic testis	Female and/or male	Female, ambiguous, or male	. . .	Pathologic mitosis in early zygote*
Deficiency of antimüllerian hormone	46,XY	Deficiency of an X chromosomal gene for antimüllerian hormone*	Testis	Female and male	Male, often cryptorchid	. . .	X chromosomal recessive gene mutation*

(continued)

TABLE 17–6.—(continued)

DISORDER	CHROMOSOMES	GENES	GONADA	DUCTS	EXTERNAL GENITALIA	HORMONES	CAUSE
Deficiency of an enzyme in steroid synthesis	46,XY	Defective gene for one of the steroid synthesis enzymes	Testis, cryptorchid-like	Male	Ambiguous	Testosterone low	Probably autosomal recessive gene mutation
5α-reductase deficiency	46,XY	Deficiency of an autosomal gene for 5α-reductase	Testis, cryptorchid-like	Male	Ambiguous	Testosterone and gonado-tropins normal	Probably autosomal recessive gene mutation
Complete testicular feminization	46,XY	Deficiency of an X-chromosomal gene for testosterone receptor	Testes	Rudimentary male	Infantile female	Testosterone normal or high, gonadotropins elevated	X chromosomal recessive mutation of the gene for testosterone receptor
Incomplete testicular feminization	46,XY	Partial deficiency of X chromosomal gene for testosterone receptor	Testes	Rudimentary or male	Ambiguous	Testosterone normal or high, gonadotropins elevated	Probably X chromosomal recessive mutant alleles of the gene for testosterone receptor
Female pseudohermaphroditism							
Adrenogenital syndromes	46,XX	Deficiency of gene(s) for adrenal steroid synthesis enzymes	Ovary	Female	Masculinized	Androgens elevated (intermediates from adrenal)	Autosomal recessive mutation of gene(s) for adrenal steroid synthesis enzymes
Nonadrenal masculinization	46,XX	. . .	Ovary	Female	Clitoral hypertrophy	. . .	Gene mutation*
Exogenous teratogens	46,XX	. . .	Ovary	Female	Masculinized	Androgens may be elevated	Aminoglutethimide; inhibits 3β-hydroxysteroid dehydrogenase Androgens from maternal tumors or medication

*The information is not yet established.
†Dashes indicate that no data available.
‡From Pelliniemi L.J., Dym M.: The fetal gonad and sexual differentiation, in Tulchinsky D., Ryan K.J. (eds.): *Maternal-Fetal Endocrinology*. Philadelphia, W.B. Saunders Co., 1980, p. 270. Used by permission.

Chapter 18

Edema and/or Oliguria

Edema in the newborn infant within the first week of life (physiologic) may not be related to any known pathologic condition. Pathologic conditions causing edema with increased interstitial fluid include decreased plasma colloid oncotic pressure, increased capillary hydrostatic pressure, and decreased tissue hydrostatic pressure. Renal or cardiac failure is the most common cause of edema in the newborn period.

I. NORMAL DATA: PHYSIOLOGIC EDEMA

When edema occurs in the newborn period without any related pathologic condition it is called physiologic edema. Normal infants expand their extracellular volume at maximum by the third day and contract by the seventh day of life. The mechanism of physiologic edema is not clear. However, without therapy, edema gradually regresses.

A. Renal Anatomy/Function in the Neonate

Renal structures in the neonate are immature. The glomeruli and tubules are incompletely developed with the juxtamedullary elements being less developed than the cortical elements. Glomerular development precedes tubular development resulting in glomerulotubular imbalance. Neonatal total renal blood flow is diminished due to increased renal blood flow resistance and a reduced fraction of the cardiac output going to the kidneys. Blood pressure increases, vascular resistance decreases, and renal blood flow increases by the third day postbirth but does not reach adult levels until the infant is 1 to 2 years of age.

Functionally, the GFR is low and the ability to concentrate and excrete a fluid challenge is diminished. The fractional reabsorption of bicarbonate, phosphate, sodium, glucose, and amino acids at the proximal tubule is incomplete. The secretion of organic acids by the proximal tubule is ineffective and NH_4 production by the distal tubule is low. Antidiuretic hormone is present in the neonate and is increased with hypoxia. Renin-angiotensin levels are increased during the neonatal period and may cause decreased GFR.

B. Normal Urine Examination (See Appendix A–34 for Normal Constituents of Urine in Neonatal Period)

Squamous epithelial cells	seen in greater than 50% of urine analyzed
Tubular epithelial cells	seen in 25% of urine analyzed
Urinary pH	5 to 7
Protein	8 to 12 mg/24 hours
Glucose	Negative
White blood cells/high power field	2 to 3
Red blood cells/high power field	0
Casts	0
Bacteria	0
Osmolality	141 to 303 mOsm/L
Specific gravity	1.003 to 1.008
Addis count	
White blood cells	Up to 100,000
Red blood cells	Up to 75,000
Casts	0

C. Urine Data

1. The first voiding (see appendix A–36, A–37)
   Ninety-three percent of normal neonates void within 24 hours of birth and 99.4% within 48 hours; 23% do so in the delivery room.
2. Frequency of voiding
   Normal neonates void two to six times per day during first 48 hours of life and subsequently 5 to 25 times daily.
3. Daily urinary volume (Appendix A–38)
   Minimal urine volume is 1.0 ml/kg/hour but well-hydrated fullterm infants 2 to 3 days of age may void considerably more.
4. Osmolality
   Osmolality is the number of particles per unit weight of a solvent. Urinary osmolality on day 1 in the well-hydrated healthy, full term infant usually ranges between 141 and 303 mOsm/L and should be maintained between 150 and 520 mOsm/L (specific gravity, 1.004 to 1.013). Urine osmolality (mOsm/L) = (specific gravity $-$ 1) $\times$ 4 $\times$ 10^4

Maximal concentration is 750 mOsm/L (specific gravity, 1.018) in premature infants and 1,000 mOsm/L (specific gravity, 1.025) in term infants.
Serum sodium concentration provides a good indication of osmolality:

$$\text{mOsm/L} = 2\ \text{Na} + \frac{\text{BUN(mg/dl)}}{2.8} + \frac{\text{Blood glucose (mg/dl)}}{18}$$

Each 18 mg/dl of glucose or 2.8 mg/dl of BUN increases the osmolality by 1 mOsm/L.
The term newborn is capable of excreting the renal solute from formulas containing an average of 100 mOsm/L.

5. Specific gravity
   Specific gravity averages 1.006 to 1.008 in the well-hydrated low-birth-weight infant. Newborns have limited ability to concentrate urine maximally. Specific gravity should be maintained between 1.004 and 1.013.
   Protein and glucose in the urine falsely increase the specific gravity. To determine the actual specific gravity when glucose or protein is present, subtract 0.003 unit of specific gravity for each gram of protein per 100 ml of urine and 0.004 unit of specific gravity for each gram of glucose per 100 ml of urine.
6. Proteinuria
   The newborn excretes 8 to 12 mg/dl of protein in the urine daily. Protein is not normally detected by conventional methods of testing, i.e., Albustix or 10% sulfosalycylic acid since 8 to 12 mg/dl is too low for detection. Highly alkaline urines or those with high concentration of urates may give false positive reactions for protein.
   Proteinuria indicates glomerular injury and may be seen with asphyxia, cardiac failure, massive doses of penicillin, dehydration, fever, radiopaque dyes, and the nephrotic syndrome (proteinuria is persistent in the nephrotic syndrome).
7. Hematuria, greater than 2 to 3 red blood cells per high power field in centrifuged urine, indicates glomerular irritation and is seen in coagulopathy, disseminated intravascular coagulation, infections, congenital malformations, nephrotoxic drugs, renal vascular accidents, cortical or medullary necrosis, obstructive uropathy, and asphyxia.
8. Pyuria, greater than 3 to 5 white blood cells per high power field in centrifuged urine, is often associated with urinary tract infection, but may be seen in glomerular injury, tubular disease, acidosis, dehydration, interstitial nephritis, or following instrumentation.
9. Urinary casts
   a. Red blood cell casts may be seen in glomerular ischemic injury usually due to renal vascular occlusion, cortical necrosis, or glomerulonephritis.
   b. White blood cell casts may be seen in infection, interstitial injury, or renal inflammation.
   c. Epithelial cell casts are seen in tubular or interstitial injury.
   d. Granular casts are seen in dehydration, interstitial injury, and tubular injury.

II. COMMON CAUSES OF EDEMA AND/OR OLIGURIA IN THE NEWBORN

A. Physiologic

B. Pathologic Causes

1. Decreased plasma colloid oncotic pressure
   Colloid oncotic pressure is determined by plasma protein concentration: one gram of protein retains 15 ml fluid intravascularly.
   a. Hypoproteinemia may be due to decreased protein intake, decreased protein synthesis, or increased protein loss as in
      1) Liver failure or zinc or copper deficiency
      2) Starvation
      3) Nephrotic syndrome
      4) Hydrops fetalis
      5) Cystic fibrosis
   b. Hypoproteinemia may be due to increased capillary permeability of colloid (protein) leaking into the extravascular space as in
      1) Prematurity
      2) Vitamin E deficiency (lack of antioxidant effect)
      3) Endothelial damage due to asphyxia, sepsis, endotoxemia, necrotizing enterocolitis, respiratory distress syndrome, meconium aspiration, transient tachypnea of the newborn
         These conditions often lead to prerenal failure.
   c. Hypoproteinemia may be due to dilutional factors as when blood volume expanders are given.
2. Increased capillary hydrostatic pressure
   The intravascular fluid is normally related to the interstitial fluid in a 1:3 ratio. When there is an increase in intravascular pressure intravascular fluid is forced into the interstitial compartment as in
   a. Congestive heart failure
   b. Acute renal failure: renal and postrenal failure (see chapter 18–IVB for causes of edema due to acute renal failure)
   c. Syndrome of inappropriate antidiuretic hormone
   d. Placental transfusion
   e. Fluid overload
   f. Excessive sodium intake in infants
   g. Decreased sodium excretion
3. Decreased tissue hydrostatic pressure or decreased lymphatic drainage as in
   a. Lymphedema
   b. Pulmonary edema due to bronchopulmonary dysplasia
   c. Turner's syndrome

III. WHAT THE PHYSICIAN SHOULD DO WHEN CONFRONTED WITH AN INFANT WITH EDEMA AND/OR OLIGURIA

A. Diagnostic Workup

1. Review the prenatal, intrapartum, and postnatal history.
   a. If asphyxia, hypoxia, hypovolemia, and/or hypotension were present, consider syndrome of inappropriate antidiuretic hormone, acute renal failure, congestive heart failure, placental transfusion, respiratory distress syndrome in prematures, fluid overload with aggressive correction of acidosis, shock, etc.
   b. If intrauterine arrhythmia was present, consider congestive heart failure.
2. Review the maternal history during the pregnancy.
   a. If the mother is diabetic, consider renal vein thrombosis.
   b. If the mother is Rh negative with rising (high) anti-Rh titers or change in optical density of amniotic fluid from zone 2 to zone 3 (or rising optical density of amniotic fluid), consider immune hydrops fetalis (see chapter 13–VII).
   c. If the mother had infection(s), consider intrauterine or congenital infection.
   d. If the mother has a history of oligohydramnios, consider renal anomalies and if there is a history of polyhydramnios, consider hydrops fetalis, congenital infection, etc.
3. Review the family history.
   If there was a history of erythroblastosis fetalis, a chromosomal aberration, cystic fibrosis in a sibling, or renal anomalies (polycystic kidney, nephrotic syndrome, etc.), consider repetitive occurrence in the same family.
4. Review the infant's history.
   a. If the infant is premature, consider deficiencies of vitamin E, copper, zinc, protein, etc.
   b. If umbilical catheterization was performed, consider renal artery thrombosis/embolus with acute renal failure.
   c. If there is a history of inadequate protein intake or loss, starvation, infection, respiratory distress, fluid or sodium overload, necrotizing enterocolitis, bronchopulmonary dysplasia, etc., consider hypoproteinemia.
   d. Review the infant's daily weight and intake and output. If the infant received excessive fluid, consider edema due to increased capillary hydrostatic pressure.
   e. If the infant has oliguria with urine output less than 1.0 ml/kg/hour, consider acute renal failure, congestive heart failure, and syndrome of inappropriate antidiuretic hormone.
   f. Review the infant's blood pressure. If the infant presently has hypertension or has had hypotension, consider renal artery thrombosis.

5. Examine the infant carefully considering the following:
   a. Tachypnea, tachycardia, pallor, hepatosplenomegaly, abdominal mass, meatal stenosis, hypospadias or epispadias, ascites, weight gain, etc.
   b. Malformations, e.g., Potter's syndrome, VATER syndrome, prune belly syndrome, Turner's syndrome, etc.
6. Obtain laboratory studies.
   a. Blood type and group and Coomb's test to determine immune hydrops fetalis
   b. Complete blood count (CBC), platelet count, peripheral blood smear for evidence of anemia, hemolysis, polycythemia to determine immune hydrops fetalis, sepsis, renal vein thrombosis, acute renal failure, congestive heart failure, etc.
   c. Blood culture if sepsis is suspected
   d. Serum electrolytes, blood urea nitrogen (BUN), creatinine, and osmolality. In acute renal failure of renal origin, the BUN and serum creatinine are elevated and the rise is proportional, i.e., the serum BUN: creatinine ratio remains 10 to 15:1. In acute renal failure of prerenal origin, the rise in BUN is disproportionate to the rise of creatinine and the ratio of 10 to 15:1 is elevated. Note the potassium level carefully. The serum potassium usually rises within 2 to 3 days of acute renal failure. The serum creatinine doubles with each 50% to 60% decrease in renal function.
   e. Serum calcium, phosphorus, protein, and albumin to determine decreased calcium, protein, or albumin or increased phosphorus
   f. Blood gas studies. Metabolic acidosis often accompanies acute renal failure, congestive heart failure, respiratory problems, sepsis, etc.
   g. Coagulation studies if there is any bleeding tendency
   h. Urinalysis, urine electrolytes and osmolality, culture and sensitivity, and creatinine. Hematuria, proteinuria, and casts are seen frequently in acute renal failure. The presence of any organism in urine obtained by suprapubic tap indicates urinary tract infection.
7. Obtain a chest x-ray film and ECG. Cardiomegaly may be seen in congestive heart failure.
8. Obtain vitamin E, copper, or zinc levels if a deficiency is suspected.
9. Obtain diagnostic radiologic, radioisotopic, and sonographic studies if acute renal failure, obstructive uropathy, hypertension, etc., are present. (See chapter 18–IV, 18–XI, 18–VI, etc.)
   a. B-mode ultrasonography (renal)
      This noninvasive procedure is valuable in analyzing structural anatomy including the renal size and anatomy of the dilated collecting system and ureters and differentiating renal cystic from solid masses. This is especially useful in patients with elevated BUN and creatinine where organic iodide compounds can not be employed to localize the lesion.
   b. The intravenous pyelogram is a major diagnostic technique for delineating multicystic kidneys, unilateral vascular occlusions, ureteric abnormalities, and other abnormalities that impinge on the renal output.

c. Voiding cystourethrogram (VCU)
This technique will demonstrate the presence of reflux and the status of the bladder and outline the lower urinary tracts. It is useful for defining obstructive lesions of the ureter, urethral diverticula, valves, and strictures. It should be performed in infants with postrenal failure.

d. Percutaneous needle puncture
Percutaneous needle puncture for culture and sensitivity and microscopic examination may be helpful. If a large fluid-filled mass is delineated, a catheter may then be threaded into the area for temporary drainage.

e. Arteriography
In the newborn intensive care unit, when an umbilical catheter is in place, direct injection of contrast material into the umbilical artery will produce an aortogram and renal arteriogram including the peripheral distribution of the vessels.

f. Retrograde urethrography
In this technique, contrast material is inserted with a syringe directly into the urethral meatus so that areas proximal to any obstructive uropathy may be outlined.

g. Computerized tomography
Computerized tomography may be utilized to delineate tumors, etc.

h. Cystoscopy
Cystoscopy is most useful in the management of prostatic urethral valves.

i. Radionucleatide scanning provides information regarding renal parenchyma, blood flow, size, shape, location, and outflow tract.

B. General Supportive Management for the Infants With Edema and/or Oliguria

1. Handle the infant gently (as always).
2. Monitor vital signs including blood pressure. Maintain the infant's temperature at a neutral thermal range (skin temperature at 36.5°C and/or rectal temperature 37°C).
3. Record intake and output strictly.
4. Weigh the infant every 8 to 12 hours to determine weight loss or gain.
5. Monitor urine electrolytes, osmolality, and/or specific gravity.
6. Maintain serum electrolytes within normal range.
7. Maintain normal acid-base balance.
8. Screen blood glucose every 2 to 4 hours to prevent or correct hypoglycemia promptly (see chapter 15–X).
9. Correct metabolic acidosis with $NaHCO_3$ (see chapter 11–IIIB12). Do not attempt to use sodium or hypertonic solutions if acute renal failure and/or overhydration is present.
10. Correct hypocalcemia with calcium gluconate, 100 to 500 mg/kg slowly (see chapter 15–IX).
11. Do not administer potassium till the infant voids adequately (see chapter 18–XVI).

12. Correct hypoalbuminemia with fresh frozen plasma or 5% salt-poor albumin. Be cautious not to overload as congestive heart failure can occur.
13. Transfuse to correct anemia (see chapter 14–III).
14. Administer Lasix 1.0 (0.5–2.0) mg/kg/dose and repeat every 6–8 hours as required.
15. See the appropriate section for the specific problem.
    See chapter 18–XIII for zinc deficiency, chapter 18–XIV for copper deficiency, chapter 18–X for congenital nephrotic syndrome, chapter 18–XII for hydrops fetalis, chapter 17–VII for cystic fibrosis, chapter 6 for prematurity, chapter 14–XV for vitamin E deficiency, chapter 16–XIX for sepsis, chapter 17–XVI for necrotizing enterocolitis, chapter 11 for respiratory problems, chapter 11–XXIX for congestive heart failure, chapter 18–IV for acute renal failure, chapter 18–XV for syndrome of inappropriate antidiuretic hormone, etc.

IV. ACUTE RENAL FAILURE

Acute deterioration in renal function is associated with reduced glomerular filtration rate (GFR), decreased urinary output (oliguria), and frequently acidosis and/or fluid and electrolyte imbalance. Acute renal failure is usually diagnosed if urinary output is less than 1 ml/kg/hour for 24 hours and serum creatinine is greater than 1.0 mg/dl or BUN is greater than 20 mg/dl. Infants with bilateral renal agenesis do not reveal signs of acute renal failure at birth since the placenta functions as an excretory organ.

A. Normal Data. See chapter 18–I

B. Who Is at Risk?

1. Prerenal failure
   a. Infants with hypovolemia due to the following:
      1) Hypoxia and/or asphyxia
      2) Hypotension
      3) Congestive heart failure
      4) Maternal or fetal/neonatal hemorrhage
      5) Dehydration
      6) Septicemia
      7) Disseminated intravascular coagulation
      8) Drugs
      9) Toxins
   b. Infants with renal arterial occlusion with or without hypertension

2. Intrinsic renal failure
   a. Nephrotoxins (e.g., aminoglycosides, cephaloridine, tolazoline, indomethacin)
   b. Renal vascular accidents
      1) Renal vein thrombosis
      2) Renal artery thrombosis/emboli
   c. Renal cortical or medullary necrosis
   d. Acute tubular necrosis from hemorrhage, shock, hypoxia, perinatal asphyxia, etc.
   e. Pyelonephritis
   f. Acute interstitial nephritis
   g. Renal hypoplasia/dysplasia/aplasia (Potter's syndrome)
   h. Infantile polycystic kidneys, multicystic kidneys
   i. Congenital nephrotic syndrome
3. Postrenal failure
   a. Neurogenic bladder
   b. Asphyxiated bladder
   c. Obstructive uropathy
      1) Bladder neck obstruction
      2) Obstructive megaureter
      3) Ectopic ureter
      4) Ureterocele
      5) Ureteropelvic junction obstruction
      6) Ureteral stricture

C. Clinical Manifestations

1. Oliguria (urinary output less than 1.0 ml/kg/hour)
2. Edema and/or abrupt weight gain. Increased or decreased blood pressure may be present.
3. Abdominal distension and/or flank mass(es)
   Abdominal and/or flank masses are most commonly renal in origin. Prune belly syndrome is associated with congenital absence of the abdominal musculature, undescended testicles, and various renal anomalies. Kidneys may be enlarged and palpable when they are edematous, hydronephrotic, infantile polycystic, multicystic, or affected by renal vascular accidents. Enlarged kidney(s) with hematuria suggests renal vein thrombosis.
4. Abdominal distension and/or distended bladder may be seen in congenital lower urinary tract obstruction.
5. Ascites may be seen in congenital lower urinary tract obstruction, congenital nephrotic syndrome, etc.
6. Seizures may be seen in severe acute renal failure associated with hyponatremia, hypocalcemia, disseminated intravascular coagulation, or systemic hypertension, etc.

7. Clinical manifestations of the primary problem causing acute renal failure such as shock, Potter's syndrome, etc., may be present.

D. Laboratory Findings

1. Azotemia (BUN greater than 20 mg/dl)
   The BUN of healthy infants at 28 to 31 weeks of gestation is 14 to 27 mg/dl on day 1 or 2 and decreases with advanced gestational age and postnatal age.
2. Increased creatinine greater than 1.0 mg/dl (see appendix A–26)
   Creatinine averages 0.6 mg/dl in the premature infants and does not increase until GFR is reduced to 60% of normal. In the preterm infant in the first few days of life, creatinine may be greater than 1 mg/dl.
3. Acidosis (pH less than 7.30)
   Metabolic acidosis (plasma bicarbonate less than 18 mEq/L)
4. Hyponatremia: serum sodium less than 130 mEq/L
5. Hyperkalemia: serum potassium greater than 6.5 mEq/L
6. Hypocalcemia: serum calcium less than 6.5 mg/dl in prematures and less than 7.0 mg/dl in term infants
7. A decreased glomerular filteration rate is seen in acute renal failure and can be measured by a clearance test using insulin, creatinine, etc.
8. Urinalysis may show increased or decreased urine osmolality and specific gravity, proteinuria, hematuria, pyuria, and urinary cast (see chapter 18–I for normal data)

E. Radiologic Features

Radiologic features are related to the underlying problem (see chapter 18–IIIA9)

F. General Supportive Management for the Infant With Acute Renal Failure

1. See chapter 18–IIIB for "general supportive management for the infant with edema and/or oliguria."
2. Measure intake and output carefully.
3. Weigh the infant every 8 to 12 hours.
4. Determine blood pressure.
   a. Hypotension, systolic blood pressure less than 40 mm Hg for a 1,000-gm infant and less than 50 mm Hg for a 3,000-gm infant, and/or hypovolemia may be the cause or result of acute renal failure. Correct hypovolemia and/or hypotension with colloid (blood, Plasmanate, etc.; see chapter 14–IIID7). If hypotension persists, a vasopressor such as dopamine may be utilized in a constant infusion.
   b. Hypertension, blood pressure greater than 90/65 in term infants and greater than 80/45 in premature infants, and/or overload may be the re-

sult of acute renal failure or renal artery thrombosis. Correct hypertension with fluid restriction (for acute stage) and/or hydralazine or other drugs (see chapter 18–VI).

5. Examine the infant carefully to see if the infant has Potter's facies, other signs of obstructive uropathy such as bladder distension, hydronephrosis, etc.
6. Obtain blood for the following tests and correct if abnormal:
   a. CBC with smear and platelet
   b. Serum sodium, chloride, potassium, BUN, creatinine, calcium, phosphorus, total protein, albumin, HCO_3^-, and plasma osmolality
   c. Blood gases
   d. Blood cultures and sensitivities
7. Obtain and follow urine for the following tests (see chapter 18–I for normal data):
   a. Osmolality and/or specific gravity
   b. Protein
   c. Glucose
   d. White and red blood cells
   e. Urinary casts
   f. pH
   g. Clearance test (insulin or creatinine)
8. Obtain the appropriate radiologic studies if obstructive uropathy is suspected by physical examination (see chapter 18–XID). Nephrosonogram is noninvasive, simple, and portable and usually is obtained prior to other tests.
9. Differentiate prerenal from intrinsic renal failure if the infant does not have obstructive uropathy.
   a. A urine/plasma osmolality ratio less than 1.0 suggests intrinsic renal failure while greater than 1.0 suggests syndrome of inappropriate antidiuretic hormone
   b. Fluid challenge test
      1) Prior to the fluid challenge test, make sure the infant does not have congestive heart failure and/or the syndrome of inappropriate antidiuretic hormone
      2) Administer normal saline or plasma, 20 ml/kg in 1 to 2 hours.
      3) If oliguria persists, give furosemide 1.0 (0.5–2.0) mg/kg/dose IV and repeat every 6–8 hours as required (furosemide may be given at the same time as the saline or plasma).
      4) Suspect prerenal failure if the infant voids in response to the fluid challenge test.
      5) Suspect intrinsic renal failure if the infant does not start to void within 1 to 2 hours after the fluid challenge test.
10. Prerenal failure
    Correct the causative problems while monitoring renal function.
    a. Continue appropriate hydration.
    b. Correct hypoxia and/or asphyxia (see chapters 11–III, 11–IV, 11–VI, and 15–IV).

c. Correct congestive heart failure (see chapter 11–XXIX).
d. Treat for sepsis, disseminated intravascular coagulation, hemorrhage as required (see chapters 16–XIX, 14–XII, and 14–III).
e. Discontinue medications that may give hypovolemia.

11. Intrinsic renal failure
 a. Restrict fluid intake to insensible water loss (see Table 6–3) composed of 10% dextrose in water plus nonrenal (GI) fluid losses and add urinary output with same electrolyte concentrations as urine.
 b. If the infant is fluid overloaded, edematous, or has congestive heart failure:
 1) Estimate the desired weight loss in percentage. For example, for an infant who should weigh 3,050 gm and now weighs 3,500 gm, the desired weight loss in percent would be 13%.
 2) Calculate the insensible water loss for the infant that day.

$$3.5 \text{ kg(weight of infant)} \times 50 \text{ ml/kg/day (insensible water loss)} = 175.0 \text{ ml/day}$$

 3) Then subtract the percent of fluid that represents the difference between the ideal weight and the edematous weight (13%).

$$175 \text{ ml} - 22.75 \text{ ml} = 152.25 \text{ ml}$$

 That is the amount of fluid to be given to the infant that day.
 c. Withhold potassium intake until the infant is voiding adequately.
 d. Eliminate protein from diet but attempt to maintain caloric intake at 100 calories/kg/24 hours using high concentrations of glucose and fat.
 e. Weigh every 8 to 12 hours. With this regimen, a daily loss of 0.5% to 1.0% of weight is expected.
 f. Increase intake and correct electrolyte losses as urinary output starts to increase.
 g. Correct metabolic acidosis with $NaHCO_3$ (see chapter 11–IIIB12). Hypernatremia may result from sodium retention.
 h. Correct hypocalcemia with calcium gluconate (see chapter 15–IX).
 i. Correct hyperkalemia (see chapter 18–XVI).
 If serum K^+ is elevated beyond 8.5 mEq/L and significant ECG changes are present (peaked T wave, wide QRS complex, ST depression, prolonged PR interval, flattened P waves), treat with 1.0 to 2.0 ml/kg of 10% calcium gluconate over 2 to 4 minutes while observing the ECG *or* administer 200 to 400 mg of glucose/kg with 0.2 units/kg of crystalline zinc insulin to promote intracellular movement of potassium. Then give 0.5 to 2 gm/kg of sodium polystyrene sulfonate (Kayexalate) in 20% sorbitol as a retention enema every 4 to 6 hours.
 j. Reduce the dosage of nephrotoxic drugs or drugs excreted through the kidneys.
 k. Severe anemia may be treated with exchange transfusion using fresh citrate phosphate dextrose (CPD) packed red blood cells to prevent hypervolemia and hyperkalemia (see chapter 13–VI).

l. Treat infection with the appropriate antibiotic therapy. Monitor the blood level of antibiotics if possible.
m. Examine the patient frequently for the development of pulmonary edema.
n. Peritoneal or hemodialysis is indicated with the following:
   1) Persistent elevated K^+ unresponsive to therapy
   2) Severe metabolic acidosis not controlled by $NaHCO_3$
   3) Intractable hypoglycemia
   4) Persistent azotemia with oliguria lasting 3 to 4 days

REFERENCES

Anand S.K.: Acute renal failure in the neonate. *Pediatr. Clin. N. Am.* 29:791, 1982.

Anand S.K., Northway J.D., Crussi F.G.: Acute renal failure in newborn infants. *J. Pediatr.* 92:985, 1978.

Leake R.D.: Perinatal nephrobiology: A developmental perspective. *Clin. Perinatol.* 4:321–349, 1977.

Nash M.A., Edelmann C.M. Jr.: The developing kidney. Immature function or inappropriate standard. *Nephron* 11:71, 1973.

V. ACUTE RENAL CORTICAL NECROSIS

Compromise of renal cortical perfusion in hemorrhagic and asphyxial shock may cause ischemic necrosis. Necrosis of other organs, i.e., liver, adrenals, intestines, or brain, frequently accompanies acute renal cortical necrosis.

A. Who Is at Risk?

Infants with severe shock, anemia, and asphyxia, e.g., fetomaternal transfusion, severe hemolytic disease, abruptio placentae, or severe perinatal asphyxia, are at risk.

B. Clinical Manifestations

Nonspecific renal findings are common and include enlarged kidneys, anemia, oliguria, and edema.

C. Laboratory Findings

1. Hematuria
2. Increased urine specific gravity and osmolality
3. Thrombocytopenia
4. Intravenous pyelogram usually shows poor renal visualization (not recommended)
5. Renal biopsy may delineate degree of necrosis
6. Associated findings include hypotension or hypertension, low hematocrit, and positive blood or stool culture.

D. Radiologic Features

Within 10 days to 2 weeks, necrotic cortical tissue becomes calcified, exhibiting a characteristic pattern of bilateral symmetric cortical calcification.

E. Supportive Therapy

See chapter 18–IIIB for "general supportive management for the infant with edema and/or oliguria" and 18–IVF for "general supportive management for the infant with acute renal failure."

F. Specific Therapy

Indications for nephrectomy or embolectomy are not clear at this time.

G. Prognosis

The prognosis is related to underlying cause and degree of renal compromise. Infants who survive have small, scarred kidneys. Chronic renal insufficiency and/or hypertension may develop.

REFERENCES

Bernstein J., Meyer R.: Congenital abnormalities of the urinary system II: Renal cortical and medullary necrosis. *J. Pediatr.* 59:657, 1961.

Nogrady M.B., Lesk D.M.: Renal papillary necrosis in the newborn. *Am. J. Roentgenol. Radium Ther. Nucl. Med.* 116:661, 1972.

VI. NEONATAL SYSTEMIC HYPERTENSION

Hypertension in the newborn has been increasingly reported perhaps due to the increased ability to detect hypertension and more awareness of elevated blood pressure, increased use of umbilical artery catheters, and the increased survival of very ill neonates. The incidence has been reported to be 2.5% of neonatal intensive care unit admissions. Blood pressure in the newborn is directly related to chronologic age and birth weight and is higher during awake states than during sleep states (see appendix A–1, Figs A–1 and A–2).

Hypertensive values:

Fullterm: Systolic blood pressure greater than 90 mm Hg
Diastolic blood pressure greater than 65 mm Hg

Premature: Systolic blood pressure greater than 80 mm Hg
Diastolic blood pressure greater than 45 mm Hg

Treatment is usually instituted when blood pressure is above 120/80 mm Hg.

A. Who Is at Risk?

Infants with (or those who have had)

1. Indwelling umbilical arterial catheters or a patent ductus arteriosus (see chapter 11–XXX)
2. Congenital adrenal hyperplasia (Table 17–5, 11 or 17 hydroxylase deficiency)
3. Congenital renal artery stenosis (thrombosis; see chapter 18–VII)
4. Renal vein thrombosis (see chapter 18–VIII)
5. Polycystic kidneys (see chapter 18–IX)
6. Coarctation of the aorta (see Table 11–3)
7. Neuroblastoma (see Table 17–4)
8. Primary hyperaldosteronism

B. Clinical Manifestations

Clinical manifestations of hypertension are nonspecific and may be due to concomitant problems.

The infant may be asymptomatic or may have the following:

1. Tachypnea, cyanosis, and signs of congestive heart failure (see chapter 11–XXIX)
2. Lethargy, coma, tremors, apnea, opisthotonos, seizures, and hemiparesis
3. Signs of peripheral vascular occlusion (e.g., decreased pulses, cool extremities, cyanosis of the digits, cutaneous mottling, etc.)
4. Clinical manifestations related to underlying disease process

C. Laboratory Findings

1. An elevated blood pressure: see hypertensive values previously mentioned
2. Hematuria from renal artery or vein thrombosis
3. Proteinuria
4. Serum creatinine usually greater than 0.7 mg/dl, BUN greater than 15 mg/dl
5. Electrolyte imbalance: hyponatremia, hypernatremia, hyperkalemia, and metabolic acidosis
6. Abnormal coagulation profile (see chapter 14 for normal values)
7. Elevated peripheral plasma renin activity
8. Increased vanilmandelic acid (VMA; normal $\leq$200 μg/kg/day) and catecholamines in a 24-hour urine sample of those infants with neuroblastoma

D. Radiologic/Sonographic Features

1. Aortography through an indwelling umbilical artery catheter or percutaneous femoral artery puncture may reveal renal artery stenosis or partial or complete thrombotic occlusion of the main renal artery or its branches.

2. Renal scan reveals the function of each kidney, but may not reveal renal arterial occlusion clearly. Percutaneous femoral angiography should be performed for the diagnosis if umbilical route is not available.

E. Supportive Management

1. See chapter 18–IIIB for "general supportive management for the infant with edema and/or oliguria" and chapter 18–IVF for "general supportive management for the infant with acute renal failure."
2. Restrict fluids.

F. Specific therapy

1. Specific therapy is directed toward correction of the cause e.g., correction of renal artery thrombosis/embolism.
2. Medical therapy
   a. For acute, life-threatening extreme elevations of blood pressure
      1) Diazoxide, 5 mg/kg/dose IV rapidly, may be given.
      2) A sodium nitroprusside drip at a dose of 1 to 5 μg/kg/minute may be started.
   b. For mild hypertension
      1) Chlorothiazide, 20 to 40 mg/kg/24 hours in four divided doses every 6 hours IV or orally
      2) Furosemide, 1 to 4 mg/kg/day IV or orally in two to four doses
      3) Hydralazine, 0.2 to 0.5 mg/kg/dose IM every 4 to 6 hours, may be used to maintain blood pressure in the physiologic range.
      4) Other oral therapies
         Hydralazine, 5 mg/kg/24 hours in divided doses every 6 hours
         Propranolol, 0.5 to 2.0 mg/kg/24 hours in divided doses given every 6 hours
3. Surgical therapy
   Unilateral nephrectomy may be used for hypertension that is not controlled with medical therapy.

G. Prognosis

Prognosis is related to the underlying disease entity.

REFERENCES

Adelman R.D.: Neonatal hypertension, *Pediatr. Clin. N. Am.* 25:99, 1978.

Rahman N., Boineau F.G., Lewy J.E.: Renal failure in the perinatal period. *Clin. Perinatol.* 8:241, 1981.

VII. RENAL ARTERY THROMBOSIS/EMBOLI

Renal artery thrombosis has been reported in infants with patent ductus arteriosus, sepsis, cardiac arrhythmias, hypercoagulable processes, and umbilical artery catheters.

A. Who Is at Risk?

Those infants with the entities previously mentioned are at risk.

B. Clinical Manifestations

Enlarged kidneys are rare. Cardiorespiratory and neurologic symptoms are seen and are related to elevated blood pressure.

C. Laboratory Findings (see chapter 18–I for normal data)

1. Elevated blood pressure
2. Hematuria, proteinuria
3. Elevated BUN, elevated creatinine
4. Electrolyte imbalance

D. Radiologic/Radionuclide Features

1. Diagnosis is made by arteriography.
2. Radionuclide or sonographic studies should be ordered to follow the infant.

E. Supportive Therapy

1. See chapter 18–IIIB for "general supportive management for the infant with edema and/or oliguria" and chapter 18–IVF for "general supportive management for the infant with acute renal failure."
2. Correct any underlying problem.
3. Treat hypertension vigorously (see chapter 18–VI).

F. Specific Therapy

1. Nephrectomy in those infants who fail to respond to antihypertensive therapy
2. Thrombectomy and anticoagulant therapy may be of value.

G. Prognosis

Mortality and morbidity may be significant.

REFERENCE

Durante D., Jones D. Spitzer R.: Neonatal renal arterial syndrome. *J. Pediatr.* 89:978, 1976.

VIII. RENAL VEIN THROMBOSIS

The occurrence of renal vein thrombosis has declined markedly in recent years perhaps due to better management of diabetes during pregnancy and better fluid management of infants.

A. Who Is at Risk?

1. Infants with asphyxia, hypoxia, clotting problems, low blood pressure, congenital heart disease, vomiting, diarrhea, polycythemia, or sepsis
2. Infants, particularly sick infants, of diabetic mothers or mothers on thiazide diuretics
3. Male infants

B. Clinical Manifestations

Infants may be dehydrated, hyperthermic, or relatively polycythemic. Renal blood flow may be low due to decreased blood pressure or hypovolemia. Abdominal distension and a palpable nontransilluminating flank mass with hematuria suggests the diagnosis of renal vein thrombosis.

C. Laboratory Findings

1. Azotemia, hyponatremia, hypernatremia, or metabolic acidosis may be present.
2. Micro or gross hematuria and/or proteinuria
3. Thrombocytopenia

D. Radiologic Features

1. A renal sonogram may show enlarged kidneys with increased echogenicity
2. A venacavogram may indicate vena cava thrombosis and/or calcification of the thrombi

E. General Supportive Management

See chapter 18–IIIB for "general supportive management for the infant with edema and/or oliguria." Treatment at the present time consists of supportive therapy and avoidance of operative therapy. Intravascular coagulation defects should be corrected. Monitor blood pressure and treat hypertension if present (see chapter 18–VI).

F. Specific Therapy

1. Rehydration and antibiotics if sepsis is suspected.
2. Anticoagulation (controversial)
3. Nephrectomy for uncontrollable renin hypertension or infection. Thrombectomy has been advocated more recently for caval obstruction and bilateral nonvisualization. Discuss with pediatric nephrologist and urologist since renal function often returns even with a clotted inferior vena cava and bilateral involvement.

G. Prognosis

Infants with renal vein thrombosis may develop hypertension and those with bilateral disease may develop reduced renal function.

REFERENCES

Rasoulpour M., McLean R.H.: Renal vein thrombosis in neonates. *Am. J. Dis. Child* 134:276, 1980.

Thompson I.M., Schneider R., Lababidi Z.: Thrombectomy for neonatal renal vein thrombosis. *J. Urol.* 113:396, 1975.

IX. CYSTIC KIDNEY DISEASE

Cystic kidney disease is detected primarily by palpation of unilateral or bilateral renal masses. Bilateral renal masses are usually associated with obstructive uropathy, bilateral multicystic kidneys, bilateral renal vein thrombosis, and bilateral renal tumors (mesoblastic nephroma). Renal cystic dysplasia is delineated into infantile polycystic disease (IPCD), adult polycystic disease (APCD), and multicystic disease. IPCD is inherited in an autosomal recessive fashion, may be sporadic, and may affect multiple members of the same family. APCD is inherited in a dominant fashion. Multicystic kidney disease has been shown to affect multiple members of the same family and is one of the most common newborn abdominal masses.

A. Who Is at Risk?

1. IPCD
   a. Infants with dystocia secondary to large abdominal masses and/or oligohydramnios are at risk.
   b. Infants with a family history of IPCD are at risk.

2. APCD
   Infants with a family history of APCD are at risk.
3. Multicystic kidney disease
   Male infants (twice the risk of females) with a family history of multicystic disease and/or Potter's syndrome.

B. Clinical Manifestations

1. IPCD
   Infants usually present with high bilateral, asymmetric, renal masses with no clinical evidence of hepatic disease, although they may have hepatic cysts and fibrosis. Potter's facies and the fetal compression syndrome may be seen. Severe renal involvement usually results in death prior to the manifestations of the liver disease. Many infants are stillborn. Respiratory distress and congestive heart failure are commonly associated.
2. APCD
   The condition is usually asymptomatic in infancy. A flank mass may be palpated. Signs of renal failure are rare. Respiratory distress has been reported.
3. Multicystic kidney disease
   Infants usually present with unilateral (80%–85%) or bilateral lobulated and cystic abdominal mass that transilluminates. In infancy unilateral type usually asymptomatic. Oligohydramnios, Potter's facies, and skeletal anomalies may be seen. Many are stillborn or die soon after birth due to hypoplastic lungs.

C. Laboratory Findings

1. IPCD
   a. Renal biopsy reveals the principal site of dilatation to be the collecting tubules with relatively little fibrosis. Periductal fibrosis and polycystic changes are also present in the liver in one third of the cases, but newborns have normal liver function tests.
   b. The ECG shows left ventricular hypertrophy and left ventricular strain pattern.
   c. BUN and creatinine are increased and hematuria may be present.
   d. Metabolic acidosis, hyperkalemia, hypocalcemia, hyperphosphatemia, and hypertension occur with time.
2. APCD
   Laboratory findings are usually normal in infancy.
3. Multicystic kidney disease
   Anuria is seen with bilateral involvement. Histologic examination reveals primitive epithelial ducts surrounded by fibromuscular collars, islands of cartilage, clusters of immature glomeruli, and regions of undifferentiated mesenchyme.

D. Radiologic/Sonographic Features

1. IPCD
   An intravenous pyelogram demonstrates poorly visualized, massively enlarged kidneys with normal contour, a sun-ray appearance, and retention of contrast medium in small cysts. Those infants with better renal function show medullary ductual ectasia. Ultrasound usually does not visualize microcysts (1–2 mm of dilated collecting ducts) but may reveal increased echogenicity in the medulla.
2. APCD
   a. Plain films of abdomen may reveal renal enlargement.
   b. The intravenous pyelogram may reveal enlarged kidneys, splaying, distortion of the calyxeal system, and persistent puddling in the compressed parenchyma. The multi cysts are best seen in delayed films of the intravenous pyelogram.
   c. Ultrasound will confirm the diagnosis.
   d. Cysts may be seen in other organs (liver, pancreas, ovary, and lung).
3. Multicystic kidney disease
   a. A "grape cluster" pattern by ultrasound is diagnostic and can be seen in utero.
   b. Excretory urogram reveals nonvisualization.
   c. Atretic proximal ureter by retrograde pyelogram and hypoplastic or absent renal artery by aortogram may be seen if these procedures are performed.
   d. Ring-like and eggshell calcifications by abdominal x-ray may be seen in older patients.

E. Supportive Management

1. IPCD, APCD, and multicystic kidney disease
   See chapters 18–IIIB for "general supportive management of the infant with edema and/or oliguria," 11–IIIB for "general supportive management for the infant with respiratory distress," 11–XX for related pulmonary hypoplasia, 18–VI for hypertension, and 18–IV for acute renal failure.
2. APCD
   Blood pressure, urine culture, and urinary findings (hematuria) should be followed during infancy. Obtain blood pressure, urinalysis, renal function studies, and sonogram of kidneys and liver of all potentially affected family members.

F. Specific Therapy

1. IPCD
   a. No specific therapy is known.
   b. Chronic renal dialysis has been attempted as has renal transplantation.

2. APCD
   No specific therapy is required during infancy.
3. Multicystic kidney disease
   Surgical resection of cystic lesion prevents future complications (e.g., hypertension, rarely malignancy).

G. Prognosis

1. IPCD and APCD
   Progressive renal failure with elevated blood pressure and progressive respiratory distress due to pulmonary hypoplasia may occur.
2. Multicystic kidney disease
   Pain, GI disturbance due to compression, infection, hypertension, malignant degeneration, and anomalies of contralateral kidney (in unilateral multicystic disease) may occur.

REFERENCES

Bengtsson U., Hedman L., Svalander C.: Adult type of polycystic disease in a newborn child. *Acta Med. Scand.* 197:447, 1975.

Resnick J., Vernier R.L.: Cystic disease of the kidney in the newborn infant. *Clin. Perinatol.* 8:375, 1981.

Stevenson R.J.: Abdominal masses. *Surg. Clin. North Am.* 65:1481, 1985.

X. CONGENITAL NEPHROTIC SYNDROME

Congenital nephrotic syndrome is a rare and, until recently, lethal disorder characterized by heavy proteinuria, edema, and hypoalbuminemia occurring in the first 3 months of life. This congenital autosomal recessive syndrome is seen mostly in infants of Finnish descent. The clinical course is less favorable than the course of idiopathic nephrotic syndrome. In Finland, the incidence is 1.2 in 10,000 live births.

A. Who Is at Risk?

1. Infants of Finnish descent (approximately 22% of infants with nephrotic syndrome)
2. Infants with microcystic disease or renal vein thrombosis
3. Infants with congenital syphilis (proliferative glomerulonephritis and epimembranous glomerulopathy), cytomegalovirus infection, toxoplasmosis, etc.
4. Infants with nail patella syndrome (onset in the first week) (see Table 9–4)
5. Infants with renal vein thrombosis (onset in the first week)

6. Infants with neuroblastoma
7. Infants with mercury toxicity

B. Clinical Manifestations

1. Premature and/or small-for-gestational-age (nearly all)
2. Breech presentation
3. Perinatal asphyxia
4. Edema within the first week in 50% and in the first 3 months of life in almost all
5. Severe growth retardation
6. Large fontanelle and widely separated cranial sutures
7. Distended abdomen
8. Symptoms of pyloric stenosis or gastroesophageal reflux are present in 7%–12% of infants with congenital nephrotic syndrome.

C. Laboratory Findings

1. Elevated levels of α-fetoprotein in utero
2. Marked proteinuria, microscopic hematuria
3. Hypoproteinemia (hypoalbuminemia)
4. Hyperlipidemia
5. Serum levels of complement and creatinine are normal in the first year of life
6. Low levels of immunoglobulin: IgG
7. High levels of α-globulin, mostly α_1-macroglobulin
8. Faulty intrauterine bone calcification
9. Laboratory findings of hydrops fetalis (see chapter 18–VII)
10. Polycythemia, hypercoagulability
11. Decreased glomerular filtration rate
12. Cystic tubular dilatation by biopsy
13. Tubular dysfunction by biopsy
14. Fusion of epithelial cell foot processes by biopsy

D. Supportive Management

1. Maintain adequate fluid and electrolyte balance by minimizing solute and fluid retention and optimizing solute and fluid excretion.
2. Use diuretics as required.
3. Follow the serum potassium carefully.
4. Restrict fluids.
5. Increase the plasma volume if hypotension is present.
6. See chapter 18–IIIB for "general supportive management of the infant with edema and/or oliguria" and chapter 18–IVF for "general supportive management of the infant with acute renal failure."

E. Specific Therapy

Most therapy is not effective; corticosteroids, immunosuppressive drugs, dialysis, and transplants have been attempted. Transplantation has been the most effective treatment. The infant must weigh more than 5 kg to qualify for transplant. The positive feedback of the transplant indicates that the problem is completely within the kidneys.

F. Prognosis and Complications

Significant bacterial infection, hypothyroidism, anemia, developmental delay, and neurologic abnormalities are common. Death in early infancy is frequent without therapy.

REFERENCES

Huttunen N.P.: Congenital nephrotic syndrome of Finnish type. Study of 75 patients. *Arch. Dis. Child.* 51:344, 1976.

Kaplan B.S., Bureau M.A., Drummond K.N.: The nephrotic syndrome in the first year of life: Is a pathologic classification possible? *J. Pediatr.* 85:615, 1974.

Mahan J.D., Mauer S.M., Sibley R.K., et al.: Congenital nephrotic syndrome: Evaluation of medical management and results of renal transplantation. *J. Pediatr.* 105:549, 1984.

Milunsky A., Alpert E., Frigoletto F.D., et al.: Prenatal diagnosis of the congenital nephrotic syndrome. *Pediatrics* 59:770, 1977.

XI. OBSTRUCTIVE UROPATHY AND HYDRONEPHROSIS

Obstructive uropathy may occur at any point in the renal system and frequently presents as part of a complex malformation syndrome. Hydronephrotic kidneys are the most or second most common palpable abdominal mass in the newborn. Unilateral hydronephrosis may be secondary to ureteropelvic obstruction (most common) from high insertion of the ureter into pelvis or ureter compression by aberrant vessels, ureterocele, paraureteral diverticulum, or ectopic distal ureter insertions. Bilateral hydronephrosis may be secondary to posterior urethral valves, meatal or urethral stenosis, reflux from neurogenic bladder (myoneural dysfunction or meningomyelocele), or prune belly syndrome. Salvage of functional renal tissue requires immediate recognition and therapy in the newborn period.

A. Who Is at Risk?

1. Infants whose mothers have had infections (e.g., rubella) during pregnancy
2. Infants of diabetic mothers
3. Infants whose mothers bled during the first trimester

4. Infants of mothers who are more than 35 years of age
5. Infants whose mothers had dystocia during labor (prolonged labor due to fetal hydronephrosis or urinary ascites)
6. Infants whose mothers had oligohydramnios due to fetal oliguria or polyhydramnios due to bilateral partial ureteral obstruction or ovarian cyst
7. Infants born by breech presentation and/or traumatic delivery
8. Infants who are small for gestational age
9. Infants with the following anomalies often have associated obstructive uropathy:
   a. Potter's syndrome
   b. VATER syndrome
   c. Pneumothorax and/or pneumomediastinum (spontaneous)
   d. Cyanotic congenital heart disease
   e. Prune belly syndrome
   f. Exstrophy of bladder or cloaca
   g. Epispadias or hypospadias
   h. Kyphosis and scoliosis with or without spina bifida or meningomyelocele
   i. Imperforate anus
   j. Single umbilical artery (controversial)
   k. Ear abnormalities
   l. Nephrogenic diabetes insipidus

B. Clinical Manifestations

1. Abdominal distension due to cystic or hydronephrotic mass and/or ascites
2. Weak, intermittent, dribbling urinary stream. (A good urinary stream does not rule out obstructive uropathy.)
3. Failure to void by 48 hours of life.
4. Gross hematuria from traumatized hydronephrotic kidney or ruptured bladder during birth (renal vein thrombosis and polycystic kidney may be associated with hematuria)
5. Failure to thrive
6. Clinical manifestations of associated anomalies are often present. See Table 9–4, chapter 11–XIV, and other appropriate sections.

C. Laboratory Findings

Significant uropathy may be present without abnormal urine findings. In the first 1 to 2 days of life, BUN and creatinine may be normal even in the absence of kidneys if the mother has normal renal function.

1. Azotemia and/or increased creatinine (see appendix A–23, A–24, A–26)
2. Electrolyte and acid-base imbalance (see appendix A–23, A–24, A–8, A–9)
3. Hematuria or bacteremia may be present (see chapter 18–I for normal data)

D. Radiologic/Sonographic Features

1. Ultrasonogram in utero or after birth may reveal hydronephrosis, polycystic (multicystic) kidney(s), hydroureter, and/or distended bladder. Ultrasonogram is of great help in infants with increased creatinine to establish diagnosis.
2. Intravenous pyelogram and/or radioisotope studies reveal delayed or nonvisualization, but tests need to be delayed until approximately 1 month of age because of poor concentrating renal function in the newborn period.
3. Percutaneous needle puncture with aspiration of fluid for culture followed by injection of contrast material may be helpful in diagnosis as well as for a decompression procedure.
4. Voiding cystourethrography and/or retrograde urethrography can demonstrate reflux to the upper urinary tract, lower tract obstruction, and the status of the bladder. Contrast material should be diluted to a less than 10% solution before instillation into the bladder.

E. Supportive Management

See chapters 18–IIIB for "general supportive management for infants with edema and/or oliguria," 18–IVF for "general supportive management for the infant with acute renal failure," 11–IV for "oxygen therapy," and 11–VI for "assisted ventilation."

F. Specific Therapy

Depending upon the infant's age and condition, disease process, the condition of contralateral kidney, and the salvageable parenchyma of the affected kidney, nephrostomy, pyeloplasty, reimplantation, valve resection, ureterostomy, vesicostomy, or nephrectomy may be done.

1. Consult specialists for associated problems, e.g., pediatric pulmonologist, cardiologist, nephrologist, cardiovascular surgeon, neurosurgeon, pediatric surgeon, and/or urologist.
2. The Crede maneuver, periodic suprapubic compression, or catheterization may be used to treat the hypotonic bladder.

G. Prognosis

There is no accurate way to predict the extent of recovery or potential for growth of an obstructed kidney. Despite early neonatal corrective surgery, renal failure may still be present throughout childhood possibly due to renal hypoplasia, dysplasia, progressive nephron loss, and/or pyelonephritic scarring. Common complications are recurrent fever, failure to thrive, urinary tract infections, etc.

REFERENCES

Evans B.B.: Obstructive uropathy in the neonate. *Clin. Perinatol.* 8:273, 1981.

Warshaw B.L., Hymes L.C., Woodard J.R.: Long term outcome of patients with obstructive uropathy. *Pediatr. Clin. North Am.* 29:815, 1982.

XII. HYDROPS FETALIS

Hydrops fetalis is defined as nonspecific generalized edema with or without ascites or pleural effusion in a fetus or a newborn at birth. Hydrops fetalis may be due to immune or nonimmune causes.

A. Who Is at Risk?

1. Infants with hematologic disorders associated with anemia
   a. Hemolytic disease due to isoimmunization (Rh, ABO, or other minor group incompatibilities)
   b. Homozygous α-thalassemia
   c. Glucose-6-phosphate dehydrogenase deficiency
   d. Acute intrauterine hemorrhage in the fetus
2. Infants with cardiovascular disorders associated with cardiac failure
   a. Structural defect (obstruction or increased work due to shunting)
      1) Premature closure of ductus arteriosus or foramen ovale
      2) Anomalies of tricuspid or pulmonic valve
      3) Other congenital heart disease with outflow obstruction or shunts
   b. Arrhythmia
      1) Heart block (familial, maternal lupus erythematosus, or others).
      2) Paroxysmal atrial tachycardia
      3) Supraventricular tachycardia
      4) Congenital atrial flutter
      5) Prolonged maternal ritodrine
   c. Myocardial dysfunction
      1) Subendocardial fibroelastosis
      2) Myocardial infarction
      3) Myocarditis
   d. Obstructive venous return
   e. Cardiac tumors including vascular tumors
3. Infants with pulmonary disorders with obstruction of venous return and/or major airway obstruction
   a. Congenital cystic adenomatoid malformation
   b. Pulmonary sequestration
   c. Pulmonary hypoplasia
   d. Diaphragmatic hernia
   e. Pulmonary lymphangiectasis

4. Infants with renal disorders
   a. Internal or external, ureteral or urethral obstruction
   b. Congenital nephrosis
5. Infants with GI and hepatic disorders
   a. GI obstruction (tracheoesophageal fistula, duodenal or jejunal atresia)
   b. Anemia, hypovolemia and/or hypoproteinemia, intrauterine volvulus, hemorrhagic infarction, or meconium peritonitis
   c. Congenital hepatitis or cirrhosis
6. Infants with congenital tumors
   a. Vascular tumors (hemangioma), Wilms' tumor, neuroblastoma
   b. Arteriovenous shunt
   c. Tumors obstructing venous return
7. Infants with chromosomal disorders
   a. Turner's syndrome
   b. Trisomy 21 or 18
8. Infants with hereditary disorders
   a. Tuberous sclerosis
   b. Storage diseases
   c. Cystic fibrosis, often with meconium peritonitis
   d. Achondroplastic and thanatophoric dwarfism
   e. Osteogenesis imperfecta
9. Infants with congenital infections
   a. Congenital syphilis
   b. Toxoplasmosis
   c. Cytomegalovirus
   d. Rubella
   e. Leptospirosis
   f. Chagas' disease
10. Infants with disorders of placenta and cord
    a. Chorioangioma of placenta
    b. Angiomyxoma
    c. Umbilical vein thrombosis
    d. Aneurysm of umbilical artery
11. Infants with gestational disorders
    a. Twin-to-twin transfusion syndrome (recipient)
    b. Fetomaternal transfusion
    c. Placental dysfunction or dysmaturity
    d. Maternal diabetes or hypertensive disease of pregnancy

B. Clinical Manifestations

1. Generalized interstitial edema
2. Pericardial or pleural effusion
3. Ascites
4. Hepatosplenomegaly

5. Tachycardia
6. Tachypnea and/or respiratory failure
7. Decreased urinary output
8. Additional physical findings depending upon the cause

C. Laboratory Findings

1. Anemia or polycythemia
2. Hypoproteinemia
3. Metabolic and/or respiratory acidosis
4. Increased edema or hypotension may occur due to decreased hydrostatic pressure (hypoproteinemia).
5. Additional laboratory findings depend upon the cause

D. Radiologic Features

1. Abnormal intrauterine ultrasound examination
   a. Placentomegaly
   b. Chorioangioma
   c. A halo if scalp edema is present
   d. The presence of pericardial, plural, or abdominal effusion

E. Supportive Management

See chapter 18–IIIB for "general supportive management for the infants with edema and/or oliguria."

F. Specific Therapy

A specific therapy depends upon the causative condition.

REFERENCE

Turkel S.B.: Conditions associated with nonimmune hydrops fetalis. *Clin. Perinatal.* 9:613, 1982.

XIII. ZINC DEFICIENCY

Zinc is a vital trace element that is part of numerous metalloenzymes including carbonic anhydrase, lactic dehydrogenase, alkaline phosphatase, and carboxypeptidase. Zinc is also a cofactor of insulin and plays a role in protein synthesis.

A. Who Is at Risk?

1. Premature infants
2. Infants with growth failure or retarded bone age
3. Infants with hepatosplenomegaly
4. Infants receiving prolonged parenteral nutrition without adequate zinc

B. Clinical Manifestations

1. Failure to thrive
2. Decreased wound healing
3. Acrodermatitis enteropathica (eczematous eruptions of the mouth, genitalia, and extremities; alopecia; irritability; paronychial lesions); Secondary *Candida* infections are common.
4. Generalized edema in prematures 5 to 9 weeks of age

C. Laboratory Findings

1. Low plasma zinc levels less than 65 to 75 μg/dl, low hair zinc less than 75 μg/dl, and low hemoglobin zinc less than 25 μg/dl
2. Questionable defect in zinc metabolism
3. Positive *Candida* lesions (frequent associated findings)
4. Reduced hematocrit; microcytic hypochromic anemia
5. Hypoproteinemia in prematures 5 to 9 weeks of age
6. Low serum alkaline phosphatase less than 68 units/L (normal range, 68 to 217 units/L)

D. Specific and Supportive Therapy

1. Oral zinc sulfate or zinc chloride
   Elemental zinc, 1 mg/kg/day for 1 to 2 months. Within few days of therapy, edema disappears and serum protein and alkaline phosphatase increase in premature infants.
2. Topical nystatin for *Candida* lesions

E. Prognosis

The response to zinc is excellent.

REFERENCES

Gordon E.F., Gordon R.C., Passal D.B.: Zinc metabolism: Basic, clinical and behavioral aspects. *J. Pediatr.* 99:341, 1981.

Henkin R.I., Schulman J.D., Schulman C.B., et al.: Changes in total, nondiffusible plasma zinc and copper during infancy. *J. Pediatr.* 82:831, 1973.

Kumar S.P., Anday E.K.: Edema, hypoproteinemia and zinc deficiency in low-birth-weight infants. *Pediatrics* 73:327, 1984.

XIV. COPPER DEFICIENCY

Cytochrome oxidase, tyrosinase, and uricase all contain copper. Copper is also important for iron utilization in hemoglobin synthesis, nerve myelination, and collagen and elastin formation. Copper deficiency has been associated with refractory iron-deficient anemia, peripheral edema, and osteoporosis. Newborns usually have good stores at birth but milk is a poor source of copper. The serum copper level increases with gestation (see appendix A–20).

A. Who Is at Risk?

1. Infants with malabsorption, e.g., cystic fibrosis, protein-losing enteropathy, kwashiorkor, or short-bowel syndrome
2. Infants who subsist on a milk diet to the exclusion of all other foods
3. Infants who have been maintained on long-term total parenteral nutrition without copper supplementation.

B. Clinical Manifestations

The disease commonly presents with edema at 7 to 9 months of age when the infants are recovering from malnutrition and are growing rapidly.

C. Laboratory Findings

1. Low serum copper (see appendix A–20 for normal values)
2. Anemia: microcytic and/or hypochromic
3. Decreased serum iron concentration (see appendix A–17 for normal values)
4. Decreased percent saturation of iron-binding protein
5. Leukopenia
6. Neutropenia
7. Hypoproteinemia
8. Variable bone marrow changes: hypochromia, erythroid hypoplasia, and immature myloid elements

D. Radiologic Features

1. Retarded bone age
2. Osteoporotic changes in the bone
3. Metaphyseal irregularities and spurring and a radiolucent zone in the metaphyses

E. Supportive Management

Support nutritional intake and improve diet.

F. Specific Therapy

Treat with copper, 400–60 μg/kg/24 hours orally.

G. Prognosis

A prompt response to copper therapy is characteristic.

REFERENCES

Cordano A., Baertl J.M., Graham G.G.: Copper deficiency in infancy. *Pediatrics* 34:324, 1964.

Henkin R.I., Schulman J.D., Schulman C.B., et al.: Changes in total, nondiffusible and diffusible plasma, zinc and copper during infancy. *J. Pediatr.* 82:831, 1973.

Karpel J.T., Peden V.H.: Copper deficiency in long-term parenteral nutrition. *J. Pediatr.* 80:32, 1972.

XV. SYNDROME OF INAPPROPRIATE ANTIDIURETIC HORMONE (SIADH)

The primary physiologic role of antidiuretic hormone (ADH) (arginine vasopressin) is its cyclic adenosine monophosphate-mediated increase in permeability of the collecting duct to water. ADH is released by the fetus during labor and by the fetus and neonate during stress, e.g., hypoxic-ischemic encephalopathy or pneumothorax. Syndrome of inappropriate antidiuretic hormone should be suspected in those infants with edema, hyponatremia, and hypoosmolality associated with hyperosmolality of the urine with continued urinary sodium excretion.

A. Who Is at Risk?

1. Infants with meningitis and/or hypoxic-ischemic encephalopathy with or without intracranial hemorrhage. There is an increase in intracranial pressure and/or stimulation of the hypothalmic-neurohypophyseal axis with continued ADH release. Increased intracranial pressure is also reported to be the reason why ADH is increased in the fetus during labor.
2. Infants with right-sided heart failure, systemic hemorrhage, or increased resistance to blood flow through the lungs (pneumothorax, bronchopulmonary dysplasia, obstructive pulmonary disease, or emphysema). Hemorrhage (decreased blood pressure) or elevated resistance to blood flow through the lungs causes reduced left atrial filling, which in turn causes baroreceptic stimulation resulting in release of ADH.
3. Infants recovering from respiratory distress syndrome
4. Infants who have had ligation of a patent ductus arteriosus

B. Clinical Manifestations

Clinical manifestations include edema, weight gain, and decreased urinary output associated with hyponatremia and hypoosmolality occurring in infants with hypoxic encephalopathy (see chapter 15–IV) or CNS hemorrhage (see chapter 15–VI, 15–VII, and 15–VIII), congestive heart failure (see chapter 11–XXIX), shock (see chapter 14–III), pneumothorax (see chapter 11–XIV), or other disorders. Symptomatology is primarily related to hyponatremia, i.e., lethargy or seizures (see chapter 15–XIV), and hypoosmolality.

C. Laboratory Findings

1. A radioimmunoassay for ADH is diagnostic.
2. Plasma hypoosmolality less than 280 mOsm/L
3. Serum hyponatremia less than 130 mEq/L
4. Urine osmolality equals or exceeds that of the plasma in the presence of hyponatremia and plasma hypoosmolality.
5. Reduced urinary output less than 1 ml/kg/hour

D. Supportive Management

1. See chapter 18–IIIB for "general supportive management for the infant with edema and/or oliguria."
2. Restrict water intake to insensible water loss (see Table 6–3) plus urinary output until plasma osmolality has increased to the normal range (285 to 295 mOsm/L).
3. In infants with severe hyponatremia and CNS symptoms, a rapid form of therapy is preferred. Administer 1.5% NaCl 20 ml/100 cal or 300 ml/sq m and furosemide 1 mg/kg/dose, one to four times daily to increase sodium concentrations (see chapter 15–XIV) and increase water diuresis.

REFERENCES

Arant B.S.: Non-renal factors influencing renal function during the perinatal period. *Clin. Perinatol.* 8:225–240, 1981.

Siegel S.R.: Hormonal and renal interaction in body fluid regulation in the newborn infant. *Clin. Perinatol.* 9:535, 1982.

XVI. HYPERKALEMIA

Release of potassium by lysed cells, decreased renal excretion of potassium, transcellular shifts of potassium, and high potassium intake can result in hyperkalemia. A serum potassium level of greater than 6.0 to 6.5 mEq/L is usually considered hyperkalemia.

A. Prevention

1. Carefully calculate potassium to be administered; requirements are 2 to 3 mEq/kg/day. Investigate all infants with high potassium levels.
2. Do not rapidly warm or transfuse red blood cells (whole blood or packed red blood cells) as hemolysis and hyperkalemia will result.
3. Monitor infants with metaboilc acidosis.
4. Prevent tissue necrosis.

B. Who Is at Risk?

1. Infants undergoing a fast hemolysis from any cause, e.g., Rh incompatibility or *Pseudomonas* sepsis
2. Infants with decreased renal excretion of potassium, e.g., acute tubular necrosis, potassium-sparing diuretics, adrenogenital syndrome, or obstructive uropathy
3. Infants who suffer transcellular movement of potassium, e.g., metabolic acidosis
4. Infants who receive high potassium intake, i.e., those who receive aged bank blood or packed cells or blood that has been overheated with resultant hemolysis
5. Infants with severe tissue necrosis

C. Clinical Manifestations

Clinical manifestations include arrhythmias, ventricular fibrillation, and asystole.

D. Laboratory Findings

1. A serum potassium greater then 6.0 to 6.5 mEq/L.
2. ECG findings of peaked T waves, a prolonged PR interval, a widened QRS complex, a sine wave, fusion of T and QRS, and ventricular fibrillation or tachycardia (see chapter 19–VII).

E. General Supportive Management

See chapter 18–IIIB for "general supportive management for the infant with edema and/or oliguria."

F. Specific Therapy

1. Restrict potassium intake; discontinue potassium administration.
2. Monitor cardiac rate and pattern carefully.

3. Administer calcium gluconate, 100 to 200 mg/kg/dose IV, or $NaHCO_3$, 2–4 mEq/kg IV.
4. As a temporary measure, administer glucose with crystalline zinc insulin. Add 6 units of regular insulin to 50 ml of 50% glucose and give 1 to 2 ml (glucose 500–1,000 mg and insulin 0.12–0.24 units); titrate with the ECG, run the ECG, and observe changes as ECG rate and pattern revert to normal.
5. Administer a sodium polystyrene sulfonate enema (Kayexalate) at a dose of 0.5 to 2 gm/kg in mineral oil. Repeat every 4 to 6 hours.
6. Peritoneal or hemodialysis may be necessary.

G. Prognosis

The outcome is good with early correction of a transient hyperkalemic state. For those infants with underlying disease, outcome depends upon resolution of the underlying disease process.

REFERENCE

Segar W.E., Chesney R.W.: Disorders of electrolyte metabolism. *Pediatr. Ann.* 10:288, 1981.

Chapter 19

Procedures Commonly Used in the Nursery

I. VESSEL PUNCTURE/CATHETERIZATION/CUTDOWN

A. Heel Puncture for Capillary Blood Specimen

This is a simple, minimally traumatic method for obtaining blood specimens for blood gas, biochemical, and cytologic analyses.

1. Wash hands thoroughly.
2. Warm the infant's foot to body temperature by immersing it in warm water or covering with warmed gauze.
   a. A temperature above 44°C may cause burns.
   b. Warming time is approximately 5 minutes.
3. Place the infant in the prone position.
4. Rub the infant's heel with 70% alcohol or Betadine (povidone-iodine) on a cotton pledget. Then dry the area.
5. Puncture the lateral or medial plantar surface of the heel perpendicularly with a Bard-Parker no. 11 blade, autolancet (less painful) or lancet sufficiently deep to obtain a free flow of blood but not deeper than 2.5 mm.
6. Wipe away the first drop of blood with a dry sponge because alcohol or Betadine causes hemolysis.
7. Do not squeeze the infant's heel because squeezing may produce hemodilution from interstitial fluid leakage.
8. Draw blood into tube by capillarity as drops form. Do not allow large drops of blood to accumulate. This tends to increase hemolysis.
9. Collect the blood in the proper capillary tubes.
10. Seal tubes with clay to a depth of 4 mm or cap securely.
11. Press a 2 by 2 gauze pad to the site and hold the foot above heart level until the bleeding stops.
12. Complications include cellulitis, osteomyelitis, abscess, calcified nodules, etc.

B. Venous Puncture for Venous Blood Specimen

Select a clearly visible and easily accessible site to obtain a venous blood sample.

1. Antecubital vein
   This site is accessible in infants, including prematures, and is well suited for blood drawing.
   a. Wash hands thoroughly.
   b. Hold the infant's arm extended.
   c. Apply a tourniquet (or rubber band) above the elbow tightly enough to compress the vein but loosely enough to allow arterial flow. Pressure is between systolic and diastolic pressure.
   d. Rub the antecubital area with 70% alcohol or Betadine with a swab or cotton pledget. Then dry the area.
   e. Wait a few minutes for the vessel to distend. Enter the vein using a 22, 23, or 25 gauge scalp-vein needle at a 25- to 45-degree angle with the bevel up and withdraw the blood slowly. Do not apply excessive negative pressure or the vessel will collapse. Direction of entry may be with or against blood flow.
   f. After obtaining the blood, release the tourniquet, withdraw the needle, and apply pressure with a dry sterile gauze for several minutes. If pressure is applied for 5 continuous minutes (without looking), a hematoma will not form and the vein may be reused.
2. Scalp vein
   This site is accessible in infants, including prematures, but is used mainly for IV infusion. Blood can be obtained if the specimen is drawn slowly with gentle negative pressure.
   a. Wash hands thoroughly.
   b. Shave the area of the infant's head surrounding the proposed puncture site. Wash the cut hairs away.
   c. Apply a rubber band around the infant's head to act as a tourniquet. Wait a few minutes for the vessel to distend. (Feel for a pulse to avoid tapping an artery.)
   d. Clean the area with 70% alcohol or Betadine on a cotton pledget.
   e. Using a 23- or 25-gauge scalp-vein needle at a shallow angle (15 to 20 degrees), puncture the vessel and withdraw the blood slowly. Do not apply vigorous suction or the vessel will collapse.
   f. After obtaining the blood, remove the rubber band, withdraw the needle, and apply pressure with a dry sterile gauze for several minutes.
3. External jugular vein
   This site is accessible in infants, including prematures, and is well suited for blood drawing. However, it should not be used in infants with respiratory distress.
   a. Wash hands thoroughly.
   b. Wrap the infant so that he or she is immobilized. An assistant is needed to hold the infant securely.
   c. Position the infant on a table in the supine position. Turn the infant's head

to one side and let the infant's head descend slightly over the table side.

d. Clean the side of the neck with 70% alcohol or Betadine on a cotton pledget.
e. Stimulate the infant to cry in order to distend the external jugular vein. Visualize the external jugular vein over the anterior border of the sternocleidomastoid muscle.
f. Puncture the vein. When entering the vein, always enter with a closed system, e.g., with a syringe attached to a scalp-vein needle, to prevent pneumothorax if pleura is punctured. Take care not to puncture the apex of the lung, which is above the clavicle in small prematures. Draw the blood slowly to prevent collapse of the vein.
g. When the needle is withdrawn, apply pressure and hold the infant upright.

4. Internal jugular vein and femoral vein
The internal jugular vein should not be used in infants, especially prematures, because of the common complications (e.g., cellulitis, pneumothorax). The femoral vein should not be used because of the common complications (e.g., femoral vein thrombosis, septic arthritis, gangrene of the foot, etc.).

C. Umbilical Vein Catheterization

This site is good for emergency vascular access for fluids and medications. Do not use if infant has omphalitis, omphalocele, necrotizing enterocolitis, or peritonitis.

1. Wash hands thoroughly.
2. Determine the proper catheter length by measuring the shoulder-umbilical length of the infant (see Fig 3–3). Note the distance in relation to the marks on the catheter. The umbilical vein catheter should be positioned inferior to the right atrium in the inferior vena cava.
3. Place the infant in a supine position under radiant heat. Restrain arms and legs loosely.
4. Don sterile gloves and cleanse the area with 70% alcohol or Betadine solution. Let dry.
5. Fill the catheter with saline and attach to a 10-ml syringe.
6. Approximately 1 cm above umbilical stump, stabilize the cord with a clamp and cut the cord with a scalpel.
7. Find the umbilical vein orifice. Remove clots with fine iris forcep.
8. Grasp the umbilical vein with a mosquito clamp and slowly push the catheter through the orifice. Advance slowly with gentle pressure. If some resistance is met at the abdominal wall, apply traction to the cord and continue gentle pressure on catheter.
9. Continue passing the catheter until the appropriate length is reached. Blood should be easily drawn out and expelled. Sometimes the catheter cores a thrombosis out of the vein. The catheter should then be removed and a second catheter should be inserted. If the catheter cannot be easily advanced to the inferior vena cava, pull it back a few centimeters and try again. If, after a few attempts, this does not succeed, pull the catheter out.

10. Secure the catheter with 000 silk and tape (see Fig 3–4).
11. Obtain anterior and lateral x-ray films to confirm the catheter's location (see Fig 3–5).
12. Complications include infection, thromboembolism, arrhythmias, pleural or pericardial effusion, necrotizing enterocolitis, hepatic necrosis, portal hypertension, etc.

D. Central Venous Catheter Placement

Central venous catheters are placed to deliver parenteral nutrition solutions into the superior or inferior vena cava proximal to the right atrium and/or to measure central venous pressure.

1. Method of placement may be cutdown or by percutaneous puncture.
2. Sterile technique is mandatory. Catheter insertion by cutdown should be performed in the operating room by an experienced physician.
3. Wash hands thoroughly. Don mask, hat and sterile gown, and gloves.
4. Select site for placement of catheter, i.e., via the internal or external jugular, innominate, basilic, or subclavian vein.
5. Shave hair at site.
6. Identify the vein, estimate the distance from the insertion site to the right atrium, and prepare the skin with Betadine followed by 70% alcohol.
7. Anesthetize with lidocaine. Make a mini-skin incision over the insertion site.
8. The muscle is split and the vein is exposed and controlled between loops of fine catgut.
9. The distal catgut is tied and the ligature is used for traction.
10. The vessel is pulled upwards, a small phlebotomy is made, and a small diameter (0.64 mm inner or outer diameter) Silastic catheter is inserted to a predetermined distance so as to lie in the superior vena cava.
11. The proximal catgut suture is then tied. Do not occlude the catheter.
12. The distal end of the catheter is tunneled subcutaneously to a remote exit behind the ear in the scalp or anterior chest wall.
13. All incisions are sutured.
14. The position of the catheter is verified by x-ray film.
15. Betadine powder, bacitracin ointment, and a dressing may be applied to the skin at the catheter entrance and exit site.
16. Two previously prepared 1-cm squares of Silastic sheeting are glued to the catheter with Silastic cement, making a dressing around the catheter at the catheter exit.
17. These dressings are changed, using sterile technique, every other day.
18. Complications include superior vena cava syndrome, pleural effusion, infection, hemorrhage, thromboembolism, vessel perforation, arrhythmia, etc.

E. Percutaneous Central Venous Catheter Placement

This route is used in infants, including prematures, for administration of total parenteral nutrition, measurement of central venous pressure when umbilical vein catheterization is unavailable, and for long-term IV access when peripheral veins are exhausted. Do not perform this procedure if infant has bleeding diathesis or local skin infection or in the presence of inadequate facilities for long-term care of the catheter. The procedure described here is for subclavian vein.

1. Place the infant supine and restrain extremities with arms at sides pulled caudally.
2. Maintain head in midline position with tape across forehead.
3. The procedure should be performed by a physician experienced with the procedure.
4. Don cap and mask.
5. Scrub hands and wrists thoroughly. Don sterile gown and gloves.
6. Prepare the insertion site with Betadine.
7. Drape the area with a sterile aperture drape.
8. Palpate the groove formed at the point where the first rib and clavicle cross. The subclavian vein passes beneath the clavicle and above the first rib.
9. Anesthetize the skin in the deltopectoral groove, 2 cm from the clavicle.
10. Use an 18- or 19-gauge venipuncture needle and insert it into the subclavian vein to serve as a catheter introducer.
11. Pass a 20- or 30-cm length Silastic catheter (with a 0.64 mm inner or outer diameter) through the introducer and advance to the superior vena cava proximal to the right atrium.
12. Withdraw and remove the introducer and attach a 25-gauge blunt-end adapter to the catheter.
13. Ascertain the location of the catheter tip radiographically by injection of 0.3 ml of radiopaque dye.
14. Apply bacitracin ointment and stabilize the catheter by placing a clear sterile polyurethane adhesive film directly over the insertion site. Secure a coil of the catheter under the adhesive film to prevent accidental dislodgment.
15. Complications include thromboembolism, infection, hemorrhage, vessel perforation, pleural effusion, etc.

F. Internal Saphenous Vein Cutdown

When percutaneous venous sites are exhausted, a venous cutdown may be used for administration of fluid.

1. Wash hands thoroughly.
2. Strap the infant's foot, leg, and thigh to a padded splint. An assistant is needed to hold the infant securely.
3. Apply a tourniquet to the midthigh or leg to be tied at a later time.
4. Using surgical aseptic technique, prepare the site with Betadine.
5. Don gloves and open the cutdown tray.
6. Fill the no. 3 or no. 4 F Silastic catheter with normal saline.
7. Isolate the area with sterile towels. Infiltrate 0.5–1.0 ml of lidocaine. Have an assistant tie the tourniquet.

8. Make a small, horizontal incision 1 cm anterior and 1 cm superior to the medial malleolus and dissect tissue to expose the internal saphenous vein.
9. Ligate the distal end of the vein and use the ligature for traction on the vein in an upward and caudad direction.
10. Pass a 0000 catgut ligature beneath the proximal segment of the vein and make a small incision into the vein with a pair of sharp scissors or a fine triangular blade.
11. Insert a no. 3 or no. 4 F Silastic catheter for a distance of 1.5 to 2.0 cm into the vein. Flush the catheter with heparinized saline. The isolated vein often contracts markedly with manipulation, but patience and gentle pressure will usually allow distention of the vessel and insertion of the catheter. Obtain a x-ray film to confirm the position of the catheter once the estimated length is inserted. Check for easy back flow of blood into catheter. A 25 to 23 gauge blunt-end adapter to the catheter may be used.
12. Secure the proximal ligature firmly around the vein and the catheter with 000 silk or 000 catgut.
13. Suture the wound with 000 silk.
    Be careful not to pull out the catheter when the dressing is applied to the wound.
14. Complications include vessel severence, infection, infiltration of infusion, etc.

G. Arterial Puncture for Arterial Blood Specimen

Arterial blood specimens are preferable to venous specimens for blood gas studies and can be obtained from radial, temporal, dorsalis pedis, posterior tibial, or bracheal (last resort) artery. Complications include distal ischemia, infection, hematoma, hemorrhage, nerve damage (median nerve from brachial, posterior tibial nerve from posterior tibial artery puncture), etc.

1. Superficial temporal artery
   a. Wash hands thoroughly.
   b. Locate by palpation the superficial temporal artery as it crosses the temporal bone slightly superiorly and anteriorly to the ear. Select frontal or parietal branch.
   c. Shave the area of the infant's head surrounding the proposed puncture site. Wash the cut hairs away.
   d. Do not apply a tourniquet. Rub the area with 70% alcohol to help distend the vessel and sterilize the skin.
   e. Attach a 23- or 25-gauge scalp-vein needle firmly to a 1-ml syringe and rinse with heparin.
   f. Puncture the superficial temporal artery at a 15- to 25-degree angle against the blood flow and withdraw the blood into the heparin-treated syringe. Be careful not to contaminate the specimen with air bubbles.
   g. Remove the needle from the scalp and apply pressure over the puncture site for approximately five minutes.

   h. Detach the syringe from the scalp-vein needle, seal the syringe, agitate the specimen, and place the specimen on ice.
   i. Complications include hematoma, infection, etc.
2. Brachial artery
   a. Wash hands thoroughly.
   b. Locate by palpation the branchial artery along the medial margin of the biceps muscle at the bend of the elbow.
   c. Sterilize the skin over the branchial artery with Betadine.
   d. Attach a 25-gauge needle firmly to a 1-ml syringe and rinse the inside of the syringe with heparin.
   e. Do not apply a tourniquet. Blood will flow without negative pressure.
   f. Insert the needle into the brachial artery with the bevel up. Withdraw the blood slowly into the heparin-treated syringe. Be careful not to contaminate the specimen with air bubbles.
   g. Withdraw the needle and apply pressure with a dry sterile gauze for several minutes.
   h. Seal the syringe, agitate the specimen, and place the specimen on ice.
   i. Complications include median nerve palsy, hematoma, infection, etc.
3. Radial aftery puncture
   a. Wash hands thoroughly.
   b. Extend the wrist in the supine position.
   c. Palpate the radial artery pulsation just proximal to the wrist. The radial artery is lateral to the flexor carpi radialis tendon. Transillumination may be of aid.
   d. Perform a modified Allen's test for collateral circulation. Occlude both radial and ulnar arteries at wrist. Release the ulnar artery. Observe color return. Do not puncture artery if color return exceeds 15 seconds.
   e. Cleanse the site with Betadine; let dry.
   f. Insert needle at a 45- to 60-degree angle (for small infants 15 to 20 degrees, bevel up), piercing the anterior and posterior walls of the artery, i.e., go through the artery. Apply negative pressure with the syringe and slowly withdraw the needle. Reentry into arterial lumen is signaled by the appearance of blood in the syringe. Occasionally, the artery can be entered as the needle is being placed.
   g. After the specimen is collected, remove the needle, place dry sterile gauze over the site, and apply firm pressure for 5 minutes. Verify adequate peripheral blood flow.
   h. Complications include gangrene of the hand, infection, etc.

H. Umbilical Artery Catheterization

1. Wash hands thoroughly
2. Insert the umbilical artery catheter as described in chapter 3–IIIC3.
3. Attach a three-way stopcock to the umbilical artery catheter so that withdrawal of the blood can be accomplished without opening the system.

4. Set aside the first milliliter withdrawn because it does not reflect the infant's true status.
5. Withdraw the specimen into a 1-ml heparin-treated syringe. Then push back the first milliliter and flush with normal saline.
6. Close the system and place the specimen on ice.

II. TAPPING VARIOUS ORGANS/CAVITIES

A. Suprapubic Bladder Tap

This method is used to obtain uncontaminated urine for culture. It should not be used if there is a skin infection at the puncture site, abdominal distention of unknown cause, bleeding disorders, dehydration, or genitourinary anomaly.

1. Wash hands thoroughly.
2. Wait at least 1 hour after urine passage. Full bladder may be confirmed by palpation or transillumination.
3. Place the infant supine on a flat surface and immobilize in a frog-leg position.
4. Use surgical gloves and aseptic technique. Don gloves and open the equipment required.
5. The site for insertion of the needle is just above the symphysis pubis at the midline.
6. Sterilize the suprapubic skin with Betadine. An assistant is needed to hold the infant securely. (The cold Betadine will frequently cause the infant to void. In a male infant, with the other gloved hand, gently apply pressure on the infant's penis thereby closing the urethra.)
7. Insert a 22- or 23-gauge, 1.5-inch needle 1 to 2 cm above the symphysis pubis at a 90-degree angle and direct the needle toward the vertebral column to approximately 3–4 cm in term infants. The urine will usually flow into the syringe with minimal negative pressure. (If not, the bladder is empty; withdraw the needle and wait another hour before repeating the procedure.)
8. After removal of the needle, apply a dry, sterile dressing.
9. Complications include transient microscopic or gross hematuria, bladder wall hematoma, bowel perforation, bacteremia, abdominal wall abscess, etc.

B. Spinal Tap

This procedure is performed to diagnose or rule out meningeal infection, subarachnoid hemorrhage, and CSF biochemical abnormality or to monitor the efficacy of antibiotic therapy or to treat communicating hydrocephalus. It should not be used if there is a skin infection, tumor, meningocele, or hematoma at the entry site or if the infant has respiratory instability or bleeding disorder.

1. Wash hands thoroughly.
2. An assistant is needed to hold the infant in a sitting or lateral decubitus

position with the spine flexed. Head need not be fully flexed. A sitting position with the back rounded is preferable for infants.

3. Monitor the infant's vital signs throughout the procedure because neck flexion can cause bradycardia and/or asphyxia. Utilize transcutaneous Po_2/Pco_2 monitor if possible. Be careful not to lower the oxygen concentration and/or temperature of the infant during the procedure.
4. Using surgical aseptic technique, open the lumbar puncture tray and don gloves.
5. Sterilize the skin, washing in enlarging circles over the lumbar spinal area with Betadine or alcohol, and isolate the area with sterile towels.
6. At the level of the iliac crest, palpate the third lumbar intervertebral space (between lumbar vertebrae 3 and 4).
7. Using a 22- or 23-gauge short spinal needle, insert the needle slowly, 0.5 to 1.5 cm into the third intervertebral space toward the sternum. As the needle passes through ligamentum flavum and dura, a "pop" with a change in resistance will be felt that signifies entry. Remove the stylet to observe the fluid. Do not rub the stylet against your gloves to check for fluid on the stylet.
8. It is incorrect and dangerous to apply negative pressure to the spinal needle.
9. When fluid is obtained, measure the pressure by attaching a manometer and three-way stopcock if required.
10. Allow the fluid to drip by gravity.
    a. Flow may be slow.
    b. If no fluid is obtained, try one interspace higher.
11. Collect fluid for diagnostic purposes. Collect 0.5 to 1.0 ml in each of three to four tubes: sample 1, bacterial culture; sample 2, cell count; and samples 3 and 4 for chemical and additional studies.
12. If tap is traumatic, look for clearing of fluid.
13. After fluid is obtained, reinsert the stylet and remove the needle.
14. Apply a dressing or collodion to the puncture site.
15. Complications include hypoxia, asphyxia, cardiopulmonary arrest, aspiration, infection, acute spondylitis, spinal subdural or epidural hematoma, intraspinal epidermoid tumor, spinal cord puncture, etc.

C. Pericardial Tap

The percutaneous introduction of a needle into the pericardial space may be used to remove fluid or air.

1. Wash hands thoroughly.
2. Place the infant supine.
3. The site should be swabbed with Betadine and then with 70% alcohol.
4. Using aseptic technique, don gloves and drape the lower chest and abdomen appropriately.
5. Sites of needle insertion. Transilluminator with sterile tip may be of aid.
    a. Subxyphoid site: Insert the needle at the left or right xiphocostal angle or below the tip of the xiphoid. Continue slightly inward and upward towards the left shoulder or tip of left scapula. This is the preferred site.

b. Triangle of safety: Insert the needle at the fifth or sixth intercostal space at the sternal margin on either side. Direct the needle inward and medially to avoid the internal mammary vessels. If there is a large pericardial effusion, use the right fifth intercostal space.
c. Apical site: If the apex beat is palpable, insert the needle 2 cm lateral to the apical beat at the fifth intercostal space. When the apical beat is not located, the point chosen should be just left of the percussion flatness.

6. Advance the needle until fluid/air is encountered.
7. Be careful not to penetrate the epicardium.
8. If no fluid/air is encountered, retract the needle a little, raise the angle of the needle and carefully advance the needle a little farther.
9. Once fluid/air is reached, clamp a hemostat across the needle barrel. Attach a 10-ml syringe with a stopcock to the needle hub.
10. Slowly aspirate the fluid/air. When the syringe is full, adjust the stopcock so that the fluid/air can be removed.
11. Water seal drainage with continuous suction can treat and prevent cardiac tamponade. Complications include hematoma, hemorrhage, cardiac or hepatic puncture, etc.

D. Thoracentesis (Needle Aspiration)

Thoracentesis is to be performed as an emergency procedure when fluid/air has accumulated in the pleural space (pneumothorax, chylothorax, or hemothorax). Pneumothorax is the most common indication for this procedure in newborns. Ascertain the diagnosis of pneumothorax with transillumination and/or chest x-ray.

1. Wash hands thoroughly. Monitor vital signs and utilize transcutaneous Po_2 and Pco_2 if possible.
2. Place the infant in supine position. An assistant is needed to hold the infant securely.
3. Select the aspiration site. The site depends on the location of the fluid/air. This is usually the second intercostal space at the midclavicular line for pneumothorax or fifth or sixth intercostal space in the anterior axillary line when a pneumothorax or effusion is drained.
4. Prepare the aspiration site with Betadine (followed by alcohol) and isolate the area with sterile towels.
5. The no. 18–21 gauge Silastic thoracentesis needle is attached to a 10-ml syringe. Insert the thoracentesis needle just over the superior margin of the rib. Take care not to go too high or intercostal vessels will be damaged. An angiocatheter may be used in lieu of a Silastic thoracentesis needle.
6. Advance the needle through the skin 2 to 3 mm until a sudden loss of resistance is felt. Then clamp the needle at the skin level to assure that it remains at the proper depth.
7. Withdraw the stylet and gently aspirate air/fluid into the syringe that is attached to the three-way stopcock.
8. If air is obtained, aspirate and allow to drain underwater by way of intrave-

nous tubing. Air coming from the pleural cavity will bubble underwater. A thoracotomy tube may be inserted (see chapter 19–IIE).

9. If no air is obtained, hold a sterile gauze sponge against the puncture site as the needle is removed. This is covered with collodion to effect an airtight seal of the chest wall.
10. Assist infant's ventilation as required.
11. Obtain an x-ray film to ensure resolution.

E. Tube Thoracotomy (Closed Intercostal Drainage)

Tube thoracotomy is performed to restore negative interpleural pressure by removing air or fluid from the interpleural space. Ascertain the diagnosis of pneumothorax with transilluminator and/or chest x-ray.

1. Wash hands thoroughly. Monitor vital signs. Utilize transcutaneous Po_2 and Pco_2 if possible.
2. Identify the site where the catheter will be placed. The second intercostal space at midclavicular line (superior) or fifth or sixth intercostal at the anterior axillary line is commonly used to evacuate air. The superior site is preferred site for pneumothorax.
3. The infant is positioned in a supine position. The operator dons mask and sterile gloves and the site is prepared as for thoracentesis.
4. Select an open-ended no. 18–21 gauge Silastic catheter with several side holes. The catheter comes with a trocar stylet. A no. 10–12 Fr polyvinyl chloride catheter may also be utilized.
5. Keeping the catheter sterile, measure the approximate length of the catheter needed to reach the desired site from the level of the entry site. Mark the tube length with a sterile 4 by 4 gauge using a clamp.
6. Clamp the end of the catheter trocar that will be inserted into the chest cavity approximately 2 cm from the tip. This will prevent the catheter with the trocar from being inserted too far.
7. For the catheters without trocar, make a small incision at the selected site and make a tunnel with curved mosquito hemostat into the pleural space.
8. Force the catheter and trocar through the chest wall. For the catheter without a trocar, insert the catheter between open tips of a hemostat in place. The infant may be taken off the ventilator to prevent lung puncture while the trocar with the catheter is forced through the chest wall. When the trocar has passed the parietal pleura, a sudden loss of resistance is felt. Work as quickly as possible. Return the infant to ventilator.
9. Remove the clamp and the trocar.
10. Aspirate gently. If air/fluid is obtained, pass the catheter into the anterior pleural cavity (for pneumothorax) or to the posterior pleural cavity (for fluid).
11. Clamp the catheter at the skin level.
12. Connect the catheter to -10 to -15 cm water seal drainage (Pleur-evac).

13. Place 000 silk, nonabsorbable sutures, through the skin and tie them around the catheter to secure the catheter.
14. Dress the site with petroleum jelly and then sterile gauze.
15. Persistent bubbling through the water seal occurs as the pneumothorax is evacuated and implies a continued air leak. Be aware that a fibrin clot may cause blockage. Multiple chest tubes may be required for bronchopleural fistula.
16. Confirm the chest tube position and resolution of pneumothorax by x-ray film.
17. Complications include lung perforation, hemorrhage, Horner's syndrome, phrenic nerve injury, infection, subcutaneous emphysema, etc.

F. Subdural Tap

This procedure is performed to obtain samples for studies to diagnose and to drain subdural collection.

This technique can be performed on any infant whose coronal sutures are sufficiently open to allow passage of a needle. Do not perform if there is a bleeding diathesis, or infection over the puncture site.

1. Wash hands thoroughly. Monitor vital signs. Utilize transcutaneous Po_2 and Pco_2 if possible.
2. Shave the infant's hair over the anterior scalp.
3. Restrain the infant securely in a sheet and place the infant in a supine position. Have an assistant hold the infant's head steady.
4. Using surgical aseptic scrub technique, wash the anterior part of the head with Betadine and isolate the area with sterile towels. Drape the field posteriorly and laterally.
5. Place a clamp on a 20- or 22-gauge spinal needle 1 cm from the tip of the needle.
6. Insert the spinal needle perpendicularly through the scalp in the lateral corner of the anterior fontanelle at least 1.0 cm from midline or in the coronal suture. Direct the needle toward the external auditory meatus into the anterior base of the lateral ventricle.
7. Advance the needle about 1.0 to 1.5 cm. Feel a "pop" to signify entry.
8. Withdraw the stylet to allow fluid to flow out.
9. Normally a drop of fluid is obtained. If the amount is more than 0.5 ml, it is significant.
10. If no fluid appears, withdraw the needle and repeat the procedure on the opposite side.
11. Send fluid for protein, sugar, culture, electrolytes, and cell count.
12. Reapply the stylet and withdraw the needle.
13. Apply collodion and a sterile 2 by 2 gauze to the puncture site.
14. Perform a spinal tap to compare fluid.
15. Complications include subdural bleeding, infection, fistula formation, trauma to cortex, subgaleal fluid accumulation, etc.

III. TRANSILLUMINATION

A. The Skull

Transillumination of the skull is used to diagnose subdural fluid collection, hydrocephalus, porencephaly and hydranencephaly.

1. Wash hands thoroughly.
2. Dark-adapt the physician's eyes. The examination should be carried out in as dark a room as possible.
3. Use a transilluminating Chun gun or fiberoptic light; apply the transilluminating light to the operator's own skin to note the maximum period of time before the light becomes too hot.
4. Hold the infant's head steady.
5. Apply the light serially to the infant's anterior, posterior, and lateral cranial vault and measure the area of transmitted light surrounding the light source (corona).
6. Repeat an opposite site and compare the corona size. Corona should be equal and symmetric: normal premature, 1 to 2 cm corona; normal fullterm, 0.5 to 1.5 cm for the two cell flashlight and 4.5 cm (occipital) to 5.4 cm (frontal) for the Chun gun or the fiberoptic light. Corona transillumination can be symmetric but excessive.
7. Factors that increase transillumination include thinner cranial bones, edema, decreased scalp thickness, decreased gestational age, increased fat in the scalp, decreased pigmented skin, sparse or blond hair, fluid in the scalp.
8. Factors that decrease transillumination include thick skull, blood or purulent fluid in the scalp, thick dark hair, and increased pigmentation of the skin.
9. In cases of subdural hematoma, the abnormal collection of fluid produces a discrete readily outlined illumination; the complete skull will "light up" with hydrocephalus or hydranencephaly.

B. The Chest

This technique is utilized for the rapid, noninvasive diagnosis of pneumothorax pneumomediastinum and pneumopericardium.

1. Wash hands thoroughly.
2. The examination should be carried out in as dark a room as possible. Dark-adapt the physician's eyes.
3. Apply the high-intensity fiberoptic light source to one's own skin to note maximum time before light becomes too hot.
4. Place the infant in a supine position. The light tip is then placed perpendicularly to the chest wall and superior to the nipple and then moved systematically around the chest.
5. Normally there is a 2 to 3-cm corona around the light tip. In the presence of a pneumothorax, the corona size will increase or the entire hemithorax will

"light up." In the presence of a pneumomediastinum, cardiac pulsations are evident in the lucent area. In the presence of a pneumopericardium, the silhouette of the beating heart and pericardial air is evident.
6. Factors that increase transillumination include air in thorax, chest wall edema, and increased subcutaneous fat.

C. The Abdomen

Transillumination of the abdomen has been useful in detecting pneumoperitonium secondary to gastrointestinal perforation.

1. Wash hands thoroughly.
2. Dark-adapt the physician's eyes. The examination should be carried out in as dark a room as possible.
3. Apply the transilluminating fiberoptic light to one's own skin to note maximum time before the light becomes too hot.
4. Apply the probe tip perpendicular to the abdominal wall to the left of the falciform ligament. Look at the abdomen from the right side. If a pneumoperitoneum is present, a very bright glow from the transillumination will be seen in the anterior abdomen.

IV. TRACHEAL INTUBATION

A. Orotracheal Intubation

See chapter 3–IIIC2a.

B. Nasotracheal Intubation

Nasotracheal intubation may be utilized when prolonged intubation is required.

1. Wash hands thoroughly.
2. Place the infant in the supine position with the head slightly flexed.
3. An assistant is needed to hold the infant securely.
4. Select a nasotracheal tube with a good natural curve (the internal diameters of the available soft straight tubes are 2.0, 2.5, 3.0, 3.5, and 4.0 mm) (see appendix A–6).
5. Insert the tube through a nostril as far as the oral pharynx.
6. Insert the laryngoscope as described previously for orotracheal intubation to expose the glottis (see chapter 3–IIIC2a).
7. Direct the nasotracheal tube by use of a McGill or Alligator forceps through the vocal cords into the larynx.
8. Insert the tube 1 to 2 cm beyond the vocal cords (see appendix Fig A–3).
9. Ascertain that the tube has not entered the right or left main bronchus or esophagus by hearing that breath sounds are equal.
10. Tape the tube to the nostril and face (see Fig 3–6).

11. Cut off excess tubing to minimize dead space.
12. Obtain a chest x-ray film to determine the position of tube.
13. Complications include tracheal perforation, hemorrhage, subglottic stenosis, perforation of nasal septum, stenosis of nasal vestibule, infection, mis-or displacement, etc.

V. FEEDING TUBE INSERTION AND TPN

A. Nasogastric Tube

Nasogastric tube may be inserted to decompress the stomach, to obtain gastric content for analysis, or to feed premature infants less than 34 weeks' gestation who have not correlated suck and swallow or for neurologically damaged infants, or infants with mild respiratory distress.

1. Wash your hands thoroughly.
2. Select a no. 5 or 8 F soft polyethylene nasogastric tube. No. 3 F tubes, though usable, frequently coil during insertion and therefore are dangerous.
3. Measure the distance from the infant's nose to the ear to the stomach. Usually, a black mark is located on the nasogastric tube and it can be used as a "guide" to judge the approximate distance between the infant's nose and stomach.
4. Do not lubricate the end of the tube because the infant's nasal secretions usually provide sufficient lubrication.
5. Hold the infant's head in the left hand and slightly flex the infant's neck while inserting tube through a nostril with the right hand. The operator should press the tip of the nose upward with the free left thumb. This will enlarge the nostril openings.
6. Slide the tube into the nostril along the base of nose, aiming towards the occiput. Do not direct the tube towards the vertex. Do not force the tube.
7. Stop when the tube has reached the premeasured site.
8. Secure the tube with tape; do not obstruct the infant's nostril with tape.
9. Ascertain that the tube is in place by listening for the flow of air over the stomach as several milliliters of air is administered into the infant's stomach and by aspirating gastric content.
10. Withdraw the tube if the infant coughs, gags, or shows any signs of respiratory distress or bradycardia. Pinch the gastric tube during removal.
11. Complications include coiling, dis- or misplacement, irritation and necrosis of nasal mucosa, apnea, bradycardia, perforation of pharynx, esophagus or stomach, etc.

B. Total or Partial Parenteral Nutrition

This technique is used when the other methods of feeding cannot be used or are inadequate. In infants, a central venous line or peripheral line can be used for total or partial parenteral nutrition. The skin-entry site must be cleaned, inspected, and dressed every other day with 70% alcohol or Betadine using a sterile technique (see chapter 19–ID and 19–IE).

VI. MISCELLANEOUS PROCEDURES

A. Tracheostomy

This operation is to create a patent airway and is utilized for upper airway obstruction (e.g., subglottic stenosis, hemangioma, macroglossia, cysts, etc.). Risks include pneumothorax, emphysema, and atelectasis.

1. Make sure that a tracheostomy set with sizes 00, 0, and 1 tracheostomy tubes is available. Suction equipment must be available. Plastic tracheostomy tubes are superior to metal tubes because they cause less tissue reaction.
2. Insert an oral or nasal endotracheal tube (see chapter 3–IIIC2a and chapter 19–IVB) because it is difficult to locate the collapsible trachea and to assure adequate ventilation during the procedure.
3. Select the incision site before scrubbing, usually the third tracheal ring, 1–1.5 cm above the sternal notch.
4. Place the infant in the supine position with the neck slightly extended.
5. Wash hands thoroughly and don sterile gloves.
6. Sterilize the skin over the selected area with Betadine and wipe with alcohol.
7. Drape the area with sterile towels.
8. Make a short, transverse skin incision. This incision is preferable to a vertical midline incision.
9. Dissect downward in the midline through the fascial planes to the thyroid isthmus until the trachea is exposed above or below the isthmus.
10. Clamp, ligate, and cut the thyroid isthmus if necessary. Use only essential dissection, keeping the surrounding tissue intact.
11. Grasp the trachea using a trachea or a thyroid hook.
12. Vertically incise the third tracheal ring in the midline. Be careful not to exert too much pressure so that the trachea is cut through.
13. Separate the edges of the tracheal incision with a hemostat.
14. Withdraw the endotracheal tube just above the incision and insert the tracheostomy tube. A correct fit must be obtained and the tube must not press on the posterior soft tracheal wall. If the plastic tracheostomy tube is too long, it can be cut to fit. Ascertain the tube position by auscultation and remove the endotracheal tube.
15. Suture the skin incision. The edges near the tube should be left open to permit drainage and prevent subcutaneous emphysema.
16. Hold the tracheal tube in place with a twill tape tied around the neck.
17. Take anteroposterior and lateral x-ray films of the neck and chest to ascertain the position of the tracheostomy tube.
18. To ascertain the patency of the tracheostomy, hold one or two strands of

cotton over the tracheostomy opening and observe the movement of the cotton in relation to the infant's respiration.
Note: Removal of the tracheostomy tube in young infants may be followed by airway obstruction secondary to necrotizing tracheobronchitis, subglottic stenosis, etc.

19. Complications include air leak syndrome, extubation, displacement, mucus plug, aerophagia, hemorrhage, T-E fistula, tracheomalasia, tracheal obstruction by granulation tissue, infection, etc.

B. Removal of Extra Digits and Skin Tags

Removal of extra digits or skin tags may be for cosmetic reasons or to prevent accidental torsion. This procedure is to be used for digits without carpal bones and with a base of 3 to 6 mm.

1. Wash hands thoroughly.
2. Leaving the ulnar side of the hand and the fifth finger exposed, restrain the hand using adhesive tape and an arm board.
3. Wipe the area with Betadine as if for a major skin preparation. Don gloves.
4. Inject 0.25 ml of a local anesthetic into the subcutaneous tissue at the base of the extra digit, if desired.
5. Without drawing up the skin, place a mosquito clamp across the base of the extra digit. For the 3–4 mm based digit, tie suture around the digit between clamp and hand, remove the clamp and place an adhesive bandage.
6. For the extra digit with base 5–6 mm in diameter, leave the clamp attached to the base of the digit for 5 to 20 minutes to seal the vessels.
7. During the waiting time, suture the subcutaneous tissue across the base, 90 degrees to the clamp. Loop, but don't tighten the sutures.
8. After the waiting period, retract the clamp slightly, keeping it parallel to the normal finger and cut away digit along the clamp. Do not cut the sutures.
9. Tighten the sutures.
10. Apply a small bandage to protect the sutures.
11. Remove the sutures in 5 to 7 days.

Small skin tags may be removed by excision or ligation using the same technique as the extra digit removal. Larger tags or those in critical areas are best left alone until after the neonatal period.

C. Blood Pressure by Doppler or Oscillometric Method

This technique is utilized to indirectly follow the infant's blood pressure by using ultrasound or oscillation to record the Doppler shift generated against the arterial walls or pulsations which are sensed in the cuff. The diastolic pressure may be slightly inaccurate.

1. Infant must be quiet and relaxed. No data indicate one position is superior to another. A pacifier may be helpful in establishing tranquility.

2. If the pressure in the brachial artery is to be measured, then the forearm is supinated and slightly flexed at the level of the heart. If the popliteal artery pressure is to be measured, the leg is slightly flexed.
3. Select an appropriate cuff. The size of the cuff utilized for the brachial artery should be 20% wider than the diameter of the upper extremity; the cuff size to measure the popliteal pressure should be 25% wider than the diameter of the thigh. The cuff also should cover two-thirds the length of upper arm or thigh. A completely encircling bladder tends to offer assurance of an accurate transmission of intrabladder pressure. Narrow cuffs are associated with the falsely high indirect values while wide cuffs may not be associated with falsely low indirect values. For a full-term or premature infant, a 2.5 to 4.0 cm width cuff is usually appropriate.
4. Coat the Doppler transducer with transmitting lubricant.
5. Wrap the sphygmomanometer cuff snugly around the bone just above area to be measured and apply the transducer to the skin directly over brachial or popliteal artery.
6. Inflate the cuff as rapidly as possible to a pressure of 20 to 30 mm Hg above the systolic pressure.
7. Deflate the cuff at 2 to 3 mm Hg/second. Read the systolic pressure at the onset of sound. Read the diastolic pressure when the sound lessens in intensity (Doppler method).
8. The flow signal may continue beyond the diastolic pressure. The diastolic measure is less accurate than the systolic.
9. The oscillometric device displays automatically systolic, diastolic, and mean blood pressure.

VII. ELECTROCARDIOGRAM

The ECG of the newborn differs from that of a child or adult because the pulmonary vascular resistance is higher in the newborn and the difference between the right and left ventricular muscle masses is smaller in the newborn.

A. Technique of Taking an ECG in the Newborn

1. Assemble the ECG equipment.
2. Wash hands thoroughly.
3. Keep the infant as quiet as possible. The infant may be given a pacifier.
4. Expose the infant's chest.
5. Provide a warm environment while taking the ECG.
6. Standardize the equipment so that a deflection of 1 centimeter represents 1 millivolt.
7. Set the speed at 25 mm/second.
8. Obtain bipolar leads I (right arm–left arm), II (right arm–left leg) and III (left arm–left leg), and unipolar leads aV_R (right arm), aV_L (left arm) and aV_F (left foot).

9. Obtain precordial leads by placing the small electrodes as follows:
   V_{4R}: Fifth right intercostal space at right midclavicular line
   V_1: Fourth right intercostal space at right sternal border
   V_2: Fourth left intercostal space at left sternal border
   V_3: Halfway between V_2 and V_4
   V_4: Fifth left intercostal space at left midclavicular line
   V_5: Fifth left intercostal space at left anterior axillary line
   V_6: Fifth left intercostal space at left midaxillary line
   V_7: Fifth left intercostal space at left posterior axillary line
10. Remove the paste from the infant's skin and electrodes after obtaining each tracing. This prevents the transmission of a false identical precordial tracing.
11. Set the speed at 50 mm/second when a more accurate and clear recording is required.
12. Obtain serial ECGs if needed.

B. Definitions of Electrocardiographic Configurations (Fig 19–1)

1. Waves

   Capital letters (Q, R, S) are utilized when the amplitude is over 5 mm and small letters (q,r,s) are utilized when the amplitude is under 5 mm.

   a. P wave: The deflection produced by atrial depolarization

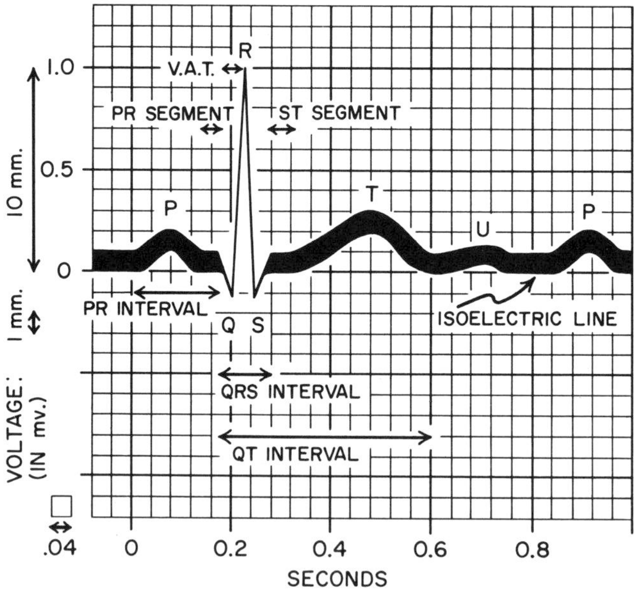

Fig 19–1.
Diagram of electrocardiographic complexes, intervals, and segments.

b. Q(q) wave: The initial negative deflection resulting from ventricular depolarization. It precedes the first positive deflection.
c. R(r) wave: The first positive deflection during ventricular depolarization
d. S(s) wave: The first negative deflection of ventricular depolarization that follows the first positive deflection (R)
e. R'(r') wave: The second positive deflection. The negative deflection following the R'(r') is termed the S'(s')
f. T wave: The deflection produced by ventricular repolarization
g. U wave: A deflection (usually positive) seen following the T wave and preceding the next P wave

2. Intervals
   a. RR interval: The distance between two successive R waves. Heart rate/minute = 10 × no. of R in 30 boxes (6 seconds) when the ventricular rhythm is regular.
   b. PP interval: The distance between two successive P waves. This will be the same as the RR interval in regular sinus rhythm.
   c. PR interval: The distance between the onset of the P wave and the beginning of the QRS complex. This measures the atrioventricular conducting time.
   d. QRS interval: The distance between the onset of the Q wave (or R if no Q is visible) and the termination of the S wave
   e. Ventricular activation time: The distance between the beginning of the Q wave and the peak of the R wave
   f. QT interval: The distance between the onset of the Q wave and the end of T wave. This interval differs in relation to the heart rate. QT_c: Corrected QT interval for a heart rate 60/minute ($QTc = QT\ interval/\sqrt{RR\ interval}$). Normal $QT_c = 0.38 \pm 0.04$.
   g. QoT interval: The distance between the onset of the Q wave and the onset of T wave. QoT interval varies in relation to the heart rate. QoTc = corrected QoT interval for a heart rate of 60/minute ($QoTc = QoT\ interval/\sqrt{RR\ interval}$). Normal values are <0.18 in fullterm and <0.20 in premature infants.
   h. ST segment: The portion of the tracing from the point at which the QRS complex ends (J) to the onset of the T wave
3. Frontal axis (see Fig 19–2)
   The net amplitude and direction of the QRS complex in any two of the three standard leads are plotted along the axis of the two standard leads, and perpendicular lines are drawn at these locations. A line drawn from the center of the reference system to the intersection of the perpendiculars represents the approximate mean QRS vector.

C. Normal Values

See appendix A–2, A–3.

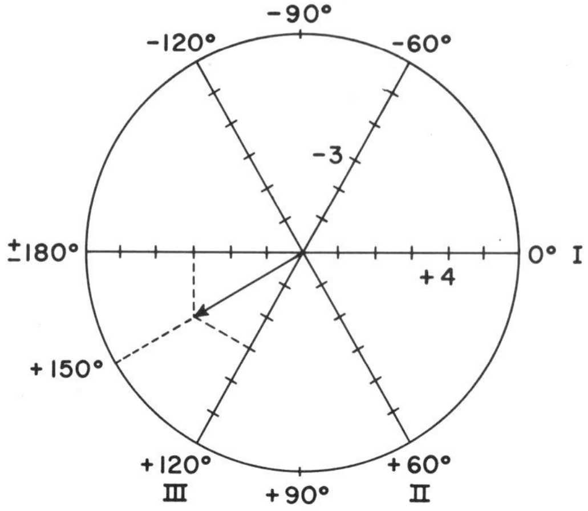

Fig 19–2.
Pediatric electrocardiography, the vector approach. (From Guntheroth W.G.: *Pediatric Electrocardiography, the Vector Approach.* Philadelphia, W.B. Saunders Co., 1965. Used by permission.)

D. Abnormal Findings

1. Right ventricular overload
   a. qR in V_1
   b. Pure R in $V_1 > 10$ mm
   c. $RV_1 > 30$ mm.
   d. $RV_{4R} > 19$ mm
   e. $SV_6 > 20$ mm after 2 days of age
   f. TV_1: positive after five days of age
   g. Right axis deviation > 180 degrees after 1 day of age
2. Left ventricular overload
   a. $SV_1 > 26$ mm
   b. $RV_6 > 15$ mm before 1 week of age and 22 mm after 1 week of age
   c. R/S $v_1 < 1.0$ mm after 2 days of age for premature infants and <0.6 mm after 7 days of age for fullterm infants
   d. $QV_6 > 3$ mm
   e. $TV_{5,6}$: inversion after 4 days of age
   f. RV_1 plus deep Q II, III, aV_F
   g. QRS axis $< +30°$
3. Combined ventricular overload
   a. Findings of right and left ventricular overload as listed above.
   b. Signs of right ventricular overload plus q 2 mm or more in left chest, sizeable though not "abnormal" RV_6, T inversion in left chest. Left axis deviation.

   c. Signs of left ventricular overload plus sizeable R or R′ in right precordial leads and marked right axis deviation
   d. Apparently normal ECG with large heart
   e. Tall R with deep S ($R + S > 60$ mm) in $V_{3,4}$
4. Right atrial enlargement
   a. Peaked, high P in I, V_1, $V_2 > 2.5$ mm in any lead
   b. Upright P in V_2
5. Left atrial enlargement
   a. Broad and/or notched P in II, III, V_5, V_6, > 0.08 seconds
   b. Biphasic and/or deep inversion of the *P* wave in V_3R or V_1
6. Combined atrial enlargement
   D4 + D5
7. RBBB (right bundle branch block)
   a. Wide S in I, V_6
   b. R(r) S(s) R′(r′) in V_1
   c. Right axis deviation
8. LBBB (left bundle branch block)
   a. Monophasic R in I
   b. Absent Q in V_6
9. Sinus arrhythmia
   Variation of the RR interval without morphological changes of P wave and QRS complex.
10. Supraventricular tachycardia
    a. Heart rate > 210/minute
    b. No P waves
    c. Wolff-Parkinson-White syndrome, prolonged QRS duration and shortened PR interval, in 20% of patients
11. PVC (premature ventricular contraction)
    Prolonged QRS complex, ST segments slope away from QRS and inverted T waves occurring before the expected P waves, often followed by a compensatory pause.
12. Congenital atrioventricular (AV) block
    Heart rate < 90/minute and usually more than 50/minute. Occasionally, heart rate less than 50–55/minute, and infants are usually symptomatic (Stokes-Adams attacks and/or dyspnea, tachypnea, peripheral cyanosis, and occasionally, congestive heart failure).
13. Myocarditis
    a. Nonspecific ST and T abnormalities (e.g., flattening T waves)
    b. Low voltage, particularly of the T waves
    c. Rhythm and conduction abnormalities are common
    d. Pathologic Q waves in I, aVL, and V_6
14. Pericarditis
    a. Elevated ST segment
    b. Varying direction of T waves during recovery stage of pericarditis
    c. Generalized low voltage

15. Effects of digoxin
    a. Therapeutic effect
        1) Prolonged RR interval
        2) Shortened QTc
        3) ST segments changes
        4) Low T wave amplitude
    b. Toxicity
        1) Bradycardia
        2) AV block
        3) Arrhythmias
        4) Hypoxia, hypokalemia, and acidosis enhance the toxicity
16. Effects of quinidine
    a. Therapeutic effect
        1) Decreased P amplitude
        2) Prolonged PR interval
        3) Prolonged QRS duration
        4) Prolonged QTc interval
    b. Toxicity
        1) Prolonged PR interval
        2) Prolonged QRS duration
        3) AV block
        4) Multifocal ventricular premature beats
17. Hyperkalemia
    a. Tall, tented, narrow T wave
    b. Depressed ST segment
    c. Widened QRS, PR, and QTc intervals
    d. Widened, flattened, finally disappearing P wave
    e. "Sine wave effect." (The QRS is widened to the extent that it blends into the T wave.)
    f. Straight ST segment
    g. Ventricular standstill
    h. Hyponatremia, hypocalcemia or acidosis enhances toxic effects.
18. Hypokalemia
    a. Prolonged QTc interval (caused by broad, flat T wave)
    b. Flattened or inverted T wave
    c. Depressed ST segment
    d. Prominent U wave
    e. Prolonged PR interval
    f. Prominent P wave
    g. Ectopic beats
19. Hypocalcemia

    Prolonged QTc interval (caused by long ST segment)
20. Hypercalcemia
    a. Shortened QTc interval (caused by shortened ST segment)
    b. Increased myocardial irritability: premature beats, paroxysmal ventricular tachycardia, and ventricular fibrillation

21. Hypomagnesemia
    Same ECG findings as hyperkalemia caused by relative hyperkalemia
22. Hypernatremia
    a. Diminished duration and amplitude of the QRS complex
    b. Lengthened QTc interval
23. Hyponatremia
    a. Increased duration and amplitude of the QRS complex
    b. Shortened QTc interval
    c. Inverted ST and T waves
24. Metabolic acidosis
    a. Increased amplitude of the P wave
    b. Prolonged PR and QRS intervals
    c. Tall and peaked T waves
25. Metabolic alkalosis
    Inverted T wave and ST segment

REFERENCES

VESSEL PUNCTURE/CATHETERIZATION/CUTDOWN

Heel Puncture

Blumenfeld T.A., Turi G.K., Blank W.A.: Optimum site and depth for newborn heel punctures. *Pediatr. Res.* 12:444, 1978.

Fenton L.J., Bertil B., Gaines J., et al.: A superior method for obtaining blood from the heel of the newborn infant. *Clin. Pediatr.* 16:815, 1977.

Harpin V.A., Rutter N.: Making heel pricks less painful. *Arch. Dis. Child.* 58:226, 1983.

Venous Puncture

Plaxico D.T., Bucciarella R.L.: Greater saphenous vein venipuncture in the neonate. *J. Pediatr.* 93:1025, 1978.

Kuhns L.R., Martin A.J., Gildersleeve S., et al.: Intense transillumination for infant venipuncture. *Radiology* 116:734, 1975.

Nabseth D.C., Jones J.E.: Gangrene of the lower extremities of infants after femoral venipuncture. *N. Engl. J. Med.* 268:1003, 1963.

Umbilical Vein Catheter

Kitterman J.A., Phibbs R.H., Tooley W.H.: Catheterization of umbilical vessels in newborn infants. *Pediatr. Clin. North Am.* 17(4):895, 1970.

Symansky M.R., Fox H.A.: Umbilical vessel catheterization: Indications, management, and evaluation of the technique. *J. Pediatr.* 80:820, 1972.

Central Venous Catheter Placement

Pereya R., Andrassy R.J., Mahour G.H.: Central venous cannulation in neonates. *Surg. Gynecol. Obstet.* 151:253, 1980.

Stewart R.D., Sanislow C.A.: Silastic intravenous catheter. *N. Engl. J. Med.* 265:1283, 1961.

Percutaneous Central Venous Catheter

Dalcourt J.L., Bose C.L.: Percutaneous insertion of Silastic central venous catheters in newborn infants. *Pediatrics* 70:484, 1982.

Loeff D.S., Matlak M.E., Black R.E., et al.: Insertion of a small central venous catheter in neonates and young infants. *J. Pediatr. Surg.* 17:944, 1982.

Internal Saphenous Vein Cutdown

Fletcher M.A., MacDonald M.G., Avery G.B. (eds.): *Atlas of Procedures in Neonatology.* Philadelphia, J.B. Lippincott, Co., 1983, p. 125.

Arterial Puncture

Shaw J.C.L.: Arterial sampling from the radial artery in premature and full-term infants. *Lancet* 2:389, 1968.

Schlueter M.A., Johnson B.B., Sudman D.A., et al.: Blood sampling from scalp arteries in infants. *Pediatrics* 51:120, 1973.

Wunderlich B., Reynolds R.N.: Arterial blood sampling in babies. *Am. J. Dis. Child.* 123:446, 1972.

Pape K.E., Armstrong D.L., Fitzhardinge P.M.: Peripheral median nerve damage secondary to bracheal artery blood gas sampling. *J. Pediatr.* 93:852, 1978.

Umbilical Artery Catheterization

Symansky M.R., Fox H.A.: Umbilical vessel catheterization: Indications, management, and evaluation of the technique. *J. Pediatr.* 80:820, 1972.

Cole A.F.D., Rolbin S.H.: A technique for rapid catheterization of the umbilical artery. *Anesthesiology* 53:254, 1980.

Gupta J.M., Robertson N.R.C., Wigglesworth J.S.: Umbilical artery catheterization in the newborn. *Arch. Dis. Child.* 43:382, 1968.

TAPPING VARIOUS ORGANS/CAVITIES

Suprapubic Tap

Abbott G.D., Shannon F.T.: How to aspirate urine suprapubically in infants and children. *Clin. Pediatr.* 9:277, 1970.

Nelson J.D., Peters P.C.: Suprapubic aspiration of urine in premature and term infants. *Pediatrics* 36:132, 1965.

Stevens D.C., Schreiner R.L., Gresham E.L.: Suprapubic bladder aspiration in the neonate. *Perinatol. Neonatol.* 5:47, 1980.

Spinal Tap

Gleason C.A., Martin R.J., Anderson J.V., et al.: Optimal position for a spinal tap in preterm infants. *Pediatrics* 71:31, 1983.

Pericardial Tap

Brans Y.W., Pitts M., Cassady G.: Neonatal pneumopericardium. *Am. J. Dis. Child.* 130:393, 1976.

Reppert S.M., Ment L.R., Todres I.D.: The treatment of pneumopericardium in the newborn infant. *J. Pediatr.* 90:115, 1977.

Lawson E.E., Gould J.B., Taeusch H.W. Jr.: Neonatal pneumopericardium: Current management. *J. Pediatr. Surg.* 15:181, 1980.

Thoracentesis

Duffy B.L.: Neonatal pneumothorax. *Pediatrics* 31:403, 1976.

Shim W.K., Philip A.G.S.: Danger of needle aspiration in pneumothorax of the newborn. *J.A.M.A.* 223:691, 1973.

Tube Thoracotomy

Ramachandra A., Russel G.: Treatment of pneumothorax in the newborn infant. *Arch. Dis. Child.* 47:464, 1972.

Rothberg A.D., Marks K.H., Maisels M.J.: Understanding the pleurevac. *Pediatrics* 67:482, 1981.

Allen R.W., Jung A.L., Lester P.D.: Effective chest tube evacuation of pneumothorax in neonate. *J. Pediatr.* 99:629, 1981.

Subdural Tap

Matson D.D.: Subdural taps. *Pediatr. Clin. North Am.* 2:239, 1955.

Rabe E.F.: Subdural effusions in infants. *Pediatr. Clin. North Am.* 14:831, 1967.

TRANSILLUMINATION

The Skull

Dodge P.R., Porter P.: Demonstration of intracranial pathology by transillumination. *Arch. Neurol.* 5:30, 1961.

Cheldelin L.V., Davis P.C., Grant W.W.: Normal values for transillumination of skull using a new light source. *J. Pediatr.* 87:937, 1975.

Shurleff D.B.: Transillumination of skull in infants and children. *Am. J. Dis. Child.* 107:14, 1964.

The Chest

Cabatu E.E., Brown E.G.: Thoracic transillumination: Aid in the diagnosis and treatment of pneumopericardium. *Pediatrics* 64:958, 1979.

Kuhns L.R., Bednarek F.J., Wyman M.L., et al.: Diagnosis of pneumothorax or pneumomediastinum in the neonate by transillumination. *Pediatrics* 56:355, 1975.

The Abdomen

Mofenson H.C., Greensher J.: Transillumination of the abdomen in infants. *Am. J. Dis. Child.* 115:428, 1968.

Wyman M.L., Kuhns L.R.: Pneumoperitoneum demonstrated by transillumination. *Am. J. Dis. Child.* 130:1237, 1976.

TRACHEAL INTUBATION

Orotracheal Intubation

Gregory G.A.: Respiratory care of newborn infants. *Pediatr. Clin. North Am.* 19:311, 1971.

Kuhns L.R., Poenanski A.K.: Endotracheal tube position in the infant. *J. Pediatr.* 78:991, 1971.

McMillan D.D., Rademaker A.W., Buchan K.A., et al.: Benefits of orotracheal and nasotracheal intubation in neonates requiring ventilatory assistance. *Pediatrics* 77:39, 1986.

Nasotracheal Intubation

Coldiran J.B.: Estimation of nasotracheal tube length in neonates. *Pediatrics* 41:823, 1968.

TUBE INSERTION TECHNIQUES

Nasogastric Tube

Pereira G.R., Lemons J.A.: Controlled study of transpyloric and intermittent gavage feeding in the small preterm infant. *Pediatrics* 67:68, 1981.

Herrell N., Martin R.J., Fanaroff A.: Arterial oxygen tension during nasogastric feeding in the preterm infant. *J. Pediatr.* 96:914, 1980.

MISCELLANEOUS PROCEDURES

Tracheostomy

Bifano E.M., Clark D.A., Pincus L.G.: Tracheostomy and decannulation in neonates. *Pediatr. Res.* 14:591, 1980.

Gibson R., Byrne J.E.T.: Tracheotomy in neonates. *Laryngoscope* 82:643, 1972.

Removal of Extra Digits and Skin Tags

Fletcher M.A., MacDonald M.G., Avery G.B. (eds.): *Atlas of Procedures in Neonatology.* Philadelphia, J.B. Lippincott, Co., 1983, p. 329.

Blood Pressure by Doppler Method

American Academy of Pediatrics: Recommendation of task force on blood pressure control in children. *Pediatrics* 59:797, 1977.

Janis K.M., Kemmerer W.T., Hagood C.O.: Doppler blood pressure measurement in infants and small children. *J. Pediatr. Surg.* 6:70, 1971.

Lagler U., Duc G.: Systolic blood pressure in normal newborn infants during the first 6 hours of life. Transcutaneous Doppler ultrasonic technique. *Biol. Neonate* 37:243, 1980.

Myerberg D.Z.: Comparison of simultaneously measured radial artery (RA), umbilical artery (UA), and dinamap pressure in sick newborns. *Pediatr. Res.* 15:673, 1981.

ELECTROCARDIOGRAM

Rowe R.D., Freedom R.M., Mehrizi A., et al. (eds.): *The Neonate With Congenital Heart Disease,* Vol. 5. *Major Problems in Clinical Pediatrics,* ed. 2. Philadelphia, W.B. Saunders, 1981, p. 65.

Appendix A

Cardiorespiratory Data
Blood Pressure

TABLE A–1.—Average Systolic, Diastolic, and Mean Blood Pressures During the First 12 Hours of Life in Normal Newborn Infants Grouped According to Birth Weight*

BIRTH WEIGHT	HOUR	1	2	3	4	5	6	7	8	9	10	11	12
1,001 to 2,000 gm	Systolic	49	49	51	52	53	52	52	52	51	51	49	50
	Diastolic	26	27	28	29	31	31	31	31	31	30	29	30
	Mean	35	36	37	39	40	40	39	39	38	37	37	38
2,001 to 3,000 gm	Systolic	59	57	60	60	61	58	64	60	63	61	60	59
	Diastolic	32	32	32	32	33	34	37	34	38	35	35	35
	Mean	43	41	43	43	44	43	45	43	44	44	43	42
Over 3,000 gm	Systolic	70	67	65	65	66	66	67	67	68	70	66	66
	Diastolic	44	41	39	41	40	41	41	41	44	43	41	41
	Mean	53	51	50	50	51	50	50	51	53	54	51	50

*From Kitterman J.A., et al.: *Pediatrics* 44:959, 1969. Used by permission.

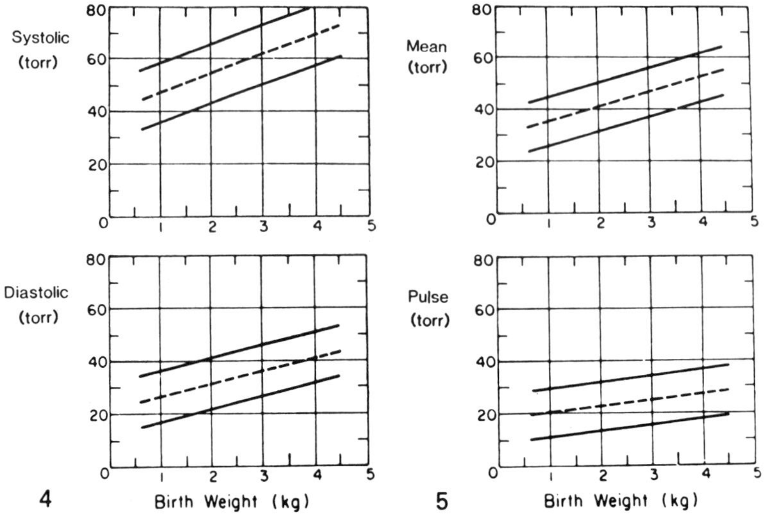

Fig A–1.

Aortic blood pressure; systolic, diastolic, mean and pulse pressure (linear regressions and 95% confidence limits) in healthy newborn infants during the first 12 hours of life. (From Versmold H.T., Kitterman J.A., Phibbs R.H., et al.: Aortic blood pressure during the first 12 hours of life in infants with birth weight 610 to 4,220 grams. *Pediatrics* 67:607, 1981. Used by permission.)

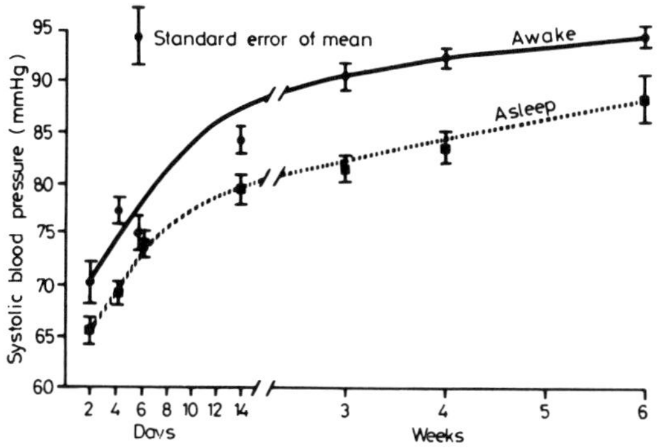

Fig A–2.
Systolic blood pressure between 2 days and 6 weeks of life in infants awake and asleep. (From Early A., Fayers P., Ng S., et al.: Blood pressure in the first 6 weeks of life. *Arch. Dis. Child.*, 55:755, 1980. Used by permission.)

TABLE A–2.—ELECTROCARDIOGRAPHIC STANDARDS IN TERM NEONATES*†

PARAMETER	AGE: 0–24 HOURS	1–3 DAYS	3–7 DAYS	7–30 DAYS
Number of patients	189	179	181	119
Heart rate (beats/min)	123 (99–148)	123 (97–149)	129 (101–161)	148 (115–177)
QRS axis (degree)	137 (91–185)	134 (93–190)	132 (91–186)	110 (76–151)
PR duration II (sec)	0.11 (0.08–0.14)	0.11 (0.09–0.13)	0.10 (0.08–0.13)	0.10 (0.08–0.13)
QRS duration V_5 (sec)	0.051 (0.034–0.069)	0.048 (0.035–0.060)	0.049 (0.034–0.063)	0.053 (0.037–0.076)
QT duration V_5 (msec)	0.29 (0.22–0.36)	0.28 (0.24–0.33)	0.27 (0.23–0.31)	0.26 (0.23–0.29)
P amplitude II (mvolts)	0.16 (0.08–0.25)	0.16 (0.05–0.25)	0.17 (0.08–0.27)	0.19 (0.09–0.29)
R amplitude V_{3R} (mvolts)	1.10 (0.42–1.86)	1.20 (0.53–2.00)	1.05 (0.16–1.82)	0.85 (0.28–1.60)
R amplitude V_1 (mvolts)	1.38 (0.62–2.36)	1.44 (0.64–2.45)	1.29 (0.50–2.14)	1.06 (0.44–1.88)
R amplitude V_5 (mvolts)	1.02 (0.25–1.88)	1.08 (0.45–1.98)	1.18 (0.45–1.94)	1.40 (0.61–2.09)
R amplitude V_6 (mvolts)	0.42 (0.03–0.96)	0.45 (0.05–0.98)	0.52 (0.08–1.05)	0.76 (0.31–1.38)
S ampitude V_{3R} (mvolts)	0.43 (0.04–1.18)	0.50 (0.04–1.20)	0.33 (0.03–0.79)	0.20 (0.02–0.55)
S amplitude V_1 (mvolts)	0.84 (0.09–1.85)	0.91 (0.14–1.90)	0.65 (0.06–1.48)	0.41 (0.04–0.95)
S amplitude V_5 (mvolts)	0.99 (0.35–1.78)	0.97 (0.20–1.58)	0.94 (0.38–1.67)	0.80 (0.26–1.35)
S amplitude V_6 (mvolts)	0.32 (0.03–0.78)	0.30 (0.03–0.75)	0.35 (0.04–0.80)	0.34 (0.04–0.84)
R/S amplitude V_{3R}	1.5 (0.3–4.8)	1.6 (0.3–4.2)	1.9 (0.2–5.8)	1.9 (0.2–4.5)
R/S amplitude V_1	2.24 (0.32–7.03)	1.96 (0.31–5.31)	2.71 (0.40–7.43)	2.85 (1.11–6.37)
R/S amplitude V_5	0.7 (0.0–7.0)	1.0 (0.0–5.0)	1.5 (0.0–5.0)	2.0 (0.0–5.1)
R/S amplitude V_6	1.97 (0.27–7.04)	2.49 (0.3–9.04)	2.15 (0.28–8.05)	3.29 (0.31–9.24)

†Mean with 5% and 95% values in parentheses.
*From Davignon A., et al.: Normal ECG standards for infants and children, in Avery M.E., Taeusch H.W., Jr. (eds.): *Diseases of the Newborn,* ed. 5. Philadelphia, W.B. Saunders Co., 1984, p. 988. Used by permission.

TABLE A–3.—NORMAL ELECTROCARDIOGRAPHIC VALUES IN FULL-TERM AND PREMATURE INFANTS*

PARAMETERS	0–24 HOURS; MEAN (5%–95%)		1–7 DAYS; MEAN (5%–95%)		8–30 DAYS; MEAN (5%–95%)	
	FULLTERM	PRETERM	FULLTERM	PREMATURE	FULLTERM	PREMATURE
HR	119 (94–145)	14[illegible] (109–173)	133 (100–175)	150 (127–182)	163 (115–190)	170 (133–200)
PR	0.10 (0.07–0.12)	. . .	0.09 (0.07–0.12)	. . .	0.09 (0.07–0.11)	. . .
P dur.	0.051 (0.040–0.065)	. . .	0.046 (0.038–0.061)	. . .	0.048 (0.040–0.057)	. . .
P in II	1.5 (0.8–2.3)	1.1 (0.5–2.0)	1.6 (0.8–2.5)	1.3 (0.5–2.0)	1.6 (0.8–2.4)	0.8 (0.3–1.5)
QRS dur.	0.065 (0.050–0.084)	. . .	0.056 (0.040–0.079)	. . .	0.057 (0.040–0.073)	. . .
QRS Axis†	135 (60–180)	127 (75–194)	125 (80–160)	121 (75–195)	110 (60–160)	80 (17–171)
T Axis†	70 (0–140)	41 (319–84)	25 (−40–80)	28 (315–60)	35 (0–60)	53 (30–75)
T in V_4	4.3 (7.2)‡	. . .	4.4 (7.7)‡	. . .	5.3 (8.1)‡	. . .
T in V_6	2.4 (3.9)‡	. . .	2.9 (4.2)‡	. . .	3.5 (5.3)‡	. . .
R in V_1	14.8 (7.0–20.0)	. . .	18.2 (9.0–27.4)	. . .	11.4 (4.2–19.8)	. . .
R in V_2	20.1 (13.0–28.1)	11.4 (3.5–21.3)	19.9 (11.7–31.1)	11.9 (5.0–20.8)	17.5 (6.8–29.0)	15.0 (8.3–21.0)
R in V_5	10.2 (4.0–18.0)	6.5 (2.0–12.6)	10.7 (3.4–19.3)	7.4 (2.6–14.9)	11.9 (3.5–27.0)	13.0 (6.2–21.6)
R in V_6	3.3 (2.3–7.0)	. . .	5.1 (2.2–13.1)	. . .	6.7 (1.7–20.5)	. . .
S in V_1	9.3 (2.5–27.0)	. . .	10.4 (4.6–18.8)	. . .	5.0 (2.5–12.8)	. . .
S in V_2	20.3 (9.0–33.8)	15.0 (2.5–26.5)	20.2 (9.3–34.1)	13.5 (2.6–26.0)	14.0 (4.2–25.7)	14.0 (5.1–26.3)
S in V_5	11.9 (0.0–24.0)	6.8 (0.06–17.6)	6.8 (3.6–16.2)	6.5 (1.0–16.0)	4.8 (2.7–12.3)	6.2 (1.2–14.0)
S in V_6	4.5 (1.6–10.3)	. . .	3.3 (0.8–9.9)	. . .	2.0 (0.6–9.0)	. . .

Dur = duration
*From Hastreiter A.R., Abella J.B.: *J. Pediatr.* 78:146, 1971, and Sreenivasan V.V., Fisher B.J., Liebman J.L., et al.: *Am. J. Cardiol.* 31:57, 1973.
†Frontal plane
‡95% value only

Blood Volume

TABLE A–4.—Relationship of Age, Total Blood Volume, and Body Weight of Infants*†

Age	Body Weight (kg) (Fiftieth Percentile)	Total Blood Volume (ml)
26 weeks	0.9	104
28 weeks	1.1	127
30 weeks	1.3	150
32 weeks	1.6	185
34 weeks	2.1	242
36 weeks	2.6	299
38 weeks	3.0	345
Birth	3.4	272–340

*From Fanaroff A.A., Martin R.J., Merkatz I.R.: *Behrman's Neonatal-Perinatal Medicine; Diseases of the Fetus and Infant,* ed. 3. St. Louis, Miss., C.V. Mosby Co., 1983, p. 1109. Used by permission.

†Based on total blood volume of (1)premature infant, 115 ml/kg, (2) newborn, 80–110 ml/kg.

Pulmonary Function

TABLE A–5.—Pulmonary Ventilation of the Infant*

Respiratory frequency, breaths/min	34–45
Tidal volume, ml/kg	6–8
Alveolar volume, ml/kg	3.8–5.8
Dead space volume, ml/kg	2.0–2.2
Minute ventilation, ml/kg/min	200–260
Alveolar ventilation, ml/kg/min	100–150
Wasted (dead space) ventilation, ml/kg/min	77–99
Dead space/tidal volume	0.27–0.37
O_2 consumption, ml/kg/min	6–8
Ventilation equivalent (alveolar ventilation/ O_2 consumption)	16–23

*From Smith C.A.: *Physiology of the Newborn* Springfield, Ill., Charles C. Thomas, Publisher, 1976, p. 209. Used by permission.

Endotracheal Tube Diameter and Length

TABLE A–6.—Endotracheal Tube Size*

INFANT WEIGHT (GM)	ENDOTRACHEAL TUBE DIAMETER	
	INSIDE	OUTSIDE
Less than 1,000	2.5 mm	12 Fr.
1,000–1,500	3.0 mm	14 Fr.
1,500–2,200	3.5 mm	16 Fr.
2,200 and over	4.0 mm	18 Fr.

*From Avery G., (ed.): *Neonatology,* ed. 2. Philadelphia, J.B. Lippincott, 1981. Used by permission.

TABLE A–7.—Insertion Distance of Endotracheal Tube*

INFANT WEIGHT (GM)	CORD-CARINA DISTANCE (CM)	INSERTION PAST CORDS (CM)
1,000–1,500	4.0	1.5–2.0
1,500–2,500	4.5	2.0
2,500–3,500	5.0	2.2
3,500–4,000	5.5	2.5

*From Avery G., (ed.): *Neonatology,* ed. 2. Philadelphia, J.B. Lippincott, 1981. Used by permission.

A

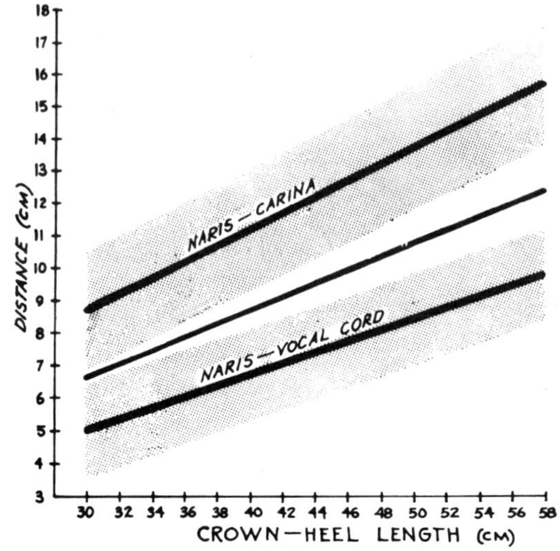

B

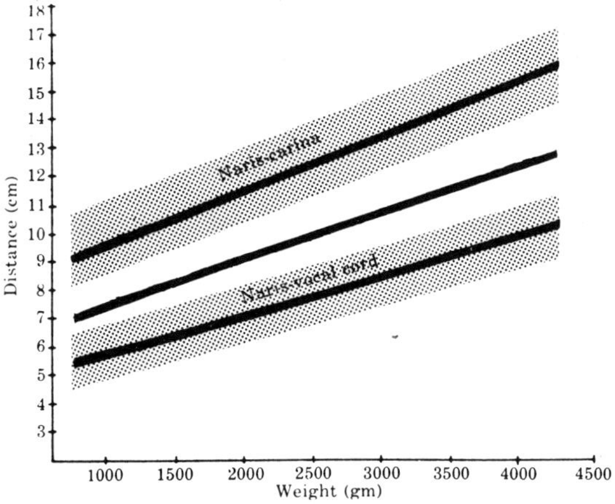

Fig A–3.
Estimation of nasotracheal tube length. (From Coldiron J.S.: Estimation of nasotracheal tube length in neonates. *Pediatrics* 41:823, 1968. Used by permission.)

TABLE A–8.—ARTERIAL BLOOD GASES AND ACID BASE BALANCE IN THE NORMAL NEWBORN*

		UMBILICAL		MINUTES				HOURS		DAYS		
		VEIN	ARTERY	5–10	20	30	60	5	24	2	4	7
pH	Mean	7.320	7.242	7.207	7.263	7.297	7.332	7.339	7.369	7.365	7.370	7.371
	Range	7.178	7.111	7.091	7.180	7.206	7.261	7.256	7.290	7.314	7.320	7.320
		7.414	7.375	7.302	7.330	7.380	7.394	7.389	7.448	7.438	7.440	7.431
P_{CO_2} mm Hg	Mean	37.8	49.1	46.1	40.1	37.7	36.1	35.2	33.4	33.1	34.3	35.9
	Range	26	35	35	31	28	28	29	27	26	27	30
		52	60	65	58	54	45	45	40	43	43	42
Pa_{O_2} mm Hg	Mean	27.4	15.9	49.6	50.7	54.1	63.3	73.7	72.7	73.8	73.3	73.1
	Range	15	7	33	31	31	38	55	54	62	60	57
		40	23	75	85	85	83	106	95	91	93	94
Standard bicarbonate mEq/L	Mean	20	18.7	16.7	17.5	18.2	19.2	19.4	20.2	19.8	20.4	21.8
	Range	15.5	14.0	12.5	14.0	15.0	16.0	16.0	18.0	16.5	17.5	18.5
		22.5	21.0	20.5	20.0	21.0	21.5	22.0	23.5	24.5	25.0	26.0
O_2-capacity ml/100 ml	Mean	19.9	20.3	22.1	23.2	22.2	22.5	23.6	22.1	21.7	20.8	20.2
	Range	16.5	16.4	18.2	19.0	17.3	19.0	19.7	16.8	16.9	16.1	14.1
		24.1	23.7	26.3	26.3	26.0	25.9	28.4	28.0	26.7	25.7	25.7
Lactate mEq/L	Mean	2.6	2.7	3.8	—	2.2	1.6	1.3	1.0	—	—	0.9
	Range	1.5	1.5	2.6	—	1.2	0.9	0.9	0.8	—	—	0.5
		3.8	4.5	4.7	—	4.3	2.7	2.0	1.2	—	—	1.4
Excess lactate mEq/L	Mean	1.0	1.2	1.7	—	0.7	—	—	0.2	—	—	—
	Range	0.9	0.8	0.6	—	0.2	—	—	0.05	—	—	—
		1.5	1.2	2.5	—	1.2	—	—	0.3	—	—	—
SO_2 %	Mean	60.0	29.5	80.9	—	88.0	92.2	95.9	96.8	—	—	96.3
	Range	33.8	9.0	57.5	—	65.0	72.1	84.5	93.9	—	—	91.6
		85.6	51.4	93.5	—	95.6	97.3	98.5	98.8	—	—	99.1
Hct %	Mean	48.3	49.9	53.0	—	54.1	54.1	52.4	54.8	53.9	51.4	51.0
	Range	39.0	40.5	40.1	—	32.1	43.1	44.4	36.4	40.7	38.5	35.8
		57.3	54.5	62.5	—	65.3	61.4	66.0	67.7	65.3	64.2	69.0

*From Koch G., Wendel H.: *Biol. Neonatol.* 12:136, 1968. Used by permission.

TABLE A–9.—Arterial Blood Gas Values in Normal Premature Infants*

		3–5 HOURS	6–12 HOURS	13–24 HOURS	25–48 HOURS	3–4 DAYS	5–10 DAYS	11–40 DAYS
pH	$\bar{x}$	7.329	7.425	7.464	7.434	7.425	7.378	7.425
	SD	±0.038	±0.072	±0.064	±0.054	±0.044	±0.043	±0.033
PCO_2, mm Hg	$\bar{x}$	47.3	28.2	27.2	31.3	31.7	36.4	32.9
	SD	±8.5	±6.9	±8.4	±6.7	±6.7	±4.2	±4.0
PO_2, mm Hg	$\bar{x}$	59.5	69.7	67.0	72.5	77.8	80.3	77.8
	SD	±7.7	±11.8	±15.2	±20.9	±16.4	±12.0	±9.6
BE,† mEq/L	$\bar{x}$	3.7	4.7	3.0	2.3	2.9	3.5	2.1
	SD	±1.5	±3.1	±3.3	±3.0	±2.3	±2.3	±2.2
SaO_2 (%)	$\bar{x}$	91.3	95.2	95.3	95.0	95.7	95.1	96.0
	SD	±1.7	±1.2	±2.1	±2.0	±1.5	±1.3	±0.6

*From Orzalesi M.M., Mendicini M., Bucci G., et al.: *Arch. Dis. Child.* 42:174, 1967. Used by permission.
†Base excess.

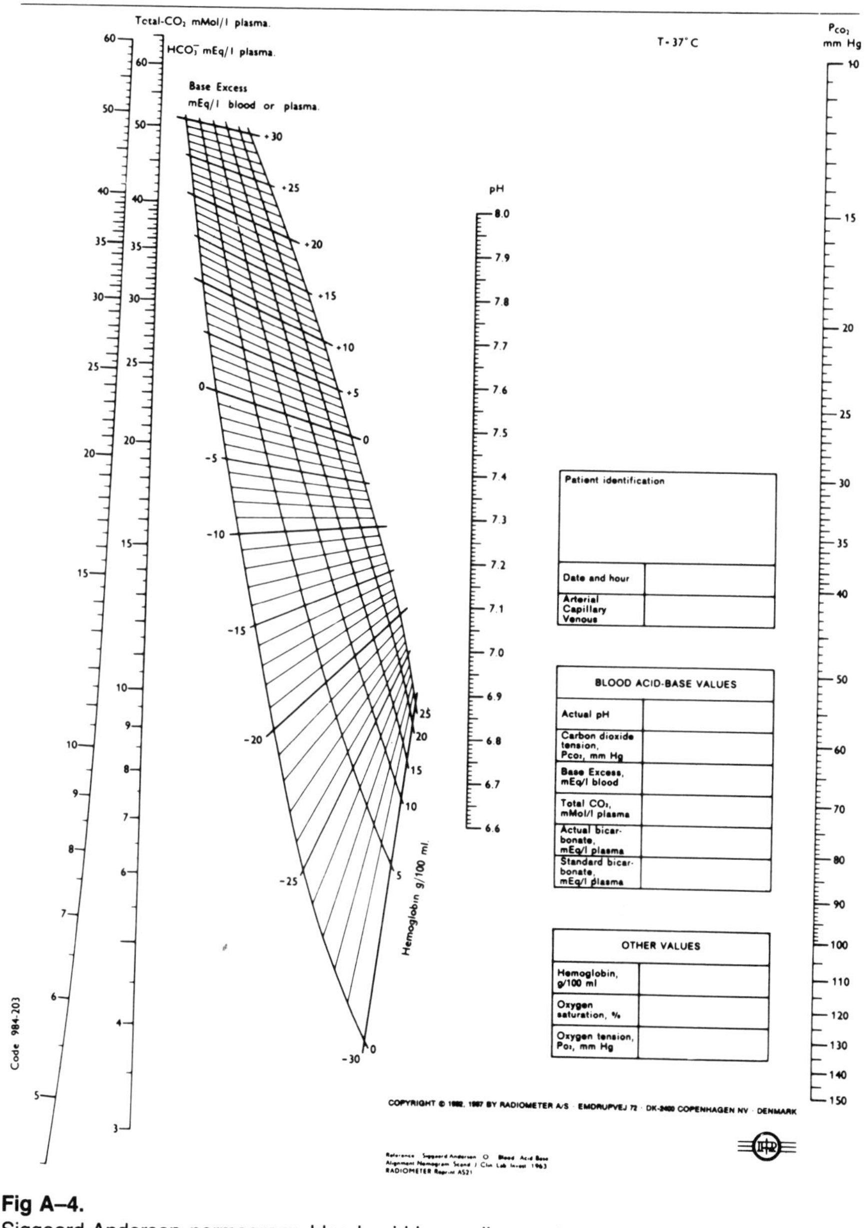

Fig A–4.

Siggaard-Andersen normogram: blood acid-base alignment normogram. (From Andersen, O.S.: Blood acid-base alignment normogram. *Scand. J. Clin. Lab. Invest.* 15:211, 1963. Used by permission.)

HEMATOLOGIC VALUES

TABLE A–10.—Normal Hematologic Values During the First 12 Weeks of Life in the Term Infant as Determined by an Electronic Cell Counter*

AGE	NO. OF CASES	HB GM/DL ± SD	RBC × 10^6 ± SD	HCT % ± SD	MCV CU μ^3 ± SD	MCHC % ± SD	RETICULOCYTES % ± SD
Days							
1	19	19.3 ± 2.2	5.14 ± 0.7	61 ± 7.4	119 ± 9.4	31.6 ± 1.9	3.2 ± 1.4
2	19	19.0 ± 1.9	5.15 ± 0.8	60 ± 6.4	115 ± 7.0	31.6 ± 1.4	3.2 ± 1.3
3	19	18.8 ± 2.0	5.11 ± 0.7	62 ± 9.3	116 ± 5.3	31.1 ± 2.8	2.8 ± 1.7
4	10	18.6 ± 2.1	5.00 ± 0.6	57 ± 8.1	114 ± 7.5	32.6 ± 1.5	1.8 ± 1.1
5	12	17.6 ± 1.1	4.97 ± 0.4	57 ± 7.3	114 ± 8.9	30.9 ± 2.2	1.2 ± 0.2
6	15	17.4 ± 2.2	5.00 ± 0.7	54 ± 7.2	113 ± 10.0	32.2 ± 1.6	0.6 ± 0.2
7	12	17.9 ± 2.5	4.86 ± 0.6	56 ± 9.4	118 ± 11.2	32.0 ± 1.6	0.5 ± 0.4
Weeks							
1–2	32	17.3 ± 2.3	4.80 ± 0.8	54 ± 8.3	112 ± 19.0	32.1 ± 2.9	0.5 ± 0.3
2–3	11	15.6 ± 2.6	4.20 ± 0.6	46 ± 7.3	111 ± 8.2	33.9 ± 1.9	0.8 ± 0.6
3–4	17	14.2 ± 2.1	4.00 ± 0.6	43 ± 5.7	105 ± 7.5	33.5 ± 1.6	0.6 ± 0.3
4–5	15	12.7 ± 1.6	3.60 ± 0.4	36 ± 4.8	101 ± 8.1	34.9 ± 1.6	0.9 ± 0.8
5–6	10	11.9 ± 1.5	3.55 ± 0.2	36 ± 6.2	102 ± 10.2	34.1 ± 2.9	1.0 ± 0.7
6–7	10	12.0 ± 1.5	3.40 ± 0.4	36 ± 4.8	105 ± 12.0	33.8 ± 2.3	1.2 ± 0.7
7–8	17	11.1 ± 1.1	3.40 ± 0.4	33 ± 3.7	100 ± 13.0	33.7 ± 2.6	1.5 ± 0.7
8–9	13	10.7 ± 0.9	3.40 ± 0.5	31 ± 2.5	93 ± 12.0	34.1 ± 2.2	1.8 ± 1.0
9–10	12	11.2 ± 0.9	3.60 ± 0.3	32 ± 2.7	91 ± 9.3	34.3 ± 2.9	1.2 ± 0.6
10–11	11	11.4 ± 0.9	3.70 ± 0.4	34 ± 2.1	91 ± 7.7	33.2 ± 2.4	1.2 ± 0.7
11–12	13	11.3 ± 0.9	3.70 ± 0.3	33 ± 3.3	88 ± 7.9	34.8 ± 2.2	0.7 ± 0.3

*Matoth Y., Zaizov R., Varsano I.: *Acta Paediatr. Scand.* 60:317, 1971. Used by permission.

TABLE A–11.—Normal Red Blood Cell Values in Term and Low-Birth Weight Infants, First 8 Weeks of Life*

Determination	Wt. (kg)	1–3 days	4–7 days	2 weeks	4 weeks	6 weeks	8 weeks
Hemoglobin (gm/100 ml)	Term	18.7 ± 3.4	17.9 ± 2.5	17.3	14.2	11.9	—
	1.2–1.5	20.2 ± 3.1	18.0 ± 1.9	17.1	12.0	9.1	8.3
	<1.2	15.6 ± 1.0	16.4 ± 1.9	15.5	11.3	8.5	7.8
Hematocrit (%)	Term	62 ± 9.3	56 ± 9.4	54	43	36	—
	1.2–1.5		53		32		
Red blood cells × 10^6/cu mm	Term	5.11 ± 0.7	4.86 ± 0.6	4.8	4.0	3.6	—
	1.2–1.5	5.2 ± 1.3	4.5 ± 1.0	4.3	3.4	2.9	2.6
	<1.2	3.4 ± 1.3	3.7 ± 0.5	4.0	3.2	2.6	2.3
Nucleated RBCs/100 WBCs	1.2–1.5	19.8	0.8	0.	0.4	1.4	1.0
	<1.2	16.7	1.1	0.1	1.0	2.7	2.0
Reticulocytes %	Term	2.8 ± 1.7	0.5 ± 0.4	0.5	0.6	1.0	—
	1.2–1.5	2.7 ± 1.6	1.2 ± 0.7	0.9	1.0	2.2	2.7
	<1.2	8.4 ± 3.9	3.9 ± 2.1	1.9	4.1	5.4	6.1

*From: Matoth Y., Zaizov R., Varsano I.: *Acta Paediatr. Scand.* 60:317, 1971, and Wolff J.A., Goodfellow A.M.: *Pediatrics* 16:753, 1955. Used by permission.

TABLE A–12.—NORMAL WHITE BLOOD CELL VALUES IN TERM AND PREMATURE INFANTS*

DETERMINATION	WT (KG)	1–3 DAYS	4–7 DAYS	2 WEEKS	4 WEEKS	6 WEEKS	8 WEEKS	10 WEEKS	12 WEEKS
Leukocytes × 10^3/cu mm	Term	18.1	12.2	11.4	10.8				
	1.2–1.5	10.8 ± 4.0	8.9 ± 2.9	14.3	11.0	10.5	9.1	—	—
	<1.2	14.8 ± 10.2	12.2 ± 7.0	15.8	13.2	10.8	9.9	11.1	9.7
Segments %	Term	52	39	34	30	—	—	—	—
	1.2–1.5	47 ± 16.9	31 ± 9.0	33	26	20	25	—	—
	<1.2	46 ± 7.1	32 ± 10.9	41	28	23	23	21	19
Bands %	Term	9	6	5.5	4.5	—	—	—	—
	1.2–1.5	11.9	10.5	5.9	3.0	1.4	2.1	1.0	3.3
	<1.2	10.7	9.7	8.0	5.9	5.8	4.4	2.4	6.0
Eosinophils %	Term	2.2	4.1	3.1	2.8	—	—	—	—
	1.2–1.5	1.3	2.2	2.5	5.1	2.6	2.3	3.5	2.3
	<1.2	0.4	6.2	1.0	3.7	2.0	3.8	5.1	5.6
Basophils %	Term	0.6	0.4	0.4	0.5	—	—	—	—
	1.2–1.5	5.1	2.4	2.7	1.8	1.7	1.6	0.3	0.3
	<1.2	2.0	3.9	5.3	3.6	2.6	2.0	0.8	2.0
Lymphocytes %	Term	31	41	48	56	—	—	—	—
	1.2–1.5	34 ± 10.3	48 ± 13.9	52	59	69	64	—	—
	<1.2	32 ± 11.2	43 ± 12.8	39	55	61	65	68	59
Monocytes %	Term	5.8	9.1	8.8	6.5	—	—	—	—
	1.2–1.5	3 ± 2.5	6 ± 4.4	3	4	5	5	—	—
	<1.2	5 ± 4.3	7 ± 4.9	5	4	6	3	3	7
Platelets × 10^3/cu mm	Term	192 ± 94	224 ± 101	—	—	—	—	—	—
	1.2–1.5	151 ± 35	134 ± 49	153	189	212	244	—	183
	<1.2	148 ± 61	163 ± 69	162	158	210	212	218	218

*From: Ablin A.R., Kushner J.H., Murphy A., et al.: *Pediatrics* 28:822, 1961, and Altman P.L., Ditter D.S.: Federation of American Societies for Experimental Biology, Washington, D.C., 1961, and Wolff J.A., Goodfellow A.M.: *Pediatrics* 16:753, 1955.

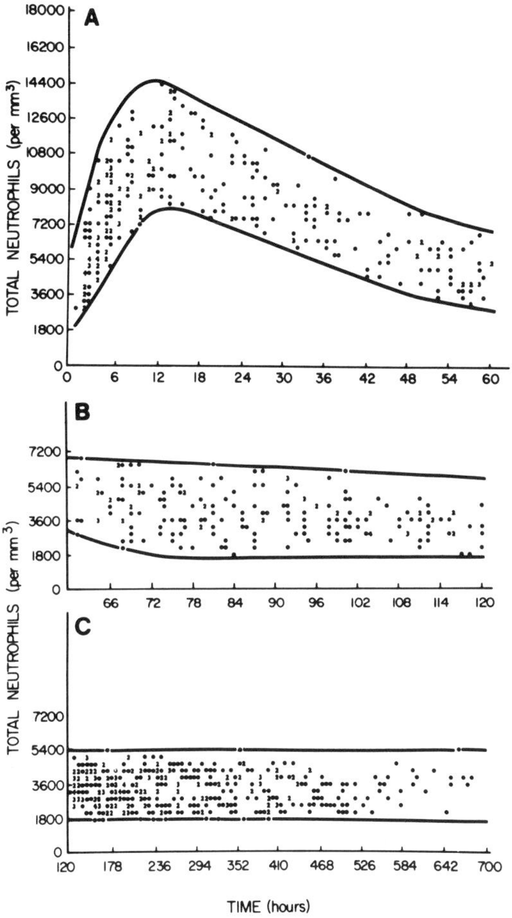

Fig A–5.
Total neutrophil count in the first 0 to 60 **(A),** 60 to 120 **(B),** and 120 to 700 (28 days) **(C)** hours of age. (From Manroe B.L., Weinberg A.G., Rosenfeld C.R., et al.: The neonatal blood count in health and disease. I. Reference values for neutrophilic cells. *J. Pediatr.* 95:89, 1979. Used by permission.)

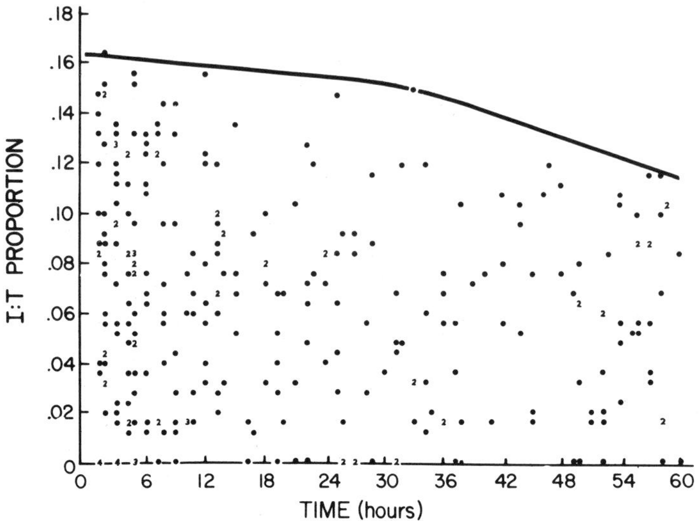

Fig A–6.
Immature (I)/total (T) neutrophils ratio in the first 60 hours of life. (From Manroe B.L., Weinberg A.G., Rosenfeld C.R., et al.: The neonatal blood count in health and disease. I. Reference values for neutrophilic cells. *J. Pediatr.* 95:89, 1979. Used by permission.)

TABLE A–13.—Platelet Counts in Normal Low-Birth-Weight Infants*

	NORMAL LOW BIRTH WEIGHT	
DAY	MEAN (cu mm)	RANGE (1,000s)
0	203,000	80–356
3	207,000	61–335
5	233,000	100–502
7	319,000	124–678
10	399,000	172–680
14	386,000	147–670
21	388,000	201–720
28	384,000	212–625

*From Appleyard W.J., Brinton A.: *Biol. Neonate* 17:30, 1971. Used by permission.

TABLE A–14.—COAGULATION FACTOR PERCENT ACTIVITY LEVELS FOR PRETERM AND TERM INFANTS

SUBJECT	I (MG/100 ML)	II	V	VII-X	VIII	IX	XI	XII	XIII	PLASMINOGEN	ANTI THROMBIN III	PREKALLIKREIN (FLETCHER FACTOR)	HMW KININOGEN
Normal adult	315 ± 60†	100	100	100	100	100	100	100	100	61–125	98 ± 9	100	100
Preterm infant 24–31 wks	282†	31†	73†	39†	87†	22†	20†	20†	. . .	. . .	27†	27†	28†
Preterm infant 27–31 wks	256 ± 70†	30 ± 8‡	91 ± 30‡	38 ± 14‡	90†	27†	. . .	27†	. . .	24 ± 8†	29 ± 3‡	. . .	. . .
Preterm infant 32–35 wks	260 ± 80‡	33 ± 11‡	90 ± 12‡	42 ± 20‡	120†	34 ± 14‡	. . .	33†	. . .	30 ± 10†	44 ± 10‡	. . .	. . .
Preterm infant 36–39 wks	230 ± 50‡	52 ± 20†	85 ± 15†	43 ± 20†	125†	43 ± 13‡	. . .	. . .	. . .	35 ± 11†	51 ± 10‡	. . .	. . .
Term infant	215 ± 35†	54 ± 15*	114 (56–200)* 99(40–150)†	56 ± 16*	97(50*–180) 168†	28* (15–42)	31*	47 ± 18*	50†	43 ± 16†	60 ± 16†	33 ± 6*	56 ± 12.5*
Older infant	340 ± 70‡ (21 days)	97 ± 4† (45–60 days)	100‡ (21 days)	92 ± 10‡ (21 days)	. . .	72 ± 15‡ (21–45 days)	. . .	100† (14 days)	100† (1 mo)	61† (6 mo)	82† (6 mo)	. . .	. . . .

Values represent smoothed means ± I standard deviation or (ranges) from cord,* venous,† or capillary ‡ samples in the first 24 hours of life. Other values are given for older infants at age when values approximate adult levels.

Hathaway W.E., Bonnar J.: *Perinatal Coagulation*. New York, Grune & Stratton, 1978. Used by permission.

TABLE A–15.—Bone Marrow Differential Count During the First Week of Life*

	0–24 HOURS (%)	7 DAYS (%)	ADULT (%)
Myeloblasts	0–2	0–3	0.3–50
Promyelocytes	0.5–6.0	0.5–7.0	1.0–8.0
Myelocytes	1.0–9.0	1.0–11.0	5.5–22.5
Metamyelocytes	4.5–25.0	7.0–35.0	13.0–32.0
Band forms	10.0–40.0	11.0–45.0	. . .
Erythroblasts	0–1.0	0–0.5	1.0–8.0
Proerythroblasts	0.5–9.0	0–0.5	2.0–10.0
Normoblasts	18.0–41.0	0–15.0	7.0–32.0
Myeloid : erythroid ratio	1.5 : 1.0	6.5 : 1.0	3.5 : 1.0

*From Oski F.A., Naiman J.L.: *Hematologic Problems in the Newborn,* ed. 3. Philadelphia, W.B. Saunders Co., 1982, p. 21; adapted from Shapiro, Bassen: *Am. J. Med. Sci.* 203:341, 1941; and Gardner D., et al.: *Arch. Dis. Child.* 27:214, 1952. Used by permission.

TABLE A–16.—Normal Percentile Values for Micro-Erythrocyte Sedimentation Rate in Low-Birth-Weight Infants at Less Than 3 and 9 to 56 Days of Age*

	LESS THAN 3 DAYS		9–56 DAYS
PERCENTILE	MALE†	FEMALE‡	BOTH SEXES
10	1.0	1.0	3.0
25	1.8	1.8	3.8
50	2.5	3.0	—
75	3.3	4.0	5.5
90	4.0	6.0	9.5
95	6.0	6.0	11.0
99	8.8	8.3	

*From Evans H., Glass L., Mercado C.: *J Pediatr.* 76:448–450, 1970. Used by permission.

†Hematocrit: median 57%, range 43% to 78%.

‡Hematocrit: median 54%, range 41% to 77%.

XHematocrit: median 35%, range 25% to 58%.

TABLE A–17.—SERUM IRON, IRON-BINDING CAPACITY IN THE NEWBORN AND MOTHER*

SERUM IRON (μG/DL)		TOTAL IRON BINDING CAPACITY (μG/DL)		
INFANT	MOTHER	INFANT	MOTHER	AUTHOR
173	98	259	470	Hagberg (1953)
147	80	226	446	Laurell (1947)
193 (145–240)	. . .	240 (147–468)	. . .	Sturgeon (1954)
159 (106–227)	. . .	. . .	. . .	Vahlquist (1941)
154 (72–237)	. . .	. . .	. . .	Weippl et al. (1973)

*From Oski F.A., Naiman J.L.: *Hematologic Problems in the Newborn,* ed. 3. Philadelphia, W.B. Saunders Co., 1982, p. 33. Used by permission.

TABLE A–18.—SERUM FOLIC ACID (mμg/ml) IN NORMAL PREMATURE INFANTS*

AGE	RANGE	MEAN ± SD
Normal premature infants		
1–4 days	7.17–52.00	29.54 ± 0.98
2–3 weeks	4.12–15.62	8.61 ± 0.55
1–2 months	2.81–11.25	5.84 ± 0.35
2–3 months	3.56–11.82	6.95 ± 0.50
3–5 months	3.85–16.50	8.92 ± 0.86
5–7 months	6.00–12.25	9.02 ± 0.74
Normal children		
1–6 years	4.12–21.25	11.37 ± 0.82

*From Klaus M.H., Fanaroff A.A.: *Care of the High Risk Neonate,* Philadelphia, W.B. Saunders Co. 1973, p. 407. Adapted from Shojania A., Gross S. *J. Pediatr* 64:323, 1964. Used by permission.

TABLE A–19.—Serum Vitamin E Levels in Term and Preterm Infants; Serum Vitamin E (mg/dl)—Mean ± (1 SD)*

WEEKS	1	2	3	4	5	6	7	8	9	10
<1,500 gm	0.40	0.30	0.25	0.25	0.25	0.25	0.25	0.25	0.35	0.45
28–32 weeks	[0.05]	[0.04]	[0.03]	[0.03]	[0.03]	[0.03]	[0.03]	[0.03]	[0.04]	[0.05]
1,500–2,000 gm	0.45	0.40	0.40	0.45	0.45	0.45	0.50	0.50	0.60	0.70
32–36 weeks	[0.05]	[0.05]	[0.05]	[0.05]	[0.05]	[0.05]	[0.05]	[0.05]	[0.06]	[0.06]
2,000–2,500 gm	0.50	0.45	0.50	0.60	0.70	0.75	0.75	0.75	0.75	0.80
36–40 weeks	[0.05]	[0.05]	[0.05]	[0.06]	[0.06]	[0.06]	[0.60]	[0.60]	[0.60]	[0.70]
>2,500 gm	0.55	0.55	0.55	0.60	0.75	0.80	0.85	0.85	0.85	0.85
Term	[0.60]	[0.60]	[0.60]	[0.60]	[0.70]	[0.70]	[0.80]	[0.80]	[0.80]	[0.80]

*From Klaus M.H., Fanaroff A.A.: *Care of the High Risk Neonate.* Philadelphia, W.B. Saunders Co., 1979. p. 408. Used by permission.

TABLE A–20.—Mean ± SD of Serum Copper Concentrations (μg/dl) by Postconceptional Age in Premature Infants*

	WEEKS OF POSTCONCEPTUAL AGE										
	25–28	29–30	31–32	33–34	35–36	37–38	39–40	41–42	43–44	45–46	47–60
Mean	28.6	27.1	31.5	36.4	39.2	47.2	52.1	59.6	70.2	65.3	81.8
Standard deviation	17.1	14.9	17.5	14.6	13.8	24.1	11.6	21.1	28.1	15.8	18.0
Number of cases	16	27	35	43	33	22	20	18	18	9	4

*From Hillman L.S.: *J. Pediatr.* 98:305, 1981. Used by permission.

TABLE A-21.—Serum Immunoglobulin Levels (mg/dl) in Newborns*

AGE	NEWBORN	1–3 MONTHS
IgG	1,031 ± 200 (645–1244)	430 ± 119 (272–762)
IgA	2 ± 3 (0–11)	21 ± 13 (6–56)
IgM	11 ± 5 (5–30)	30 ± 11 (16–67)

*From Stiehm E.R., Fudenberg H.H.: *Pediatrics* 37:715, 1966. Used by permission.

TABLE A–22.—MEAN COMPLEMENT LEVELS OF SERA OF NEWBORN INFANTS OF DIFFERENT BIRTH WEIGHTS AND THE MATERNAL SERA, COMPARED WITH A NORMAL ADULT STANDARD SERUM*

	COMPLEMENT COMPONENT LEVELS (MEAN ± 1 STANDARD ERROR OF MEAN)								
	RATIO TO STANDARD SERUM						MG/100 ML		
GROUP	CH_{50}†	C1q	C2	$C3(B_{1C})$	C4	$C4(B_{1E})$	C1q	B_{1C}	B_{1E}
<1,000 gm	0.6 ± 0.1 (7)‡	0.5 ± 0.1 (7)	1.2 ± 0.1 (2)	0.6 ± 0.1 (7)	0.5 ± 0.1 (7)	0.6 ± 0.2 (7)	1.1 ± 0.2	89 ± 16	9 ± 3
1,000–1,500 gm	0.7 ± 0.1 (7)	0.4 ± 0.02 (9)	0.4 ± 0.2 (3)	0.7 ± 0.1 (9)	1.4 ± 0.3 (7)	0.8 ± 0.1 (9)	1.1 ± 0.1	94 ± 10	12 ± 2
1,500–2,000 gm	0.7 ± 0.3 (5)	0.7 ± 0.1 (8)	1.2 ± 0.5 (4)	0.9 ± 0.2 (7)	1.0 ± 0.6 (4)	1.0 ± 0.3 (8)	1.6 ± 0.3	141 ± 24	15 ± 4
2,000–2,500 gm	0.9 ± 0.2 (5)	0.8 ± 0.1 (5)	1.0 ± 0.2 (5)	1.0 ± 0.2 (5)	1.2 ± 0.4 (5)	1.4 ± 0.3 (5)	1.9 ± 0.3	151 ± 33	21 ± 5
>2,500 gm	0.9 ± 0.1 (8)	0.9 ± 0.5 (11)	1.0 ± 0.2 (6)	1.0 ± 0.1 (11)	1.4 ± 0.2 (7)	1.0 ± 0.1 (11)	2.2 ± 0.1	160 ± 13	16 ± 2
Mother	1.5 ± 0.1 (24)	0.9 ± 0.04 (25)	1.2 ± 0.2 (18)	1.8 ± 0.1 (27)	1.9 ± 0.2 (23)	2.3 ± 0.1 (26)	2.3 ± 0.1	254 ± 12	35 ± 2
Normal standard	1.0	1.0	1.0	1.0	1.0	1.0	2.5	145.2	15.2

*From Sawyer M.K., Forman M.L., Kuplic L.S., et al.: *Biol. Neonate* 19:148, 1971. Used by permission.
†Total hemolytic complement expressed in 50% hemolytic units.
‡Number in parenthesis refers to number in group.

BLOOD CHEMISTRY VALUES

TABLE A–23.—NORMAL BLOOD CHEMISTRY VALUES FOR TERM INFANTS*

DETERMINATION	CORD	5 HOURS	18 HOURS	36 HOURS	48 HOURS
Sodium, mEq/L	147 (126–166)	143 (124–156)	146 (132–159)	148 (134–160)	149 (139–162)
Potassium, mEq/L	7.8 (5.6–12)	6.8 (5.1–7.5)	6.3 (5.3–8.9)	6.0 (5.2–7.3)	5.9 (5.0–7.7)
Chloride, mEq/L	103 (98–110)	100.7 (90–111)	103 (87–114)	102 (92–114)	103 (93–112)
Calcium, mg/dl	9.3 (8.2–11.1)	8.4 (7.3–9.2)	7.8 (6.9–9.4)	8.0 (6.1–9.9)	7.9 (5.9–9.7)
Phosphorus, mg/dl	5.6 (3.7–8.1)	6.1 (3.5–8.6)	5.7 (2.9–8.1)	5.9 (3.0–8.7)	5.8 (2.8–7.6)
Blood urea, mg/dl	29 (21–40)	27 (8–34)	33 (9–63)	32 (13–77)	31 (13–68)
Total protein, g/dl	6.1 (4.8–7.3)	6.6 (5.6–8.5)	6.6 (5.8–8.2)	6.9 (5.9–8.2)	7.2 (6.0–8.5)
Glucose, mg/dl	73 (45–96)	63 (40–97)	63 (42–104)	56 (30–91)	59 (40–90)
Lactic acid, mg/dl	19.5 (11–30)	14.6 (11–24)	14.0 (10–23)	14.3 (9–22)	13.5 (7–21)

*From Acharya P.T., Payne W.W.: *Arch. Dis. Child.* 40:430, 1965. Used by permission.

TABLE A–24.—NORMAL BLOOD CHEMISTRY VALUES IN LOW-BIRTH-WEIGHT INFANTS, FIRST DAY OF LIFE*

DETERMINATION	1,000 GM OR LESS	1,001–1,500 GM	1,501–2,000 GM	2,001–2,500 GM
Sodium, mEq/L	137 (135–139)	133 (130–136)	135 (127–139)	134 (127–144)
Potassium, mEq/L	6.4 (5.5–7.2)	6.1 (5.0–7.6)	5.3 (4.6–6.3)	5.6 (4.5–9.0)
Chloride, mEq/L	100 (95–106)	101 (93–113)	105 (93–112)	104 (92.3–115)
Total CO_2, mEq/L	19 (14.3–22.1)	20 (10.7–24.6)	20 (11.1–26.8)	20 (14.5–27.2)
Urea, mg/100 ml	22 (14–27)	21 (9–60)	15 (8–36)	16 (7–32)
Total protein gm/dl	4.8	4.8	5.2	5.3

*From Pincus J.B., Gittleman I.F., Saito M., et al.: *Pediatrics* 18:39, 1956. Used by permission.

TABLE A–25.—NORMAL BLOOD CHEMISTRY VALUES IN LOW-BIRTH-WEIGHT INFANTS*

DETERMINATION	CORD	1–3 DAYS	6–10 DAYS	12–18 DAYS	20–25 DAYS
Creatinine, mg/100 ml	1.12 (0.86–1.42)	1.56 (0.76–2.84)	1.17 (0.62–1.54)	1.23 (0.62–2.26)	1.06 (0.67–1.58)
Calcium, mg/100 ml	9.3 (8.58–10.76)	7.10 (5.1–9.10)	8.10 (5.40–9.82)	8.62 (7.23–9.89)	8.9 (7.56–10.7)
Phosphorus, mg/100 ml	6.79 (5.32–7.52)	8.13 (5.88–10.2)	8.91 (6.8–11.9)	8.90 (6.84–9.25)	8.0 (6.4–9.64)
Total protein, gm/100 ml	. . .	6.3 (4.46–8.01)	6.0 (4.82–7.34)	5.9 (5.24–6.87)	4.76 (4.54–4.85)
Magnesium, mg/100 ml	2.1 ± 0.1 (8 hours)	2.2 ± 0.1	. . .	. . .	. . .
Osmolarity, mOsm/L	282 (265–295)	295 (231–352)	285 (237–326)	288 (277–310)	289 (269–315)
Glucose, mg/100 ml	50 ± 3 (8 hours)	58 ± 3	. . .	. . .	. . .

*From: Smith F.G., Scrivens B., Borden M.: *J. Pediatrics* 66:997, 1965, and Tsang R.C., Oh W.: *Pediatrics* 45:773, 1970.

TABLE A–26.—PLASMA CREATININE VALUES IN FIRST MONTH OF LIFE*

GESTATION (WEEKS)		POSTNATAL AGE (DAYS) 2 ALL BABIES	2 BREATHING SPONTANEOUSLY	2 VENTILATED	7 ALL BABIES	14	21	28
28	μmol/L ± 2SD	116 ± 40	108 ± 20	121 ± 45	84 ± 32	72 ± 32	60 ± 33	58 ± 24
	mg/dl ± 2SD	1.31 ± 0.45	1.22 ± 0.23	1.37 ± 0.51	0.95 ± 0.36	0.81 ± 0.36	0.68 ± 0.37	0.66 ± 0.27
29–32	μmol/L ± 2SD	104 ± 38	100 ± 32	115 ± 43	83 ± 41	69 ± 32	59 ± 32	52 ± 33
	mg/dl ± 2SD	1.18 ± 0.43	1.13 ± 0.36	1.30 ± 0.49	0.94 ± 0.46	0.78 ± 0.36	0.67 ± 0.36	0.59 ± 0.37
33–66	μmol/L ± SD	93 ± 39	94 ± 39	87 ± 46	68 ± 44	55 ± 36	50 ± 37	35 ± 24
	mg/dl ± SD	1.05 ± 0.44	1.06 ± 0.44	0.98 ± 0.52	0.77 ± 0.50	0.62 ± 0.41	0.56 ± 0.42	0.40 ± 0.27
37–42	μmol/L ± SD	75 ± 38	75 ± 38	—	50 ± 36	38 ± 20	35 ± 20	30 ± 18
	mg/dl ± SD	0.85 ± 0.43	0.85 ± 0.43	—	0.56 ± 0.41	0.43 ± 0.23	0.40 ± 0.23	0.34 ± 0.20

*From Rudd P.T., Hughes E.A., Placzek M.N., et al.: *Arch. Dis. Child.* 58:212, 1983. Used by permission.
Conversion SI to traditional units: 1 μmol/L = 0.0113 mg/100 ml.

TABLE A–27.—TRUE BLOOD SUGAR LEVELS IN NORMAL TERM AND LOW-BIRTH-WEIGHT INFANTS*

MATERNAL STATUS	DELIVERY TYPE	AGE, HOURS						
		0	½	1	2	4	6	24
No fluid	Vaginal	66	55	55	48	55	47	—
administration		44–84	34–90	35–89	22–73	30–71	27–78	—
Saline, IV	Cesarean section	64	75	76	70	60	57	54
administration		38–90	58–107	34–136	45–108	47–101	35–76	43–76
Glucose, IV	Cesarean section	109	69	66	56	58	52	68
administration		61–204	31–125	31–111	35–85	27–86	32–77	35–91
Glucose, IV	Vaginal	89	54	47	41	50	51	—
administration		54–163	27–98	16–82	19–71	34–80	29–80	—

*From Cornblath M., et al.: *Pediatrics* 27:378, 1961. Used by permission.

TABLE A–28.—SERUM TOTAL PROTEIN AND ELECTROPHORESIS FRACTIONS IN NEWBORNS (GM/DL)*

FRACTION	CORD BLOOD	AGE: AT BIRTH	1 WEEK	1–3 MONTHS
Total protein	4.78–8.04	4.6–7.0	4.4–7.6	3.64–7.38
Albumin	2.17–4.04	3.2–4.8	2.9–5.5	2.05–4.46
Alpha-1	0.25–0.66	0.1–0.3	0.09–0.25	0.08–0.43
Alpha-2	0.44–0.94	0.2–0.6	0.30–0.46	0.40–1.13
Beta	0.42–1.56	0.3–0.6	0.16–0.60	0.39–1.14
Gamma	0.81–1.61	0.6–1.2	0.35–1.3	0.25–1.05

*Data from Meites S.: Pediatric clinical chemistry a survey of normals, methods and instruments. Washington, D.C., American Association for Clinical Chemistry, 1981, p. 381, and Ellis E.F., Robbins J.B.: Children are different. Columbus, Ohio, Ross Laboratories, p. 188, 1978.

TABLE A–29.—SERUM ENZYMES IN NEWBORNS*

ENZYMES (IU/L at 37° C)	CORD	1–3 DAYS	0–1 MONTH
Acid phosphatase	—	—	7.4–19.4
Alanine amino transaminase (SGPT)	5.5 ± 2.5	1–25	—
Alkaline phosphatase	—	95–368	—
Aspartate amino transaminase (SGOT)	15.1 ± 4.1	16–74	—
Creatinine phosphokinase (CPK)	—	40–474	—
Gamma glutamyl transpeptidase (GGTP)	—	—	12–271
Lactate dehydrogenase (LDH)	330 ± 82	40–348	—

*From O'Brien D., Rodgerson D.O.: Interpretation of biochemical values, in Kempe C.H., Silver H.K., O'Brien D. (eds.): *Current Pediatric Diagnosis and Treatment,* ed. 4. Los Altos, Cal., Lange Medical Publications, 1982, p. 1062, and King J., Morris M.B.: *Arch. Dis. Child.* 36:604, 1961.

TABLE A–30.—NORMAL SERUM THYROID HORMONE VALUES IN FULL-TERM AND HEALTHY PREMATURE NEWBORNS*

		BIRTH	24 HOURS	48 HOURS	72 HOURS	1 WEEK	2 WEEKS	4 WEEKS
T_4 (μg/dl)	Fullterm	11.2 (6.9–16.7)		← 11–23 →			← 9–18 →	
	Premature	6.5 ± 1.2	9.7 ± 1.12	8.8 ± 1.31	7.1 ± 1.10	8.9 ± 1.02	9.4 ± 0.91	. . .
T_3 (ng/dl)	Fullterm	50 (15–88)	. . .	. . .	. . .	185 (115–285)	. . .	. . .
	Premature	39 ± 12	76 ± 10	68 ± 11	56 ± 14	88 ± 11	130 ± 16	. . .
TSH (μU/ml)	Fullterm	8.38 (3–22)	17.1 ± 3	12.8 ± 1.9	. . .	. . .	1–10	. . .
	Premature	5.6 ± 0.80	10.5 ± 3.12	5.1 ± 0.74	3.7 ± 0.51	3.6 ± 0.26	3.4 ± 0.19	. . .
PBI (μg/dl)	Fullterm	4.3–9.5	7.3–12.9	9.6–16.8	. . .	7.3–14.5	4.0–11.0	4.0–11.0
BEI (μg/dl)	Fullterm	5.5 (4.5–6.5)	. . .	. . .	. . .	9.8 (7.8–12.0)	7.8 (7.0–8.2)	4.8 (4.0–5.5)
TBG (mg/dl)	Fullterm	2.9 (1.9–3.9)		← 2.7 (1.4–4.1) →			← 2.6 (1.5–3.9) →	
FT_4 (ng/dl)	Fullterm				← 1.3–3.8 →			

*Modified from Meites S. (ed.): *Pediatric Clinical Chemistry: A Survey of Normals, Method, and Instruments.* Washington, D.C., American Association for Clinical Chemistry, 1977, and Fisher D.A., in Oppenheimer J.J. (ed.): *Thyroid Today: Hypothyroidism in Childhood,* Vol. 1, No. 8, June 1978, p. 3, and Uhrmann S., Marks, K.H., Maisels, M.J., et al.: Thyroid function in the preterm infant: A longitudinal assessment. *J. Pediatr.* 92:968, 1978.

T_4 = thyroxine; T_3 = triiodothyronine; TSH = thyroid-stimulating hormone; PBI = protein bound iodine; BEI = butanol extractive iodine; TBG = tyroxine-binding globulin; FT_4 = free thyroxine. Values are means ± S.E.M. or means (range).

TABLE A–31.—HORMONES AND STEROID METABOLITES IN THE HEALTHY NEWBORN (PLASMA AND SERUM)*

	AGE	MALE	FEMALE
Follicle-stimulating hormone (IU/L)	0–6 months	<30	<75
Luteinizing hormone (IU/L)	0–3 months	<45	<40
Testosterone (ng/dl)	0–2 weeks	<190	<30
Human growth hormone (ng/dl)	Newborn (fasting)	15–40 response to provocation variable	
	After newborn (fasting resting)	0–5 ng/ml, response to natural and artificial provocation (i.e., arginine, insulin, hypoglycemia) >8 ng/ml	
17-Hydroxyprogesterone	<4 days	<15 μg/L	
	>4 days	< 5 μg/L	
Cortisol (μg/dl)	Newborn	5–25 (morning) 5–15 (evening)	

*From Meites S. (ed.): *Pediatric Clinical Chemistry: A Survey of Normals, Methods and Instruments, With Commentary,* ed. 2. Washington, D.C., American Association for Clinical Chemistry, 1981, and O'Brien D., Rodgerson D.O.: Interpretation of biochemical values, in Kempe C.H., Silver H.K., O'Brien D. (eds.): *Current Pediatric Diagnosis and Treatment,* ed. 4. Los Altos, Cal., Lange Medical Publications, 1982.

TABLE A–32.—AMINO ACID CONCENTRATIONS (μMOL/L)*

	MOLECULAR WEIGHT	TERM AMNIOTIC FLUID	UMBILICAL ARTERIAL PLASMA	7TH DAY CAPILLARY PLASMA
Taurine	125·2	63–283	48–304	9–155
Urea	60·1	865–8200	560–2321	938–4986
Aspartic acid	133·1	6–31	3–117	11–114
Hydroxyproline	131·1	9–25	6–48	13–93
Threonine	119·1	38–153	95–584	65–340
Serine	105·1	19–75	68–284	58–347
Asparagine	132·1	3–21	8–53	7–28
Glutamic acid	147·1	7–42	19–813	99–629
Glutamine	145·1	64–598	276–825	113–385
Proline	115·1	56–243	52–225	134–669
Glycine	75·1	67–233	133–433	53–583
Alanine	89·1	56–270	133–557	138–368
Citrulline	175·1	1–8	4–36	7–34
α-Amino-n butyric acid	103·1	1–11	4–30	9–37
Valine	117·2	19–77	30–413	55–438
Cystine	240·3	28–107	13–119	3–89
Methionine	149·2	2–10	12–31	18–63
Cystathionine	222·0	tr–2	1–3	2–61
Isoleucine	131·2	5–15	26–107	32–145
Leucine	131·2	9–29	46–220	21–273
Tyrosine	181·2	8–27	27–120	85–300
Phenylalanine	165·2	9–33	23–97	26–200
β-Alanine	89·0	tr	—	—
β-Amino-iso butyric acid	103·1	tr	—	—
γ-Amino-butyric acid	103·1	tr–3	tr–4	2–16
Tryptophan	204·2	2–10	4–106	6–54
Ethanolamine	61·1	25–244	2–43	6–47
Ornithine	132·2	13–39	38–176	28–354
Lysine	146·2	35–183	147–643	51–341
Histidine	155·2	16–75	61–280	29–196
1-Methylhistidine	169·0	1–13	tr–3	tr–18
3-Methylhistidine	169·0	1–5	tr–5	4–16
Arginine	174·2	6–23	35–159	16–78

To convert values in μmol/L to mg/100 ml, multiply by the molecular weight, then divide by 10,000, i.e.,

$$\frac{\mu\text{mol/L} \times \text{molecular weight}}{10{,}000} = \text{mg/100 ml}$$

Tr = trace.
*From Cockburn F., Drillien C.H.: *Neonatal Medicine.* Edinburgh, Blackwell Scientific Publications, 1974, p. 792. Used by permission.

TABLE A–33.—NORMAL BLOOD CHEMISTRY VALUES OF NEWBORNS*

CONSTITUENT	AGE	VALUES
Ammonia (plasma)	Newborn	90–150 μg/dl (53–58 μmol/L) (higher in prematures)
α-Fetoprotein (plasma, serum)	Newborn	0–10 mg/dl (decrease with increasing gestation)
Cholesterol (plasma, serum)	Premature, cord blood	47–98 mg/dl (1.2–2.5 mmol/L)
	Fullterm, cord blood	45–98 mg/dl (1.2–2.5 mmol/L)
	Fullterm, newborn	45–167 mg/dl (1.2–4.3 mmol/L)
	3 days–1 year	69–174 mg/dl (1.8–4.5 mmol/L)
Lipids (serum)		
Total lipids	Newborn	
	1st day	126–330 mg/dl
	>5 days	300–650 mg/dl
Free nonesterified fatty acids	Newborn	250–1000 μEq/L
Neutral fat (glycerides)	Newborn	10–54 mg/dl
Phospholipids	Newborn, cord blood	75–150 mg/dl
	Newborn, 1st week	170–250 mg/dl
Lipoproteins		
Alpha	Newborn	71–176 mg/dl
Beta	Newborn	51–158 mg/dl
Omega (chylomicrons)	Newborn	48–106 mg/dl
Total	Newborn	170–440 mg/dl

*From O'Brien D., Rodgerson D.O.: Interpretation of biochemical values, in Kempe C.H., Silver H.K., O'Brien D. (eds.): *Current Pediatric Diagnosis and Treatment,* ed. 3, Los Altos, Cal., Lange Medical Publications, 1974, p. 970, and Karlson B.W., Bergstrand C.G., Ekelund H., et al.: *Acta Paediatr. Scand.* 61:133, 1972, and Cockburn F., Drillien C.H.: *Neonatal Medicine.* Edinburgh, Blackwell Scientific Publications, 1974, p. 798.

URINE AND STOOL

TABLE A–34.—NORMAL CONSTITUENTS OF URINE IN THE NEONATAL PERIOD*

	TERM 1 DAY	TERM ≥7 DAYS	PRETERM
α Amino nitrogen (mg/kg/24 hours)	3–9		6–18
Ammonia (mEq/kg/24 hours)	0.02–0.50	0.26–0.86	
Calcium (mg/24 hours)	0.1–0.3	1.8–3.4	
Chloride (mEq/kg/24 hours)	0.1–0.8	0.1–4.1	
Clearance (ml/min/1.73 sq m)			
Creatinine	40–65		
Urea	8.5–33		3.5–17
Creatine (mg/kg/24 hours)	15–36		0.3–4.3
Creatinine (mg/kg/24 hours)	10–20		
Fructose (mg/dl)		<70	
Galactose (mg/dl)		<25	
Glucose (mg/dl)		<25	
Glucuronic acid (mg/kg/24 hours)	12–20	5–12 (2–7 w)	
Homovanillic acid (HVA, μg/mg creatinine)	Up to 15		
5-Hydroxyindole acetic acid			
(μg/24 hrs)	120	100–900	
(5-HIAA, μg/mg creatinine)		10–20	
Lactose (mg/dl)	<120	<10	
Magnesium (mg/24 hours)	0–0.04	0–1	
Nitrogen (mg/kg/24 hours)	2–76	66–150	
Osmolality (mOsm/L)	141–303	150–250	
pH	5.1–6.8	5.1–6.8	
Phosphorus (mg/kg/24 hours)	0.06–0.18	0.07	
Potassium (mEq/kg/24 hours)	0.08–0.64	0.00–2.25	
Protein (mg/24 hours)	8–12		
Sodium (mEq/kg/24 hours)	0.11–0.39	0.0–4.4	
Steroids (mg/24 hours)			
17-Oxysteroids	0–0.5		
17-Hydroxycorticosteroids	1.1–6.8		
Pregnanetriol (μg/24 hours)	200–300		
11-Deoxysteroids/ 11-Oxysteroids	<.5	<.8	
Titrable acidity (μEq/min/1.73 sq m)	45–110		0–120
Urea (mg/24 hours)	139	266	
(mg/kg/24 hours)	39	73	
Urea nitrogen (mg/24 hours)	68	124	
(mg/kg/24 hours)	18	34	
Uric acid (mg/kg/24 hours)	4.8		
Vanilmandelic acid (μg/kg/24 hours)	<200		

*Adapted from Cockburn F., Drillien C.H.: *Neonatal Medicine.* Edinburgh, Blackwell Scientific Publications, 1974, p. 802. Used by permission.

TABLE A–35.—Urine Amino Acids in Normal Infants (1 Month–3 Years)*

Amino Acid	μmol/L
Phosphoethanolamine	3–39
Taurine	0–228
Asparagine	0–80
Aspartic acid	0–45
Threonine	0–73
Serine	0–164
Glutamic acid	0–19
Proline	0–22
Glycine	0–335
Alanine	0–183
α-Aminoadipic acid	0–41
α-Amino-*n*-butyric acid	0–18
Valine	0–29
Cystine	0–33
Methionine	0–34
Isoleucine	0–20
Tyrosine	0–87
Phenylalanine	0–46
β-Aminoisobutyric acid	0–91
Citrulline	0–4
Ornithine	0–11
Lysine	0–95
1-Methylhistidine	0–95
3-Methylhistidine	0–60
Carnosine	0–145
β-Aminobutyric acid	0–91
Cystathionine	0–17
Arginine	0–10
Histidine	0–338
Leucine	0–25

*Adapted from Meites S., (ed.): *Pediatric Clinical Chemistry: A Survey of Normals, Methods and Instruments.* Washington, D.C., American Association for Clinical Chemistry, 1981, p. 86. Used by permission.

TABLE A–36.—Time of Passage of First Stool and First Voiding by 500 Full-term Infants*

	Age (hours)	0	12	12–24	24–48	over 48
Stool	%	27.2	41.8	25.0	5.8	0.2
	Cumulative %	27.2	69.0	94.0	99.8	100
Voiding	%	17.0	50.6	24.8	7.0	0.6
	Cumulative %	17.0	67.6	92.4	99.4	100

*From Sherry S.N., Kramer I.: *J. Pediatr.* 46:158, 1955. Used by permission.

TABLE A–37.—Time of Passage of First Stool and First Urine in 200 Premature Infants*

Age (Hours)		0	0–12	12–24	24–48	48
Stool	%	13.0	31.5	35.5	14.0	6.0
	Cumulative %	13.0	44.5	80.0	94.0	100.0
Voiding	%	21.5	43.0	26.0	9.5	
	Cumulative %	21.5	64.5	90.5	100.0	

*From Kramer I., Sherry S.N.: *J. Pediatr.* 51:373, 1957. Used by permission.

TABLE A–38.—Urinary Volume in the First Weeks of Life*

Day	Volume (ml)	Range
1	20	0–68
2	21	0–82
3	36	0–96
4	65	5–180
5	103	1–217
6	125	42–268
7	147	40–302
10	190	106–320
12	227	207–246

*From Thomson J.: *J. Arch. Dis. Child.* 19:169, 1944. Used by permission.

CENTRAL NERVOUS SYSTEM

TABLE A–39.—Normal Values for Cerebrospinal Fluid in Healthy Term Infants*

Age	0–24 Hours	1 Day	7 Days
Color	Clear or xanthochromic	Clear or xanthochromic	Clear or xanthochromic
Red blood cells/cu mm	9 (0–1070)	23 (0–620)	3 (0–48)
Polymorphonuclear leukocytes/cu mm	3 (0–70)	7 (0–26)	2 (0–5)
Lymphocytes/cu mm	2 (0–20)	5 (0–16)	1 (0–4)
Protein (mg/dl)	63 (32–240)	73 (40–148)	47 (27–65)
Sugar (mg/dl)	51 (32–78)	48 (38–64)	55 (48–62)

*From Naidoo B.T.: *S. Afr. Med. J.* 42:933, 1968. Used by permission.

TABLE A–40.—NORMAL VALUES FOR CEREBROSPINAL FLUID IN HEALTHY PREMATURE INFANTS*

AGE (DAYS)	1–7	8–19	21–40
White blood cell/cu mm	27 (4–112)	20 (3–56)	17 (2–70)
Protein (mg/dl)	150 (57–292)	110 (74–189)	86 (55–166)

*From Gyllensward A., Malmstorm S.: *Acta Paediatr. Scand.* (suppl.) 135:54, 1962. Used by permission.

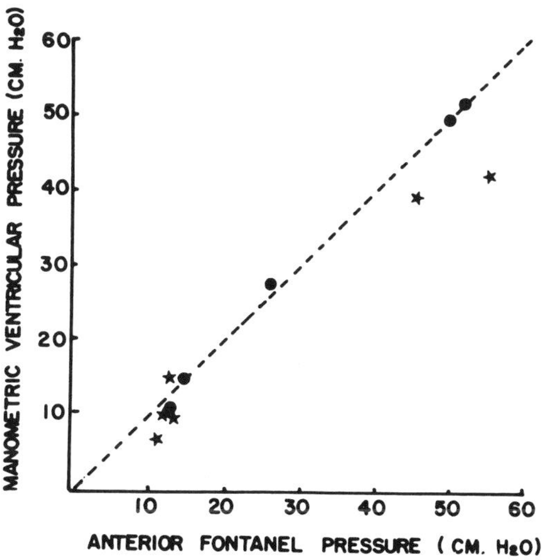

Fig A–7.
Correlation of fontanel pressure with manometric ventricular pressure. (From Donn S.M., Philip A.G.S.: Early increase in intracranial pressure in preterm infants. *Pediatrics* 61:904, 1978. Used by permission.)

TABLE A–41.—LEVELS OF INNERVATION OF MUSCLES OF LOWER LIMBS USED IN TESTING FOR SPINA BIFIDA*

SPINAL LEVEL	SPINAL SEGMENTS	MUSCLES INNERVATED
Thoracic	8–10	Abdomen, upper
	11–12	Abdomen, lower
Lumbar	1–2	Psoas
	3–4	Adductors
	3–4	Quadriceps
	4	Tibialis anterior
Lumbosacral	5–1	Extensor hallucis longus
	5–1	Extensor digitorum longus
	5–1	Hamstrings, medial
	5–1	Abductors
	5–1	Peronei
Sacral	1–2	Calf
	1–2	Hamstrings, lateral
	1–2	Gluteus maximus
	1–2	Flexor hallucis longus
	1–2	Flexor digitorus longus
	2–3	Intrinsics of foot

*From Cockburn F., Drillien C.M.: *Neonatal Medicine,* Oxford, Blackwell Scientific Publications, 1974, p. 591. Used by permission.

MISCELLANEOUS

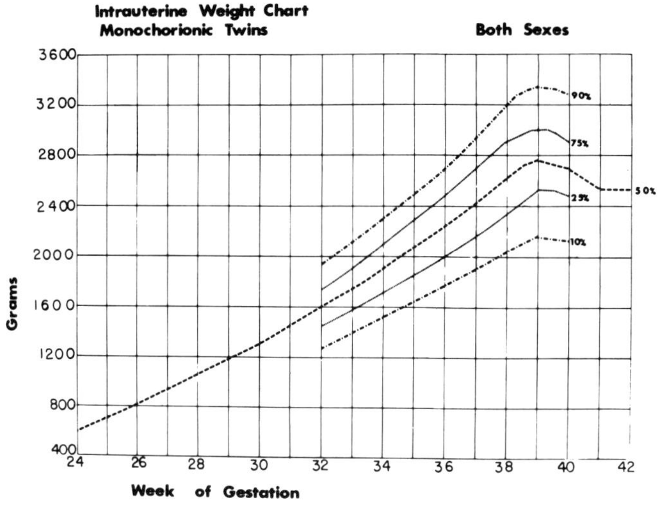

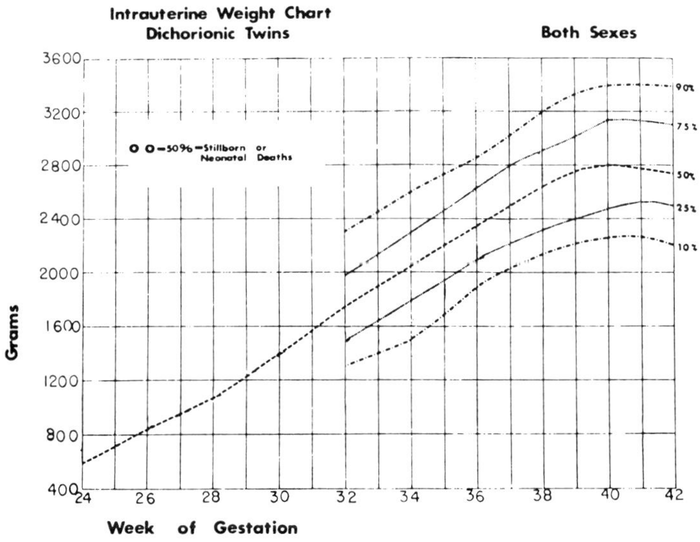

Fig A–8.
Intrauterine growth charts for monochorionic **(top)** and dichorionic **(bottom)** twins. (From Naeye R.L., Benirschke K., Hagstrom J.W.C., et al.: Intrauterine growth of twins as estimated from live birth-weight data. *Pediatrics* 37:409, 1966. Used by permission.)

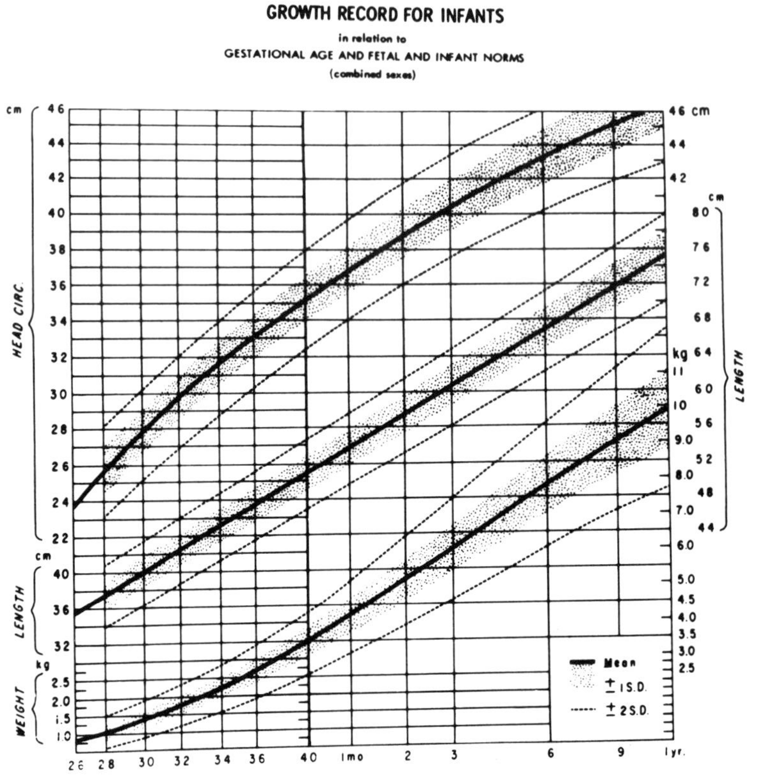

Fig A–9.
A fetal-infant growth graph for infants of varying gestational ages to be used for plotting growth from birth until one year of age after "term" has been reached. (From Babson S.G., Benda G.I.: Graphs for the clinical assessment of infants of varying gestational age. *J. Pediatr.* 89:814, 1976. Reproduced by permission.)

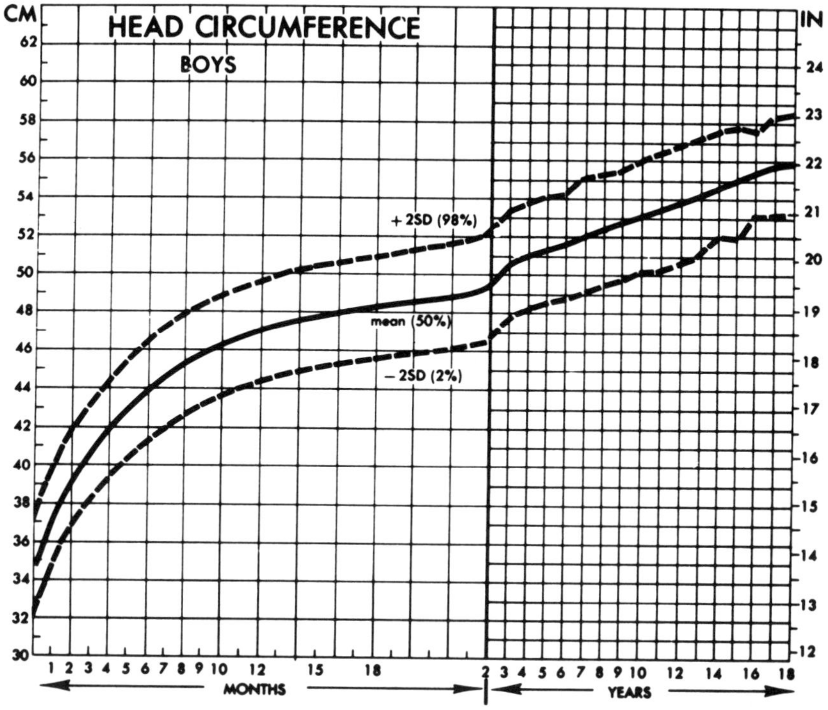

Fig A–10.
Head circumference (boys). (From Nellhaus G.: Head circumference from birth to eighteen years. Practical composite international and interracial graphs. *Pediatrics* 41:106, 1968. Reproduced by permission.)

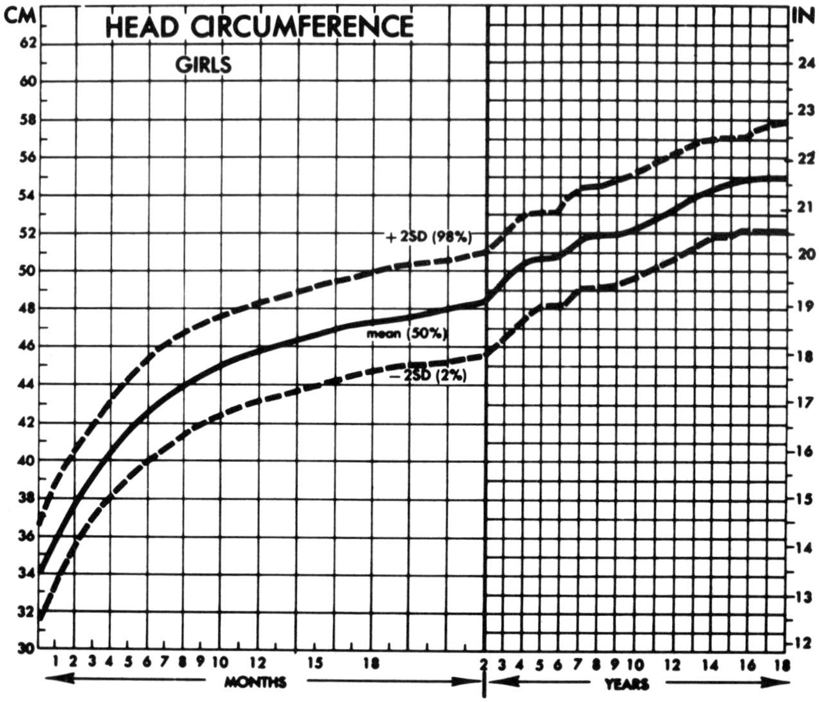

Fig A–11.
Head circumference (girls). (From Nellhaus G.: Head circumference from birth to eighteen years. Practical composite international and interracial graphs. *Pediatrics* 41:106, 1968. Reproduced by permission.)

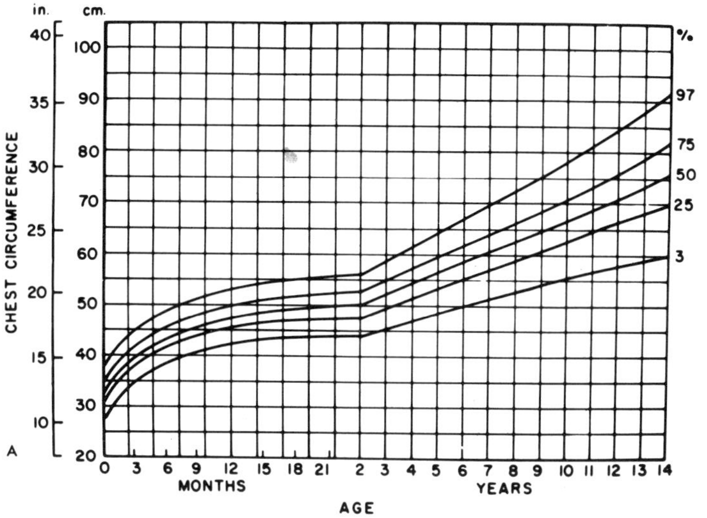

Fig A–12.
Chest circumference. (From Feingold M., Bossert W.H.: Normal values for selected physical parameters: An aid to syndrome delineation. *Birth Defects* 10(13):1, 1974. Used by permission.)

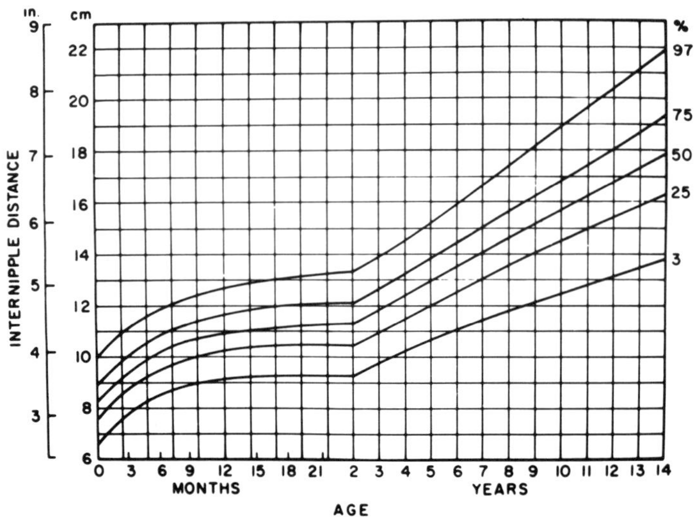

Fig A–13.
Internipple distance. (From Feingold M., Bossert W.H.: Normal values for selected physical parameters: an aid to syndrome delineation. *Birth Defects* 10(13):1, 1974. Used by permission.)

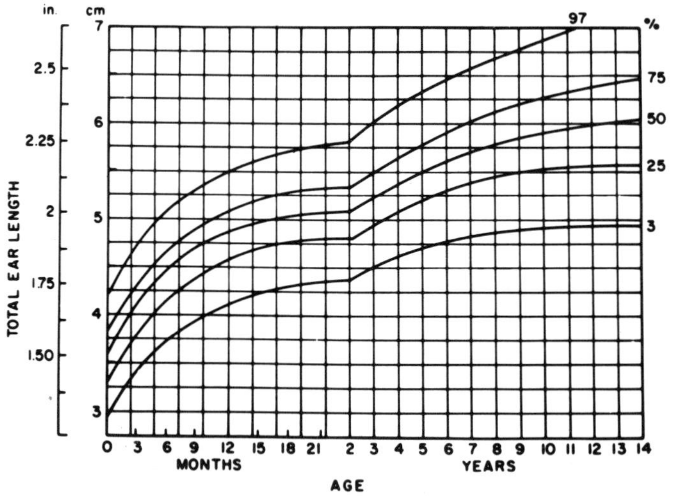

Fig A–14.
Ear length. (From Feingold M., Bossert W.H.: Normal values for selected physical parameters: An aid to syndrome delineation. *Birth Defects* 10(13):1, 1974. Used by permission.)

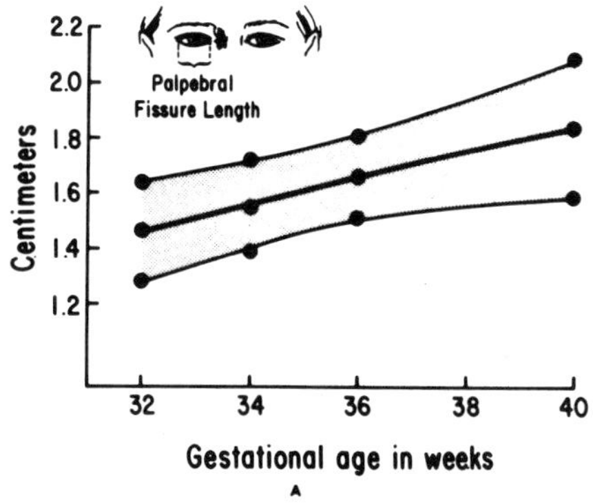

Fig A–15.
Palpebral fissure length in newborn infants. (From Jones K.L., Hanson J.W., Smith D.W.: Palpebral fissure size in newborn infants. *J. Pediatr.* 92:787, 1978. Used by permission.)

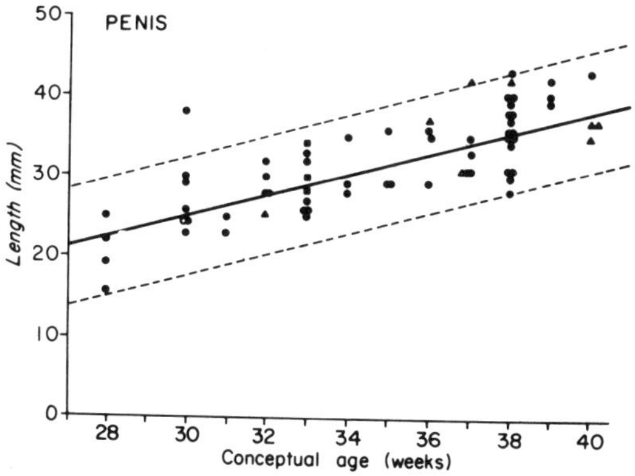

Fig A–16.
Penile stretched length. (From Feldman K.W., Smith D.W.: Fetal phallic growth and penile standards for newborn male infants. *J. Pediatr.* 86:395, 1975. Used by permission.)

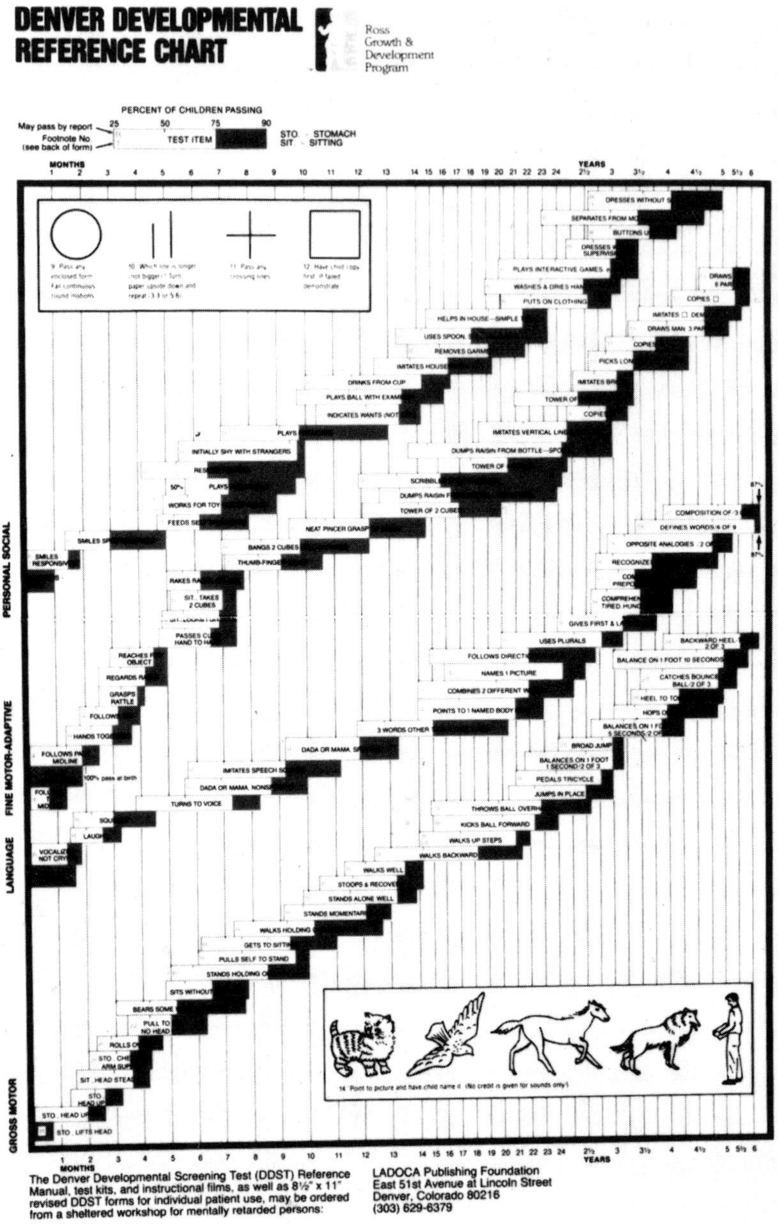

Fig A–17.
Denver Developmental Reference Chart is based on developmental data provided by William K. Frankenburg, M.D., John F. Kennedy Child Development Center, University of Colorado Health Sciences Center, Denver. Directions appear on facing page. (© 1981 by W.K. Frankenburg. Used by permission of Ross Laboratories, Columbus, Ohio.)

DIRECTIONS FOR DENVER DEVELOPMENTAL REFERENCE CHART

This Denver Developmental Reference Chart has been developed as a parent counseling aid to parallel a smaller version of the Denver Developmental Screening Test, which helps to determine whether or not a given child's developmental status falls within established norms. Health professionals need to administer and interpret each item on the Screening Test according to standardized procedures and then plot the development of each child in their practice on a separate form. They then may use this Reference Chart, which has been designed in size and format for this purpose, as an office aid to discuss a child's development with the parents.

1. Try to get child to smile by smiling, talking, or waving to him or her. Do not touch him or her.
2. When child is playing with toy, gently pull it away from him or her. Pass if he or she resists.
3. Child does not have to be able to tie shoes or button in the back.
4. Move yarn slowly in an arc from one side to the other, about 6″ above child's face. Pass if eyes follow 90° to midline. (Past midline; 180°)
5. Pass if child grasps rattle when it is touched to the backs or tips of fingers.
6. Pass if child continues to look where yarn disappeared or tries to see where it went. Yarn should be dropped quickly from sight from tester's hand without arm movement.
7. Pass if child picks up raisin with any part of thumb and a finger.
8. Pass if child picks up raisin with the ends of thumb and index finger using an overhand approach.
9, 10, 11, 12. (See directions on face of chart. When giving items 9, 11, and 12, do not name the forms. Do not demonstrate 9 and 11)
13. When scoring, each pair (2 arms, 2 legs, etc.) counts as one part.
14. (See directions on face of chart).
15. Tell child to: Give block to Mommie; put block on table; put block on floor. Pass 2 of 3. (Do not help child by pointing, moving head or eyes.)
16. Ask child: What do you do when you are cold? . . . hungry? . . . tired? Pass 2 of 3.
17. Tell child to: Put block *on* table; *under* table; *in front of* chair; *behind* chair. Pass 3 of 4. (Do not help child by pointing, moving head or eyes.)
18. Ask child: If fire is hot, ice is _____? Mother is a woman, Dad is a _____(man)? A horse is big, a mouse is _____? Pass 2 of 3.
19. Ask child: What is a ball? . . . lake? . . . desk? . . . house? . . . banana? . . . curtain? . . . ceiling? . . . hedge? . . . pavement? Pass if defined in terms of use, shape, what it is made of, or general category (such as banana is fruit, not just yellow). Pass 6 of 9.
20. Ask child: What is a spoon made of? . . . a shoe made of? . . . a door made of? . . . (No other objects may be substituted.) Pass 3 of 3.
21. When placed on stomach, child lifts chest off table with support of forearms and/or hands.
22. When child is on back, grasp his or her hands and gently pull him or her to sitting. Pass if head does not hang back.
23. Child may use wall or rail only, not person. May not crawl.
24. Child must throw ball overhand 3 feet to within arm's reach of tester.
25. Child must perform standing broad jump over width of test sheet (8½ inches).
26. Tell child to walk forward, heel within 1 inch of toe. Tester may demonstrate. Child must walk 4 consecutive steps, 2 out of 3 trials.
27. Bounce ball to child who should stand 3 feet away from tester. Child must catch ball with hands, not arms, 2 out of 3 trials.
28. Tell child to walk backward, toe within 1 inch of heel. Tester may demonstrate. Child must walk 4 consecutive steps, 2 out of 3 trials.

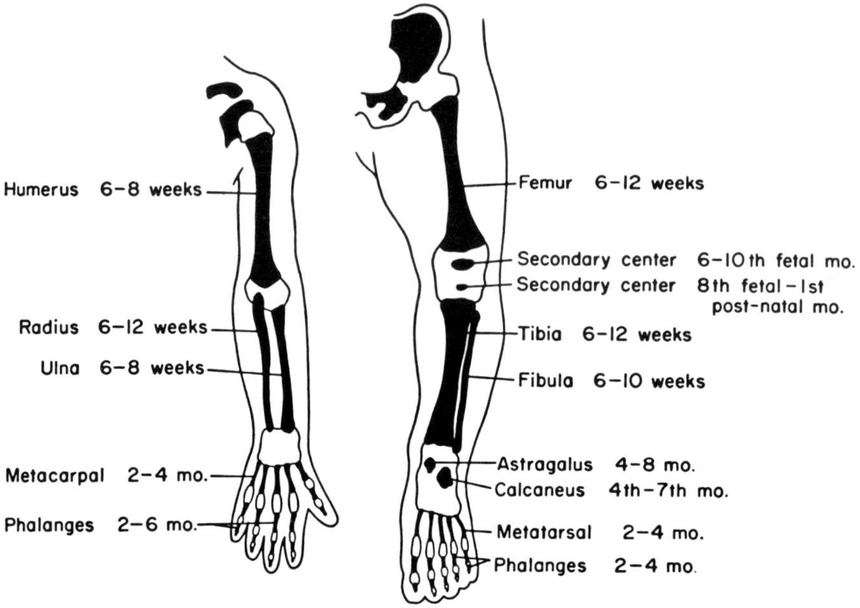

Fig A–18.
Time schedule for the appearance of the primary ossification centers in the shafts of the long bones and in the tarsal bones during fetal life. (From Caffey J.: *Pediatric X-ray Diagnosis, ed. 5.* Chicago, Year Book Medical Publishers, Inc. 1967, p. 716. Used by permission.)

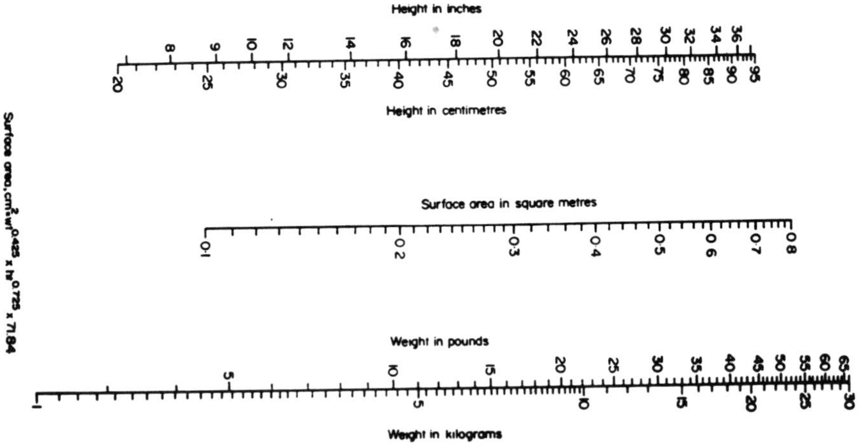

Fig A–19.
Normogram for the determination of body surface area of children. (From DuBois E.F.: *Basal metabolism in Health and Disease.* Philadelphia, Lea and Febiger, 1936.) Used by permission.)

CONVERSION TABLES

TABLE A–42.—POUNDS AND OUNCES TO GRAMS

OUNCES	0 LB	1 LB	2 LB	3 LB	4 LB	5 LB	6 LB	7 LB	8 LB	9 LB	10 LB	11 LB	12 LB
	GRAMS												
0	0	454	907	1361	1814	2268	2722	3175	3629	4082	4536	4990	5443
1	28	482	936	1389	1843	2296	2750	3204	3657	4111	4564	5018	5471
2	57	510	964	1418	1871	2325	2778	3232	3686	4139	4593	5046	5500
3	85	539	992	1446	1899	2353	2807	3260	3714	4167	4621	5075	5528
4	113	567	1021	1474	1928	2381	2835	3289	3742	4196	4649	5103	5557
5	142	595	1049	1503	1956	2410	2863	3317	3771	4224	4678	5131	5585
6	170	624	1077	1531	1985	2438	2892	3345	3799	4252	4706	5160	5613
7	198	652	1106	1559	2013	2466	2920	3374	3827	4281	4734	5188	5642
8	227	680	1134	1588	2041	2495	2948	3402	3856	4309	4763	5216	5670
9	255	709	1162	1616	2070	2523	2977	3430	3884	4337	4791	5245	5698
10	283	737	1191	1644	2098	2552	3005	3459	3912	4366	4819	5273	5727
11	312	765	1219	1673	2126	2580	3033	3487	3941	4394	4848	5301	5755
12	340	794	1247	1701	2155	2608	3062	3515	3969	4423	4876	5330	5783
13	369	822	1276	1729	2183	2637	3090	3544	3997	4451	4904	5358	5812
14	397	851	1304	1758	2211	2665	3119	3572	4026	4479	4933	5386	5840
15	425	879	1332	1786	2240	2693	3147	3600	4054	4508	4961	5415	5866

To convert: 1 pound = 453.59237 grams; 1 ounce = 28.349523 grams; 1,000 grams = 1 kilogram. Example: To obtain grams equivalent to 6 pounds, 8 ounces, read "6" on top scale, "8" on side scale; equivalent is 2948 grams.

TABLE A–43.—OUNCES TO MILLILITERS

1	fl oz	=	30	ml
½	fl oz	=	15	ml
2–½	fl dr	=	10	ml
2	fl dr	=	8	ml
1–¼	fl dr	=	5	ml
1	fl dr	=	4	ml
45	min	=	3	ml
30	min	=	2	ml
15	min	=	1	ml
12	min	=	0.75	ml
10	min	=	0.6	ml
8	min	=	0.5	ml
5	min	=	0.3	ml
4	min	=	0.25	ml
3	min	=	0.2	ml
1–½	min	=	0.1	ml
1	min	=	0.06	ml
¾	min	=	0.05	ml
½	min	=	0.03	ml

TABLE A–44.—GRAINS TO MILLIGRAMS AND GRAMS

GRAINS		MILLIGRAMS		GRAMS
30	=	2000	=	2
15	=	1000	=	1.0
10	=	600	=	0.6
7–½	=	500	=	0.5
5	=	300	=	0.3
4	=	250	=	0.25
3	=	200	=	0.2
2–½	=	150	=	0.15
2	=	120	=	0.12
1–½	=	100	=	0.1
1	=	60	=	0.06
¾	=	50	=	0.05
½	=	30	=	0.03
⅜	=	25	=	0.025
⅓	=	20	=	0.02
¼	=	15	=	0.015
⅙	=	10	=	0.010
⅛	=	8	=	0.008
1/10	=	6	=	0.006
1/15	=	4	=	0.004
1/20	=	3	=	0.003
1/30	=	2	=	0.002
1/40	=	1.5	=	0.0015
1/60	=	1	=	0.0010
1/100	=	0.6	=	0.0006
1/120	=	0.5	=	0.0005

(continued)

GRAINS		MILLIGRAMS		GRAMS
1/150	=	0.4	=	0.0004
1/200	=	0.3	=	0.0003
1/250	=	0.25	=	0.00025
1/500	=	0.12	=	0.00012
1/600	=	0.1	=	0.0001
1/1000	=	0.06	=	0.00006

TABLE A–45.—INCHES TO CENTIMETERS

INCHES	0	10	20	30	40
0	0	25.4	50.8	76.2	101.6
½	1.3	26.7	52.1	77.5	102.9
1	2.5	27.9	53.3	78.7	104.1
1½	3.8	29.2	54.6	80.0	105.4
2	5.1	30.5	55.9	81.3	106.7
2½	6.4	31.8	57.2	82.6	108.0
3	7.6	33.0	58.4	83.8	109.2
3½	8.9	34.3	59.7	85.1	110.5
4	10.2	35.6	61.0	86.4	111.8
4½	11.4	36.8	62.2	87.6	113.0
5	12.7	38.1	63.5	88.9	114.3
5½	14.0	39.4	64.8	90.2	115.6
6	15.2	40.6	66.0	91.4	116.8
6½	16.5	41.9	67.3	92.7	118.1
7	17.8	43.2	68.6	94.0	119.4
7½	19.1	44.5	69.9	95.3	120.7
8	20.3	45.7	71.1	96.5	121.9
8½	21.6	47.0	72.4	97.8	123.2
9	22.9	48.3	73.7	99.1	124.5
9½	24.1	49.5	74.9	100.3	125.7

To convert: 1 inch = 2.54 centimeters.

To obtain centimeter equivalent to 14½ inches read "10" in the top scale and "4½" on the side scale; equivalent is 36.8 centimeters.

TABLE A–46.—CENTIGRADE (C) TO FAHRENHEIT (F)

°C	°F	°C	°F	°C	°F	°C	°F
25.0	77.0	29.0	84.2	33.0	91.4	37.0	98.6
25.2	77.4	29.2	84.6	33.2	91.8	37.2	99.0
25.4	77.7	29.4	84.9	33.4	92.1	37.4	99.3
25.6	78.1	29.6	85.3	33.6	92.5	37.6	99.7
25.8	78.4	29.8	85.6	33.8	92.8	37.8	100.0
26.0	78.8	30.0	86.0	34.0	93.2	38.0	100.4
26.2	79.2	30.2	86.4	34.2	93.6	38.2	100.8
26.4	79.5	30.4	86.7	34.4	93.9	38.4	101.1
26.6	79.9	30.6	87.1	34.6	94.3	38.6	101.5
26.8	80.2	30.8	87.4	34.8	94.6	38.8	101.8
27.0	80.6	31.0	87.8	35.0	95.0	39.0	102.2
27.2	81.0	31.2	88.2	35.2	95.4	39.2	102.6
27.4	81.3	31.4	88.5	35.4	95.7	39.4	102.9
27.6	81.7	31.6	88.9	35.6	96.1	39.6	103.3
27.8	82.0	31.8	89.2	35.8	96.4	39.8	103.6
28.0	82.4	32.0	89.6	36.0	96.8	40.0	104.0
28.2	82.8	32.2	90.0	36.2	97.2	40.2	104.4
28.4	83.1	32.4	90.3	36.4	97.5	40.4	104.7
28.6	83.5	32.6	90.7	36.6	97.9	40.6	105.1
28.8	83.8	32.8	91.0	36.8	98.2	40.8	105.4

To convert C to F: $\frac{9}{5} \times$ temperature + 32
Example: To convert 40°C to F
$\frac{9}{5} \times 40 = 72 + 32 = 104$°F
to convert F to C: (Temperature − 32) $\times \frac{5}{9}$
Example: To convert 98.6°F to C
$98.6 - 32 = 66.6 \times \frac{5}{9} = 37$°C

Appendix B

TABLE B–1.—COMPOSITION OF FREQUENTLY USED FORMULAS

	MATURE HUMAN MILK 22 kcal/oz	SMA (WYETH) W/WO IRON 20 kcal/oz		ENFAMIL (MEAD JOHNSON) W/WO IRON 20 kcal/oz		SIMILAC (ROSS) W/WO IRON 20 kcal/oz	
PROTEIN	Lactalbumin: 65% Casein: 35% (% of total N_2)	Nonfat milk and demineralized whey		Nonfat milk and reduced minerals, whey		Nonfat milk (skim) Casein: 18% Whey: 82%	
FAT (OILS)	High in olein Low in volatile fatty acids E/PUFA ratio: 0.4	Oleo: 33% Oleic: 25% Coconut: 27% Soy: 15%		Coconut oil: 53% Soy oil: 47%		Coconut oil: 40% Soy oil: 60% E/PUFA ratio: 1.0	
CARBOHYDRATE	Lactose	Lactose		Lactose		Lactose	
CONSTITUENTS	PER LITER	PER LITER	PER 100 KCAL	PER LITER	PER 100 KCAL	PER LITER	PER 100 KCAL
Energy (kcal)	730	676	—	676	—	676	
Protein (gm)	11	15	2.2	15	2.2	15	2.22
Fat (gm)	45	36	5.3	38	5.6	36.3	5.37
Carbohydrate (gm)	71	72	10.6	70	10.3	72.3	10.7
Water (gm)	—	904	134	909	134	900	133
Linoleic acid (mg)	—	3,300	500	7,370	1,100	8,790	1,300
Ash (gm)	—	2.5	0.4	3.1	0.46	3.3	0.48
Vitamin A (IU)	2,500	2,000	300	2,100	310	2,030	300
Vitamin D (IU)	22	400	60	420	62	410	60
Vitamin E (IU)	1.8 (mg)	9.5	1.4	21	3.1	20	3.0
Vitamin K (mcg)	20	55	8	58	8.6	54	8
Thiamine (vitamin B_1) (mcg)	140	670	100	520	78	680	100
Riboflavin (vitamin B_2) (mcg)	370	1,000	150	1,050	156	1,010	150
Vitamin B_6 (mcg)	110	420	62.5	420	62	410	60

Vitamin B_{12} (mcg)	0.46	1.3	0.2	1.5	0.23	1.7	0.25
Niacin (mcg)	1,800	5,000	750	8,400	1,250	7,100	1,050
Folic acid (folacin) (mcg)	52	50	7.5	105	15.6	100	15
Pantothenic acid (mcg)	2,300	2,100	315	3,100	470	3,040	450
Biotin (mcg)	—	15	2.2	15.4	2.3	10.4	1.5
Vitamin C (ascorbic acid) (mg)	52	55	8.5	54	8.1	60	9
Choline (mg)	—	100	15	105	15.6	47	7.0
Inositol (mg)	—	—	—	31	4.7	27	4.0
Taurine (mg)	—	40	5.9	40	5.9	45	6.7
Carnitine (mg)	—			36.25	5.4	14	2.1
Calcium (mg)	330	420	63	460	69	510	75
Calcium (mEq)	17	20.9	3.1	23	3.4	25.5	3.8
Phosphorus (mg)	150	280	42	320	47	390	58
Phosphorus (mEq)	—	18.1	2.7	18	2.6	22.7	3.4
Magnesium (mg)	40	45	7	52	7.8	41	6
Magnesium (mEq)	—	3.7	0.6	4.3	0.64	3.4	0.5
Iron (mg)	0.21	12.0/1.5*	1.8/0.2*	1.3/1.1*	1.9/0.16*	12/1.5*	1.8/0.2*
Zinc (mg)	1.6	5	0.8	5.2	0.78	5.1	0.75
Manganese (mcg)	7–15.0	150	22	105	15.6	34	5
Copper (mcg)	240	470	70	630	94	610	90
Iodine (mcg)	30	60	9	68	10.2	100	15
Sodium (mg)	180	150	22	186	27	220	32
Sodium (mEq)	8	6.5	1.0	8.0	1.17	9.6	1.4
Potassium (mg)	530	560	83	720	108	810	120
Potassium (mEq)	14	14.3	2.1	18.4	2.8	20.7	3.1
Chloride (mg)	390	375	55.5	420	62	510	75
Chloride (mEq)	11	10.6	1.6	11.9	1.8	14.4	2.1
Est. ren. sol. load (mOsm)	77	91.2	13.5	100	14.5	105	15
Osmolality (mOsm/kg H_2O)	300	300	300	300		290	

*w/wo = with/without.

(continued)

TABLE B–1 *(cont.)*.

	SIMILAC PM 60/40 (ROSS) 20 kcal/oz		NUTRAMIGEN (MEAD JOHNSON) 20 kcal/oz		PREGESTIMIL (MEAD JOHNSON) 20 kcal/oz	
PROTEIN	Demineralized whey: 60%, calcium, sodium caseinate: 40%		Hydrolyzed casein		Hydrolyzed casein	
FAT (OILS)	Coconut oil: 40% Soy oil: 60%		Corn oil		Corn oil, MCT oil	
CARBOHYDRATE	Lactose		Corn syrup solids, corn starch		Corn syrup solids, corn starch	
CONSTITUENTS	PER LITER	PER 100 KCAL	PER LITER	PER 100 KCAL	PER LITER	PER 100 KCAL
Energy (kcal)	676		676	—	678	—
Protein (gm)	15.8	2.34	19	2.8	19	2.8
Fat (gm)	37.6	5.56	26.4	3.9	27	4.1
Carbohydrate (gm)	69	10.2	91	13.4	91	13.4
Water (gm)	910	134	900	134	858	127
Linoleic acid (mg)	8,790	1,300	13,520	2,000	9,222	1,360
Ash (gm)	2.2	0.33	4.5	0.66	5.0	0.72
Vitamin A (IU)	2,030	300	2,096	310	2,120	310
Vitamin D (IU)	410	60	419	62	424	62
Vitamin E (IU)	20	3.0	21	3.1	15.9	2.3
Vitamin K (mcg)	54	8	106	15.6	106	15.6
Thiamine (vitamin B_1) (mcg)	680	100	527	78	530	78
Riboflavin (vitamin B_2) (mcg)	1,010	150	635	94	636	94
Vitamin B_6 (mcg)	410	60	419	62	424	62
Vitamin B_{12} (mcg)	1.7	0.25	2.0	0.3	2.1	0.3
Niacin (mcg)	7,100	1,050	8,450	1,250	8,500	1,250

Folic acid (folacin) (mcg)	100	15	105	15.6	106	15.6
Pantothenic acid (mcg)	3,040	450	3,177	470	3,200	470
Biotin (mcg)	30	4.5	53	7.8	53	7.8
Vitamin C (ascorbic acid) (mg)	60	9	55	8.1	55	8.1
Choline (mg)	81	12	90	13.3	90	13.3
Inositol (mg)	162	24	32	4.7	32	4.7
Taurine (mg)	45	6.7	40	6.0	40	6.0
Carnitine (mg)	14	2.1	13	1.9	13	1.9
Calcium (mg)	380	56	635	94	630	94
Calcium (mEq)	19	2.8	32	4.7	31	4.7
Phosphorus (mg)	190	28	419	62	420	62
Phosphorus (mEq)	11.1	1.6	24	3.5	24	3.5
Magnesium (mg)	41	6	74	10.9	74.0	10.9
Magnesium (mEq)	3.4	0.5	5.6	0.8	6.0	0.9
Iron (mg)	1.5	0.22	12.7	1.88	12.7	1.88
Zinc (mg)	5.1	0.75	5.3	0.78	4.2	0.62
Manganese (mcg)	34	5	210	31	212	31
Copper (mcg)	610	90	635	94	636	94
Iodine (mcg)	41	6	47	7	48	7
Sodium (mg)	160	24	318	47	318	47
Sodium (mEq)	7	1.0	13.8	2	14	2
Potassium (mg)	580	86	737	109	742	109
Potassium (mEq)	14.8	2.2	18.8	2.6	19	2.8
Chloride (mg)	400	59	581	86	583	86
Chloride (mEq)	11.3	1.7	16.4	2	16	2.4
Est. ren. sol. load (mOsm)	95	14	134	19.8	125	18.4
Osmolality (mOsm/kg H_2O)	260		320		350	

(continued)

TABLE B–1 *(cont.)*.

	PORTAGEN (MEAD JOHNSON)		LOFENALAC (MEAD JOHNSON)	
PROTEIN	Sodium caseinate		Casein hydralysate	
FAT (OILS)	Corn oil, MCT oil		Corn oil	
CARBOHYDRATE	Corn syrup solids, sucrose		Corn syrup solids, modified tapioca starch	
CONSTITUENTS	PER LITER	PER 100 KCAL	PER LITER	PER 100 KCAL
Energy (kcal)	678	—	676	—
Protein (gm)	23	3.5	22	3.3
Fat (gm)	32	4.8	26	3.9
Carbohydrate (gm)	78	11.5	88	13.1
Water (gm)	910	134	890	133
Linoleic acid (mg)	2,332	350	13,520	2,000
Ash (gm)	5.3	0.78	5.0	0.75
Vitamin A (IU)	5,300	780	1,690	250
Vitamin D (IU)	530	78	420	62
Vitamin E (IU)	21	3.1	10.6	1.56
Vitamin K (mcg)	106	15.6	106	15.6
Thiamine (vitamin B_1) (mcg)	1,100	160	500	80
Riboflavin (vitamin B_2) (mcg)	1,300	190	600	90
Vitamin B_6 (mcg)	1,400	210	400	60
Vitamin B_{12} (mcg)	4.2	0.62	2,100	0.31

Niacin (mcg)	13,700	2,100	8,500	1,250
Folic acid (folacin) (mcg)	106	15.6	106	15.6
Pantothenic acid (mcg)	7,100	1,050	3,200	470
Biotin (mcg)	53	7.8	53	7.8
Vitamin C (ascorbic acid) (mg)	55	8.1	55	8.1
Choline (mg)	90	13.3	90	13.3
Inositol (mg)	Trace	Trace	32	4.7
Taurine (mg)	40	6.0		
Carnitine (mg)				
Calcium (mg)	630	94	630	94
Calcium (mEq)	31	4.7	32	4.7
Phosphorus (mg)	480	70	480	70
Phosphorus (mEq)	27	3.9	28	4.1
Magnesium (mg)	137	20	74	10.9
Magnesium (mEq)	11.3	1.65	6.2	0.9
Iron (mg)	12.7	1.88	12.7	1.88
Zinc (mg)	6.3	0.94	4.2	0.62
Manganese (mcg)	800	125	1,060	157
Copper (mcg)	1,100	156	630	93
Iodine (mcg)	48	7	48	7
Sodium (mg)	340	50	320	47
Sodium (mEq)	13.9	3.2	13.9	2.0
Potassium (mg)	850	125	690	102
Potassium (mEq)	22	3.2	17.6	2.6
Chloride (mg)	580	86	480	70
Chloride (mEq)	16	2.4	13.5	2.0
Est. ren. sol. load (mOsm)	148	22	133	20
Osmolality (mOsm/kg H_2O)	220		360	

(continued)

TABLE B–1 *(cont.)*.

	SMA-13 (WYETH) W/WO IRON		ENFAMIL (MEAD JOHNSON) W/WO IRON 13 kcal/oz		SIMILAC (ROSS) W/WO IRON 13 kcal/oz	
PROTEIN	Nonfat milk and demineralized whey		Nonfat milk and reduced minerals, whey		Nonfat milk Casein: 18% Whey: 82%	
FAT (OILS)	Oleo: 33% Oleic: 25% Coconut: 27% Soy: 15%		Coconut oil: 55% Soy oil: 45%		Coconut oil: 40% Soy oil: 60%	
CARBOHYDRATE	Lactose		Lactose		Lactose	
CONSTITUENTS	PER LITER	PER 100 KCAL	PER LITER	PER 100 KCAL	PER LITER	PER 100 KCAL
Energy (kcal)	439.4		440	—	440	—
Protein (gm)	9,75	2.2	10	2.2	11.9	2.71
Fat (gm)	23.4	5.3	25	5.6	23.2	5.27
Carbohydrate (gm)	46.8	10.6	45	10.3	46.2	10.5
Water (gm)	936.4	134	920	134	940	213
Linoleic acid (mg)	2,145	500	4,790	1,100	5,720	1,300
Ash (gm)	1.63	0.4	2.0	0.46	2.6	0.59
Vitamin A (IU)	1,300	300	1,378	310	1,320	300
Vitamin D (IU)	260	60	420	62	260	60
Vitamin E (IU)	6.2	1.4	21	3.1	13	3.0
Vitamin K (mcg)	35.8	8	58	8.6	35	8
Thiamine (vitamin B_1) (mcg)	435.5	100	520	78	440	100
Riboflavin (vitamin B_2) (mcg)	650	150	1,050	156	660	150
Vitamin B_6 (mcg)	273	62.5	420	62	260	60
Vitamin B_{12} (mcg)	0.85	0.2	1.5	0.23	1.1	0.25

Niacin (mcg)	3,250	750	8,400	1,250	4,620	1,050
Folic acid (folacin) (mcg)	32.5	7.5	105	15.6	66	15
Pantothenic acid (mcg)	1,365	315	3,100	470	1,980	450
Biotin (mcg)	9.8	2.2	15.4	2.3	6.6	1.5
Vitamin C (ascorbic acid) (mg)	35.8	8.5	54	8.1	40	9
Choline (mg)	65	15	105	15.6	30	7.0
Inositol (mg)		—	31	4.7	18	4.0
Taurine (mg)	26	5.9	26	5.9	29	6.7
Carnitine (mg)	—		23.5	5.4	11	2.5
Calcium (mg)	273	63	307	69	400	90
Calcium (mEq)	13.6	3.1	15	3.4	20	4.5
Phosphorus (mg)	182	42	212	47	310	70
Phosphorus (mEq)	11.8	2.7	12	2.7	18.0	4.1
Magnesium (mg)	29.3	7	34	7.8	31	7
Magnesium (mEq)	2.4	0.6	3.0	0.68	2.6	0.6
Iron (mg)	7.8/1.0*	1.8/0.22*	8.2/0.7*	1.9/0.16*	7.9/1.0*	1.8/0.22*
Zinc (mg)	3.3	0.8	3.4	0.78	3.3	0.75
Manganese (mcg)	97.5	22	68.9	15.6	22	5
Copper (mcg)	305.5	70	413	94	400	90
Iodine (mcg)	39	9	45	10.2	66	15
Sodium (mg)	97.5	22	121	27	190	43
Sodium (mEq)	4.2	1.0	5.2	1.18	8.3	1.9
Potassium (mg)	364	83	477	108	590	135
Potassium (mEq)	9.3	2.1	12.3	2.8	15.1	3.4
Chloride (mg)	243.8	55.5	276	62	400	90
Chloride (mEq)	6.9	1.6	8	1.8	11.3	2.5
Est. ren. sol. load (mOsm)	59.6	13.5	70	14.5	82	19
Osmolality (mOsm/kg H_2O)	191		180		190	

*w/wo = with/without

(continued)

TABLE B–1 (*cont.*).

	"PREEMIE" SMA-24 (WYETH)		ENFAMIL PREMATURE FORMULA (MEAD JOHNSON) 24 kcal/oz		SIMILAC SPECIAL CARE 24 (ROSS) 24 kcal/oz	
PROTEIN	Nonfat milk and demineralized whey		Nonfat milk and demineralized whey		Nonfat milk and demineralized whey (whey/casein: 60/40)	
FAT (OILS)	MCT: 10% Oleo: 20% Oleic: 25% Coconut: 27% Soy: 18%		MCT: 40% Coconut oil: 20% Soy oil: 40%		MCT: 50% Coconut oil: 20% Soy oil: 30%	
CARBOHYDRATE	Lactose: 50% Glucose polymers: 50%		Lactose: 40% Maltodextrins: 60%		Lactose: 50% Corn syrup solids: 50%	
CONSTITUENTS	PER LITER	PER 100 KCAL	PER LITER	PER 100 KCAL	PER LITER	PER 100 KCAL
Energy (kcal)	810	—	812	—	812	—
Protein (gm)	20	2.4	24	3	22.0	2.71
Fat (gm)	44	5.4	41	5.1	44.1	5.43
Carbohydrate (gm)	86	10.5	89	11	86.1	10.6
Water (gm)	880	108	880	108	890	109
Linoleic acid (mg)	4,000	500	8,150	1,000	5,680	700
Ash (gm)	4.00	0.5	5.2	0.64	6.5	0.80
Vitamin A (IU)	2,400	300	9,768	1,200	5,520	680
Vitamin D (IU)	480	60	2,686	330	1,220	150
Vitamin E (IU)	15	1.9	37	4.6	32	4.0
Vitamin K (mcg)	70	8.6	106	13	100	12
Thiamine (vitamin B_1) (mcg)	800	100	2,035	250	2,030	250

Riboflavin (vitamin B_2) (mcg)	1,300	160	2,850	350	5,030	620
Vitamin B_6 (mcg)	500	60	2,035	250	2,030	250
Vitamin B_{12} (mcg)	2	0.3	2.4	0.3	4.5	0.55
Niacin (mcg)	6,300	750	32,560	4,000	40,600	5,000
Folic acid (folacin) (mcg)	100	12.5	285	35	300	37
Pantothenic acid (mcg)	3,600	450	9,768	1,200	15,430	1,900
Biotin (mcg)	18	2.2	16.3	2	300	37
Vitamin C (ascorbic acid) (mg)	70	8.6	285	35	300	37
Choline (mg)	127	16	62	7.6	81	10
Inositol (mg)	32	4	38	4.7	45	5.5
Taurine (mg)	51	6.3	49	6.0	54	6.7
Carnitine (mg)			73.5	9.1	48	5.9
Calcium (mg)	750	90	950	117	1,460	180
Calcium (mEq)	37.4	4.5	47	5.8	73	9.0
Phosphorus (mg)	400	50	476	59	730	90
Phosphorus (mEq)	25.8	3.2	27	3.3	42.5	5.2
Magnesium (mg)	70	8.6	40.0	4.9	100	12
Magnesium (mEq)	5.8	0.7	7.0	0.9	8.3	1.0
Iron (mg)	3	0.38	2.0	0.25	3.0	0.37
Zinc (mg)	8	1	8.1	1.0	12.2	1.5
Manganese (mcg)	200	25	106	13	100	12
Copper (mcg)	700	86	1,300	160	2,030	250
Iodine (mcg)	83	10	64	7.9	160	20
Sodium (mg)	320	40	317	39	410	50
Sodium (mEq)	13.9	1.7	14	1.7	17.8	2.2
Potassium (mg)	750	90	898	111	1,140	140
Potassium (mEq)	19.2	2.3	23	2.8	29.1	3.6
Chloride (mg)	530	66	687	85	730	90
Chloride (mEq)	14.9	1.8	19	2.4	20.6	2.5
Est. ren. sol. load (mOsm)	128	15.8	220	26	156	20
Osmolality (mOsm/kg H_2O)	280	280	300		300	

(continued)

TABLE B–1 *(cont.)*.

	"PREEMIE" SMA-20 (WYETH)		ENFAMIL PREMATURE FORMULA (MEAD JOHNSON) 20 kcal/oz		SIMILAC SPECIAL CARE (ROSS) 20 kcal/oz	
PROTEIN	Nonfat milk and demineralized whey		Nonfat milk and reduced minerals, whey		Nonfat milk and demineralized whey (whey/casein: 60/40)	
FAT (OILS)	MCT: 10% Oleo: 20% Oleic: 25% Coconut: 27% Soy: 18%		MCT: 40% Coconut oil: 20% Soy Oil: 40%		MCT: 50% Soy oil: 30% Coconut oil: 20%	
CARBOHYDRATE	Lactose: 50% Glucose polymers: 50%		Lactose: 40% Maltodextrins: 60%		Lactose: 50% Glucose polymers: 50%	
CONSTITUENTS	PER LITER	PER 100 KCAL	PER LITER	PER 100 KCAL	PER LITER	PER 100 KCAL
Energy (kcal)	676	—	676	—	676	—
Protein (gm)	20	3.0	20	3	18.3	2.71
Fat (gm)	35	5.2	34	5.1	36.7	5.43
Carbohydrate (gm)	70	10.4	74	11	71.7	10.6
Water (gm)	904	133	898	108	900	133
Linoleic acid (mg)	3,300	485	6,700	1,000	4,730	700
Ash (gm)	3.4	0.5	4.3	0.64	5.4	0.80
Vitamin A (IU)	3,200	475	8,139	1,200	4,600	680
Vitamin D (IU)	510	75	2,220	330	1,010	150
Vitamin E (IU)	15	2.2	31	4.6	27	4.0
Vitamin K (mcg)	70	10.5	88	13	81	12
Thiamine (vitamin B_1) (mcg)	800	120	1,690	250	1,690	250
Riboflavin (vitamin B_2) (mcg)	1,300	190	2,325	350	4,190	620

Vitamin B_6 (mcg)	500	75	1,690	250	1,690	250
Vitamin B_{12} (mcg)	2	0.3	2.0	0.3	3.7	0.55
Niacin (mcg)	6,300	930	27,482	4,000	33,800	5,000
Folic acid (folacin) (mcg)	100	15	238	35	250	37
Pantothenic acid (mcg)	3,600	530	800	1,200	12,840	1,900
Biotin (mcg)	18	2.5	13.6	2	250	37
Vitamin C (ascorbic acid) (mg)	70	10.5	232	35	250	37
Choline (mg)	127	19	51	7.6	68	10
Inositol (mg)	30	4.4	32	4.7	37	5.5
Taurine (mg)	51	7.5	40	6.0	45	6.7
Carnitine (mg)			61.2	9.1	40	5.9
Calcium (mg)	750	110	793	117	1,220	180
Calcium (mEq)	37.4	5.5	39	5.8	61	9.0
Phosphorus (mg)	380	55	400	58.5	610	90
Phosphorus (mEq)	25.8	3.5	23	3.3	35.5	5.2
Magnesium (mg)	70	10.5	34.0	4.9	81	12
Magnesium (mEq)	5.8	0.9	6.0	0.9	6.8	1.0
Iron (mg)	3	0.45	1.7	0.25	2.5	0.37
Zinc (mg)	8	1.2	6.8	1.0	10.1	1.5
Manganese (mcg)	200	30	88	13	80	12
Copper (mcg)	700	105	1,078	160	1,690	250
Iodine (mcg)	83	12	54	7.9	140	20
Sodium (mg)	320	47	264	39	340	50
Sodium (mEq)	13.9	2.0	11	1.7	14.8	2.2
Potassium (mg)	750	110	750	110	950	140
Potassium (mEq)	19.2	2.8	19	2.8	24.3	3.6
Chloride (mg)	530	80	570	85	610	90
Chloride (mEq)	14.9	2.3	16	2.4	17.2	2.5
Est. ren. sol. load (mOsm)	128	18.9	170	26	129	20
Osmolality (mOsm/kg H_2O)	268	268	244		250	

(continued)

TABLE B–1 *(cont.)*.

	NURSOY (WYETH)		PROSOBEE LIQUID (MEAD JOHNSON)		ISOMIL 20 (ROSS)	
PROTEIN	Soy protein isolate		Soy protein isolate		Soy protein isolate: 100%	
FAT (OILS)	Oleo: 33% Oleic: 25% Coconut: 27% Soy: 15%		Coconut oil: 55% Soy oil: 45%*		Coconut oil: 40% Soy oil: 60%	
CARBOHYDRATE	Sucrose		Corn syrup solids		Corn syrup: 50% Sucrose: 50%	
CONSTITUENTS	PER LITER	PER 100 KCAL	PER LITER	PER 100 KCAL	PER LITER	PER 100 KCAL
Energy (kcal)	676	—	676	—	676	
Protein (gm)	21	3.1	20	3	18.0	2.66
Fat (gm)	36	5.3	36	5.3	36.9	5.46
Carbohydrate (gm)	69	10.2	68	10	68.3	10.1
Water (gm)	898	133	900	134	900	133
Linoleic acid (mg)	3,300	500	9,400*	1,000*	8,790	1,300
Ash (gm)	3.5	0.5	4.0	0.6	3.8	0.56
Vitamin A (IU)	2,000	300	2,100	310	2,030	300
Vitamin D (IU)	400	60	420	62	410	60
Vitamin E (IU)	9.5	1.4	21	3.1	20	3.0
Vitamin K (mcg)	100	15	106	15.6	100	15
Thiamine (vitamin B_1) (mcg)	670	100	530	78	410	60
Riboflavin (vitamin B_2) (mcg)	1,000	150	630	94	610	90
Vitamin B_6 (mcg)	420	62.5	420	62	410	60
Vitamin B_{12} (mcg)	2	0.3	2.1	0.3	3.0	0.45
Niacin (mcg)	5,000	750	8,500	1,250	9,130	1,350

Folic acid (folacin) (mcg)	50	7.5	106	15.6	100	15
Pantothenic acid (mcg)	3,000	450	3,200	470	5,070	750
Biotin (mcg)	35	5.5	53	7.8	30	4.5
Vitamin C (ascorbic acid) (mg)	55	8.5	55	8.1	60	9
Choline (mg)	85	13	53	7.8	54	8
Inositol (mg)	27	4.1	32	4.7	34	5
Taurine (mg)	40	5.9	40	5.9	45	6.7
Carnitine (mg)	8.5	1.3	13	1.9	14	2.1
Calcium (mg)	600	90	630	93	710	105
Calcium (mEq)	29.9	4.5	31	4.6	35.5	5.2
Phosphorus (mg)	420	63	500	74	510	75
Phosphorus (mEq)	27.1	4.1	29	4.3	29.7	4.4
Magnesium (mg)	67	10	740	109	51	7.5
Magnesium (mEq)	5.5	0.8	6.0	0.9	4.2	0.6
Iron (mg)	11.5	1.7	12.7	1.88	12	1.8
Zinc (mg)	5	0.8	5.3	0.78	5.1	0.75
Manganese (mcg)	200	30	210	31	200	30
Copper (mcg)	470	70	630	93	510	75
Iodine (mcg)	60	9	69	10.2	100	15
Sodium (mg)	200	30	243	36	320	47
Sodium (mEq)	8.7	1.3	10.4	1.5	13.9	2.0
Potassium (mg)	700	105	820	122	950	140
Potassium (mEq)	17.9	2.7	21	3	24.3	4.3
Chloride (mg)	375	55.5	560	83	440	65
Chloride (mEq)	10.6	1.6	16	2.4	12.4	1.8
Est. ren. sol. load (mOsm)	122.2	18.0	129	19	122	18
Osmolality (mOsm/kg H_2O)	296	296	200		250	

Table B–1 modified from *Product Handbook,* Ross Laboratories, Columbus, Ohio, 1985; *Infant Formulas Handbook,* Mead Johnson and Company, Evansville, Ind., 1985; Manufacturer data, Wyeth Laboratories, Philadelphia, Penn., 1986.

(continued)

TABLE B–2.—PHARMACOPEIA FOR THE NEWBORN*

DRUG	ROUTE	DOSE	DIVIDED INTO NO. OF DOSES	TOXICITY AND COMMENTS
Acetaminophen (Tempra, Tylenol) 80 mg/0.8 ml	PO	0–3 mo.: 40 mg/dose 3 mo.–1 yr: 60–80 mg/dose Repeat every 4–6 hr as needed		
Acetazolamide (Diamox) 125 mg/vial	PO, IM, IV	20 mg/kg/day For diuretic: For glaucoma:	 3 3	Metabolic acidosis Hypokalemia with chronic use
ACTH (aqueous) 40 unit/ml	IV, IM	3–5 units/kg/day for hypoglycemia (1 mg/unit)	4	Same as for cortisol Steroid complications
Acyclovir	IV	30 mg/kg/day	3	
Adrenaline (epinephrine) 1:10,000 aqueous solution 0.1 mg/ml	SC, IV IC, IT	0.1–0.2 ml/kg/dose Repeat in 2–4 hr as needed May repeat as early as in 15 min for 3–4 doses 0.5–1.00 μg/kg/min (may be given as IV drip in 5% Dextrose in water)		Tachycardia Arrhythmia Dilute 1 ml (1:1000) units/9 ml saline if not diluted Use as inotropics vasoconstrictives
Albumin, 5% (or 25%) 1 gm/20 ml (1 gm/4 ml)	IV	1 gm (20 ml)/kg/day or 0.2 gm/kg/dose Repeat as needed		Pulmonary edema, heart failure, hypervolemia
Amikacin 50 mg/ml 100 mg/ml	IM, IV	<7 days: PT: 15 mg/kg/day FT: 20 mg/kg/day PT <28 wks: 7.5 mg/kg/day >7 days: 20–30 mg/kg/day	2 2 2 or 3	Nephrotoxicity, ototoxicity Maintain 10–25 μg/ml of peak blood level (<40 μg/ml) Adjust dose and frequency according to renal function
Aminophylline 25 mg/ml (IV) 21 mg/ml (PO) (70%–85% of theophylline)	IV, PO	Loading: 3–7 mg/kg Maintenance: 2–6 mg/kg/day	 2–3	Tachycardia, abdominal distention, GI hemorrhage, jitteriness, or seizures;

				Give by slow IV and keep blood level of theophylline at 10–15 μg/ml
Amoxicillin 125, 250 mg/5 ml	PO	20–30 mg/kg/day	3	Nephrotoxic, vitamin K depletion, distal renal tubular acidosis
				Flushing, febrile reaction
Amphotericin B	IV	0.1–1.00 mg/kg/day Slow IV drip diluted to 1 mg/10 ml	1	Nephrotoxicity, hepatotoxicity
Ampicillin 125, 250, 500 mg/ vial	IM, IV	Meningitis: <7 days: PT: 100 mg/kg/day FT: 200 mg/kg/day >7 days: 300 mg/kg/day Sepsis: <7 days: PT: 50–100 mg/kg/day FT: 100–150 mg/kg/day >7 days: 100–150 mg/kg/day	 2 2 3 2 2 3	Rare; increased transaminase: eosinophilia; irritability
Atropine sulfate (dilute to 0.1 mg/ml)	SC, IV, IT	0.01–0.03 mg/kg/dose every 2–4 hr as needed		Tachycardia, urine retention, hyperthermia
Bacitracin	Top	500 units/gm ointment	3–4	IM not recommended because of nephrotoxicity. For resistant organisms only
Belladonna, tincture 0.3 mg atropine/ml	PO	0.1 ml/kg/dose (0.03 mg atropine) every 4–6 hr, 10–30 min before feeding Increase cautiously to flushing		Hyperthermia, dry secretions, and flushing Maximum: 3.5 ml/day
Bicarbonate (administer as 0.5 mEq/ml: 4.2%)	IV	1–2 mEq/kg/dose (for emergency) Maximum: 7 mEq/day Wt (kg) × base deficit (mEq) × 0.3 to infuse ½ dose slowly 0.5 mEq/min, then ½ later		Transient hyperosmolarity (1 mOsm/ml), alkalosis, and hypernatremia Must have normal P_{CO_2} before use
Blood (whole)	IV	10–20 ml/kg/day (repeat as required)	1–2	Administer slowly
Blood (packed cells)	IV	5–10 ml/kg/day (repeat as required)	1–2	Administer slowly

(continued)

TABLE B–2.—*(continued)*

DRUG	ROUTE	DOSE	DIVIDED INTO NO. OF DOSES	TOXICITY AND COMMENTS
Caffeine citrate	IV, PO	Loading: 10 mg/kg Maintenance: 2.5–5.0 mg/kg/day	 1	Keep serum caffeine 10–15 μg/ml Tachycardia, seizures, and abdominal distension
Calcium gluconate (10% calcium gluconate: 100 mg/ml)	IV	Loading: 100–500 mg/kg/dose over 5 min		Bradycardia, sloughing, and calcification with infiltration. Potentiates digitalis effect
	IV, PO	Maintenance: 400–1,000 mg/kg/day	4–6	Gastric irritation, necrosis Administer slowly
Calcium lactate (13% calcium)	PO	500 mg/kg/day	4	May potentiate digitalis effect and cause arrhythmia and gastric irritation
Carbenicillin (Dilute to 50–100 mg/ml with sterile water)	IM, IV	<7 days: PT: 200 mg/kg/day FT: 250 mg/kg/day >7 days: 300–400 mg/kg/day	2 3 4	Hypernatremia, sloughing with infiltration Transaminase elevation, platelet dysfunction
Cephalothin (Keflin) (Dilute to 100 mg/ml with sterile water)	IM, IV	<7 days: 50 mg/kg/day >7 days: 100 mg/kg/day	3 4	Nephrotoxicity, neutropenia, false positive Coombs' test, allergic rash, poor passage blood-brain barrier
Cefazolin (25, 50 mg/ml)	IM, IV	<7 days: 25–50 mg/kg/day >7 days: 25–60 mg/kg/day	2 3	Neutropenia, thrombocytopenia, false positive Coombs' test, transient transaminase elevation
Chloral hydrate (500 mg/5 ml)	PO, PR	10–30 mg/kg/dose Repeat every 6–8 hr as needed		Gastric irritation, paradoxical excitement

Chloramphenicol (Chloromycetin)	IV, PO	<7 days: PT: 25 mg/kg/day FT: 50 mg/kg/day >7 days: 50 mg/kg/day	2 2 4	May cause "gray baby syndrome" with toxic level; potentiates Dilantin effect, reversible bone marrow depression Maintain peak plasma level 10–20 μg/ml
Chlorpromazine		See Thorazine		
Chlorothiazide (Diuril) (250 mg/5 ml)	PO	20–40 mg/kg/day	2–4	Hyperglycemia, hypokalemia, hyponatremia, alkalosis IV use is not usually recommended Monitor serum electrolytes carefully
Cholestyramine (Questran)	PO	240 mg/kg/day (administer with feeding)	4–6	Steatorrhea, GI dysfunction, malabsorption of fat soluble vitamins; metabolic acidosis
Cimetidine (Tagamet) (300 mg/5ml or /2 ml vial)	PO, IV	10–20 mg/kg/day over 15–20 minutes	4	H_2 antagonist (limited experience in newborns)
Colistin (Colistimethate) (25 mg/5 ml suspension, 150 mg/ vial)	PO, IM	<7 days: 5.0 mg/kg/day >7 days: 7.5 mg/kg/day	2 3	Nephrotoxicity (dose dependent) Respiratory arrest may occur with IM injection with impaired renal function Ototoxicity
Cortisone (25, 50 mg/ml)	PO, IM	Replacement: 1.0 mg/kg/day Pharmacologic: 2–10 mg/kg/day withdraw slowly	4	Infection, hypertension, salt retention, adrenal suppression, hypokalemia

(continued)

TABLE B–2.—*(continued)*

DRUG	ROUTE	DOSE	DIVIDED INTO NO. OF DOSES	TOXICITY AND COMMENTS
Desoxycorticosterone acetate (DOCA) (5 mg/ml)	IM	1 mg/kg/day	1	Check electrolytes carefully
Dexamethasone (Decadron) (0.5 mg/5 ml Elixir 4 mg/ml)	PO, IV	Loading: 0.2–0.5 mg/kg Maintenance: 0.1–0.4 mg/kg/day	3–4	Same as cortisone
Dextran (10% solution)	IV	Up to 2 gm/kg/day (low molecular weight)	1	Avoid circulatory overload
Diazepam (Valium) (5 mg/ml)	IV	Status epilepticus: 0.1–1.0 mg/kg/dose Do not exceed 2 mg/kg/dose	3–4	Sodium benzoate dilutent; competes with bilirubin for albumin binding sites Respiratory depression, hypotension
Diazoxide (Hyperstat) (15 mg/ml)	IV	5 mg/kg/dose in 30 sec Repeat every 4–8 hr as needed		Hypotension, hyperglycemia, sodium and water retention
Dicloxacillin (125 mg/5 ml)	PO	16–32 mg/kg/day	4	Penicillin sensitivity
Digoxin (Lanoxin) (elixir, 0.05 mg/ml; injection, 0.1 mg/ml)	PO	*PO digitalizing dose:* PT: 20–40 μg/kg (0.02–0.04 mg/kg) *Weight (gm)* — *Dose (μg/kg)* 501–1000 — *20* 1,001–1,500 — *25* 1,501–2,000 — *30* 2,001–2,500 — *35* FT to 1 mo. — *40–60* 1 mo. to 2 yrs. — *50–70*		Toxicity: bradycardia, vomiting, arrhythmias, poor feeding (>2 mg/ml) Monitor ECG serially Initial digitalizing: ½ dose stat ¼ dose in 6–8 hr ¼ dose in 12–16 hr from first dose

	IV	IV dose is 75% of IM or PO dose (e.g., 15–20 μg/kg for PT and 25–35 μg/kg for FT therapeutic level: 1–2 mg/ml		Maintenance: ¼ total digitalizing dose/day divided into two doses Begins 12 hr after last digitalization dose
Diphtheria antitoxin	IM, IV	20,000–50,000 units/day for 3 days		Hypersensitivity reaction
Dopamine Hcl (Inotropin) (40 mg/ml)	IV	Inotropic and vasoconstrictive dose: 2–20 μg/kg/min in 5% D/W (Dilute to a concentration of 10 mg/dl, 100 μg/ml)		Monitor blood pressure; may cause pulmonary vasoconstriction, keep phantolamine (Regitine) at bedside (antidote for peripheral ischemia) Necrosis with infiltration
Edrophonium		See Tensilon		
Epinephrine (1:1000)		See adrenalin		
Erythromycin (5 mg/drop) (50 mg/ml)	PO, IV	< 7 days: 40 mg/kg/day > 7 days: 40 mg/kg/day	2 3–4	May potentiate theophylline effect; contraindicated with impaired liver function IV solution is unstable and painful Antagonist of clindamycin
Ethacrynic Acid (Edecrin) (50 mg/vial)	PO, IV	1(0.5–3.0) mg/kg/dose diluted with 5% D/W given over 5–10 min. Repeat every 8 hr as needed		Ototoxicity when used with aminoglycoside; Hypokalemia, alkalosis, and hyponatremia Dosage for infants not well established
Ferrous sulfate (25 mg Fe/ml)	PO	See iron		
Fibrinogen	IV	50 mg/kg/dose as needed		Monitor clotting time
Fluorocytosine	IV, PO	100–150 mg/kg/day	3–4	Hepatotoxicity
Folic acid (5 mg/ml) (1 mg/tab)	IM PO	FT: 50 μg/day or 5 mg/dose every 7–14 days PT: 1 mg/dose weekly		

(continued)

TABLE B–2.—*(continued)*

DRUG	ROUTE	DOSE	DIVIDED INTO NO. OF DOSES	TOXICITY AND COMMENTS
Furosemide (Lasix) (10 mg/ml)	PO, IV, IM PO, IV	1.0(0.5–2.0) mg/kg/dose Repeat every 6–8 hr as needed 1–4 mg/kg/day for hypertension	2 2–4	Hypokalemia, hyponatremia, hypochloremia, alkalosis, dehydration, ototoxicity with aminoglycosides, renal calcifications. Enhance nephrotoxicity of cephaloridine
γ-Globulin (165 mg/ml)	IM	Preventive: 0.22 ml/kg Attenuating: 0.05 ml/kg agammaglobulinemia: 100 mg (0.6 ml)/kg every 2–4 wk		Discomfort, pain
Gentamicin (40 mg/ml)	IV, IM	<7 days: 5 mg/kg/day PT < 28 wks: 2.5 mg/kg/day >7 days: 7.5 mg/kg/day	2 3	Nephrotoxicity, ototoxicity Maintain trough level at 1–3 μg/ml (peak not more than 10 μg/ml)
Gentian violet	Top (skin, mouth)	1% solution	2	
Glucagon (1 unit/1 mg/vial)	SC, IV or IM	50–300 μg/kg/dose May repeat every 20–30 min (maximum dose: 1 mg/day)		Rebound hyperglycemia Infants of diabetic mothers may require 300 μg/kg
Heparin sodium (1000 unit/ml)	IV	Loading: 50 units/kg/dose Maintenance: 10–20 units/kg/hour as a continuous infusion		Aim to obtain 20–30 min clotting time or 2–3 times preheparin clotting time Intractable bleeding (reversible with protamine)
Hepatitis B immune globulin	IM	0.5 ml single dose at birth		
Hepatitis B vaccine	IM	0.5 ml at birth, one month and 6 months		

Hydralazine HCl (Apresoline) (20 mg/ml)	IM, IV	0.5–1.0 mg/kg/day	4–6	May cause hypotension or tachycardia
	PO	Increase gradually (maximum: 7.5 mg/kg/day) 5 mg/kg/day	4	
Hydrocortisone sodium succinate (Solu-Cortef) (100 mg MIX-O-VIAL)	IV	Initial dose for shock: 35–50 mg/kg q30 min, maximum ×4 then 50–75 mg/kg/day Physiologic replacement: 1 mg/kg/day 5 mg/kg/day for hypoglycemia	4	Withdraw slowly Hypertension, salt retention, leukocytosis, adrenal suppression, immune suppression
Indomethacin (Indocin) (1.0 mg/vial)	IV, PO	Dosage (mg/kg) Age at 1st dose: 1st / 2nd / 3rd < 48 hours: 0.2 / 0.1 / 0.1 2–7 days: 0.2 / 0.2 / 0.2 > 7 days: 0.2 / 0.25 / 0.25 May be repeated up to 2 courses	1–2	Infants with successful closure of patent ductus arteriosus usually >30 wk gestational age and <14 days of age Transient renal and liver dysfunction, decreased platelet aggregation (bleeding problems), hyponatremia, hyperkalemia, hypoglycemia
Insulin	SC IV SC	Hyperglycemia: 0.25 units/kg/dose or 0.01–0.1 units/kg/hr continuous Hyperkalemia: 1–2 ml of solution containing 6 units of regular insulin in 50 ml of 50% glucose	4–6	Titrate rate of infusion to achieve desired glucose concentration Monitor ECG while infusing for hyperkalemia
Iron (elemental) (Feosol Elixer: 44 mg Fe/5 ml) (Fer-In-Sol: 25 mg Fe/ml)	PO	Therapeutic: 6 mg/kg/day Prophylaxis: 1–2 mg/kg/day	3 2–3	
Isoniazid (50 mg/5 ml)	PO	Prophylaxis: 10 mg/kg/day Therapeutic: 10–20 mg/kg/day	1 1	Give pyridoxine supplement and follow liver functions after newborn period Newborns do not require pyridoxine supplement

(continued)

TABLE B–2.—*(continued)*

DRUG	ROUTE	DOSE	DIVIDED INTO NO. OF DOSES	TOXICITY AND COMMENTS
Isoproterenol (1:5000) (0.2 mg/ml)	IV	0.05–0.50 μg/kg/min diluted with 5% D/W to 1.0 mg/dl (10 μg/ml) until effect is obtained.		Marked inotropic effect, hypotension, arrhythmia Follow heart rate, ECG, and blood pressure
Kanamycin (75 mg/2 ml)	IM, IV	<7 days: PT: 15 mg/kg/day FT: 20 mg/kg/day	2	Nephrotoxicity, ototoxicity
		>7 days: 20–30 mg/kg/day	3	
Kayexalate (polystyrene sulfonate) [3.5 gm/1 tsp, 100 mg (4.1 mEq) Na/gm]	PO, PR	0.5–2.0 gm/kg/dose every 4–6 hours Give as a 20%–25% sorbitol		Binds 1 mEq K^+ per gm of resin Hypocalcemia or hypomagnesemia may occur
Levothyroxine (Synthroid) (50, 70, 100 μg/tab)	PO	25–50 μg/kg/day Starting dose: 10 μg/kg/day Increase by 12.5–25 μg/24 hours every two weeks	1	Adjust dosage biweekly by clinical response and T_4, TSH levels
Lidocaine HCl (0.5%: 5 mg/ml)	IV	0.5 mg/kg/dose every 5–10 min as needed. Maintenance: 10–50 μg/kg/min.		Hypotension, seizures, respiratory arrest, asystole
Magnesium sulfate (50%: 500 mg/ml)	IV, IM	0.1–0.2 ml/kg/dose of a 50% solution every 6–12 hr		Hypotension, CNS depression Calcium gluconate should be available as an antidote
Mannitol	IV	0.25–2.0 gm/kg/dose Infusion over 1–6 hr as 15%–20% solution after 200 mg/kg IV test dose Repeat every 8–12 hr as needed		Rebound edema and/or circulatory overload
Mecholyl (25 mg/ampule)	SC	0.2 mg/kg/dose increased by 25% Repeat every 15 min until desired effect (for paroxysmal tachycardia)		Cardiac arrest (antidote: atropine)

Meperidine HCl (Demerol) (25 mg/ml)	PO, IM IV, SC	1.0–1.5 mg/kg/dose 6 mg/kg/day	4–6	CNS and respiratory depression, reversible with naloxone
Methicillin (Staphcillin) (500 mg/ml)	IV, IM	<7 days: PT: 50–100 mg/kg/day FT: 100–150 mg/kg/day >7 days: 100–200 mg/kg/day	2 2–3 3–4	Nephrotoxicity (interstitial nephritis) Transaminase elevations
Methyldopa (Aldomet) (250 mg/5 ml)	PO, IV	5–10 mg/kg/day Increase every 2 days gradually as needed to maximum of 65 mg/kg/day	2–3	Hypotension, hemolytic anemia, positive Coomb's test, leukopenia, liver damage
Methylene blue (1% solution) (10 mg/ml)	IV slowly	1–2 mg/kg/dose over 5 min 0.1–0.2 mg/kg/dose for methemoglobinemia		Reducing agent: May decrease hemoglobin O_2 capacity
Methylprednisolone (SoluMedrol) (40 mg/ml)	IV, IM	10–30 mg/kg/dose every 6 hr for severe shock		Hydrocortisone preferred for physiologic replacement
Morphine sulfate (0.5 mg/ml)	IM, IV, SC	0.05–0.2 mg/kg/dose every 3–4 hr as needed		Respiratory and CNS depression Antidote: naloxone (Narcan)
Moxalactam (Moxam) (100 mg/ml)	IV, IM	<7 days: PT: 50–100 mg/kg/day FT: 100 mg/kg/day >7 days: 150 mg/kg/day Loading dose for gram-negative meningitis: 200 mg/kg	2 2 3	Thrombocytopenia, platelet dysfunction, hypothrombinemia, good penetration into CSF
Mycostatin (100,000 units/ml)	PO	100,000–200,000 units/dose every 6 hr.	4	Not used in systemic infections
Naloxone HCl (Narcan) (0.02 mg/ml)	IM, IV	0.005–0.01 mg/kg/dose Repeat every 10–15 min as needed		Tachycardia, hypertension, tremors, seizures
Neo-Calglucon (calcium glubionate, 23 mg calcium/ml)	PO	500 mg/kg/day for therapy 150 mg/kg/day for supplement (every 3–4 hr in each feeding)	6–8	High osmatic load may cause diarrhea

(continued)

TABLE B–2.—*(continued)*

DRUG	ROUTE	DOSE	DIVIDED INTO NO. OF DOSES	TOXICITY AND COMMENTS
Neomycin (125 mg/ml)	PO	<7 days: PT: 50 mg/kg/day FT: 100 mg/kg/day >7 days: 100 mg/kg/day	4 4 4	Nephrotoxicity, ototoxicity
Neutra-Phos-K (250 mg, 14.25 mEq phosphorus/75 ml)	PO	75 mg/kg/day	4–6	Used to supplement phosphorus intake Large amount causes a laxative effect Increase gradually
Nitroprusside (Nipride) (50 mg/5 ml)	IV drip	1–5 (0.5–8.0) μg/kg/min Begin with low dose and increase gradually to control blood pressure		Monitor blood pressure, heart rate continuously Follow cyanide levels. Hypotension, tachyphylaxis Thiocyanate toxicity with long-term use
Oxacillin (Prostaphlin) (250 mg/5 ml)	IV	<7 days: PT: 50–100 mg/kg/day FT: 100–150 mg/kg/day >7 days: 100–200 mg/kg/day	2 2–3 3–4	Penicillin sensitivity, nephrotoxicity
Pancreatin 2400 mg/tab.	PO PR colostomy	0.3–0.5 gm with each feeding 0.3–0.5 gm in sufficient liquid		For meconium ileus
Pancuronium bromide (Pavulon) (1,2 mg/ml)	IV	0–1 wk: 30 μg/kg/dose 1–2 wk: 60 μg/kg/dose 2–4 wk: 90 μg/kg/dose Repeat every 1–4 hr as needed until paralyzed		Curare-like voluntary muscle paralysis Has very short half-life Edema, common
Paraldehyde (5 ml/ampule)	PO, PR, IV (slow)	0.1–0.2 ml/kg/dose as 4% solution every 4–6 hr		Cardiopulmonary depression, CNS depression, pulmonary edema Avoid plastic containers, photodecomposition can occur

Paregoric (0.4 mg morphine/ml)	PO	0.2–0.5 ml/dose every 3–4 hr Increase by 0.05 ml (to 1 ml) cautiously		Titrate until clinical improvement is apparent
Penicillin G aqueous Pencillin G potassium, (1,000,000 units, 1.7 mEq k^+ and 0.3 mEq Na/vial) penicillin G Na: (5 million units, 2.0 mEq Na/vial)	IV, IM	For meningitis: <7 days: PT: 150–200,000 units/kg/day FT: 150–250,000 units/kg/day <7 days: 100,000 units/kg/day >7 days: 100,000 units/kg/day For Gonococcal ophthalmia: 50,000 units/kg/day	2 2 2 3	Dilute to provide 100,000 μ/ml Higher dose for GBS meningitis and sepsis For 7 days Single dose for prophylaxis
Penicillin (procaine) (300,000 units, 500,000 units/ml)	IM	For congenital neurosyphilis: 50,000 units/kg/day single dose		For neurosyphilis, for 10 days For prophylaxis, single dose
Phenobarbital (20 mg/5 ml elixir, 65 mg/ml/vial)	IV PO, IM, IV	Loading: 15–20 mg/kg (max) Maintenance: 3–5 mg/kg/day For sedation: 5–12 mg/kg/day	2–3	CNS depression with respiratory arrest with overdose Therapeutic serum level: 20–40 μg/ml
Phenytoin (Dilantin, Di-phenylhydantoin (50 mg/ml vial, 30 mg/5 ml elixir)	IV PO, IV	Loading: 15–20 mg/kg Do not exceed 50 mg/min Maintenance: 4–5 mg/kg/day	2–3	Bone marrow depression, nystagmus Therapeutic level: 10–20 μg/ml
Pitressin (aqueous) (20 units/ml)	SC	0.3–1.0 ml/day	3	Fluid overload, electrolyte imbalance
Polymyxin B (10,000 units/mg)	IM, IV Intrathecal	3–4 mg/kg/day 1.0 mg total dose for 3 days	3 1	Nephrotoxicity, neurotoxicity
Potassium triplex (3 mmole/ml)	PO	2.1 mmole/kg/day	3	
Prednisone (5 mg/5 ml)	PO	1–3 mg/kg/day	4	Infection, hypertension, salt retention, adrenal suppression

(continued)

TABLE B–2.—*(continued)*

DRUG	ROUTE	DOSE	DIVIDED INTO NO. OF DOSES	TOXICITY AND COMMENTS
				Every other day therapy advisable to minimize growth retardation
Procainamide (Pronestyl) (100 mg/ml)	IV	1.5–2.5 mg/kg/dose over 10–30 min may be repeated in 30 min		For PVC
	PO	40–60 mg/kg/day	4	
Propranolol HCl (Inderal) (1 mg/ml)	IV	For arrhythmias: Starting: 0.05–0.15 mg/kg/dose over 10 min		Atropine for excess bradycardia
		Maintenance: 0.5–1.0 mg/kg/day	4	
	PO	For hypertension/hyperthyroidism 1 (0.5–2) mg/kg/day	4	
Prostigmin (0.25, 0.5 mg/ml)	IM	For test for myasthenia gravis: 0.1–0.2 mg for test		Respiratory failure cardiovascular collapse
		For treatment of myasthenia gravis: 0.1–0.2 mg every 6 hr for 6 wk for transient form		
Protamine Sulfate (10 mg/ml)	IV	1 mg/100 units heparin in past 4 hr Maximum dose: 50 mg		
Pyridoxine (Vitamin B_6) 25, 50 mg/tab	IV	Test for dependency: 50 mg IV stat	1	For vitamin B_6 dependent seizures
	PO	Therapy: 2–5 mg/day	4	
Pyrimethamine (Daraprim) (25 mg/tab)	PO	1.0 mg/kg/day for first 3–4 days Then, 0.5 mg/kg/day for 3–4 wk	2	Folic acid deficiency, bone marrow depression
Quinidine gluconate (330 mg/tab.)	PO	4–10 mg/kg/dose every 6 hr until desired effect		Discontinue if QRS is > 0.10 sec
Silver nitrate (1% solution)	Top	Prophylaxis for gonorrheal opthalmia: 1 drop 1% solution in each eye	1	Chemical conjunctivitis

Spironolactone (Aldactone) (25 mg/tab.)	PO	1.5–3.0 mg/kg/day	1	Do not use in hyperkalemia, IV alimentation, renal failure
Streptomycin sulfate (200, 250 mg/ml)	IM	20 mg/kg/day for tuberculosis	1	Nephrotoxicity, ototoxicity, cardiovascular collapse
Sulfadiazine (100 mg/ml for PO 400 mg/ml for IV)	PO IV	50–100 mg/kg/day 60 mg/kg/day	4 4	Contraindicated first 3 wk or in presence of jaundice
Sulfisoxazole (Gantrisin) (100 mg/ml)	PO SC	100 mg/kg/day 150 mg/kg/day	4 2	Contraindicated first 3 wk or in presence of jaundice
Tensilon (Edrophonium) (10 mg/ml)	SC, IM	0.5–1.0 mg (0.05–0.1 ml) for test for myasthenia		Test for myasthenia gravis: clinical improvement in 30 min Profuse tracheal secretion Diarrhea that may require atropine Cardiac arrhythmias
Tetanus antitoxin	IM, IV	10,000–20,000 units/day for 2 days		Optimal dosage not established for newborns.
Tetanus immune globulin	IM	3,000–6,000 units single dose		
Tetracycline ophthalmic ointment	Top	At birth to prevent gonococcal ophthalmia		
THAM (tris-hydroxymethylamino methane) (0.3M solution: 0.3 mEq/ml)	IV	Total dose (ml) = kg (wt) × base deficit × 1.1 Give ¼ over 2–5 min. Rest according to response Maximum: 40 ml/kg/day		Hypoglycemia, apnea, hyperkalemia, sclerosing Equivalent acid buffering to equal mmole of $NaHCO_3$
Theophylline (80 mg/15 ml for PO)	PO	Loading: 5.5 mg/kg Maintenance: 1.1 mg/kg/6–8 hr	3–4	Maintain blood level to 10–15 µg/ml
Thorazine (Chlorpromazine) (10 mg/5 ml for PO, 25 mg/ml for IV, IM)	IV, IM, PO	2.2 mg/kg/day	3–4	Hypotension, hypothermia rare, liver disease and bone marrow depression Potentiate narcotics
Thyroxine Thyroid (dessicated)	PO	See levothyroxine		

(continued)

TABLE B–2.—*(continued)*

DRUG	ROUTE	DOSE	DIVIDED INTO NO. OF DOSES	TOXICITY AND COMMENTS
Ticarcillin (dilute to 200 mg/ml)	IV, IM	<7 days: PT: 150 mg/kg/day FT: 150 mg/kg/day >7 days: 225–300 mg/kg/day	2 3 3–4	Bleeding problems, hypernatremia
Tobramycin sulfate (40 mg/ml)	IV, IM	<7 days: PT: 4 mg/kg/day FT: 5 mg/kg/day >7 days: 7.5 mg/kg/day	2 2 3	Nephrotoxicity, ototoxicity
Tolazoline (Priscoline) (25 mg/ml)	IV	Loading: 1–2 mg/kg over 10 min Maintenance: 0.28 mg/kg/hr		Follow blood pressure carefully for hypotension (Rx: epinephrine drip 2 μg/kg/min) Pulmonary, GI hemorrhage (may be related to histamine effect), renal dysfunction
Tubocuranine chloride (Curare)	IV	0.25–0.6 mg/kg/dose as needed		Voluntary muscle paralysis hypotension, histamine-like effect
Vancomycin (50 mg/ml)	PO, IV	<7 days: 30 mg/kg/day >7 days: 45 mg/kg/day	2 3	Nephrotoxicity, ototoxicity histamine-like response
Verapamil (5 mg/2 ml)	IV	0.1–0.2 mg/kg over 2 min (for supraventricular tachycardia) Repeat in 30 min if needed		Monitor ECG for sinus bradycardia, AV blockage, or asystole Not well studied for newborns
Vidarabine (adenine arabinoside) (200 mg ml)	IV	15–30 mg/kg/day	1	Bone marrow depression
Vitamin K_1 oxide (Aquamephyton) (1 mg/0.5 ml)	IM	Prevention: 0.5–1.0 mg single dose Therapy: 1–2 mg every 6–12 hr as needed, not more than four times		Follow prothrombin time
Zosterimmune globulin (ZIG)	IM	0.1 ml/kg 1.25 ml, single dose of varicella ZIG		

*PO, by mouth; PR, by rectum; IM, intramuscularly; IV, intravenously, SC, subcutaneously; Top, topically; IC, intracardiac; IT, intratracheal; PT, preterm; FT, fullterm.

Index

F

G

H

J

K

Q

R

S

T

U

V